HEREDITARY
BREAST
CANCER

HEREDITARY BREAST CANCER

Edited by

Claudine Isaacs
Georgetown University
Washington, DC, USA

Timothy R. Rebbeck
University of Pennsylvania School of Medicine
Philadelphia, Pennsylvania, USA

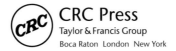

CRC Press
Taylor & Francis Group
Boca Raton London New York

CRC Press is an imprint of the
Taylor & Francis Group, an **informa** business

CRC Press
Taylor & Francis Group
6000 Broken Sound Parkway NW, Suite 300
Boca Raton, FL 33487-2742

First issued in paperback 2019

© 2008 by Taylor & Francis Group, LLC
CRC Press is an imprint of Taylor & Francis Group, an Informa business

No claim to original U.S. Government works

ISBN-13: 978-0-8493-9022-7 (hbk)
ISBN-13: 978-0-367-38862-1 (pbk)

A CIP record for this book is available from the British Library.

Library of Congress Cataloging-in-Publication Data available on application

Visit the Taylor & Francis Web site at
http://www.taylorandfrancis.com

and the CRC Press Web site at
http://www.crcpress.com

Foreword

The timing of this book's publication is ideal given the public health, medical, molecular genetic implications, and the world-wide magnitude of breast cancer. This field is impacted heavily by significant advances in screening and management opportunities, which can be lifesaving. These challenges are particularly evident when directed toward high-risk groups where certainty of risk status can often be established through molecular genetic testing, particularly *BRCA1* and *BRCA2* germline mutations.

The table of contents reads like a *Who's Who* of the world's most outstanding clinicians and scientists who are committed to greater elucidation of the many mysteries that continue to exist in breast cancer's etiopathogenesis. Hereditary breast cancer's epidemiology is covered by a true pioneer, Doug Easton; his subject matter appropriately merges into risk prediction by Lisa Walker, followed by the bioethics of genetic testing by Beth Peshkin. Ken Offit and Peter Thom discuss the nitty-gritty of how we can obtain optimum breast and ovarian cancer risk certainty once the deleterious mutation is identified. At that point, we are able to delve deeply into the litany of other molecular genetic breast cancer risk disorders, as evidenced by the discussion of Cowden syndrome by Zbuk and Eng, and Li-Fraumeni syndrome by Louise Strong.

It might appear that we have advanced significantly up the proverbial "learning curve" for this disease. However, we must hold our breath, since we still have a vast amount to learn. This is evidenced in the chapter by Nathanson which elucidates some of the rare causes of this disorder in families.

PATHOLOGY

Painstaking research (1–3) has shown distinctive differences in the histopathology of breast cancers in *BRCA1* mutation carriers which are more likely medullary or poorly differentiated, have a low rate of carcinoma in situ, and lower estrogen receptor and progesterone receptor positivity. In contrast, *BRCA2* breast cancer shows a higher frequency of lobular and tubulo-lobular breast cancer, and it is now judged to be more similar to the so-called "typical" or "common" type of breast cancer. Llamas and Brody provide additional insight into the biology of these mutations, while Foulkes and Akslen further our knowledge about breast cancer's pathology in the hereditary setting. The pathology of the "second tumor of high risk," namely, ovarian cancer, is addressed by Penault-Llorca and Lakhani.

GENETIC COUNSELING

Genetic counseling strategies, particularly focusing on whom to test, are discussed in depth by two extremely well-known representatives of the genetic counseling community, Stopfer and Schneider. The important and related topic of *BRCA* testing is discussed by Tavtigian. When interpreting breast-cancer-prone pedigrees, the genetic counselor must constantly keep in mind that there will be *BRCA1/BRCA2* mutation positive individuals who will live into their 70s, 80s, or even longer, and never manifest carcinoma of the breast. Yet some of their first-degree relatives, i.e., sisters, brothers, progeny, mother or father, as well as second-degree relatives, may be mutation carriers, a subset of whom will develop early-onset breast and/or ovarian cancer. Therefore, when interpreting such pedigrees with reduced penetrance, one often asks, "What is really happening that is responsible for these gaps in cancer occurrence in the family?" Often, the relatively inexperienced clinician may not appreciate the fact that the genetic issue is not "skipping a generation" but, rather, he or she may be dealing with the phenomenon of reduced penetrance. Fortunately, Pharoah discusses this evidence in the scientific depth which it deserves.

But how do you deliver the so-called "good news" (absence of a *BRCA* mutation) vs. the "bad news" (presence of the mutation) when providing genetic counseling? This is a crucial issue, since many factors impact heavily upon its delivery. These include the perception of insurance and/or employment discrimination; further confounders include fear and anxiety about receiving this "dreaded news" of being a mutation carrier, which will entail lifelong screening and decisions about prophylactic surgery. How will this news affect marital relations, decisions about pregnancy and cancer risk to children, and potential stereotyping by close family members? These complex concerns are discussed by Graves and Schwartz.

How do we clinically manage a typical hereditary breast-ovarian cancer (HBOC) family wherein DNA testing proves to be negative, an issue that may impact as many as 30% to 40% of so-called "classical" HBOC families? In my career as a cancer geneticist/ medical oncologist, I have insisted that, in the interest of caution, these mutation-negative but family-history-positive patients receive the same type of genetic counseling and education about HBOC's natural history as is given to *BRCA* mutation carriers should they be participants in our rigorous screening and management program (4). Noah Kauff deals convincingly with this key concept.

OVARIAN CANCER

What may perhaps be the more deadly tumor in *BRCA* mutation carriers, ovarian cancer, must be reckoned with. The clinical issue boils down to "How do we screen for this disease?" (unfortunately, the answer is *very poorly*). The next "bombshell" for the patient to consider is the issue of "do or don't" with respect to the preventive option of prophylactic oophorectomy, once her family is completed. This important subject is discussed by Lu and Skates. Similar options exist with respect to breast screening and prophylactic surgery, as discussed by Smith and Isaacs.

GENOTYPIC/PHENOTYPIC HETEROGENEITY

Why is there such phenotypic heterogeneity in *BRCA* mutation carriers? Is it due to risk modifiers, as discussed by Milne and Chenevix-Trench? Or is there something comparable in *BRCA* mutations to the situation that exists in *APC* germline mutations in familial adenomatous polyposis (FAP) which give rise to genotype-phenotype correlations? For example, a well-known model is attenuated FAP, which is characterized by only occasional colonic adenomas with as many as 25 or 50 but rarely approaching 100. This phenomenon is attributed to mutations before codon 157, after codon 1595, as well as in the alternatively spliced region of exon 9. Other variations in the polyposis expression occur, including patients with more than 1000 adenomas due to mutations between codons 1250 and 1464; and even congenital hypertrophy of the retinal pigment epithelium and desmoid tumors which have been found to correlate with mutations between codons 311 and 1444 and after 144 respectively (5). Clearly, the *BRCA* mutation situation deserves comparable molecular genetic scrutiny.

THERAPY

In spite of the diagnostic measures available clinically that offer the potential for early diagnosis, our increased ability to determine an individual's risk status (significantly abetted through the family history), the increasing body of knowledge regarding hereditary cancer syndromy, and the power of molecular genetics, many high-risk patients will regrettably fall through the cracks and manifest cancer. This can occur even in the case of a skilled and knowledgeable clinician treating a highly compliant patient. This clearly leads us to consider treatment disciplines, namely surgery, chemotherapy, and radiation therapy, which are covered in the discussions of local treatment issues by Ben-David and Pierce. Systemic chemotherapy is explored in the chapter by Robson.

DISPARITIES

Funme Olopade discusses *BRCA1* and *BRCA2* mutation carriers among underserved and special populations. This issue is extremely important when considering how ethnic and racial differences in cancer's clinical and molecular genetic expression may impact screening and management.

HISTORICAL PERSPECTIVE

Finally, from a historical perspective, it is personally very moving to me to realize that so much has been accomplished since Paul Broca, the eminent French surgeon, published a description of his wife's family in 1866 (6). This family certainly qualified as the *first* hereditary breast-cancer-prone family to be documented in the medical literature. Then, a century later, Lynch and colleagues (7–9) described for the first time the HBOC syndrome. This hereditary disorder posed an exceedingly difficult "sell job" to the breast/ovarian cancer research community. However, thanks to the discovery of *BRCA1* and *BRCA2* mutations, its existence has been confirmed beyond doubt.

READERSHIP

Who should read this book? Frankly, it should be on the shelf of all physicians who deal, however infrequently, with hereditary breast cancer and its differing syndromes. It should be a precious item on the shelves of all medical libraries. Genetic counselors need to have this book constantly in their possession. Family members may also find the book useful to them, although they may need to discuss some of the more complicated aspects of the science with their genetic counselor and/or cancer specialist. It is clear to me that this tome will prove to be of great value and should even merit translation into different languages.

Henry T. Lynch
Creighton University
Omaha, Nebraska, U.S.A.

REFERENCES

1. Lynch H, Marcus JN, Watson P, Page D. Distinctive clinicopathologic features of BRCA1-linked hereditary breast cancer. Proc Am Soc Clin Oncol 1994; 13:56.
2. Marcus JN, Watson P, Page DL, et al. Hereditary breast cancer: pathobiology, prognosis, and BRCA1 and BRCA2 gene linkage. Cancer 1996; 77:697–709.
3. Marcus JN, Page DL, Watson P, Narod SA, Lenoir GM, Lynch HT. BRCA1 and BRCA2 hereditary breast carcinoma phenotypes. Cancer 1997; 80(suppl):543–556.
4. Lynch HT, Marcus JN, Lynch JF, Snyder CL, Rubinstein WS. Breast cancer genetics: heterogeneity, molecular genetics, syndrome diagnosis, and genetic counseling. In: Bland KI, Copeland EMI, editors. The Breast: Comprehensive Management of Benign and Malignant Disorders. 3 ed. St. Louis, MO: Saunders; 2004 p. 376–411.
5. Nieuwenhuis MH, Vasen HFA. Correlations between mutation site in APC and phenotype of familial adenomatous polyposis (FAP): A review of the literature. Crit Rev Oncol Hematol 2007; 61:153–161.
6. Broca PP. Traité des tumeurs. Paris: Asselin; 1866.
7. Lynch HT, Krush AJ. Carcinoma of the breast and ovary in three families. Surg Gynecol Obstet 1971; 133(4):644–648.
8. Lynch HT, Krush AJ. Genetic predictability in breast cancer risk: surgical implications. Arch Surg 1971; 103:84–88.
9. Lynch HT, Krush AJ, Lemon HM, Kaplan AR, Condit PT, Bottomley RH. Tumor variation in families with breast cancer. JAMA 1972; 222:1631–1635.

Preface

The existence of hereditary breast cancer has been recognized for centuries. Hereditary breast cancer was first described in detail in 1866 by the French surgeon Paul Broca (1), who characterized the pattern of breast and other cancers in members of his wife's family. This early description of a hereditary syndrome involving breast cancer was refined in the subsequent 100 years to firmly establish that hereditary breast cancer occurs in a small but significant percentage of the population, that some discrete syndromes involving breast cancer exist, and that these syndromes are explained by mutations in single genes. Within the past three decades, the underlying genetic causes of hereditary breast cancer have been identified and characterized. These genes include *TP53* (in Li-Fraumeni Syndrome), *PTEN* (in Cowden Syndrome), *BRCA1* and *BRCA2* (in hereditary breast/ovarian cancer syndrome), *LKB1* (in Peutz-Jeghers Syndrome), and others.

Research regarding hereditary breast cancer is now sufficiently developed to provide a strong understanding of the basic biology and epidemiology underlying hereditary breast cancer, and to allow translation of this knowledge into clinical practice. Building on the tremendous recent growth in our knowledge and application of genetic information in understanding and managing hereditary breast cancer, we have designed this volume to provide an overview of our accumulated knowledge of hereditary breast cancer, and as a guide to the current state of clinical practice. While a number of specialized referral centers exist, there has also been a growing interest in the use of genetic risk assessment, testing, and counseling for breast cancer in the wider medical community, including primary care physicians, gynecologists, oncologic surgeons, radiation oncologists, and medical oncologists. Thus, there is a critical need to better understand the epidemiology of hereditary breast cancer, apply cancer risk assessment models, and implement cancer prevention and screening options for individuals with hereditary breast cancer. A major goal of this text is to disseminate information in a comprehensive way to both specialist researchers and clinicians as well as the wider community of individuals with interests in hereditary breast cancer.

To accomplish this goal, we present a volume organized in five sections. In the first section, we provide an overview of genetic epidemiology, risk assessment models, and ethical considerations for genetic testing in hereditary breast cancer. In the second section, we present a comprehensive overview of hereditary breast cancer syndromes with known etiologies, including those associated with *BRCA1* or *BRCA2* mutations, Cowden Syndrome, Li-Fraumeni Syndrome, other rare syndromes involving breast cancer, and those that may be associated with low-penetrance genetic variants. In the third section, we present more detailed information about *BRCA1* and *BRCA2*, which comprise the most common explanations for hereditary breast cancer. This section includes discussion of the biology of *BRCA1*- and *BRCA2*-associated breast cancer, genetic testing and counseling issues, molecular diagnosis, modifiers of risk, issues for underserved populations, and psychological impact of genetic testing. In the final two sections, we present a comprehensive discussion of the cancer screening, prevention, and treatment options for *BRCA1*- and *BRCA2*-associated breast and ovarian cancers.

We believe this volume provides a timely reference for the current state of knowledge regarding hereditary breast cancer and the clinical application of genetic risk assessment, counseling, testing, and management that will be of value to a wide range of clinicians and researchers.

We would like to acknowledge the families who have generously contributed their time and information to the generation of the research that is summarized in this volume.

Finally, we would like to express our appreciation to our families for their support, encouragement and patience: Claudine Isaacs' husband Steve Riskin and sons Jeffrey and Timmy; and Tim Rebbeck's wife Jill Stopfer and daughters Alanna and Sophie.

Claudine Isaacs
Timothy R. Rebbeck

REFERENCE

1. Broca PP. 1866. *Traité des tumeurs*. Vol. 1, 2. Paris: Asselin.

Contents

SECTION 4: SCREENING AND PREVENTION OF HEREDITARY BREAST CANCER

SECTION 5: CLINICAL MANAGEMENT OF HEREDITARY BREAST CANCER

Contributors

Lars A. Akslen   The Gade Institute, Section for Pathology, Haukeland University Hospital, University of Bergen, Bergen, Norway

Antonis C. Antoniou   Cancer Research U.K. Genetic Epidemiology Unit, University of Cambridge, Cambridge, U.K.

Merav A. Ben-David   Department of Radiation Oncology, Comprehensive Cancer Center, University of Michigan, Ann Arbor, Michigan, U.S.A.

Lawrence C. Brody   Molecular Pathogenesis Section, Genome Technology Branch, National Human Genome Research Institute, Bethesda, Maryland, U.S.A.

Wylie Burke   Department of Medical History and Ethics, University of Washington, Seattle, Washington, U.S.A.

Georgia Chenevix-Trench   Queensland Institute of Medical Research, Brisbane, Queensland, Australia

Douglas F. Easton   Cancer Research U.K. Genetic Epidemiology Unit, University of Cambridge, Cambridge, U.K.

Rosalind Eeles   The Institute of Cancer Research & Royal Marsden NHS Foundation Trust, Surrey, U.K.

Charis Eng   Genomic Medicine Institute, Lerner Research Institute and Taussig Cancer Center, Cleveland Clinic Foundation, and Department of Genetics and Case Comprehensive Cancer Center, Case Western Reserve University School of Medicine, Cleveland, Ohio, U.S.A.

William D. Foulkes   Departments of Medicine, Human Genetics, and Oncology, McGill University, Montreal, Quebec, Canada

Kristi Graves   Cancer Control Program, Lombardi Comprehensive Cancer Center, Georgetown University, Washington, D.C., U.S.A.

Claudine Isaacs   Fisher Center for Familial Cancer Research, Lombardi Comprehensive Cancer Research, Georgetown University, Washington, D.C., U.S.A.

Noah D. Kauff   Clinical Genetics and Gynecology Services, Memorial Sloan-Kettering Cancer Center, New York, New York, U.S.A.

Sunil R. Lakhani   Molecular and Cellular Pathology, School of Medicine, University of Queensland, Queensland Institute of Medical Research & The Royal Brisbane & Women's Hospital, Herston, Queensland, Australia

Florence LeCalvez-Kelm   International Agency for Research on Cancer, Lyon, France

Jenny Llamas   Molecular Pathogenesis Section, Genome Technology Branch, National Human Genome Research Institute, Bethesda, Maryland, U.S.A.

Karen H. Lu   Department of Gynecologic Oncology, University of Texas M.D. Anderson Cancer Center, Houston, Texas, U.S.A.

Roger Milne   Queensland Institute of Medical Research, Brisbane, Queensland, Australia

Katherine L. Nathanson   University of Pennsylvania School of Medicine, Philadelphia, Pennsylvania, U.S.A.

Kenneth Offit   Clinical Genetics Service, Department of Medicine, Memorial Sloan-Kettering Cancer Center, New York, New York, U.S.A.

Olufunmilayo I. Olopade   Section of Hematology/Oncology, Department of Medicine, University of Chicago, Chicago, Illinois, U.S.A.

Frédérique Penault-Llorca   Département de Pathologie, Centre Jean Perrin, Clermont-Ferrand Cedex, France

Beth N. Peshkin   Lombardi Comprehensive Cancer Center, Fisher Center for Familial Cancer Research, Georgetown University, Washington, D.C., U.S.A.

Paul D. P. Pharoah   Department of Oncology, University of Cambridge, Cambridge, U.K.

Lori J. Pierce   Department of Radiation Oncology, Comprehensive Cancer Center, University of Michigan, Ann Arbor, Michigan, U.S.A.

Mark Robson   Clinical Genetics Service, Memorial Sloan-Kettering Cancer Center, New York, New York, U.S.A.

Katherine Schneider   Dana Farber Cancer Institute, Boston, Massachusetts, U.S.A.

Marc D. Schwartz   Cancer Control Program, Lombardi Comprehensive Cancer Center, Georgetown University, Washington, D.C., U.S.A.

Steven J. Skates   Biostatistics Center, Massachusetts General Hospital, Boston, Massachusetts, U.S.A.

Karen Lisa Smith   Washington Cancer Institute, Washington Hospital Center, Washington, D.C., U.S.A.

Jennifer Stein   Genomic Medicine Institute, Lerner Research Institute, Cleveland Clinic Foundation, Cleveland, Ohio, U.S.A.

Jill Stopfer   Abramson Cancer Center, University of Pennsylvania, Philadelphia, Pennsylvania, U.S.A.

Louise C. Strong   University of Texas M.D. Anderson Cancer Center, Houston, Texas, U.S.A.

Sean V. Tavtigian   International Agency for Research on Cancer, Lyon, France

Peter Thom   Clinical Genetics Service, Department of Medicine, Memorial Sloan-Kettering Cancer Center, New York, New York, U.S.A.

Deborah Thompson   Cancer Research U.K. Genetic Epidemiology Unit, University of Cambridge, Cambridge, U.K.

Vickie Venne   Huntsman Cancer Center, University of Utah, Salt Lake City, Utah, U.S.A.

Lisa Walker   Department of Clinical Genetics, The Churchill Hospital, Oxford, U.K.

Kevin M. Zbuk   Genomic Medicine Institute, Lerner Research Institute, Cleveland Clinic Foundation, Cleveland, Ohio, U.S.A.

Bifeng Zhang   Section of Hematology/Oncology, Department of Medicine, University of Chicago, Chicago, Illinois, U.S.A.

SECTION 1: OVERVIEW OF HEREDITARY BREAST CANCER

1

The Genetic Epidemiology of Hereditary Breast Cancer

Douglas F. Easton, Antonis C. Antoniou, and Deborah Thompson
Cancer Research U.K. Genetic Epidemiology Unit, University of Cambridge, Cambridge, U.K.

INTRODUCTION

A family history of breast cancer is one of the most well-established risk factors for the disease. It has been recognized for hundreds of years that the disease can occur in an unusually high frequency in some families. Such anecdotal evidence of familial aggregation has been supported by many systematic epidemiological studies, showing that breast cancer is about twice as common in the women with an affected relative with the disease than it is in the general population (1). Since the mid-1990s, some of the genes that underlie this familial clustering of breast cancer have been identified, and testing for mutations in these genes is now an important part of clinical cancer genetics.

What Is Hereditary Breast Cancer?

It is worth stating at the outset that the term "hereditary breast cancer," while in widespread usage, is somewhat problematic. Hereditary implies that the propensity to disease in that individual has been inherited. Thus, the implication is that breast cancer can be dichotomized into those cases where susceptibility is inherited and those where it is not. This concept arose from consideration of cancers with a simpler genetic basis such as retinoblastoma and Wilm's tumor, which can be usefully categorized in this way (2,3). As we shall see, the situation is much more complex for breast cancer. There are many different susceptibility genes for breast cancer, and a substantial fraction (in fact the majority) of breast cancer cases occur in women who are predisposed in some way. It is also worth emphasizing here that there is no known pathologically distinct type of breast cancer that is hereditary (although certain pathological features are more common in *BRCA1* carriers), so it is not sensible to think of "hereditary" breast cancer as a distinct disease entity.

In clinical genetics, "hereditary" cancer is often used in a more practical sense to denote cases with a strong family history of the disease, consistent with the inheritance of a single dominant gene. This is often distinguished from "sporadic" cancer, meaning no family history and "familial" cancer, meaning any family history of the disease. Familial by itself is a rather loose concept in that it depends on how detailed a family history has been taken. Since breast cancer is a common disease, some family history of breast cancer will be found in most women if the pedigree is extended far enough. However, if restricted to first-degree relatives, approximately 10% of breast cancer cases would be considered "familial." The proportion of women with a strong family history (say two affected first-degree relatives) is much smaller, but again it depends on how comprehensive a family history is available.

Distinguishing women with a strong family history is useful in practice, since such individuals are at higher risk of the disease and may be managed differently. However, it is important to emphasize though that "hereditary" is a misleading term for this group. Even a strong family history does not necessarily imply the presence of a high-risk disease-causing mutation (although it makes it more likely). Conversely, carriers of high-risk mutations may have no apparent family history, for example, if the mutation was inherited through their father.

A more rational approach to the management of women at increased risk of breast cancer is to categorize them according to their level of risk. Such information is the basis for management guidelines in several countries. This risk will depend on their family history and other risk factors and, increasingly, their genotype at known predisposition genes.

Historical Context

The aggregation of breast cancer in families has been recognized for hundreds of years (4). In the mid-20th century, more systematic attempts were made to document high-risk families, such as that described by Gardner and Stephens (5), leading to the hypothesis that a subset of breast cancer may have a strong hereditary component. Subsequently, the study of such families led to the idea of distinct family cancer syndromes, such families with a high risk of breast and ovarian cancer described by Lynch et al. (6) and the Li-Fraumeni syndrome (7).

At the same time, population-based epidemiological studies began to quantify the effect of family history on the risk of the disease; particularly important examples were the studies conducted in Utah and Iceland (8,9). The genetics and epidemiology came together with the systematic studies to define the genetic models for breast cancer (10). Some, though not all such studies, found evidence of a major dominant gene component, providing impetus to studies finding the causative genes themselves.

With the development of methods for typing large numbers of genetic markers, attempts began in the late 1980s to map breast cancer susceptibility genes by genetic linkage analysis in multiple case families. These studies bore fruit with the identification of linkage to chromosome 17 (11), one of the first loci for a genetically complex disease to be mapped. This subsequently led to the identification of the *BRCA1* gene (12). Subsequent similar studies led to the identification of the *BRCA2* gene on chromosome 13 (13,14). Further genetic linkages have not been successful at identifying further high-penetrance susceptibility genes and interest has shifted to association studies to find commoner low-penetrance variants (15,16).

EPIDEMIOLOGICAL STUDIES OF FAMILIAL BREAST CANCER

Much of the impetus for breast cancer genetics has come from observations of families with extraordinary numbers of cases of the disease (5). These families have often been critical to the identification of the high-risk susceptibility genes. They are, however, less useful for evaluating the risks associated with a family history of breast cancer or with any particular gene, because they are not collected in a systematic fashion. To provide useful information for genetic counseling, risk estimates from epidemiological studies are required. Fortunately, many such studies have been conducted. Most are case-control studies that compare the family history of breast cancer in cases with the family history in controls. Other studies are cohort studies of relatives of breast cancer patients. These latter studies include those based on record linkage with national records, notably those done in Sweden, Iceland, and Utah, and they provide estimates that are free from any potential recall bias (8,9,17).

The largest systematic analysis of the risks associated with a family history of breast cancer was a combined analysis of 52 studies by the Collaborative Group on Hormonal Factors in Breast Cancer (1). The results from this study are broadly consistent with the results of other studies, but because the Collaborative Group study is larger, the risk estimates are more reliable. One potential concern is that most of these studies were retrospective case-control studies, raising the possibility that some of the difference is due to differential reporting of family history. However, very similar effects have been observed in cohort studies (8,9,17,18).

The Collaborative Group study estimated that a first-degree family history of breast cancer is associated with an approximately twofold risk of breast cancer. The relative risks associated with an affected mother and an affected sister were very similar (indicating little evidence for any recessive breast cancer susceptibility loci). An important observation was that the relative risk increases progressively with the number of affected first-degree relatives (Table 1).

For women with one affected relative, the risk is inversely related to the age at diagnosis of the breast. Note, however, that the increased risk is present at all ages, and there is no particular age below which the risk is more markedly increased. These observations are consistent with a model in which some predisposition genes confer higher relative risks at young ages.

Table 1 Estimated Risk Ratios for Breast Cancer

		Risk ratio (95% FCI)
Number of affected relatives	None	1.0 (0.97–1.03)
	1	1.80 (1.70–1.91)
	2	2.93 (2.37–3.63)
	3 or more	3.90 (2.03–7.49)
Age at diagnosis	<35	2.91 (2.05–4.13)
	35–39	2.53 (1.97–3.23)
	40–44	2.13 (1.76–2.57)
	45–49	1.84 (1.55–2.17)
	50–54	1.99 (1.71–2.32)
	55–59	1.53 (1.29–1.80)
	60–64	1.46 (1.23–1.74)
	65–69	1.61 (1.37–1.89)
	70–74	1.64 (1.36–1.99)

Abbreviation: FCI, floating confidential internal.
Source: From Ref. 1.

A limitation of the Collaborative Group study is that it was only able to consider first-degree family history. However, the cohort studies from Utah and Iceland provide reliable data on more distant relatives and show a progressive decline in the risk with degree of relationship, so that the relative risk of breast cancer is approximately 1.5 for second-degree relatives of cases for example (19). This relationship is consistent with the hypothesis that the familial aggregation is driven by one or more susceptibility genes (20).

These risks are used as the basis for classifying women for management purposes. For example, according to the National Institute for Clinical Excellence guidelines in the United Kingdom, women with a first-degree relative affected below age 40, or two affected relatives at any age, are considered to be at "moderate" risk. Women with two affected first-degree relatives diagnosed under age 50 are considered to be at "high risk."

There is little consistent evidence that familial risks of breast cancer vary by histological type or grade. Some studies have suggested a strong familial association for lobular breast cancer, but this has not been substantiated (17). The familial risks extend to both ductal and lobular carcinoma in situ (21). There is also a strong familial association between breast cancer in males and breast cancer in the female relatives (22).

There is surprisingly little consistent evidence for the familial aggregation of breast cancer with other cancers, indicating that, to a large extent, susceptibility to breast cancer is site specific. The clearest evidence for clustering with another cancer type is for ovarian cancer for which the risk is approximately 30% higher in mothers and sisters of breast cancer cases (18). This clustering probably reflects the effects of mutations in the *BRCA1* and *BRCA2* genes that predispose to both these cancer types. Associations between breast cancer and colorectal cancer have been suggested but not proven.

Twin Studies and Bilateral Breast Cancer

In principle, the familial aggregation of breast cancer may be due either to genetic factors or to lifestyle or environmental factors that are shared among relatives. The latter possibility is unlikely in that no lifestyle risk factors that are sufficiently strong to materially affect familial aggregation of the disease have been identified. More formal evidence that familial aggregation has a genetic basis comes from twin studies. Based on an analysis of population-based twin registers from the Nordic studies, Lichtenstein et al. (23) found that the risk of breast cancer in the monozygotic (MZ) twins of cases was about twice as great as the risk in the dizygotic (DZ) twins. Using a particular multifactorial model, this study estimated that about 27% of the variation in breast cancer risk was genetic. This particular estimate should be viewed cautiously since it does depend on the model used and on how one defines the variation in breast cancer risk, but it does point to a substantial genetic component.

This evidence of a higher risk of the disease in MZ twins of cases was supported by the study of Peto and Mack (24), who estimated that the risk of breast cancer in the MZ twins of cases was 1.4% per annum. They noted that this risk was approximately twice the incidence rate of contralateral breast cancer in affected women. This is consistent with the hypothesis that the increased risk of a second breast cancer is primarily due to genetic susceptibility, but with only one breast at risk. Peto and Mack also hypothesized that the relative constancy in the risk of contralateral breast cancer might imply that much of breast cancer occurred in women who had reached a high risk of the disease, and that genetic susceptibility might effect the age at which women became high risk rather than (as in more standard models of susceptibility) the actual risk of the disease.

BREAST CANCER SUSCEPTIBILITY AND OTHER RISK FACTORS

An important and largely unresolved question is the relationship between genetic and lifestyle risk factors for breast cancer. The combined analysis by the Collaborative Group examined the effect of several important risk factors on the familial risk of breast cancer, including parity, age at first full-term pregnancy, and ages at menarche and menopause. In each case, they found that the relative risks conferred by these risk factors were similar in women with and without a family history (1). These results imply that such risk factors can be assumed to multiply the familial risks of breast cancer (an assumption made in the Tyrer et al. and Gail models). It also suggests that such risk factors are largely independent of genotype. Whether this is true for specific susceptibility genes, in particular *BRCA1* and *BRCA2*, is less clear however. Several studies have examined the effects of these risk factors in *BRCA1/2* carriers but many of the results are contradictory, perhaps reflecting small sample sizes and the difficulty of obtaining unbiased data in high-risk families. There is reasonably convincing evidence that early oophorectomy is protective in carriers, but the effect of parity, for example, is much less clear, with some studies showing a protective effect comparable to that in the general population and other studies showing no effect or even an increased risk (25–29).

Another interesting factor is that some other risk factors for breast cancer themselves have a heritable basis. The most important is mammographic breast density. Twin studies have estimated that approximately 65% of breast density is heritable. Boyd et al (30). have estimated that about 5% to 10% of the familial aggregation of breast cancer is attributable to the breast density (30). Other risk factors that also have a heritable basis include age and menarche, age at menopause, and body mass index.

MODELS OF BREAST CANCER SUSCEPTIBILITY

Several models have been developed to derive estimates of risk to women with a family history of breast cancer or to estimate the probability of carrying a mutation in the *BRCA1* or *BRCA2* gene. These models can be broadly categorized as "empirical models" and "genetic models." Empirical models are based summarily on measures of family history, such as the number of affected relatives and other risk factors. Perhaps the most widely used model of this kind is the Gail model, which incorporates a variety of breast cancer risk factors in addition to the number of affected relatives (31). Such a model is useful in the general population context, for example, in selecting women for prevention trials but is less useful in high-risk families where the nuances of the family history cannot be captured well.

Genetic models seek to model the familial aggregation of the disease in terms of the effects of specific genes or other familial risk factors. These models are developed from population-based studies of pedigrees using the statistical technique of segregation analysis. One best most well-known model of this kind is that of Claus et al. (32), based on an analysis of the Cancer and Steroid Hormone (CASH) study. This model postulated a single major gene, with an allele frequency of 0.3%, conferring a breast cancer risk of about 80% by age 80. This study found no evidence of any additional polygenic component, so that all the familial aggregation of breast cancer could be explained by a single gene. According to this model, approximately 5% of breast cancer cases would be attributable to this postulated gene. (The model is thus largely responsible for spawning the misleading statements that "about 5% of breast cancer is hereditary.") Other segregation analyses have also been conducted, some of which found other models of disease susceptibility, including models with a recessive component (33). However, the CASH model became widely accepted and used in genetic counseling, perhaps in part because it conformed to the general impression that high-risk families appeared to be dominant, and because it provided a straightforward way of classifying individual risk. And, to an extent, the model was vindicated by the identification of the *BRCA1* and *BRCA2* genes.

In reality, however, the situation is more complex. Mutations in the *BRCA1* and *BRCA2* genes do confer high risks of breast cancer comparable to those suggested by the model, but they do not explain all the familial aggregation of the disease. Since the identification of *BRCA1* and *BRCA2*, more recent models have sought to model the effects of these genes. One of the most widely used is called BRCAPRO (34,35). It models the effects of *BRCA1* and *BRCA2* mutations and can therefore be used to obtain mutation carrier probabilities and age-specific cancer risks. However, it does not account for the effects of other genes and therefore tends to overpredict carrier probabilities. From population-based series and high-risk families from the United Kingdom, Antoniou et al. (36) found that the best fitting model was one incorporating the effects of *BRCA1*, *BRCA2*, and a polygenic component, the effect of many additional genes of small effect. This model, Breast and Ovarian Analysis of Disease Incidence and Carrier Estimation Algorithm (BOADICEA), has been shown to model accurately the familial risks of breast cancer and the prevalence of *BRCA1* and *BRCA2* mutations in population-based series (36). An alternative model was devised by Tyrer et al. (37), which incorporates the effects of *BRCA1*, *BRCA2*, and a third major gene.

There are additional reasons for believing that the polygenic model is reasonable. The frequency of *BRCA1* and *BRCA2* in breast cancer families is strongly dependent on the degree of family history, so that the majority of families with a strong family history (for example, six or more cases) harbor a mutation in one of these genes. This suggests strongly that most other breast cancer genes will confer lower risks. In addition, further genetic linkage studies in multiple case families have not found evidence of any further susceptibility loci, suggesting that if other high-risk susceptibility loci do exist, the alleles are likely to be rare (15,38). The recent identification of some low-penetrance breast cancer loci is further confirmation that susceptibility to breast cancer does have a substantial polygenic component.

The polygenic model has quite different implications to single-gene models like that of Claus et al. (32). Although the latter model classifies everyone as either low or high risk, the polygenic model implies a virtually continuous distribution of risk, such that an individuals' risk is determined by the combination of high-risk alleles that they carry. Under this model, a much higher fraction of breast cancer cases can occur in "high-risk" individuals. Using this model, for example, Pharoah et al. (39) have estimated that about half of all breast cancer cases occur in women in the top 12% of the risk distribution.

Another prediction of the polygenic BOADICEA model is that the "polygenes" will also alter the risk in *BRCA1* and *BRCA2* carriers. Evidence in support of this is provided by the fact that estimates of the risk of breast cancer *BRCA1/2* carriers have generally been higher than those estimated from studies of unselected breast cancer cases (40,41).

BRCA1 AND *BRCA2*

Four genes are known to predispose to a high lifetime risk of breast cancer (Table 2).

Table 2 Known High-Risk Breast Cancer Susceptibility Genes

Gene	Location	Population carrier frequency[a] (Ref.)	Risk of breast cancer by age 70 (95% confidence interval)[b] (Ref.)	Other cancers associated with mutations	Attributable breast cancer incidence (%)	Attributable familial breast cancer risk (%)
BRCA1	17q	1 in 860 (36)	65% (44–78%) (41)	Ovarian, fallopian tube, peritoneum, pancreatic, prostate (29)	1–2	8
BRCA2	13q	1 in 740 (36)	45% (31–56%) (41)	Ovarian, fallopian tube, male breast, prostate, pancreatic, gallbladder, and bile duct (27,28)	1–2	8
TP53	17p	1 in 5000 (45)	≈50–60% by age 45 (46)	Li–Fraumeni Syndrome, including sarcomas, brain tumors and leukemias	<1	<1
PTEN	10q	1 in 250,000 (47)	30–50% (47)	Cowdens disease (multiple hamartomas, thyroid cancer, mucocutaneous lesions) or Bannayan–Riley–Ruvalcaba Syndrome	<<1	<1

[a]Estimated frequency in the United Kingdom. May not be applicable to populations with significant founder mutations (see text).
[b]Risks are based on available large studies but may depend on mutation type and context (e.g., degree of family history).

The most important, numerically, are *BRCA1* and *BRCA2*. Mutations in these genes confer a high risk of both breast cancer and ovarian cancer (40,41). *BRCA2* mutations also confer increased risks of prostate and pancreatic cancer and perhaps also head and neck cancer and melanoma (42,43). *BRCA1* mutations may also predispose to prostate and pancreatic cancer (although with lower risks than for *BRCA1*) and perhaps also to endometrial and cervical cancer (44).

Despite their similarities and the fact that these genes have related roles in the repair of double-strand DNA breaks, there are important differences between *BRCA1* and *BRCA2* in terms of cancer predisposition. Although the lifetime risk of breast cancer is similar in carriers of mutations in *BRCA1* and *BRCA2*, the risk of breast cancer is higher in *BRCA1* carriers at younger ages. The risk of ovarian cancer is markedly higher in *BRCA1* carriers, and the disease tends to occur earlier (in the 35–49 age group). Conversely, the risk of male breast cancer is much higher in *BRCA2* carriers (although *BRCA1* carriers are still at increased risk). As a result, families with multiple cases of breast and ovarian cancer are more likely to harbor a mutation in *BRCA1*, whereas families with multiple cases of breast cancer without ovarian cancer, and particularly those with male breast cancer, are more likely to harbor a *BRCA2* mutation. The higher risks of prostate and pancreatic cancer in *BRCA2* carriers are also a useful diagnostic feature.

Another important difference that has emerged between *BRCA1* and *BRCA2* is in the cancer pathology. The large majorities of *BRCA1*-related breast cancers are estrogen-receptor (ER), progesterone-receptor, and human-epidermal-growth-factor-receptor-2 (HER2) negative and have been shown to stain positive for "Basal" markers such as cytokeratin 5/6 and 14. *BRCA2* tumors, on the other hand, have a more heterogeneous distribution of histopathology, similar to that in noncarriers, with the majority being ER positive.

Founder Mutations

Most mutations in *BRCA1* and *BRCA2* are rare and have arisen relatively recently [typically less than 100 generations ago (48,49). This is presumably because they confer a selective disadvantage perhaps relating to the risk during childbearing age or nonviability of homozygotes (this is even more true of *TP53* mutations owing to the high risk of childhood cancer). Mutations therefore tend to be population specific, so that the spectrum of mutations in, for example, England is different from that in France or the Netherlands. In large populations such as the United Kingdom or the United States, there are many individually rare mutations. Some mutations are found in multiple families, usually because they are descended from a common founder, but no mutation accounts for a high fraction of all families. In some population isolates, however, individual mutations can be quite common, owing to the effects of population bottlenecks and genetic drift. Important examples are the *185delAG* mutation in *BRCA1* and *6174delT* mutation in *BRCA2*, each of which have frequencies of approximately 1% in the Ashkenazi Jewish population (50), and the *999del5* mutation, which has a frequency of approximately 0.5% in the Icelandic population (51). The *5382insC* mutation in *BRCA1* is also quite common in Ashkenazi Jews and also in many populations in East Europe. In Poland, there are three relatively common *BRCA1* mutations. In each of these cases, the known founder mutations appear to explain the large majority of *BRCA1* or *BRCA2* families in these populations. This allows cheaper mutation screening based on the founder mutations, which is reasonably complete. Significant founder mutations have been found in many other populations, for example, in the Netherlands.

Penetrance of *BRCA1* and *BRCA2* Mutations

The cancer risks associated with *BRCA1* and *BRCA2* mutations are critical for genetic counseling and have been the subject of considerable controversy. Ultimately, estimates of penetrance based on prospective followup of unaffected carriers should become available, but current estimates are derived from retrospective data. Penetrance estimates have been derived from high-risk families (the so-called maximum logarithm of (LoD score) odds score approach) and from population-based studies based on the incidence of cancer inrelatives of carriers identified in a series of cases, unselected for family history (the "kin-cohort" approach). Estimates based on high-risk families are directly relevant to that type of family but may overestimate the risk to randomly selected carriers in the population. Population studies may give results that are more applicable to the majority of mutation carriers, but a degree of selection remains since the cohort are all, by definition, relatives of cancer patients. The low frequency of mutations means that even large studies often detect only a small number of carriers, resulting in imprecise estimates. Straightforward case-control studies avoid the potential selection due to other familial factors but are also severely limited by the low frequency of mutations. They are only possible in populations with founder mutations, and even then, the estimates lack precision.

Since mutations are relatively rare, penetrance estimates from individual studies lack precision. Perhaps the best estimates are those derived by Antoniou et al. (41), based on a combined analysis of 22 population studies (Fig. 1).

The cumulative risks of both breast and ovarian cancer are lower in *BRCA1* carriers than *BRCA2* carriers, but the difference is more marked for ovarian cancer (39% vs. 11% by age 70). The difference is also more marked for breast cancer at younger ages. This is a consequence of the fact that *BRCA1* breast cancer incidence rates rise steeply to approximately 3% to 4% per annum in the 40 to 49 age group and are roughly constant thereafter, whereas the *BRCA2* rates show a pattern similar to that in the general population (though approximately 10-fold higher), rising steeply up to age 50 and more slowly thereafter. Ovarian cancer risks in *BRCA1* carriers are very low below age 40, rising thereafter to 1% to 2% per annum, whereas *BRCA2* risks are very low below age 50 but then increase sharply.

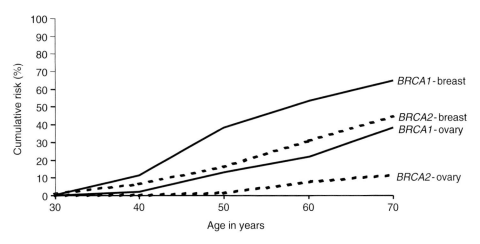

Figure 1 *BRCA1* and *BRCA2* breast and ovarian cancer penetrance estimates, based on a meta-analysis of 22 population-based studies (41).

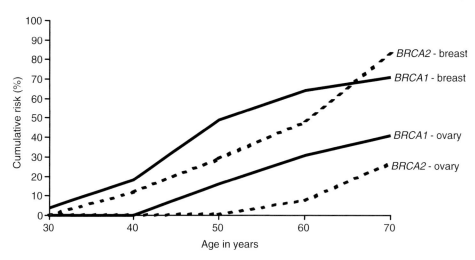

Figure 2 *BRCA1* and *BRCA2* breast and ovarian cancer penetrance estimates, based on high-risk BCLC families (40,52). *Abbreviation*: BCLC, Breast Cancer Linkage Consortium.

For comparison, Figure 2 shows the corresponding penetrance estimates derived from two Breast Cancer Linkage Consortium (BCLC) collaborative studies of high-risk families (40,52).

It is notable that the risks are somewhat higher than those in the Figure 1, especially the breast cancer risks for *BRCA2* carriers. Although it has become generally accepted that penetrance estimates from population-based studies are lower than estimates based on high-risk families, one more recent study based on New York Ashkenazi Jewish breast cancer patients, unselected for age or family history of cancer, found risks of breast cancer by age 80 of 81% and 85% for *BRCA1* and *BRCA2* mutation carriers, respectively, and ovarian cancer risks of 54% and 23%, respectively, by age 80 years (53), more similar to the estimates from high-risk families.

The New York Ashkenazi Jewish study found that the risk of breast cancer by age 50 in carriers of a *BRCA1* or *BRCA2* founder mutation was 24% in women born prior to 1940 but 67% in those born after this date (53). The meta-analysis of population-based studies also found the relative risk of breast cancer associated with a *BRCA1* mutation to be significantly higher for more recent birth cohorts (the same trend was seen for *BRCA2* but was not statistically significant) (41). This could reflect less accurate reporting of cancers in the earlier decades. However, changes in a wide range of lifestyle factors, including diet, exercise, reproductive factors such as age at first pregnancy, family size, breast-feeding preferences, and oral contraceptive use, or in other environmental factors, might also be contributory factors.

The above estimates assume that all mutations confer the same cancer risks. Although most reported deleterious mutations are protein truncating, some expression is still present in the majority of cases, and it is plausible that gene-products truncated to differing degrees may confer different cancer risks. The clearest evidence for such genotype–phenotype correlation is for *BRCA2*, where mutations in a central region referred to as the "Ovarian Cancer Cluster Region" (OCCR; nucleotides 3035–6629; Fig. 1) appear to be associated with a lower breast cancer risk and a higher ovarian cancer risk than other *BRCA2* mutations (54,55). This association may be explained by the fact that the OCCR is coincident with the RAD51-binding domain of *BRCA2*.

There is also some evidence that *BRCA1* mutations in a central region of the gene (nucleotides 2401–4191) confer a lower breast cancer risk than other mutations, whereas mutations toward the 3' end confer a lower risk of ovarian cancer (Fig. 1) (56,47). These mutation-specific effects are not, however, sufficiently large to explain the higher risk of breast cancer in multiple case families. A more likely explanation is that the breast cancer risk in carriers is modified by other genetic factors or lifestyle risk factors in families.

Risks of Other Cancers in *BRCA1/BRCA2* Carriers

In addition to the marked excess of breast and ovarian cancer in *BRCA1* and *BRCA2* carriers, there is also evidence of more moderate risks of other cancer types. The largest study of cancer risks in *BRCA1* carriers, based on 699 carrier families, found an overall cancer risk in male carriers very close to that in the general population, but the risk of cancers other than breast or ovarian in female carriers was increased by approximately twofold (44). Specifically, significant excesses were seen for cancers of the corpus uteri, the cervix, the fallopian tubes, and the peritoneum. There was also some evidence of a twofold relative risk of pancreatic cancer in carriers of both sexes and prostate cancer below age 65.

In a parallel study based on 173 *BRCA2* families, the risk of other cancers was approximately twofold in both male and female carriers (42). The largest excess risk was for prostate cancer, with an estimated 4.7-fold relative risk, increasing to sevenfold in men below age 65. A 3.5-fold risk of pancreatic cancer was also found, and significant excesses were also seen for cancers of the stomach, buccal cavity and pharynx, gallbladder and bile duct, and fallopian tube and for melanoma. A more recent study from the Netherlands also found increased risks of prostate, pancreatic cancer, and head and neck cancer (43).

Other studies have also demonstrated an association between prostate cancer and *BRCA2* mutations. For example, two Icelandic studies found relative risks of prostate cancer between three and five among the first-degree relatives of *BRCA2* mutation carriers (58,59). In addition, a study of 263 prostate cancer cases diagnosed below age 56 years, unselected for family history, estimated a *BRCA2* carrier frequency of nearly 3% (60).

OTHER BREAST CANCER GENES

High-Risk Breast Cancer Genes

Breast cancer is involved in two other hereditary syndromes, for which causative genes have been identified. The Li–Fraumeni syndrome is characterized by childhood sarcoma and early-onset breast cancer, brain tumors, and a variety of other cancers. Most families with Li–Fraumeni syndrome appear to be due to germline mutations in the *TP53* gene. *TP53* mutations confer a very high risk of breast cancer (approaching 100% by age 50) but are much rarer than *BRCA1* or *BRCA2* mutations (45,46). Cowden's syndrome is a rare syndrome characterized by hamartomas, multiple hamartomas, thyroid cancer, and mucocutaneous lesions and is due to germline mutations in *PTEN* (61). The risk of breast cancer associated with Cowden's syndrome has not been well estimated, but it is of the order of 30% to 50% lifetime (47).

Low-Risk Breast Cancer Genes

A growing list of genes is associated with more moderate risks of breast cancer. The first such gene to be identified was *ATM*. Mutations in this gene cause the recessive condition Ataxia-Telangiectasia (A-T) (62). Studies dating back over 30 years have suggested that relatives of A-T patients were at increased risk of breast (and perhaps other) cancer (63). This was long regarded as controversial because the studies were small. However, more recent national cohort studies, and direct studies of *ATM* mutations in breast cancer families and controls, have confirmed that *ATM* mutations confer an approximately twofold risk of breast cancer (with perhaps a higher relative risk at young ages) (64–67).

Another important low-risk susceptibility gene is *CHEK2*, another DNA repair gene that acts downstream of *ATM*. Mutations in this gene were first identified in patients with a family history reminiscent of Li–Fraumeni syndrome, and it was therefore suspected that this was another high-risk susceptibility gene (68). It was subsequently shown, however, that a single mutation in *CHEK2*, *1100delC*, that is present at frequencies of ½% to 1% in European populations, confers an approximately twofold risk of breast cancer (69,70). There is no evidence of any high-risk mutations in this gene. *CHEK2 1100delC* appears to be the predominant disease-causing mutation in Western Europe, but other mutations in Poland and in Ashkenazi Jews, conferring similar risks, have been found. More recently, it has been shown that rare mutations in two other DNA repair genes, *BRIP1* and *PALB2*, also confer similar risks of breast cancer (71–73).

Only one common variant identified through candidate gene studies has been unequivocally linked to breast cancer risk. An amino acid substitution D302H in the *CASP8* gene, with an allele frequency of 13% in Europeans, has been estimated to confer a relative risk of 0.89 in heterozygotes and 0.74 in homozygotes (74). Recently, gene wide association studies have identified six further breast cancer loci (75,76). Many other associations between common genetic variants and breast cancer risk have been reported but most have been refuted (75). However, several genome-wide association studies are currently in progress, and it seems likely that further susceptibility loci will be identified soon.

CONTRIBUTION OF KNOWN GENES TO BREAST CANCER INCIDENCE

The frequency of *BRCA1* and *BRCA2* mutations in breast cancer cases has been estimated by a number of studies. By pooling data from a number of population-based studies, Thompson and Easton (78) estimated that the prevalences of *BRCA1* and *BRCA2* mutations among breast cancer patients diagnosed below their mid-30s were approximately 4.6% and 3.5%, respectively. In contrast, the Anglian Breast Cancer Study (the largest population-based study to date) found the prevalences among cases diagnosed between 45 and 54 years of age to be just 0.3% and 1.0%, respectively (79). These studies underestimate the true prevalence of mutations because studies use methods that are not fully sensitive. Indeed, the fraction of mutations that are detected by such studies is somewhat uncertain because some variants in *BRCA1* and *BRCA2* are of uncertain significance and may or may not be associated with risk. Nevertheless, overall fraction of breast cancer patients in outbred populations carrying *BRCA1* and *BRCA2* mutations is probably close to 1% to 2% for each gene. As noted above, the frequency can be significantly higher in founder populations (see Table 3).

TP53 and *PTEN* mutations are very rare and account for much less than 1% of breast cancer cases. Mutations in *ATM*, *CHEK2*, *BRIP1*, and *PALB2* are also uncommon and also each account for 1% or less of cases. The *CASP8* 302H allele, however, is common, and the estimated attribution fraction is 8% while the attributable fractions for

Table 3 Low Risk Breast Cancer Susceptibility-Genes

Gene	Population frequency of mutations (%)[b]	Relative risk (Refs.)		Attributable risk (%)[c]	Contribution to familial risk of breast cancer (%)[c]
		Carriers:			
ATM	0.3	~2.3 (66,67)		0.8	0.7
CHEK2	0.5[a]	~2.2 (69,70)		1	1
BRIPI	0.1	2.1 (71)		0.1	0.1
PALB2	0.1	2.3 (72)		0,3	0.2
		Hct[d]	Horn[e]		
CASP8 D302H	13 (0)	0.89	0.74 (74)	8.0	0.2
FGFR2 (rs2981582)	38 (30)	1.23	1.63 (75)	16.6	2.0
TNCR9/LOC643714 (rs3803662)	25 (60)	1.23	1.39 (75)	10.0	1.0
MAP3K1 (rs889312)	28 (54)	1.13	1.27 (75)	6.9	0.4
LSP1 (rs3817198)	30 (14)	1.06	1.17 (75)	3.9	0.16
8q (rs13281615)	40 (56)	1.06	1.18 (75)	5.4	0.22
2q (rs13387042)	50 (12)	1.11	1.44 (76)	14.2	1.3

[a] Frequency of the 1100delC mutations that is predominant in Western Europeans. Other mutations have been reported at significant frequency in Poland and in Ashkenazi Jews.

[b] Estimated frequency of mutation carrier or, for common polymorphisms, of the minor allele in European populations, For common polymorphisms, frequency of the corresponding allele in East Asian populations given in brackets.

[c] Estimates based on frequencies in European populations.

[d] Relative risk in heterozygotes.

[e] Relative risk to homozygotes of the minor allele in Europeans.

the loci identified through the genome scans range from 3.9–16.6%. Attributable fraction is, however, not a particularly useful concept for low-penetrance alleles. These risks cannot be avoided, and as more alleles are identified, these fractions are likely to add up to much more than 100%.

CONTRIBUTION OF KNOWN GENES TO FAMILIAL BREAST CANCER

An important question is the extent to which the known susceptibility genes can explain the familial aggregation of breast cancer. The simplest assessment of this is the proportion of the familial risk to first-degree relatives of cases that is explicable by each gene. We might term this the familial attributable fraction of each gene. These estimates can then be added over genes, on the assumption that the genes interact either additively or combined on a log scale, if the genes interact multiplicatively. Unlike the population-attributable fraction, the contribution of known genes to the familial risk cannot exceed 100%, so that it provides an assessment of how much genetic variation remains to be explained and is a much more useful concept. Note, however, that this does not reflect the contribution of these genes to larger multiple case families, which are largely explained by *BRCA1* and *BRCA2* mutations.

In the case of *BRCA1* and *BRCA2*, the familial attributable fraction can be estimated using data from population-based studies that have performed mutation screening, based on the proportion of cases with a family history that have a mutation. Two studies in the United Kingdom have used this approach and obtained very similar estimates—15% to 16% (79,80). Thus, although the proportion of high-risk families that harbor a mutation is high, the fraction of all familial breast cancer due to *BRCA1* and *BRCA2* is quite low. Note, however, that this estimate does depend on the frequency of mutations in the population. It is higher in founder populations such as Ashkenazi Jews and Iceland, for example, and would be expected to be higher in Poland than in the United Kingdom. Because they are rare, the contribution of *TP53* and *PTEN* mutations to the familial risk is likely to be very small—less than 1% (45,47).

The contribution of low-risk genes to the familial aggregation of breast cancer can be estimated more directly from the estimated frequency of the risk allele and the relative risk it confers (Table 3).

Because the relative risks are low, these estimated contributions are small. The rarer variants contribute about 2%, while the common polymorphans identified so far contribute further 5%.

Thus, taken, together, the known genes probably explain approximately 20% to 25% of the familial risk of breast cancer in outbred populations such as those in the United Kingdom or the United States. Thus, the large majority of familial breast cancer remains to be explained. A combination of large genome-wide association studies and resequencing studies to find rarer variants, will be required to find the remaining susceptibility loci.

REFERENCES

1. Beral V, Bull D, Doll R, Peto R, Reeveg G, Familial breast cancer: collaborative reanalysis of individual data from 52 epidemiological studies including 58209 women with breast cancer and 101986 women without the disease. Lancet 2001; 358(9291):1389–1399.
2. Cavenee WK, Dryja TP, Phillips RA, et al. Expression of Recessive All eles by Chromosomal Mechanisms in Rctinoblastoma. Nature 1983; 305(3937):779–784.
3. Pritchard-Jones K, Molecular genetic pathways to Wilms tumour. Critical Reviews Oncogenetics 1997; 8(1):1–27.
4. Broca PP. Traites des Tumeurs, Paris, Asselin, 1886.
5. Gardner EJ, Stephens FE. Breast cancer in 1 family group. Am J Hum Genet 1950; 2(1): 30–40.
6. Lynch HT, Guirgis HA, Albert S, et al. Familial association of cancer of the breast and ovary. Surg Gynecol Obstet 1974; 138(5):717–724.
7. Li FP, Fraumeni JF Jr. Soft-tissue sarcomas, breast cancer and other neoplasms: a familial syndrome? Ann Intern Med 1969; 71(4):747–752.
8. Goldgar DE, Easton DF, Cannon-Albright LA, et al. Systematic population-based assessment of cancer risk in first-degree relatives of cancer probands. J Natl Cancer Inst 1994; 86(21): 1600–1608.
9. Tulinius H, Sigvaldason H, Olafsdottir G, et al. Epidemiology of Breast-Cancer in Families in Iceland. J Mod Genet 1992; 29(3):158–164.
10. Williams WR, Anderson DE. Genetic epidemiology of breast cancer: segregation analysis of 200 Danish pedigrees. Genetic Epidemiol 2007; 1(1):7–20.

11. Hall JM, Lee MK, Newman B, et al. Linkage of Early-Onset Familial Breast-Cancer to Chromosome-17Q21. Science 1990; 250(4988): 1684–1689.
12. Miki Y, Swensen J, Shattuck-Eidens D, et al. A strong candidate for the breast and ovarian cancer susceptibility gene BRCA1. Science 1994; 266(5182):66–71.
13. Wooster R, Neuhausen SL, Mangion J, et al. Localization of A Breast-Cancer Susceptibility Gene, Brca2, to Chromosome 13ql2-l3. Science 1994; 265(5181): 2088–2090.
14. Wooster R, Bignell G, Lancaster J, et al. Identification of the breast cancer susceptibility gene BRCA2. Nature 1995; 378(6559):789–792.
15. Smith P, McGuffog L, Easton DF et al. A genome wide linkage search for breast cancer susceptibility genes. Genes Chromosomes Cancer 2006; 45(7):646–655.
16. Pharoah PDP, Dunning AM, Ponder BAJ, et al. Association studies for finding cancer-susceptibility genetic variants. Nature Rev Cancer 2004; 4(11):850–860.
17. Hemminki K, Vaittinen P. Familial breast cancer in the family-cancer database. Int J Cancer 1998; 77(3):386–391.
18. Peto J, Easton DF, Matthews FE, et al. Cancer mortality in relatives of women with breast cancer: the OPCS Study. Int J Cancer 1996; 65(3):275–283.
19. Slattery ML, Kerber RA. A Comprehensive Evaluation of Family History and Breast-Cancer Risk - the Utah Population Database. JAMA 1993; 270(13):1563–1568.
20. Risch N, Linkage Strategies for Genetically Complex Traits . 1, Multilocus Models. Am J Hum Genet 1990; 46(2):222–228.
21. Claus EB, Stowe M, Carter D. Family history of breast and ovarian cancer and the risk of breast carcinoma in situ. Breast Cancer Res Treat 2003; 78(1):7–15.
22. Weiss JR, Moysich KB, Swede H. Epidemiology of male breast cancer. Cancer Epidemiol Biomarkers Prevention 2005; 14(1):20–26.
23. Lichtenstein P, Holm NV, Vcrkasalo PK et al. Environmental and heritable factors in the causation of cancer - Analyses of cohorts of twins from Sweden, Denmark, and Finland. N Engl J Med 2000; 343(2):78–85.
24. Peto J, Mack TM. High constant incidence in twins and other relatives of women with breast cancer. Nature Genet 2000; 26(4):411–414.
25. Jemstrom H, Lerman C, Gbadirian P, et al. Pregnancy and risk of early breast cancer in carriers of BRCAl and BRCA2. Lancet 1999; 354(9193):1846–1850.
26. Hartge P, Chatterjee N, Wacholder S, et al. Breast cancer risk in Ashkenazi BRCAl/2 mutation carriers: effects of reproductive history. Epidemiol 2002; 13(3):255–261.
27. Tryggvadottir L, Olafadottir EJ, Gudlaugsdottir S, et al. BRCA2 mutation carriers, reproductive factors and breast cancer risk. Breast Cancer Res 2003; 5(5):R121–R128.
28. Narod SA, Goldgar D, Cannon-Albright L, et al. Risk modifiers in carriers of BRCAl mutations. Int J Cancer 1995; 64(6):394–398.
29. Andrieu N, Goldgar DE, Easton DF, et al. Pregnancies, breast-feeding, and breast cancer risk in the International BRCA1/2 Carrier Cohort Study (IBCCS). J Natl Cancer Inst 2006; 98(8): 535–544.
30. Boyd NF, Rommens JM, Vogt K et al. Mammographic density as an intermediate phenotype for breast cancer. Lancet Oncol 2005; 6(10):798–808.
31. Gail MH, Brinton LA, Byar DP, et al. Projecting individualized probabilities of developing breast cancer for white females who are being examined annually. J Natl Cancer Inst 1989, 81(24):1879–1886.
32. Claus EB, Risch N, Thompson WD. Genetic-Analysis of Breast-Cancer in the Cancer and Steroid-Hormone Study. Am J Hum Genet 1991; 48:232–242.
33. Goldstein AM, Hailc RW, Hodge SE, et al. Possible heterogeneity in the segregation pattern of breast cancer in families with bilateral breast cancer. Genet Epidemiol 1988; 5(2):121–133.
34. Berry DA, Parmigiani G, Sanchez J, et al. Probability of carrying a mutation of breast-ovarian cancer gene BRCA1 based on family history. J Natl Cancer Inst 1997; 89(3):227–238.
35. Parmigjani G, Berry DA, Aguilar O, Determining carrier probabilities for breast cancer-susceptibility genes BRCA1 and BRCA2. Am J Hum Genet 1998; 62(1):145–158.

36. Antoniou AC, Pharoah PDP, Smith P et al. The BOADICEA model of genetic susceptibility to breast and ovarian cancer. Br J Cancer 2004; 91(8):1580–1590.

37. Tyrer J, Duffy SW, Cuzick J, A breast cancer prediction model incorporating familial and personal risk factors. Stat Med 2004; 23(7):1111–1130.

38. Huusko P, Gillanders E, Vahteristo P et al. Genome-wide scanning for linkage in Finnish breast cancer families. Am J Hum Genet 2001; 69(4):205.

39. Pharoah PDP, Antoniou A, Zimmern R, et al. Polygenic susceptibility to breast cancer and implications for prevention. Nature Genet 2002; 31(1):33–36.

40. Ford D, Easton DF, Stratton MR, et al. Genetic heterogeneity and penetrance analysis of the BRCA1 and BRCA2 genes in breast cancer families. The Breast Cancer Linkage Consortium. Am J Hum Genet 1998; 62(3):676–689.

41. Antoniou A, Pharoah PDP, Narod S, et al. Average risks of breast and ovarian cancer associated with mutations in BRCA1 or BRCA2 detected in case series unselected for family history: a combined analysis of 22 studies. Am J Hum Genet 2003; 72(5):1117–1130.

42. The Breast Cancer Linkage Consortium. Cancer risks in BRCA2 mutation carriers. J Nat Cancer Inst 1999; 91(15):1310–1316.

43. van Asperen CJ, Brohet RM, Meijers-Heijboer EJ, et al. Cancer risks in BRCA2 families: estimates for sites other than breast and ovary. J Med Genet 2005; 42(9):711–719.

44. Thompson D, Easton DF, Breast Cancer Linkage Consortium. Cancer Incidence in BRCA1 Mutations, J Natl Cancer Inst 2002; 94(18):1358–1365.

45. Lalloo F, Varley J, Ellis D, et al. Prediction of pathogenic mutations in patients with early-onset breast cancer by family history. Lancet 2003; 361(9363):1101–1102.

46. Chompret A, Brugicres L, Rensin M, et al. p53 germline mutations in childhood cancers and cancer risk for carrier individuals. Brit J Cancer 2000; 82(12):1932–1937.

47. Ball S, Arolker M, Purushotham AD. Breast cancer, Cowden disease and PTEN-MATCHS syndrome. Eur J Surg Oncol 2001; 27(6):604–606.

48. Neuhausen SL, Mazoyer S, Friedman L, et al. Haplotype and phenotype analysis of six recurrent BRCA1 mutations in 61 families: results of an international study. Am J Hum Genet 1996; 58(2):271–280.

49. Neuhausen SL, Godwin AK, Gershoni-Baruch R, et al. Haplotype and phenotype analysis of nine recurrent BRCA2 mutations in 111 families: results of an international study. Am J Hum Genet 1998; 62(6):1381–1388.

50. Fodor FH, Weston A, Bleiweiss U, et al. Frequency and carrier risk associated with common BRCA1 and BRCA2 mutations in Ashkenazi Jewish breast cancer patients. Am J Hum Genet 1998; 63(1):45–51.

51. Johannesdottir G, Gudmundsson J, Bergthorsson JT, et al. High prevalence of the 999del5 mutation in Icelandic breast and ovarian cancer patients. Cancer Res 1996; 5 (16):3663–3665.

52. Easton DF, Ford D, Bishop DT, Breast Cancer Linkage Consortium, Breast and ovarian cancer incidence in BRCA1 mutation carriers. Am J Hum Genet 1995; 56(1):265–271.

53. King MC, Marks JH, Mandell JB. Breast and ovarian cancer risks due to inherited mutations in BRCA1 and BRCA2. Science 2003; 302(5645):643–646.

54. Gayther SA, Mangion J, Russell P, et al. Variation of risks of breast and ovarian cancer associated with different germline mutations of the BRCA2 gene. Nat Genet 1997; 15(1):103–105.

55. Thompson D, Easton D, Breast Cancer Linkage Consortium. Variation in cancer risks, by mutation position, in BRCA2 mutation carriers. Am J Hum Genet 2001; 68(2):410–419.

56. Gayther SA, Warren W, Mazoyer S, et al. Germline mutations of the BRCA1 gene in breast and ovarian cancer families provide evidence for a genotype-phenotype correlation. Nat Genet 1995; 11(4):428–433.

57. Thompson D, Easton D, Breast Cancer Linkage Consortium. Variation in BRCA1 cancer risks by mutation position. Cancer Epidemiol Biomarkers Prev 2002; 11(4):329–336.

58. Thorlacius S, Sigurdsson S, Bjamedottir H, et al. Study of a single BRCA2 mutation with high carrier frequency in a small population. Am J Hum Genet 1997; 60(5):1079–1084.

59. Sigurdsson S, Thorlacius S, Tomasson J, et al. BRCA2 mutation in Icelandic prostate cancer patients. J Mol Med 1997; 75(10):758–761.

60. Edwards SM, Kote-Jarai Z, Meitz J, et al. Two percent of men with early-onset prostate cancer harbor germline mutations in the BRCA2 gene. Am J Hum Genet 2003; 72(1):1–12.

61. Liaw D, Marsh DJ, Li J, et al. Germline mutations of the PTEN gene in Cowden disease, an inherited breast and thyroid cancer syndrome. Nat Genet 1997; 16(1):64–67.

62. Savitsky K, BarShira A, Gilad SA, et al. Single Ataxia-Telangicctasia Gene with A Product Similar to Pi-3 Kinasc. Science 1995; 268(5218):1749–1753.

63. Swift M, Morrell D, Massey RB et al. Incidence of Cancer in 161 Families Affected by Ataxia-Telangiectasia. New Engl J Med 1991; 325(26):1831–1836.

64. Olsen JH, Hahnemann JM, Borresen-Dale AL, et al. Cancer in patients with ataxia-telangiectasia and in their relatives in the Nordic countries. J Natl Cancer Inst 2001; 93(2): 121–127.

65. Janin N, Andrieu N, Oasian K, et al. Breast cancer risk in ataxia telangiectasia (AT) heterozygotes: haplotype study in French AT families, Brit J Cancer 1999; 80(7):1042–1045.

66. Renwick A, Thompson D, Seal S, et al. ATM mutations that cause ataxia-telangiectasia are breast cancer susceptibility alleles. Nat Genet 2006; 38(8):873–875.

67. Thompson D, Duedal S, Kirner J, et al. Cancer risks and mortality in heterozygous ATM mutation carriers. J Natl Cancer Inst 2005; 97(11):813–822.

68. Bell DW, Varley JM, Szydlo TE, et al. Heterozygous germ line hCIIK2 mutations in Li-Fraumeni syndrome. Science 1999; 286(5449):2528–2531.

69. Meijers-Heijboer H, van den Ouweland A, Klijn J et al. Low-penetrance susceptibility to breast cancer due to CHEK2*1100delC in noncarriers of BRCA1 or BRCA2 mutations. Nat Genetics 2002; 31(1):55–59.

70. The CHEK2 Breast Cancer Case-Control Consortium. CHEK2*1l00delC and susceptibility to breast cancer: A collaborative analysis involving 10,860 breast cancer cases and 9,065 controls from ten studies. Am J Hum Genet 2004; 74(6):1175–1182.

71. Seal S, Thompson D, Renwick A, et al. Truncating mutations in the Faneoni anemia J gene BRIPl are low-penetrance breast cancer susceptibility alleles. Nat Genet 2006; 38(11): 1239–1241.

72. Rahman N, Seal S, Thompson D, et al. PALB2, which encodes a BRCA2-interacting protein, is a breast cancer susceptibility gene. Nat Genets 2007; 39(2):165–167.

73. Erkko H, Xia B, Nikkila J. et al. A recurrent mutation in PALB2 in Finnish cancer families. Nature 2007; 446(7133):316–319.

74. Cox A, Dunning AM, Garcia-Closas M et al. A common coding variant in CASP8 is associated with breast cancer risk. Nat Genet 2007; 39(3):352–358.

75. Easton DF, Pooley KA, Dunning AM, et al. Genome-wide association study identifies novel breast cancer susceptibility loci. Nature 2007; 447(7148):1087–1093.

76. Staccy SN, Manoleseu A, Sulem P, et al. Common variants on chromosomes 2q35 and 16ql2 confer susceptibility to estrogen receptor-positive breast cancer. Nat Genet 2007; 39(7): 865–9.

77. Breast Cancer Association Consortium. Commonly studied SNPs and breast cancer: negative results from 12,000 - 32,000 cases and controls from the Breast Cancer Association Consortium. J Nat Cancer Inst 2006; 98(19):1382–1396.

78. Thompson D, Easton DF. The BRCA1 and BRCA2 genes. In: RA Eeles, DF Easton, BAJ Ponder, C Eng eds. Genetic predisposition to cancer, 2nd ed. London: Arnold, 2004:256–276.

79. Anglian Breast Cancer Study Group. Prevalence of BRCA1 and BRCA2 mutations in a population-based series of breast cancer caaea. Br J Cancer 2000; 83(10):1301–1308.

80. Peto J, Collins N, Barfoot R, et al. Prevalence of BRCAl and BRCA2 gene mutations in patients with early-onset breast cancer. J Natl Cancer Inst 1999; 91(11):943–949.

2

Risk Prediction in Breast Cancer

Lisa Walker

Department of Clinical Genetics, The Churchill Hospital, Oxford, U.K.

Rosalind Eeles

The Institute of Cancer Research & Royal Marsden NHS Foundation Trust, Surrey, U.K.

INTRODUCTION

Individuals with a family history of breast and ovarian cancer are often seen in cancer genetics clinics, as they are worried about their chances of developing these and other types of cancer. Clinical management of these individuals involves assessment of the degree of risk due to the family history, often in conjunction with genetic testing. The first risk estimation to be made is the chance that a familial cluster is due to genetic predisposition. This is called the prior probability of a cancer predisposition gene being present in a family. This estimation can be based upon published data or clinical experiences when published data are lacking, which unfortunately is often the case with rare genetic conditions. In the case of hereditary breast and ovarian cancer, however, we are in the fortunate position of having several risk prediction models. The primary function of these is to try to evaluate the prior probability of a high-risk gene being present in the family. The second part of risk evaluation in the cancer genetics clinic is the risk that a specific individual will go on to develop a malignancy. This is also facilitated by some, but not all, of the risk prediction models currently available.

A number of genes have been identified, which confer increased susceptibility to breast cancer. The main genes are *BRCA1* and *BRCA2* (1,2), but others include *CHEK2* (3), *ATM* (4), *TP53* (5), and *PTEN* (6). These known genes are estimated to account for 20% to 25% of the observed familial cases of breast cancer, indicating that other genes remain to be identified. Recently, several rare low-risk genes have been reported (7,8), but these only account for about 2% of the familial risk.

Since the most common genes known to be involved in hereditary breast and ovarian cancer are *BRCA1* and *BRCA2*, the risk assessment models, which have been developed have focused on these two genes. Management of *BRCA1/2* mutation carriers is complex and may involve screening, chemoprevention, or risk-reducing surgery. It is therefore important to identify these individuals at the highest risk in order that such strategies may be targeted appropriately.

This chapter will be devoted to the different models used to establish the risk to an individual. The way in which the risk is conveyed to the individual is, however, vital. It is of no use conveying information that "you are at 43% risk of carrying a

BRCA1/2 mutation" to an individual whose sociodemographic and educational background means that he/she has no idea of the significance and implications of that statement. The optimal format for conveying risk information is unknown. Currently, risk estimates tend to be given as a percentage risk or a "1 in *x*" value and followed up with a written summary, incorporating this risk estimate, to the individual attending the genetics consultation. Unfortunately, there are data that suggest that women prefer not to have, or remember, numerical information. For example, 98% of women attending a cancer family clinic because of a family history of breast cancer could not remember their percentage annual risk, even when this was given both verbally in the clinic and by follow-up letter. More importantly though, they were able to report the qualitative category of their risk (low, medium, high) with reasonable accuracy, but this did not relate to their perception that they were more or less likely to get cancer (9). This suggests that clients have a poor understanding of the risk information being given. Green and Brown (10) have suggested that the qualitative aspect of risk is more important than the quantitative aspect. However, this finding contrasts with that of Josten et al. (11) who report from a cancer family clinic in Wisconsin, U.S.A. that "clients say that a number gives them boundaries rather than having an ambiguous sense of being high risk." The main problem with the quantitative approach is that one person's high risk is another's moderate risk.

Genetic testing can, in some cases, refine risk; however, it is expensive and has been shown to be associated with adverse psychological effects in some studies (12,13). In particular, the psychological stress of predictive genetic testing for *BRCA* mutations in unaffected individuals has been well documented. However, this seems to be temporary and the overall psychological status is not worsened three to five years after genetic testing (14).

The effect of genetic testing on insurance policies is also important, as this varies in different countries. The social implications of the ability to purchase life and medical insurance, mortgages, and a possible effect on employment opportunities may be just as important as, if not more important than, the personal and familial implications. At present, effects on employment are theoretical. Following a recent statement from the Association of British Insurers in March 2005, an individual may apply for a total of up to £500,000 of life insurance and £300,000 of any class of insurance without having to disclose to the insurer the results of any predictive genetic test previously taken (15). This moratorium is currently scheduled to remain in place until 2011 at least and breast cancer genetic tests are not included on the list with these restrictions at present. In the United States, however, the effect of genetic testing on insurance policies varies from state to state.

In order to provide an effective clinical genetics service to patients at risk of carrying mutations in the *BRCA1* and *BRCA2* genes, therefore, it is important to target genetic testing to those individuals at the highest risk. To assess the risk to an individual conferred by a family history, however, is complex and requires consideration of several independent factors. Mathematical models have been developed to try to provide consistent and effective risk assessment. These differ in their methods of analysis and also in their ease of use in the clinical setting. This last factor is vital if a model is to become widely used in genetic clinics, as the majority of cancer genetics clinicians who see patients in clinics are not, themselves, mathematicians. The models and computer programs also need to be user friendly in a busy clinical setting. It is important, therefore, that clinicians retain a sense of perspective with regard to the likelihood of a family history being high risk, independent of any mathematical models that are used. Hopefully, this will prevent errors due to incorrect entering of information into the model and/or errors due to the limitations of the various models.

It is likely that other factors contribute to the risk of breast cancer in individuals from these families. Assessment of these possible "lifestyle" factors, together with other modifying genes, will become increasingly important. It is likely that future models will incorporate these additional factors to a greater extent.

The models themselves have been developed over the last 17 years. Several of them are logistic regression models that utilize descriptive measures of family history, and these are useful in cancer genetics because other, nongenetic risk factors can readily be incorporated. One disadvantage of this type of analysis, however, is that it does not deal adequately with complex family histories. None of the models used currently consider a history of risk-reducing surgical procedures (e.g., prophylactic mastectomy or salpingo-oophorectomy), which are important for more accurate risk assessment and this should be thoroughly ascertained by the clinician. The other factor that is not currently dealt with by any of the models [although Breast and Ovarian Analysis of Disease Incidence and Carrier Estimation Algorithm (BOADICEA) does have plans to include it in the near future] is pathological data, which can have a bearing on the likelihood of a family history corresponding to a mutation in a high-risk gene.

In this chapter, we will describe the most commonly used models for risk assessment in breast and ovarian cancer. Each model will be described briefly, together with its advantages and limitations. We will use clinical examples to illustrate this where possible.

CLAUS MODEL

This was one of the first of the risk prediction models to be developed. It was derived from the Cancer and Steroid Hormone ("CASH" or "Claus") study (16). This was a study of 4700 women with breast cancer, who had their family history taken. A statistical model (Claus model, named after the author of the study) was developed that estimated the chance that a cancer-predisposition gene was present in a family. The model dates from before the *BRCA1* and *BRCA2* genes were identified. The complex segregation analysis used to derive the model assumes that a single, rare, dominantly inherited gene accounts for genetic susceptibility to breast cancer in the general population. The penetrance of this gene is assumed to be 95% by the age of 80. This model can be used to generate the curves in Figure 1, which can be used easily in a genetics clinic to estimate risk.

For example, if an individual has two first-degree relatives with breast cancer at 45 years there is a 60% chance that there is a breast cancer–predisposition gene present.

Although this model remains one of the most widely used, it has obvious limitations given the extent to which knowledge about genes conferring susceptibility to breast cancer has accumulated since its development. The major limitation is that we now know there are several high-risk genes with varying degrees of penetrance.

Moreover, the limited validation data available regarding the Claus model suggest that it has poor sensitivity and specificity. It also has been found to significantly underestimate breast cancer risk and does not take into account ovarian cancer or male breast cancer. It is surprising that such limited validation data are available for this model, given its long-standing widespread use.

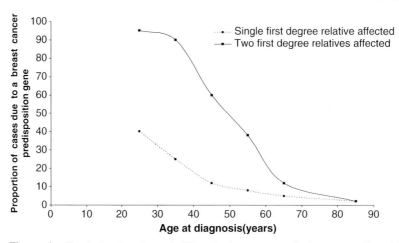

Figure 1 Graph showing the probability that breast cancer is due to a predisposition gene by age at diagnosis of breast cancer (16). *Source*: Graph courtesy of Prof. D.T. Bishop.

SHATTUCK–EIDENS MODEL

This model was one of many developed by Myriad Genetics, Inc., (Salt Lake City, U.S.A.) to predict the likelihood of a given individual having a mutation in one of the breast cancer predisposing genes *BRCA1* or *BRCA2*. This was one of the earliest such models to be developed (17,18), and it only involved prediction of mutations in *BRCA1*. The authors used full sequencing data from 798 unrelated individuals, who had been selected for testing because of a family history comprising multiple cases of breast and/or ovarian cancer. For 75% of the patients (where complete family information was available), the family history comprised only breast cancers. The authors found that the most useful factors to predict whether or not an individual was likely to have a mutation in *BRCA1* were younger age, bilateral breast cancer, individuals with both breast and ovarian cancer and Ashkenazi Jewish ancestry. These factors were then used in logistic regression analysis. Data from this model are presented as graphs of risk correlating with a specific family history. Separate graphs are presented for the Ashkenazi Jewish population, owing to the high incidence of two common mutations in *BRCA1* in this community.

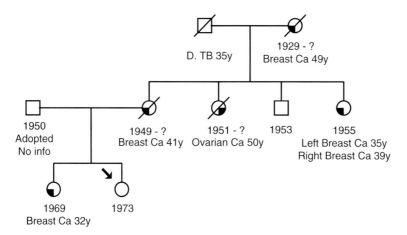

Figure 2 Proband is arrowed. Quarter filled in symbol indicates affected with cancer.

The "full sequencing" that was undertaken to produce the model in this case does, however, have limitations. Only coding regions and intronic sequences adjacent to exons were sequenced. There may be other mutations in unsequenced regions of introns, which adversely affect RNA processing or splicing, and these would not be detected by the method used in this analysis. The sequencing method would also not detect intragenic deletions or duplications, and it is not known what percentage of mutations in *BRCA1* is accounted for by such rearrangements, although this is thought to be around 8%.

Another limitation of this model is that only *BRCA1* analysis was performed. It is now known that a proportion of individuals who were found not to have mutations in *BRCA1* in this analysis are likely to have mutations in *BRCA2*.

Finally, this model does not take into account the presence of multiple affected relatives. A woman aged 45 years with one sister affected with breast cancer aged 40 would be designated as having the same likelihood of having a mutation in *BRCA1* as a woman aged 45 with four sisters affected with breast cancer aged 40. The model is also based on the prior probability of a *BRCA1* mutation being present in an individual rather than the prior probability that there is a *BRCA1* mutation present in the family. Different family members may therefore be designated as being at different risk, even though they have the same family history. This may, of course, be entirely appropriate, for example, if two sisters are the only known affected individuals in one family: one diagnosed with breast cancer aged 55, and the other diagnosed with ovarian cancer aged 45 and then breast cancer aged 50, it would follow that there would be an increased likelihood that the woman diagnosed with ovarian and breast cancer had a mutation in *BRCA1* over her sister, who may be a phenocopy. This method, however, does give risk figures for affected women with no family history, unlike previously produced models in this field.

BRCAPRO

The BRCAPRO model was initially produced in 1998 (19) and subsequently validated in a publication of 2002 (20). Unlike most other models described in this chapter, the BRCAPRO model utilizes Bayesian calculations to derive prior probability data for both *BRCA1* and *BRCA2*. It also incorporates data regarding published *BRCA1* and *BRCA2* mutation frequencies, together with information about the first- and second-degree relatives of the proband, cancer status of relevant individuals, and cancer penetrance in known mutation carriers. It does utilize data regarding bilateral breast cancer and male breast cancer and may also be used to calculate risks of developing breast cancer. A separate program has been developed for the analysis of family histories from the Ashkenazi Jewish population by these authors.

Because the data are primarily based on large families in which multiple members have been affected by breast and/or ovarian cancer (in 71% of the families analyzed, there were three or more cases of breast and ovarian cancer), the model's predictive power may be somewhat biased toward these families. As a result, the estimates of likelihood of *BRCA1/2* mutations given by the BRCAPRO model tend to be somewhat higher than for other models. This model, therefore, tends to perform well in families clinically seen to be at very high risk such as that in Figure 2, Pedigree 1. The lower risk families would be more likely to have misleading data generated by this model. The model discriminates relatively well between mutation carriers and noncarriers, but the discrimination between *BRCA1* and *BRCA2* mutation carriers is poor. In particular, it tends to overestimate the *BRCA1* carrier probability and underestimate the *BRCA2* carrier probability (21). A second problem is that only first- and second-degree relatives are considered in the analysis. Different prior probability risk figures may, therefore, be generated depending on which individual in the family is used in the analysis. It is therefore necessary to optimize the consideration of which individual to use in the analysis before embarking upon it.

Data entry for BRCAPRO requires the use of computer-generated software. This data entry is not always straightforward and may therefore be time consuming. For this reason, BRCAPRO is often felt to be less user friendly than some of the other risk-prediction models. There are many studies comparing the data generated by BRCAPRO with that generated by other prior probability risk prediction models, and the results of analysis done on these data consistently indicate that BRCAPRO performs relatively well in the highest risk families but is a less consistent discriminator of prior probability where the family history is more equivocal (22,23). BRCAPRO also tends to underestimate breast cancer risk in unaffected individuals in the single study that has been undertaken (24). For these reasons, it is not used in many genetics clinics in the United Kingdom as high-risk families can be assessed easily whereas the more difficult families to assess are those where the risk is not so high risk.

BREAST AND OVARIAN ANALYSIS OF DISEASE INCIDENCE AND CARRIER ESTIMATION ALGORITHM (BOADICEA)

BOADICEA is one of the latest of the carrier prediction models to be developed (25). It used a U.K. population–based series of 2200 breast cancer cases, 156 multiple case families, and 429 *BRCA1/2* carrier families. All were tested for *BRCA1/2* mutations. The complex segregation analysis used resulted in a model that allows for the simultaneous effects of *BRCA1* and *BRCA2*. It also takes into account the effect of many low-penetrance genes that are likely to have multiplicative effects on the breast cancer risk. The effects of genetic modifiers that cluster within families and are likely to alter breast cancer risks in *BRCA1* and *BRCA2* carriers can also be incorporated.

BOADICEA is able to compute any exact family relationship, and any size of family, in contrast to many of the other models, which will only consider a certain number of first- and second-degree relatives. BOADICEA also allows for the variable sensitivity of mutation testing. This is especially important for the United Kingdom and some other countries where whole gene sequencing of *BRCA1* and *BRCA2* has only become available relatively recently, and prior to this, targeted analysis of mutation hot spots in both genes was the only available testing, which has reduced sensitivity.

BOADICEA will calculate the probability of developing breast or ovarian cancer and also the probability of carrying a *BRCA1/2* mutation. It also allows for the "cohort effect," which is not considered by other models. The cohort effect reflects the fact that breast cancer is becoming relatively more common in the general population. If a woman was born in 1925, her risk of getting breast cancer by age 70 is lower than that if she was born in 1955. This cohort effect also holds true for *BRCA* carriers.

There are few limitations of BOADICEA in its current form. Those that do exist come from the relatively broad age categories by which the genotype-specific incidence rates are computed. For example, these would then be deemed constant over the age period 30 to 34 but would differ from that at age 29 and that at age 35. At present, the "risk of developing cancer" only gives a risk of the first incidence of either breast or ovarian cancer. BOADICEA is being updated to address this. The model does not as yet take into consideration data regarding the pathology of breast tumors found, but this is planned. This is reported to differ between *BRCA* carriers and noncarriers and also between *BRCA1* carriers and *BRCA2* carriers (26). Extension of the model to incorporate nongenetic risk factors, e.g., parity, breast feeding, and age at menopause may be possible when the contribution of these factors to the overall risk to *BRCA* carriers has been more comprehensively assessed by long-term studies such as Epidemiological Study of Familial Breast Cancer (EMBRACE) (27).

There have been two studies thus far to validate BOADICEA. The first (22) compared the current version of BOADICEA with BRCAPRO using 188 French Canadian families. BOADICEA was found to be more accurate, and this was thought to result from the increased data gathered by BOADICEA because of the consideration of more relatives in the calculations. The other study used an older version of BOADICEA, which was found to be comparably accurate with BRCAPRO, Myriad, and the Manchester scoring system in non-Ashkenazi Jewish families. BOADICEA was found to be the most accurate in the Ashkenazi Jewish families (23).

Software to facilitate the implementation of the BOADICEA model by clinicians is still in its final development stage, but the authors have thus far produced an extremely user-friendly web-based interface, which is undergoing β-testing in the clinical setting.

MANCHESTER

The Manchester scoring system was developed by Evans et al. in 2004. Its aim was to provide a quick accurate method of assessing whether genetic testing for *BRCA1* or *BRCA2* is appropriate given a family history of breast and ovarian cancer, and if so, which of the two genes should be tested first.

Development of the scoring system used a dataset of 422 non-Jewish families with a history of breast and/or ovarian cancer. These were subsequently screened for mutations in *BRCA1*, and a subset was then screened for mutations in *BRCA2* using a whole gene approach. Using the family history data in conjunction with the mutation data on these individuals, a scoring system was developed that highlights those factors most likely to indicate *BRCA1/2* mutation status in a particular family.

The model was specifically designed to estimate a pretest probability of 10% of carrying a mutation in *BRCA1/2*. This would then enable the practicing clinician to prioritize families appropriately for genetic testing. Different factors are more likely to be responsible for mutations in *BRCA1* versus *BRCA2*. This is reflected by differential scoring between the two genes. For example, male breast cancer below age 60 scores 8 in *BRCA2* but 5 in *BRCA1* (assuming *BRCA2* has been tested), and female breast cancer scores 6 in *BRCA1* but 5 in *BRCA2*. This model also takes into consideration other cancers commonly seen in *BRCA*-carrier families. *BRCA2* families are known to have a higher incidence of young onset prostate cancer and pancreatic cancer than the general population. This is reflected by the inclusion of scoring data for these cancers in the criteria for *BRCA2*. Originally, the authors of the Manchester scoring system stated that a score of 10 represented a 10% likelihood of finding a *BRCA1/2* mutation in a given family. This has now been updated, however (28), and a combined Manchester score of 15 is now taken to be the 10% threshold for initiating *BRCA* testing. This update resulted from the more extensive genetic analysis for the original dataset and those subsequently used to validate the original data.

The Manchester scoring system is extremely useful in the clinical setting, and it has been validated on many families with and without known mutations in the *BRCA* genes. It does have some limitations in its current form, however. It would not allow for genetic testing of an isolated case of male or female breast cancer, whatever the age, despite consensus that this may be worthwhile in females with Grade 3 estrogen-receptor negative breast cancer aged less than 35 years. The scoring system does not actually produce a carrier probability: it simply computes a threshold above which testing should be initiated. It is therefore difficult to compare it with other models in this respect. The scoring system is likely to have limitations in extremely small families, which are unlikely to reach the threshold for testing unless the family history is extremely powerfully suggestive of the presence of a *BRCA1/2* mutation. The algorithm also does not include data from the Ashkenazi Jewish community and, clearly, this may need to be addressed in areas where large Ashkenazi populations are present, as it has not been validated for this population. Ideally, other factors could be added to the Manchester scoring system to make it more precise. The authors have already alluded to differences encountered in mutation data given different ovarian pathology but similar pedigree data. The use of breast cancer pathology data may also be useful, together with data concerning risk-reducing surgery as this becomes more prevalent in these families.

Validation of the Manchester scoring system has been done in a study by Evans et al. (21). This involved 258 low-risk families from the United Kingdom, whose *BRCA1/2* mutation status was known. The scoring system performed best in a test of discrimination and sensitivity, when compared with the Myriad model, Frank and BRCAPRO, but its specificity is not as good. This reflects the fact that the best use of this model is as a screening test to decide who should be put forward for *BRCA1/2* genetic analysis.

FRANK/MYRIAD

There have been several risk prediction models produced by Myriad Genetics, Inc. The latest of these is known as the Frank model or the Myriad model. The original work used 216 U.S. breast cancer patients who were diagnosed at below 50 years of age, with at least one first- or second-degree relative with breast cancer diagnosed at less than 50 years of age or ovarian cancer at any age. It involved logistic regression analysis, which identified the following factors as likely to be predictive of *BRCA1/2* mutation status: breast cancer below 50 years and ovarian cancer and bilateral breast cancer (29).

The current Frank model was updated in Spring 2005, using data from a retrospective analysis of 10,000 individuals whose *BRCA1/2* genes had been analyzed at Myriad Genetics, Inc., and may be found on the Myriad website (www.myriadtests.com/provider/mutprev.htm) (30). It takes the form of two tables, one involving Ashkenazi Jewish individuals, the other for non-Jewish individuals. Data are presented as a percentage likelihood of having a mutation in *BRCA1/2*. The model does not separate the two genes in terms of likelihood of having a mutation. This may, of course, be influenced by commercial considerations, given that Myriad are themselves involved in the provision of genetic testing for *BRCA1* and *BRCA2* mutations. Furthermore, the family history given on the test request forms for Myriad genetics is not very detailed, particularly for second and more distantly related relatives.

The Frank model is extremely useful since it is the only one to provide percentage probability estimates for the Ashkenazi Jewish population separately. As more Jewish families become aware of the high prevalence of *BRCA1/2* mutations within their community, it is likely that more of the risk prediction models will produce data for this community, as more mutation data are likely to become available in the next few years.

The sample families used to derive the Frank model originally were all high-risk families. Because of this, the percentage probabilities generated by the model tend to be higher than those found in the other models. This problem is also encountered in BRCAPRO. The table format is user friendly, and the data are clearly presented. This is important if a model is to be used in the clinical setting. Many visitors to the Myriad website are, however, family members curious about their risk of breast and ovarian cancer. Presentation of the data in this way facilitates its use by these non-specialists, but this may not be optimal, for reasons outlined below.

Like the original Myriad model, (the Shattuck–Eidens model), this model calculates the *BRCA1/2* mutation probability data based on one individual, rather than for the family as a whole. This has advantages and disadvantages: clearly, mutation probability may vary between individuals within a family, and it is prudent to test the individual with the highest probability where possible. This phenomenon may, however, prove difficult to explain to families where multiple members are being seen together for genetic counseling. The model is not applicable to an unaffected individual with a family history of breast and ovarian cancer. Another difficulty with this model is that the categories used are somewhat broad. Age 50 is taken as the cutoff, indicating that a woman with breast cancer at the age of 49 confers the same *BRCA1/2* mutation probability risk on her family members as a woman of 32 with the same diagnosis which is clearly not the case. A woman with breast cancer diagnosed at the age of 51, strictly speaking, would not confer any additional risk to her family members at all. The age of onset of ovarian cancer is also not considered in this model, and no other cancers (e.g., prostate, melanoma, and pancreas) are used in the calculation.

For example, a woman presenting with breast cancer at 45 years, with a family history of a male breast cancer in her father at 60 years and one case of melanoma and one of pancreatic cancer in his two brothers would only have the first two malignancies considered by this model. The male breast cancer would not have the increased significance usually afforded to this diagnosis in these families, simply because he is not the proband. The other two cancers would not be considered in the analysis despite the fact that, in the context of this family history, they would make this diagnosis of a *BRCA2* mutation significantly more likely.

Again, as with the other models reviewed, no pathological data are taken into consideration by this model.

A recent comparison of Frank/Myriad with the Manchester scoring system, using 267 families (31), gave the Myriad model a relatively high sensitivity but a low specificity. Preliminary data suggest that this model may be better at predicting *BRCA1* mutations than *BRCA2* mutations. This may be because of the criteria used, the relative absence of other cancers such as prostate, melanoma, pancreas in *BRCA2* families, and the earlier presentation of *BRCA1* tumors.

TYRER–CUZICK (INTERNATIONAL BREAST CANCER INTERVENTION STUDY)

This is the most recently developed of the breast cancer risk assessment models (32). It was developed using published data regarding *BRCA1* and *BRCA2* mutation carrier frequencies from a study of mother-daughter pairs (33) and penetrance estimates from the Breast Cancer Linkage Consortium (34) rather than one specific dataset. There are two parts to the model's calculations: a "genetic" part and a "personal risk factors" part. Like the BRCAPRO model, International Breast Cancer Intervention Study (IBIS) uses Bayesian calculations as a basis for the genetic part of the model. The Bayesian variables used are *BRCA1* mutation, *BRCA2* mutation, and "other genetic risk factor," an as yet unknown low-penetrance gene that is assumed to follow an autosomal-dominant inheritance pattern. Like BOADICEA, IBIS can incorporate exact family relationships and is not restricted to a certain number of first- and second-degree relatives in order to make its assessment. It is also capable of dealing with bilateral breast cancer but only in first-degree relatives of the proband. The cancers considered, however, are only breast and ovarian, like many of the other models previously discussed in this chapter.

Uniquely, at present, however, IBIS incorporates personal risk factors into its calculation. A number of risk factors have long been known to influence an individual's risk of breast and ovarian cancer in the general population. These are primarily related to hormonal and reproductive factors. Research is currently under way via the EMBRACE study to ascertain whether these known risk factors also influence the likelihood of breast and/or ovarian cancer developing in *BRCA1/2* mutation carriers.

The personal risk factors incorporated into the IBIS model are the ages at menarche, first childbirth and menopause, parity, height, and body mass index, and two diagnoses associated with increased risk, namely atypical hyperplasia and lobular carcinoma in situ. Both these diagnoses are known to be associated with at least a fourfold increase in risk in the general population (35,36). Some risk factors have not yet been included. These are the administration of exogenous hormones such as the oral contraceptive pill and hormone replacement therapy and the presence of ductal carcinoma in situ.

In using the model, the genetic risks are calculated first, and then the personal risk factors are used to modify the genetic risk to create a personal calculation for the individual. Calculations of the likelihood of carrying a *BRCA1/2* mutation and of developing breast or ovarian cancer are possible.

IBIS is such a new risk assessment model that it has not yet been comprehensively validated. In one study of prediction of cancer risks, involving 3170 women in the United Kingdom, IBIS outperformed other models such as BRCAPRO and Claus (24). Like many of the other models available, IBIS is computer based. It remains to be seen whether it is user friendly in the clinical setting.

EXAMPLES OF THESE MODELS IN USE

For the examples below, we have decided to use some of the models discussed on three sample pedigrees. The pedigrees are not real pedigrees but are based on real histories given by families seen in our cancer genetics clinics, and the mutation status of each family is known. They have been selected to illustrate the various strengths and weaknesses of the models. We have, in addition to the models themselves, incorporated an assessment by an "experienced clinician." This reflects the opinion of a recognized cancer geneticist with many years' experience in the clinical setting.

The family history evident from Figure 2 Pedigree 1, on assessment by an experienced clinician, would yield a high expectation that a *BRCA* mutation is present in the family. Because of the young ages of onset and multiple affected individuals with breast cancer in this family, this would be more likely to be *BRCA1* on first inspection. Analysis of *BRCA1/2* by full sequencing and multiplex ligation-dependent probe amplification (MLPA) showed a *BRCA1* mutation to be present in the family, and, on predictive testing, this was shown to be present in the unaffected proband.

Figure 3 Pedigree 2 is more complicated because of the presence of cancers other than breast and ovarian in the family history. These other cancers are not considered by many of the risk assessment models, and the result is that the estimates of *BRCA1/2* carrier probability are extremely variable in this family. An experienced clinician, however, would rate this family as being highly likely to carry a *BRCA2* mutation and rather less likely to carry a *BRCA1* mutation. Genetic analysis by the methods detailed above did show a *BRCA2* mutation to be present in this family. It was found to be present in the unaffected proband on predictive testing.

Figure 4 Pedigree 3 is a low-risk family on initial assessment. It was included in order that the discriminatory strengths of the models could be demonstrated. No mutations were found in this family.

The following table summarizes the results for Pedigree 1:

Model used	*BRCA1* risk	*BRCA2* risk
Manchester scoring system	26 (score)	23 (score)
Myriad	12.2%	12.2%
Breast and Ovarian Analysis of Disease Incidence and Carrier Estimation Algorithm	38.1%	8.4%
IBIS	27.1%	17.1%
BRCAPRO	47.4%	1%
Experienced clinician	High risk (test first)	High risk

Even in this obviously high-risk breast/ovarian cancer family, the models produce widely differing results. There are a total of six cancers in this family in first- and second-degree relatives to the proband. The fact that the proband is unaffected by cancer herself means that her individual risk on the Myriad tables is much lower than one would expect looking at this pedigree. If the Myriad tables are consulted regarding the proband's sister, however, a risk of 39.2% of carrying a *BRCA1/2* mutation is seen. Interestingly, however, not all affected relatives are involved in the calculation by the Myriad tables, and the extremely young ages of onset, which would lead the experienced clinician to their "high-risk" assessment, (when taken together with the pattern of inheritance in the family and the number of relatives affected), are not considered by the Myriad tables to be relevant. Both BOADICEA and BRCAPRO give this pedigree a much lower risk of *BRCA2* than *BRCA1*. The extremely low risk given by BRCAPRO illustrates its tendency to overestimate *BRCA1* risk and underestimate *BRCA2* risk. The IBIS data here also agree that the likelihood is of a *BRCA1* mutation over a *BRCA2* mutation; however, lifestyle factors were not used in this analysis. The Manchester scoring system gives a high-risk score to each gene, slightly higher for *BRCA1* than for *BRCA2*. Using data to convert the Manchester score into a percentage chance of a *BRCA1* or a *BRCA2* mutation being present, however, the probabilities are 21% for *BRCA1* and 14% for *BRCA2*.

The following table summarizes the results for Pedigree 2:

Model used	*BRCA1* risk	*BRCA2* risk
Manchester	12 (score)	11 (score)
Myriad	12.2%	12.2%
Breast and Ovarian Analysis of Disease Incidence and Carrier Estimation Algorithm	10.6%	15%
IBIS	6.5%	4.6%
BRCAPRO	14.9%	1.1%
Experienced clinician	High risk	High risk (test first)

This case highlights the shortcomings of all the models when a family history falls outside the strict remit of the model. The family history depicted in the pedigree is strongly suggestive of a mutation in *BRCA2* to the experienced clinician, given the additional prostate cancer and melanoma on a background of early-onset breast cancer and ovarian cancer. Both these types of cancer have been found to be associated with *BRCA2* mutations rather than *BRCA1* mutations in recent studies [EMBRACE, unpublished, Thompson et al. (37)]. Out of the models above, only the Manchester scoring system and BOADICEA consider the additional cancers, and neither of them incorporates melanoma into their calculations yet. It is unexpected that the Myriad risk assessment for this family is identical to that for the family in Pedigree 1. This reflects the limitations of that model in terms of the number of relatives it assesses and the cancers it will consider. This pedigree also serves to demonstrate further the shortcomings of BRCAPRO in terms of its overestimation of *BRCA1* at the expense of *BRCA2*. The IBIS model also performs poorly in this assessment, probably due to not incorporating the other cancers into its calculations.

The following table summarizes the results for Pedigree 3:

Model used	*BRCA1* risk	*BRCA2* risk
Manchester	5 (score)	5 (score)
Myriad	4.5%	4.5%
Breast and Ovarian Analysis of Disease Incidence and Carrier Estimation Algorithm	1%	1.6%
IBIS	1.8%	1.3%
BRCAPRO	1.5%	0.7%
Experienced clinician	Moderate risk (no test)	Moderate risk (no test)

The results for Pedigree 3 demonstrate that the models are all capable of discriminating between families that are clearly low risk and families that may require testing. All the models rated Pedigree 3 as low risk, and this family would not have warranted genetic testing under current UK National Institute for Clinical Excellence (NICE) guidelines (38).

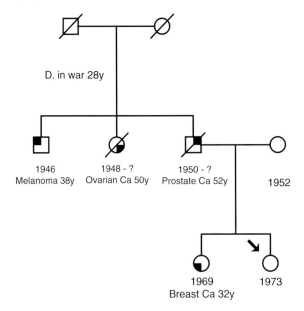

Figure 3 Pedigree 2.

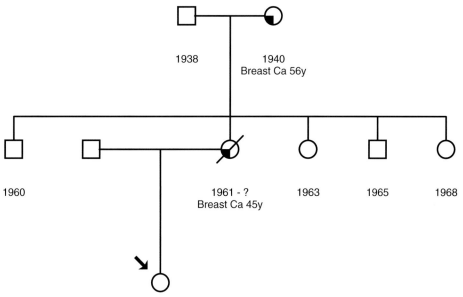

Figure 4   Pedigree 3.

SUMMARY

We have reviewed the major risk assessment models available for determination of the likelihood of *BRCA1/2* gene mutations being present in families with a history of breast and ovarian cancer. With current available data, it is not clear which model is the most effective; however, a large study is currently under way in the United Kingdom to assess the efficacy of the models. It is hoped that the resulting data will resolve this question and result in consistency in risk assessment and equity of access to genetic testing. Until this time, the experienced clinician's assessment is adequate to determine test thresholds and performs superiorly when complex pedigrees with other cancers other than breast and ovarian cancer are present. Recently more common lower penetrance alleles have been identified (39,40) and as more evidence is accrued regarding their precise risks these will need to be incorporated into risk assessment and the models will have to be adjusted to accommodate this.

REFERENCES

1. Miki Y, Swensen J, Shattuck-Eidens D, et al. Isolation of *BRCA1*, the 17q-linked breast and ovarian cancer susceptibility gene. Science 1994; 266:66–71.
2. Wooster R, Bignell G, Lancaster J, et al. Identification of the breast cancer susceptibility gene, *BRCA2*. Nature 1995; 378:789–792.
3. Meijers-Heijboer H, van de Ouweland A, Klijn J, et al. The CHEK2–Breast Cancer Consortium. Low-penetrance susceptibility to breast cancer due to CHEK2 1100delC in noncarriers of *BRCA1* or *BRCA2* mutations. Nat Genet 2002; 31:55–59.
4. Swift M, Reitnauer PJ, Morrell D, et al. Incidence of cancer in 161 families affected by ataxia telangiectasia. N Engl J Med 1991; 325:1831–1836.
5. Malkin D, Li FP, Strong LC, et al. Germ line *p53* mutations in a familial syndrome of breast cancer, sarcomas, and other neoplasms. Science 1990; 250:1233–1238.

6. Eng C. Genetics of Cowden's syndrome: through the looking glass of oncology. Int J Cancer 1998; 12:701–710.

7. Seal S, Thompson D, Renwick A, et al. Truncating mutations in the Fanconi anemia J gene *BRIP1* are low-penetrance breast cancer susceptibility alleles. Nat Genet 2006; 38(11): 1239–1241.

8. Reid S, Schindler D, Hanenberg H, et al. Biallelic mutations in PALB2 cause Fanconi anemia subtype FA-N and predispose to childhood cancer. Nat Genet 2007; 39(2):162–164.

9. Lloyd S, Watson M, Waites B, et al. Familial breast cancer: a controlled study of risk perception, psychological morbidity and health beliefs in women attending for genetic counselling. Brit J Cancer 1996; 74:482–487.

10. Green H, Brown RA. Counting lives. J Occ Accid 1978; 2:55.

11. Josten DM, Evans AM, Love RR. The cancer prevention clinic: a service program for cancer-prone families. J Psych Oncol 1985; 3:5–20.

12. Kash KM, Holland JC, Halper MS, Miller DG. Psychological distress and surveillance behaviours of women with a family history of breast cancer. J Natl Cancer Inst 1991; 84:24–30.

13. Lerman C, Daly M, Masny A, Balshem A. Attitudes about genetic testing for breast-ovarian cancer susceptibility. J Clin Oncol 1994; 12:843–850.

14. Watson M, Foster C, Eeles R, et al. Psychosocial impact of breast/ovarian (*BRCA1/2*) cancer-predictive genetic testing in a UK multi-centre clinical cohort. Brit J Cancer 2004; 91(10): 1787–1794.

15. www.abi.org.uk

16. Claus EB, Risch NJ, Thompson WD. Genetic analysis of breast cancer in the cancer and steroid hormone study. Am J Hum Genet 1991; 48:232–242.

17. Shattuck-Eidens D, McClure M, et al. A collaborative study of 80 mutations in the *BRCA1* breast and ovarian cancer susceptibility gene. J Am Med Assoc 1995; 273:535–541.

18. Shattuck-Eidens D, Oliphant A, McClure M, et al. *BRCA1* sequence analysis in women at high risk for susceptibility mutations. J Am Med Assoc 1997; 278:1242–1250.

19. Parmigiani G, Berry D, Aguilar O. Determining carrier probabilities for breast cancer-susceptibility genes *BRCA1* and *BRCA2*. Am J Hum Genet 1998; 62(1):145–158.

20. Berry DA, Iversen ES. Jr, Gudbjartsson DF, et al. BRCAPRO validation, sensitivity of genetic testing of *BRCA1/BRCA2*, and prevalence of other breast cancer susceptibility genes. J Clin Oncol 2002; 20(11):2701–2712.

21. Evans DGR, Eccles DM, Rahman N, et al. A new scoring system for the chances of identifying a *BRCA1/2* mutation, outperforms existing models including BRCAPRO. J Med Genet 2004; 41:474–480.

22. Antoniou AC, Durocher F, Smith P, et al. *BRCA1* and *BRCA2* mutation predictions using the BOADICEA and BRCAPRO models and penetrance estimation in high-risk French-Canadian families. Breast Cancer Res 2006; 8(1):R3.

23. Barcenas CH, Hosain GM, Arun B, et al. Assessing BRCA carrier probabilities in extended families. J Clin Oncol 2006; 24(3):354–360.

24. Amir E, Evans DG, Shenton A, et al. Evaluation of breast cancer risk assessment packages in the family history evaluation and screening programme. J Med Genet 2003; 40(11):807–814.

25. Antoniou AC, Pharoah PP, Smith P, Easton DF. The BOADICEA model of genetic susceptibility to breast and ovarian cancer. Brit J Cancer 2004; 91(8):1580–1590.

26. Breast Cancer Linkage Consortium. Pathology of familial breast cancer: differences between breast cancers in carriers of *BRCA1* or *BRCA2* mutations and sporadic cases. Lancet 1997; 349(9064):1505–1510.

27. www.srl.cam.ac.uk/genepi/embraceindex.htm.

28. Evans DG, Lalloo F, Wallace A, Rahman N. Update on the Manchester Scoring System for *BRCA1* and *BRCA2* testing. J Med Genet 2005; 42(7):e39.

29. Frank TS, Deffenbaugh AM, Reid JE, et al. Clinical characteristics of individuals with germline mutations in *BRCA1* and *BRCA2*: analysis of 10,000 individuals. J Clin Oncol 2002; 20(6):1480–1490.

30. www.myriadtests.com/provider/mutprev.htm.

31. Gerdes AM, Cruger DG, Thomassen M, et al. Evaluation of two different models to predict *BRCA1* and *BRCA2* mutations in a cohort of Danish hereditary breast and/or ovarian cancer families. Clin Genet 2006; 69(2):171–178.

32. Tyrer J, Duffy SW, Cuzick J. A breast cancer prediction model incorporating familial and personal risk factors. Stat Med 2004; 23:1111–1130.

33. Anderson H, Bladstrom A, Olsson H, et al. Familial breast and ovarian cancer: a Swedish population-based register study. Am J Epidemiol 2000; 152(12):1154–1163.

34. Ford D, Easton DF, Stratton M, et al. Genetic heterogeneity and penetrance analysis of the *BRCA1* and *BRCA2* genes in breast cancer families. The Breast Cancer Linkage Consortium. Am J Hum Genet 1998; 62:676–689.

35. Li CI, Malone KE, Saltzman BS, et al. Risk of invasive breast carcinoma among women diagnosed with ductal carcinoma in situ and lobular carcinoma in situ, 1988–2001. Cancer 2006; 106(10):2104–2112.

36. Hartmann LC, Sellers TA, Frost MH, et al. Benign breast disease and the risk of breast cancer. N Engl J Med 2005; 353(3):229–237.

37. Thompson D, Easton D. Breast Cancer Linkage Consortium. Cancer risks, by mutation position, in *BRCA2* mutation carriers. Am J Hum Genet 2001; 68(2):410–419.

38. National Institute for Clinical Excellence (UK) Guidelines on Familial Breast Cancer, 2004. (www.nice.org.uk)

39. Stacey SN, Manolescu A, Sulem P, et al. Common variants on chromosomes 2q35 and 16q12 confer susceptibility to estrogen receptor-positive breast cancer. Nat Genet 2007; 39(7): 865–869.

40. Easton DF, Pooley KA, Dunning AM, et al. Genome-wide association study identifies novel breast cancer susceptibility loci. Nature 2007; 447(7148):1087–1093.

3

Bioethics of Genetic Testing for Hereditary Breast Cancer

Beth N. Peshkin

Lombardi Comprehensive Cancer Center, Fisher Center for Familial Cancer Research, Georgetown University, Washington, D.C., U.S.A.

Wylie Burke

Department of Medical History and Ethics, University of Washington, Seattle, Washington, U.S.A.

INTRODUCTION

In the mid-1990s, the cloning of two major breast cancer genes, *BRCA1* and *BRCA2*, became a harbinger for a new era in genetic medicine. Despite the complexities, uncertainties, and potential risks associated with predictive genetic testing, over 100,000 individuals have undergone testing for breast cancer susceptibility (1). By far, most of the information available to clinicians about the attitudes of those undergoing testing and the impact of testing has been gathered in the context of comprehensive research programs. But as genetic testing diffuses into mainstream clinical practice, it is important that we continue to examine and address the ethical, legal, and social issues that are part and parcel of this new technology. In this chapter, we begin by providing a general framework for examining ethical issues in clinical cancer genetics. Then, we present a detailed analysis of some common themes that arise in this field, such as provider roles and service delivery issues, informed consent, genetic discrimination, family communication and duty to warn, predictive testing in children, and preimplantation and prenatal testing. Each section will conclude with some pointers for anticipating and addressing these issues in clinical practice.

ETHICS FRAMEWORK FOR CLINICIANS

In their seminal textbook, Beauchamp and Childress propose a useful, overarching framework known as principlism that can be applied to the examination of many ethical issues in the biomedical field (2). The four main principles they espouse are respect for persons, beneficence, nonmaleficence, and justice (Table 1).

Respect for persons, or *autonomy*, entails respect for a person's right to make decisions based on his or her own values, beliefs, and preferences (2). To make fully autonomous decisions, a person must have access to sufficient information (e.g., about the potential implications, limitations, benefits, and risks of genetic testing) and be able to act

Table 1 Ethical Principles and Applications to Cancer Genetic Counseling (2–5)

Principle	Definition	Cancer genetics examples
Autonomy	Respect for persons	Ensuring fully informed consent for genetic testing
		Protecting patient privacy regarding genetic risk or genetic test results
Beneficence/ nonmaleficence	Provision of benefits to ensure patient welfare and minimization of harm	Eliciting and interpreting adequate clinical and family history to identify individuals at high risk of cancer
		Providing comprehensive genetic counseling and/or follow-up as needed or providing appropriate referrals
Justice	Equal access to services and healthcare	Advocating on behalf of patients to obtain financial assistance when needed for genetic counseling, testing, and/or cancer risk management services
		Exploration of alternatives to traditional genetic counseling service delivery to meet the needs of underserved populations

without undue influence. In the genetics setting, where the counseling and testing processes are invariably linked to the larger family context, the latter point is one to which clinicians need to be especially sensitive. For instance, at-risk (unaffected) women are frequently the first in their family to inquire about genetic testing for hereditary breast/ovarian cancer. If the family history suggests that genetic testing is appropriate, they are often advised to approach a relative who has had breast or ovarian cancer to ask if she would be willing to undergo testing first, to maximize the chance of yielding informative results. Affected relatives may feel obligated to be tested for the sake of the family, but providers must ensure that they do so willingly and with full appreciation of the potential implications for their own health and well-being. Another possible scenario raising concerns about autonomy is a parental request to test a minor child for an adult onset condition, such as hereditary breast/ovarian cancer attributable to a *BRCA1* mutation.

These scenarios also invoke concerns about the related principles of beneficence and nonmaleficence. *Beneficence* refers to the clinician's obligation to provide benefit to patients, which involves contributing to and protecting their welfare, as well as seeking solutions that balance benefits and harms (2). The related construct, *nonmaleficence*, refers to the avoidance of harm, or at the very least, the minimization of harm. Although genetic counseling and testing are not generally associated with physical harm, attention must be paid to the potential for adverse psychological effects, discrimination, stigmatization, and breaches of confidentiality. Exposure to unnecessary or unproven treatment may also be a consideration.

Finally, the principle of *justice* involves the equitable and fair distribution of available resources and the associated benefits and risks of healthcare services (2). This principle is highly relevant when considering issues such as access of underserved or uninsured individuals to genetic counseling and testing or the accessibility of newer technologies (such as preimplantation diagnosis) to the general public. Another example of the justice principle is related to participation in cancer genetics research. For instance, limited success in recruitment of minority participants has restricted the extent to which some clinically relevant findings may be extrapolated to these populations, including data about cancer risks associated with *BRCA1/2* mutations, risk modifiers, and the psychosocial impact of testing (6,7).

Although these four principles provide a framework for identifying relevant concerns, they do not provide a specific approach for addressing ethical dilemmas that arise when the principles appear to generate competing ethical obligations. For example, if a patient does not want to disclose genetic risk information relevant for specific relatives, a clinician may be faced with a conflict between upholding patient autonomy and providing benefit or minimizing harm to family members. Various moral or ethical theories may be helpful in balancing competing ethical claims (2). For example, a utilitarian approach considers which resolution to an ethical conflict benefits the most people whereas a Kantian (deontological) approach considers that some actions must be performed out of obligation, determined in part by the universal implications of such actions (2). For example, what would be the implications of overriding patient autonomy to inform a patient's relatives of positive genetic test results? Would such an action cause family disruption or undermine the trust of future patients—or would it promote the ultimate well-being of all family members?

Often the specific medical details of a particular case, and other contextual factors, play an important role in resolving dilemmas of this kind. The case-based analysis suggested by Jonsen et al. (8) offers a method for applying moral reasoning to clinical dilemmas. In this approach, the case is defined by questions in four domains: medical indications, patient preferences, quality-of-life considerations, and any relevant social, legal, or other contextual factors. Weighting of the different factors in the case is aided by consideration of paradigmatic cases—that is, cases bearing a similarity to the case in question, but in which the resolution is clear. Thus, it could be argued that patient autonomy should not be overruled to inform family members about a genetic risk if the risk is small and no action can be taken to avert risk. Conversely, an obligation to inform family members could be argued to be present if the risk is imminent and preventable (9). Often a consideration of bioethical principles helps to clarify the central ethical question and relevant paradigmatic cases. Other theories and approaches to moral reasoning may also provide insight, such as the communitarian perspective, which focuses on community values and the rights of others, which may override the rights of an individual, and the ethics of care, which is a relationship-oriented theory that considers emotional parameters in care giving, such as responsibility, trust, and sensitivity, and also takes into account power relationships in determining the appropriate resolution of a case (2). Like virtue ethics, this theory considers how one performs his or her actions in resolving dilemmas and whether there is genuine motivation to promote positive outcomes (2). Efforts to expand the reach of genetic counseling, especially to underserved populations, may be driven by these ideals.

When confronted with ethical dilemmas in clinical practice, the broad approaches mentioned above may provide a general framework for analysis and the four principles may be used as a "checklist" of considerations. Indeed, many authors have utilized the four principles in their examination of ethical issues in cancer genetics (3–5). Ultimately, the goal is to identify an appropriate resolution to the case at hand that fits within a consistent and coherent approach to similar dilemmas. Difficult cases often also have legal implications, which may represent an important contextual element. Thus, when complex conflicts arise, both ethical and legal analyses may be needed, and consultation with an ethics consultant or committee may provide an effective means for further deliberation and resolution.

GENETIC COUNSELING: PROVIDER ROLES, SERVICE DELIVERY, AND INFORMED CONSENT

One of the primary obligations of healthcare providers is the identification of individuals for whom genetic counseling, and possibly testing, is indicated. Since the cloning of *BRCA1* and *BRCA2*, position statements and other resources have been developed to assist clinicians with the identification and management of high-risk individuals (10–13). In addition, educational materials are widely available to assist clinicians with the recognition and management of hereditary breast cancer syndromes (14,15).

Given the complex nature of interpreting family histories and test results and the evolving literature about cancer risks and management options as well as the potentially life-changing implications of testing, comprehensive pre- and post-test genetic counseling is recommended when testing for a highly penetrant cancer syndrome is considered (16,17). Counseling can help to ensure that patients make autonomous decisions that are based on adequate information and which are consistent with their values and preferences (3,4,10,13). Anxiety and inflated risk perceptions sometimes drive patient interest in testing (18,19). Even if the objective risk of cancer or carrying a gene mutation is low, patients may still benefit from genetic counseling to gain a better understanding of their risk and available options. In general, research has demonstrated that genetic counseling results in improved knowledge and does not have significant adverse psychological effects (20). However, one of the benefits of the genetic counseling process is that risk factors for distress can be identified, and individuals can be referred for additional supportive counseling, if needed (21). These considerations underscore the justice concerns that arise when availability of genetic services is limited, or services are poorly reimbursed.

Informed consent is the process of engaging patients in a two-way discussion about the potential benefits, limitations, and risks of a proposed intervention, such as testing for cancer risk (16,17,22). When a genetic test is highly predictive, as is the case with most clinically available cancer genetic tests, written consent prior to genetic testing is also advisable, in both clinical and research settings. The consent and decision-making process may be enhanced with other supplementary resources such as detailed booklets or pamphlets, videotapes, and interactive videos/computer programs, which have been assessed in preliminary research trials (23–25).

A pervasive issue and one which will become more pressing as additional genetic tests become available is how to meet increasing demand for services in a way that ensures that patients obtain the greatest benefits from counseling and testing. Given the limited number of genetics service providers such as genetic counselors and genetic nurse specialists, particularly outside the United States, it is sometimes unclear which professional should provide these services and what the prevailing standard of care is (26,27). These questions have legal implications (28,29). Numerous studies have highlighted knowledge deficits of primary care and specialist physicians in the area of cancer genetics as well as the limited time available to devote to patient education and counseling (27,30). In addition, because of the increasing awareness about testing and subsequent consumer interest in testing, alternatives to traditional modes of service delivery are being utilized. These include the use of telephone counseling, both before and after testing, and direct-to-consumer availability of testing through the Internet (31,32). Whereas the former still affords the opportunity for thorough genetic counseling, the latter may allow motivated consumers to bypass it altogether. Proponents of these alternative modes of service delivery argue that in the interest of justice and patient autonomy, such options are beneficial because they extend the reach and accessibility of genetic counseling and testing. However, data are lacking at present regarding how these services will affect psychological outcomes, medical decision-making, and patient satisfaction.

Providers within various specialties such as primary care, gynecology, surgery, and oncology clearly play different roles in the identification and management of high-risk patients. For example, primary care physicians and gynecologists often have an integral role in identifying patients at risk and facilitating adherence with a high-risk management plan. Breast surgeons and oncologists are likely to see women who have a new diagnosis of breast cancer or who are followed routinely after a diagnosis of cancer. The decision to have genetic testing may be more imminent for some of these patients who may use the information for definitive surgical decisions (33). Research has shown that physician recommendation for genetic testing and management can be a significant predictor in patient decision-making and adherence rates (33,34). Thus, a balance has to be struck between giving patients firm recommendations about certain aspects of risk management (e.g., recommendations for breast cancer screening or for prophylactic oophorectomy in *BRCA1/2* carriers after childbearing is completed) and remaining value-neutral about choices that are more subjective and dependent on patient preferences (e.g., decisions about genetic testing and prophylactic mastectomy) (4).

Although a uniform "standard of care" delineating obligations to high-risk patients has not been established, practice guidelines establish the importance of identifying high-risk individuals, the efficacy of specific management options, and the benefits of genetic testing (10,12,13). Knowledge about the field is evolving at a rapid pace, and for optimal care, patients need to have access to state-of-the-art information. Thus, providers are encouraged to maintain a level of expertise and competence to fulfill their professional and fiduciary responsibilities to their patients, and also to recognize their limitations. It is thus helpful to establish partnerships among the cancer genetics community, primary care providers and other medical specialties, to assure that the needs of high-risk patients are met.

Another related issue concerns the duty to recontact patients with new information (35). Although not all research developments immediately translate into clinical practice, many are significant enough that providers need to consider the appropriateness of notifying specific patients. For example, clinicians practicing over the last 15 years have had to consider recontacting patients about the identification of new cancer susceptibility genes, reclassification of indeterminate *BRCA1/2* results, the availability of more sensitive methods of genetic testing, revised data about cancer risks and risk modifiers, and information about the efficacy existing or new methods of screening and risk-reducing measures. There is no uniform standard of care or any directly relevant legal precedents to guide clinicians. As predicted by a case-based analysis, ethical perspectives on this issue often vary with the clinical significance of the information. Clinicians need to balance obligations for beneficence with the possibility that some patients may not want to be informed of new developments.

In sum, practical advice for providers is summarized below:

1. Obtain a family history sufficient to identify individuals who may potentially benefit from genetic counseling and testing for cancer risk (especially those at risk for hereditary cancer syndromes). It is important to update the family history periodically and reassess, as needed.
2. Stay informed about current guidelines and educational resources through professional organizations and continuing educational opportunities.
3. Maintain a network of colleagues in various specialties to whom patients may be referred for appropriate counseling, testing, and/or for follow-up.

4. Discuss expectations with patients about ongoing management and future notification of research developments. Consider providing recommendations to patients about specific time frames when they could contact the clinic for possible updates and remind them to ensure that the provider's office has current contact information for them. It may also be appropriate to encourage patients to take a proactive role in reviewing available resources and contacting the provider as needed (35). In this regard, it is helpful to provide patients with a list of reliable resources (e.g., support groups and websites) that they can check periodically.

GENETIC DISCRIMINATION

Is there such a thing as "genetic exceptionalism"? In other words, although genetic information shares many features with other types of predictive medical information, do the unique privacy issues raised by such information render it different and subject to special protection? As we will explore in the next section, individuals may have high expectations about the privacy of their genetic information within their own families, let alone its use by other entities such as insurers and employers. The latter is of particular concern in countries like the United States that lack universal access to healthcare. Although cases of genetic discrimination in insurance and employment settings in the United States and abroad have been reported, relative to the number of people tested, the instances are few and often anecdotal (36–39). Nevertheless, fear of such discrimination may result in decreased utilization of genetic services, including genetic counseling (40,41).

In the United States, although there is no comprehensive federal law that provides protections against genetic discrimination with respect to health insurance and employment, some safeguards are in place. For example, the Health Insurance Portability and Accountability Act (HIPAA) of 1996 extends protection to those with group health insurance such that a positive genetic test result, for example, cannot be considered as a preexisting condition and insurance cannot be denied or individual premiums increased for those who qualify (42). However, several loopholes exist within this legislation in that it does not (*i*) preclude increasing everyone's premiums in a small group environment; (*ii*) protect those with individual insurance; (*iii*) address issues related to disability or life insurance. In 2001, the HIPAA Privacy Rule went into effect, requiring covered entities to limit disclosure of information about genetic test results and family history information (43). Protection against employment discrimination is less clear, although the Americans with Disabilities Act is applicable to individuals who are "regarded as" disabled (44). Pending legislation that provides more extensive protection in group and private insurance markets and the workplace has been pending in Congress for several years (45). In addition, various state laws provide a patchwork of protections (45). For research participants, genetic information and other data collected as part of a research protocol may be protected from third parties or compelled disclosure (e.g., subpoena) by a Certificate of Confidentiality, issued by the National Institutes of Health (46). However, individuals who use their insurance company to pay for testing, the results of which are collected as part of the research, may still be required to comply with requests to share that information (e.g., with their insurer). In April 2007, the United States House of Representatives passed the Genetic Information Nondiscrimination Act of 2007 (H.R. 493) (45). This Act will protect individuals against health insurance and employment discrimination based on their genetic information. The Act provides more broad based protections than those afforded by HIPAA. For example, protections apply to people in the group and individual health insurance market, and there would be prohibitions against requesting or requiring genetic testing by health insurers or employers. As of June 27, 2007, a vote in the Senate is pending.

Internationally, there are various regulatory frameworks that exist to protect people against genetic discrimination, ranging from legislation that provides some safeguards to complete moratoria on the use of genetic information by third parties (47). A common concern among insurers is the potential for adverse selection, which would occur if at-risk individuals "load up" on insurance prior to undergoing genetic testing or seeking medical management, or after discovering their risk status. Limited data on this phenomenon are conflicting, so it is unclear how significant this issue will be in the future (48,49).

Another aspect of genetic discrimination which receives less attention in the literature is the phenomenon of group or individual social stigmatization related to genetic risk. For example, after the identification of *BRCA1/2* founder mutations in the Ashkenazi Jewish population, concerns were raised about members of this ethnic group being singled out by insurers (50). On the other hand, many individuals in Jewish communities have rallied to participate in research which has provided critical data about mutation prevalence and cancer risk (51). On an individual level, however, it is not uncommon for people to ask the unanswerable question, "why me?" or as a manifestation of survivor guilt, "why not me?" It can be helpful to elicit these perceptions throughout the course of genetic counseling to help patients explore their motivation for and responses to risk information.

In sum, part of upholding patients' autonomy entails protecting their privacy, although there may be practical limitations in doing so. Suggestions for addressing this issue with patients are as follows:

1. Be familiar with current regulations in your country or region, and provide resources for patients to learn more about these protections.
2. Elicit patient concerns about genetic discrimination in insurance and employment and dispel misconceptions if necessary.
3. Written informed consent for genetic testing is advisable for tests that have the potential to reveal genotypes conferring high risk; this document should summarize how medical and family history information and genetic test results will be kept private as well as who is lawfully allowed access to the information. The potential risks of genetic discrimination should be summarized. These risks will vary depending on local circumstances and may include loss or denial of insurance (health, disability, life) or other insurance issues such as increased premiums or lack of coverage for certain services and potential employment issues (e.g., compromised hiring decisions with small employers). When writing consent documents, it may be helpful to review sample language from existing clinical consent forms about the risks of testing (52) as well as general descriptions of content (10,53). Of note, "boilerplate" language required by some institutions regarding the risks of genetic research or testing may need to be adapted to more accurately reflect the small risk of discrimination and the current availability of some legal protections (54).
4. When patients are referred to research studies, they should be encouraged to ask about the protections in place to protect the privacy and confidentiality of the genetic data collected.

FAMILY COMMUNICATION ISSUES AND THE DUTY TO WARN

The desire to obtain risk information for relatives often motivates individuals to obtain genetic testing (55). Indeed, one of the distinguishing features of genetic tests compared with other medical tests is that the results may have implications for biological relatives. However, rates of disclosure to at-risk relatives are surprisingly variable. Recent surveys of genetic counselors and medical geneticists, most of whom practiced in prenatal and pediatric settings, revealed that patients frequently refuse to notify at-risk relatives of genetic information (56,57). In the area of breast cancer genetics, studies have shown that the rate of disclosure to adult, at-risk relatives by *BRCA1/2* mutation positive probands is generally high for first-degree relatives, especially sisters, but is overall quite variable (58–60). The reasons why individuals choose not to notify relatives may include estrangement or emotionally distant relationships, concerns about insurance or employment discrimination, and worries about the impact on family dynamics, but these explanations may never become transparent to clinicians (57,58,60,61). However, for a variety of reasons, including the desire to uphold patient autonomy, concerns about liability, lack of awareness of published guidelines, or ambiguity about how to apply the guidelines, less than 1% of the professionals surveyed went on to notify at-risk relatives without patient consent (56,57).

As genetic testing for common, preventable conditions becomes more pervasive, with cancer susceptibility tests leading the way, there has been substantial discussion and debate in the literature about whether clinicians have a duty to warn family members about a shared genetic risk, and if they do, how this should be accomplished (62). Although a standard of care has not been established, public health mandates, case law, and policy statements from major medical organizations provide a framework for examining the relevant considerations for clinicians.

In the public health sector, breaches of confidentiality may be permissible to curtail the spread of preventable communicable diseases (63). With respect to case law, the well-known *Tarasoff* ruling established a provider's obligation to breach confidentiality in order to warn a third party of imminent and preventable harm (64). In this 1976 case, a psychotherapist failed to warn a woman about his patient's intention to kill her, which he eventually did. Almost 20 years later, the duty to warn was tested in the courts as it applies to the threat of genetically transmissible diseases within families. Two cases in U.S. state appellate courts are relevant. In *Pate v Threlkel*, the Florida court ruled in 1995 that the physician's duty to warn relatives about a genetic condition (i.e., medullary thyroid cancer) is fulfilled by notifying the patient who is affected by the condition of the responsibility to inform relatives of their risk (65). In *Safer v Estate of Pack*, the New Jersey appeals court reversed the trial court's decision for dismissal of the plaintiff's complaint against her father's doctor for not warning her about the hereditary nature of her father's colon condition (familial adenomatous polyposis) (66). The court also upheld a physician's duty to warn and that it is not necessarily fulfilled by warning the affected patient; moreover, "reasonable steps" had to be undertaken to ensure that at-risk relatives were duly warned of genetic risk (66). The logistical difficulties and impracticalities inherent in requiring physicians to "seek out" and notify family members about their genetic risk was acknowledged, as well as what standards apply to maintaining confidentiality after a patient is deceased (66). The court remanded the case for further proceedings and it was ultimately settled out of court (4,66).

In the absence of clear legal precedents and standards, various professional and policy organizations around the world have developed statements which provide some guidance to clinicians (67). The positions espoused by these groups are highly variable and based primarily on expert opinion; nonetheless, each provides a useful framework for considering the indications, process, and implications of a clinician's duty to warn about genetic risk. In general, many statements acknowledge the importance of maintaining patient confidentiality as well as the obligation of providers to inform patients about risk to relatives. However, the primary considerations that may justify overriding patient confidentiality to warn relatives are (*i*) the seriousness and immediacy of the risk to relatives, (*ii*) the ability to identify relatives at risk and the practicality of contacting these individuals, and (*iii*) the potential benefit of disclosing versus the harm of not disclosing (9,67,68). For example, the American Society of Human Genetics statement outlines circumstances that permit such disclosure, such as if the disease in question is highly likely to occur and can be prevented or adequately treated (9). While notification about risk for a progressive neurological condition such as Huntington disease would not meet these criteria, it could be argued that potential female carriers of a major breast cancer susceptibility gene such as *BRCA1* or *BRCA2* could avail themselves of efficacious means of early detection or risk reduction, such as breast magnetic resonance imaging (MRI) exams, prophylactic mastectomy, or prophylactic oophorectomy (69). On the other hand, some may argue that the penetrance and age of onset for *BRCA1/2* mutations are so variable (70) that these stipulations are not met. Perhaps in light of this subjectivity, organizations such as the American Society of Clinical Oncology and the American Medical Association (AMA) encourage clinicians to discuss risk to relatives and notification of such risk with their patients (consistent with the *Pate* ruling), and the AMA also suggests that physicians facilitate the communication process whenever possible (10,68). One important legal consideration is that in the United States, the HIPAA Privacy Rule prohibits disclosure of "individually identifiable health informa-tion," which includes genetic information (43). However, consistent with public health mandates, confidentiality can be overridden when there exists "serious and imminent threat to the health or safety of a person . . ." (63). As noted in the qualitative language of many position statements, it is unclear whether the risk posed by probabilistic genetic information meets this criterion.

From an ethics perspective, the dilemma about whether to supersede patient confidentiality in order to warn at-risk relatives comes down to whether the clinician's prima facie obligation rests with upholding patient autonomy (including the right to privacy and the right of at-risk relatives to not know) versus beneficence (whether the information about genetic risk is beneficial to relatives and would allow the avoidance of harm). In many families, it is in fact the at-risk relative(s) who will approach a family member with breast or ovarian cancer to be tested first, to maximize the likelihood that testing will be informative. Even so, probands may understandably feel overwhelmed with the responsibility of being the "gatekeeper" of what is often emotionally charged, highly technical information. Studies suggest that carriers of *BRCA1/2* mutations may experience distress when voluntarily communicating with relatives about their result (71). A provocative case report documents the complex emotional response by a patient who deliberately deceived family members about her positive *BRCA1* test and the ensuing ethical and legal conundrums faced by the study team, who ultimately decided to uphold her confidentiality (72). Thus, the potential for psychological harm needs to be factored in to discussions about family notification, and involuntary disclosure by the provider may exacerbate these responses. It is also important to remember that individuals vary in terms of the timeframe in which they want to share information and may also not have regular contact with relatives, particularly distant ones. The legal cases addressed only the duty to warn one's children, but in reality, the number of relatives who are at risk could be significant. It is not realistic to expect that each of these relatives is going to be notified by the tested individual, even if he or she feels a moral obligation to do so. Although one could argue that healthcare providers of family members also have an obligation to elicit their family history, assess risk, and offer genetic testing, if such information is not shared within a family, risk assessment is likely to be inaccurate.

Clinicians may never be privy to the reasons for selective communication or noncommunication preferences. Maintaining patients' trust is a fiduciary responsibility of providers, and one way to do so is to take the time to elicit these reasons, as some barriers may be overcome with time (60). Multiple strategies have been posited in the literature to facilitate family communication. For example, one approach would be to encourage a "family covenant" prior to the initiation of genetic testing in any one person (73). Such an agreement would involve contracting with family members about how and to whom information will be disseminated. Although some have proposed that primary care and family physicians undertake this process with their patients (73), it is unlikely that this will ever become a reality in the current healthcare climate owing to the lack of physician knowledge and experience with genetics and counseling (74). However, in the genetic counseling context, it is not unprecedented to meet with multiple family members simultaneously for pre- and post-test educational sessions (75). Another approach that is being evaluated is a six-step communication skills–building exercise for probands undergoing *BRCA1/2* testing (76). Ongoing research is exploring novel methods of genetic counseling and its adjuncts.

The issues outlined above underscore the complexity of family communication and the lack of clarity about the provider's responsibility and role in facilitating relative notification. Therefore, to assist clinicians with this important task, some practical guidance is summarized below:

1. Prior to undergoing genetic testing, discuss with patients what implications their genetic test results may have to their relatives (e.g., identification of other relatives at risk, specific cancer risks, management strategies) and what their plan is for disclosing the information. If it is possible that multiple relatives will be seen by the same clinician (e.g., the at-risk daughters or sisters of a breast cancer patient who has tested positive but did not disclose her test result), discuss expectations ahead of time in terms of how communication about family history and genetic testing will be handled and under what circumstances, if any, confidentiality may be breached.

2. If it is mutually agreed upon that the clinician will notify relatives of the patient about their genetic risk, express written consent should be obtained.

3. As part of a comprehensive risk assessment, a detailed pedigree should be obtained, which includes information about unaffected at-risk relatives including the patient's children, and the extended family. If positive genetic test results are obtained, it is especially important to provide written information to the patient about which family members should be notified about their risk. This documentation may also detail what those risks are and the relevant medical implications. Resources for local genetics service providers should also be made available.

4. Consider including language in consent forms that explains the importance of patients' notifying their at-risk relatives about the implications of the family history and/or genetic test results, especially positive results.

5. Provide resources for the patient to assist with family communication. This may include referrals to other providers (e.g., genetic counselors, psychologists) or support groups. In addition, patients may find it useful to have extra copies of educational materials to distribute to relatives or may want sample language to include in a letter or email to notify relatives.

6. If a situation arises in which the clinician believes it may be necessary to override a patient's wishes regarding notification of relatives, consultation with a hospital or organizational ethics committee or consultant and/or legal counsel may be appropriate.

PREDICTIVE TESTING IN CHILDREN

As genetic testing for cancer susceptibility becomes more pervasive, another issue that arises with increased frequency concerns the testing of minor children. Guidelines from various professional organizations outline a number of important points to consider before extending testing to minors, mainly that the medical benefits of testing must accrue in childhood (10,77,78). Indeed, there are several well-described cancer syndromes for which testing in childhood is clearly indicated because effective screening or prevention exists (e.g., sigmoidoscopy and colectomy for familial adenomatous polyposis; prophylactic thyroidectomy for multiple endocrine neoplasia 2) (3,79). However, of the breast cancer syndromes discussed in this book, the issue of testing children most frequently arises in families with Li-Fraumeni syndrome and those with documented *BRCA1/2* mutations. The tumor spectrum in Li-Fraumeni syndrome includes cancers that affect young children such as sarcomas, adrenocortical tumors, brain tumors, and leukemias (79). Although cancer screening guidelines are available for children at risk for Li-Fraumeni syndrome, no approach for early detection or risk reduction has been proven effective (79). Nevertheless, a case for testing children could be made so that screening measures could be considered, or if negative, parents could be spared worry as well as costly and frequent check-ups and lab tests.

With respect to *BRCA1/2* testing, there are no medical implications to males or females age 18 or under; for this reason, offering testing to individuals in this age range has been discouraged (80). However, mutation positive mothers often share their positive genetic test results with their adolescent children (81) and it is not uncommon during genetic counseling sessions for them to ask about the possibility of testing their minor children. Indeed, limited research suggests that parents support the idea of testing minor children and that many practitioners may grant that wish (82–84). Aside from medical indications, other considerations must be factored in to the decision as to whether to grant such a request from a parent, or in particular a "mature minor." For example, it is important to weigh the potential psychological benefits or harms to the child or family unit, the child's competence to make decisions about his or her healthcare and implications for future autonomy, family agreement or disagreement about testing the child, and whether the child provides assent to testing (77,78,85–87). Clearly the child's age is relevant because the decision-making capacity and maturity of younger adolescents is likely to be significantly different from that of older adolescents; however, age alone is not the sole factor on which the child's maturity and ability to make an informed decision should be determined (85,86). When all of these factors are considered, it may be appropriate and beneficial to provide genetic counseling and possibly *BRCA1/2* testing to minor children on a case by case basis. Nevertheless, it is likely that testing minors for *BRCA1/2* mutations will remain a rare event.

In summary, subsequent to a request to test minor children, practical issues to consider are as follows:

1. Often the question of testing adolescents arises after a parent has received a positive genetic test result. Therefore, the plans for disclosure of such results to adolescent children (and other relatives) can be integrated into the genetic counseling session(s).

2. It is important to recognize that parents have the authority to act in the best interests of their child; however, when evaluating a competent, minor adolescent, it is critical to elicit his or her preferences and motivations with respect to genetic testing. Several counseling sessions, with a multidisciplinary team of professionals can help the family explore together the *family context* of the genetic diagnosis, which may help defuse any potential conflict between the parental and child's autonomy and help all parties involved to look at the broader implications of their decisions (88). It is also worthwhile to consider the involvement of a psychologist on the team, who may use formal assessment tools to gauge the child's competence in decision-making, self-esteem, coping styles, and relationship with his or her parents.

3. The above evaluations should not replace the usual, comprehensive components of pre- and post-test genetic counseling for the parent(s) and if appropriate, for the minor child. Information should be imparted to everyone involved about carrier probability, medical implications, and potential risks and benefits of testing. If the decision is made to test the child, his or her assent should be obtained before proceeding (if age appropriate) and it is important to agree ahead of time on a plan for disclosure, and follow-up.

4. In instances where there is no medical benefit to the child, there is discord between the parent(s) and child, the balance of benefits and harms is not clear, and/or the healthcare professional does not believe it is in the best interest of the child to provide testing, there is not an obligation to provide testing at that time. In these circumstances, it may be worthwhile to seek the input of an ethics committee or consultant.

PREIMPLANTATION AND PRENATAL TESTING FOR HEREDITARY BREAST CANCER

Another emerging issue concerns the use of preimplantation genetic diagnosis (PGD) (89) and prenatal diagnosis for hereditary cancer syndromes. A recent review of this issue cited 55 reports of testing for these purposes (90). Both technologies have been utilized in families with Li-Fraumeni syndrome, and PGD has been used by parents at risk for having a child with a *BRCA1/2* mutation (90). The ethical issues raised by these procedures share some similarities but also have some unique features. The option of prenatal diagnosis raises the question of appropriate use of this technology. In most developed countries, the offer of prenatal diagnosis and selective termination is generally considered acceptable when the condition is a childhood onset disorder with significant morbidity and premature mortality. In contrast, the application of prenatal diagnosis to a disorder such as hereditary breast/ovarian cancer syndrome is controversial. In the case of PGD, the strongest argument in favor of its utilization is one of parental autonomy, as with other reproductive choices within parents' purview. However, this technology is expensive and is cost prohibitive for many individuals, thus raising the issue of justice and fair access (90). One approach taken in countries outside the United States is to create oversight committees that review requests for PGD and determine acceptable use of PGD and prenatal diagnosis. Recently, the Human Fertilisation and Embryology Authority (HFEA) in the U.K. approved PGD for *BRCA1* and *BRCA2* mutations (91). In the United States, however, these services are unregulated, with use determined primarily by professional standards and the preferences of parents who have the ability to pay for such services. In countries without regulation, ethical resolutions are left largely to individual discretion.

Offit et al. raise the thorny issue of whether healthcare providers have a legal obligation to explain options for assisted reproduction to individuals with gene mutations associated with cancer syndromes, as part of their "duty to warn" (90). For example, it has been recommended that *BRCA2* testing be offered to Ashkenazi Jewish reproductive-age partners of an individual with a *BRCA2* mutation because of the observation that two deleterious mutations in this gene may be associated with Fanconi anemia, early onset brain tumors, and other malignancies (92). It is unclear whether there would be legal implications around the issue of wrongful birth if patients were not informed of available means to identify and potentially avoid the birth of a child with a cancer predisposition syndrome (90).

Although prenatal and preimplantation testing for hereditary cancer syndromes are not highly in demand at present, and it is not standard practice to offer these options, clinicians should be prepared to discuss options available to individuals and couples when the question arises and to help them clarify their values and preferences with respect to reproductive decision-making.

CONCLUSION

Genetic counseling and testing for hereditary breast cancer risk afford many potential benefits to individuals and their families. As clinical cancer genetics has evolved, identifying and managing those at increased risk of cancer continue to be complex and challenging. In addition, as the impact and importance of risk information become realized, we are faced with ethical, legal, and social dilemmas that do not lend themselves to uniform or straightforward solutions. Patient values, preferences, coping abilities, and communication styles contribute to the multifaceted dimensions that must be considered in the context of decision-making and ethical problem solving. Cancer genetic counseling is a work in progress, and what we learn will help establish paradigms for other forms of predictive genetic testing that will share center stage in the future. In the long term, however, the goals remain consistent, which are to maximize the access, potential benefits, and utility of genetic testing for all individuals while minimizing the prospect of harm and adverse outcomes.

REFERENCES

1. Myriad Genetics 2006 Annual Report. Available at: www.myriad.com/downloads/ MYGN_AR2006.pdf (accessed June 2007).
2. Beauchamp TL, Childress JF. Principles of Biomedical Ethics. 5th ed. Oxford: Oxford University Press, 2000.
3. Burke W, Press N. Ethical obligations and counseling challenges in cancer genetics. J Natl Compr Canc Netw 2006; 4(2):185–191.
4. Burke W, Press N. Genetics as a tool to improve cancer outcomes: ethics and policy. Nat Rev Cancer 2006; 6(6):476–482.
5. Offit K. Psychological, ethical, and legal issues in cancer risk counseling. In: Offit K, ed. Clinical Cancer Genetics: Risk Counseling and Management. New York: Wiley-Liss, 1998: 287–316.
6. Halbert CH, Kessler LJ, Mitchell E. Genetic testing for inherited breast cancer risk in African Americans. Cancer Invest 2005; 23(4):285–295.
7. Oloparde OI. Genetics in clinical cancer care: a promise unfulfilled among minority populations. Cancer Epidemiol Biomarkers Prev 2004; 13(11 Pt 1):1683–1686.

8. Jonsen AR, Siegler M, Winslade WJ. Clinical Ethics: A Practical Approach to Ethical Decisions in Clinical Medicine. 5th ed. New York: McGraw-Hill, 2002.

9. The American Society of Human Genetics Social Issues Subcommittee on Familial Disclosure, ASHG Statement. Professional disclosure of familial genetic information. Am J Hum Genet 1998; 62(2):474–483.

10. American Society of Clinical Oncology. Policy statement of the American Society of Clinical Oncology Update: genetic testing for cancer susceptibility. J Clin Oncol 2003; 21(12): 2397–2406.

11. Hampel H, Sweet K, Westman JA, et al. Referral for cancer genetics consultation: a review and compilation of risk assessment criteria. J Med Genet 2004; 41(2):81–91.

12. National Comprehensive Cancer Network. Genetic/familial high-risk assessment: breast and ovarian. Clin Pract Guidelines Oncol 2007; 1:1–30. Available at: http://www.nccn.org/ professionals/physician_gls/PDF/genetics_screening.pdf (accessed June 2007).

13. U.S. Preventive Services Task Force. Genetic risk assessment and BRCA mutation testing for breast and ovarian cancer susceptibility: recommendation statement. Ann Intern Med 2005; 143(5):355–361. Erratum in: Ann Intern Med 2005; 143(7):547.

14. GeneTests: Medical Genetics Information Resource (database online). Copyright, University of Washington, Seattle. 1993–2007. Available at: http://www.genetests.org (accessed June 2007).

15. Offit K, Garber J, Grady M, et al. ASCO Curriculum: Cancer Genetics and Cancer Predisposition Testing. 2nd ed. Alexandria, VA: ASCO Publishing, 2004.

16. McKinnon WC, Baty BJ, Bennett RL, et al. Predisposition genetic testing for late-onset disorders in adults. A position paper of the National Society of Genetic Counselors. JAMA 1997; 278(15):1217–1220.

17. Trepanier A, Ahrens M, McKinnon W, et al. Genetic cancer risk assessment and counseling: recommendations of the national society of genetic counselors. J Genet Couns 2004; 13(2): 83–114.

18. Andrews L, Meiser B, Apicella C, et al. Psychological impact of genetic testing for breast cancer susceptibility in women of Ashkenazi Jewish background: a prospective study. Genet Test 2004; 8(3):240–247.

19. Bluman LG, Rimer BK, Berry DA, et al. Attitudes, knowledge, and risk perceptions of women with breast and/or ovarian cancer considering testing for BRCA1 and BRCA2. J Clin Oncol 1999; 17(3):1040–1046.

20. Braithwaite D, Emery J, Walter F, et al. Psychological impact of genetic counseling for familial cancer: a systematic review and met-analysis. J Natl Cancer Inst 2004; 96(2): 122–133.

21. Grosfeld FJM, Lips CJM, Beemer FA, et al. Who is at risk for psychological distress in genetic testing programs for hereditary cancer disorders? J Genet Couns 2000; 9(3):253–266.

22. Geller G, Botkin JR, Green MJ, et al. Genetic testing for susceptibility to adult-onset cancer. The process and content of informed consent. JAMA 1997; 277(18):1467–1474.

23. Cull A, Miller H, Porterfield T, et al. The use of videotaped information in cancer genetic counselling: a randomized evaluation study. Br J Cancer 1998; 77(5):830–837.

24. Green MJ, Peterson SK, Baker MW, et al. Effect of a computer-based decision aid on knowledge, perceptions, and intentions about genetic testing for breast cancer susceptibility: a randomized controlled trial. JAMA 2004; 292(4):442–452.

25. Skinner CS, Schildkraut JM, Berry D, et al. Pre-counseling education materials for BRCA testing: does tailoring make a difference? Genet Test 2002; 6(2):93–105.

26. Culver JO, Hull JL, Dunne DF, et al. Oncologists' opinions on genetic testing for breast and ovarian cancer. Genet Med 2001; 3(2):120–125.

27. Pichert G, Dietrich D, Moosmann P, et al. Swiss primary care physicians' knowledge, attitudes and perception towards genetic testing for hereditary breast cancer. Fam Cancer 2003; 2(3–4):153–158.

28. Reutenauer JE. Medical malpractice liability in the era of genetic susceptibility testing. Quinnipiac Law Rev 2000; 19:539.

29. Severin JM. Genetic susceptibility for specific cancers: medical liability for the clinician. Cancer 1999; 86(8):1744–1749.

30. Wideroff L, Vadaparampil ST, Greene MH, et al. Hereditary breast/ovarian and colorectal cancer genetics knowledge in a national sample of US physicians. J Med Genet 2005; 42(10): 749–755.

31. Helmes AW, Culver JO, Bowen DJ. Results of a randomized study of telephone versus in-person breast cancer risk counseling. Patient Educ Couns 2006; 64(1–3):96–103.

32. Wolfberg AJ. Genes on the web—direct-to-consumer marketing of genetic testing. N Engl J Med 2006; 355(6):543–545.

33. Schwartz MD, Lerman C, Brogan B, et al. Impact of *BRCA1/BRCA2* counseling and testing on newly diagnosed breast cancer patients. J Clin Oncol 2004; 22(10):1823–1829.

34. Tinley ST, Houfek J, Watson P, et al. Screening adherence in *BRCA1/2* families is associated with primary physicians' behavior. Am J Med Genet A 2004; 125(1):5–11.

35. Hunter AGW, Sharpe N, Mullen M, et al. Ethical, legal, and practical concerns about recontacting patients to inform them of new information: the case in medical genetics. Am J Med Genet 2001; 103(4):265–276.

36. National Partnership for Women and Families on behalf of the Coalition for Genetic Fairness. Faces of Genetic Discrimination: How Genetic Discrimination Affects Real People. July 2004. Available at: http://www.geneticalliance.org/ksc_assets/documents/facesofgeneticdiscrimination.pdf (Accessed June 2007).

37. Kass NE, Hull SC, Natowicz MR, et al. Medical privacy and the disclosure of personal medical information: the beliefs and experiences of those with genetic and other clinical conditions. Am J Med Genet A 2004; 128(3):261–270.

38. Lapham EV, Kozma C, Weiss JO. Genetic discrimination: perspectives of consumers. Science 1996; 274(5287):621–624.

39. Otlowski MF, Taylor SD, Barlow-Stewart KK. Genetic discrimination: too few data. Eur J Hum Genet 2003; 11(1):1–2.

40. Apse KA, Biesecker BB, Giardiello FM, et al. Perceptions of genetic discrimination among at-risk relatives of colorectal cancer patients. Genet Med 2004; 6(6):510–516.

41. Armstrong KA, Calzone K, Stopfer J, et al. Factors associated with decisions about clinical *BRCA1/2* testing. Cancer Epidemiol Biomarkers Prev 2000; 9(11):1251–1254.

42. Health Insurance Portability and Accountability Act 42 USC Sec 300gg-300gg-2, 1996.

43. Hustead JL, Goldman J. Genetics and privacy. Am J Law Med 2002; 28(2–3):285–307.

44. Americans with Disabilities Act. 42 USC Sec 12101-12213, 1990.

45. National Human Genome Research Institute. Legislation on Genetic Discrimination. http://genome.gov/10002077#2 (accessed September 2006).

46. Earley CL, Strong LC. Certificates of confidentiality: a valuable tool for protecting genetic data. Am J Hum Genet 1995; 57(3):727–731.

47. Godard B, Raeburn S, Pembrey M, et al. Genetic information and testing in insurance and employment: technical, social and ethical issues. Eur J Hum Genet 2003; 11(suppl 2): S123–S142.

48. Armstrong K, Weber B, FitzGerald G, et al. Life insurance and breast cancer risk assessment: adverse selection, genetic testing decisions, and discrimination. Am J Med Genet A 2003; 120 (3):359–364.

49. Smith KR, Zick CD, Mayer RN, et al. Voluntary disclosure of *BRCA1* mutation test results. Genet Test 2002; 6(2):89–92.

50. Willner J. Hadassah opposes genetic test discrimination. Washington Jewish Week 1997 March 6:1.

51. Struewing JP, Hartge P, Wacholder S, et al. The risk of cancer associated with specific mutations of *BRCA1* and *BRCA2* among Ashkenazi Jews. N Engl J Med 1997; 336(20): 1401–1408.

52. Myriad Genetic Laboratories. Informed Consent for Hereditary Cancer Genetic Testing. Available at: http://www.myriadtests.com/doc/Myriad_Informed_Consent_Form.pdf (accessed October 2006).

53. Durfy SJ, Buchanan TE, Burke W. Testing for inherited susceptibility to breast cancer: a survey of informed consent forms for *BRCA1* and *BRCA2* mutation testing. Am J Med Genet 1998; 75(1):82–87.

54. Hamvas A, Madden KK, Nogee LM, et al. Informed consent for genetic research. Arch Pediatr Adolesc Med 2004; 158(6):551–555.

55. Lerman C, Narod S, Schulman K, et al. *BRCA1* testing in families with hereditary breast-ovarian cancer. A prospective study of patient decision making and outcomes. JAMA 1996; 275(24):1885–1892.

56. Dugan RB, Wiesner GL, Juengst ET, et al. Duty to warn at-risk relatives for genetic disease: genetic counselors' clinical experience. Am J Med Genet C Semin Med Genet 2003; 119(1): 27–34.

57. Falk JM, Dugan RB, O'Riordan MA, et al. Medical geneticists' duty to warn at-risk relatives for genetic disease. Am J Med Genet A 2003; 120(3):374–380.

58. Hughes C, Lerman C, Schwartz M, et al. All in the family: evaluation of the process and content of sisters' communication about *BRCA1* and *BRCA2* genetic test results. Am J Med Genet 2002; 107(2):143–150.

59. Julian-Reynier C, Eisinger F, Chabal F, et al. Disclosure to the family of breast/ovarian cancer genetic test results: patient's willingness and associated factors. Am J Med Genet 2000; 94(1): 13–18.

60. McGivern R, Everett J, Yager GG, et al. Family communication about positive *BRCA1* and *BRCA2* genetic test results. Genet Med 2004; 6(6):503–509.

61. Wilson BJ, Forrest K, van Teijlingen ER, et al. Family communication about genetic risk: the little that is known. Community Genet 2004; 7(1):15–24.

62. Offit K, Groeger E, Turner S, et al. The "duty to warn" a patient's family members about hereditary disease risk. JAMA 2004; 292(12):1469–1473.

63. United States Code of Federal Regulations, Title 45 § 164.512. Available at: http://a257.g. akamaitech.net/7/257/2422/13nov20061500/edocket.access.gpo.gov/cfr_2006/octqtr/ pdf/45cfr164.512.pdf (accessed June 2007).

64. Tarasoff v the Regents of the University of California, 551 P 2d 334 (Cal 1976).

65. Pate v Threlkel, 661 So 2d 278 (Fla 1995).

66. Safer v Estate of Pack, 677 A2d 1188 (NJ App), appeal denied, 683 A2d 1163 (NJ 1996).

67. Godard B, Hurlimann, Letendre M, et al. Guidelines for disclosing genetic information to family members: from development to use. Fam Cancer 2006; 5(1):103–116.

68. American Medical Association. Code of Medical Ethics: Opinion E-2.131: Disclosure of Familial Risk in Genetic Testing. Available at: http://www.ama-assn.org/ama/pub/category/ print/11963.html (accessed July 2006).

69. Peshkin BN, Isaacs C. Evaluation and management of women with *BRCA1*/2 mutations. Oncology (Williston Park) 2005; 19(11):1451–1459.

70. Antoniou A, Pharoah PD, Narod S, et al. Average risks of breast and ovarian cancer associated with *BRCA1* or *BRCA2* mutations detected in case series unselected for family history: a combined analysis of 22 studies. Am J Hum Genet 2003; 72(5):1117–1130. Erratum in: Am J Hum Genet 2003; 73(3):709.

71. Costalas Wagner J, Itzen M, Malick J, et al. Communication of *BRCA1* and *BRCA2* results to at-risk relatives: a cancer risk assessment program's experience. Am J Med Genet C Semin Med Genet 2003; 119(1):11–18.

72. Loud JT, Weissman NE, Peters JA, et al. Deliberate deceit of family members: a challenge to providers of clinical genetics services. J Clin Oncol 2006; 24(10):1643–1646.

73. Doukas DJ, Berg JW. The family covenant and genetic testing. Am J Bioeth 2001; 1(3): 3–10.

74. Stock G. The family covenant: a flawed response to the dilemmas of genetic testing. Am J Bioeth 2001; 1(3):17–18.

75. Lynch HT. Family information service and hereditary cancer. Cancer 2001; 91(4):625–628.

76. Daly MB, Barsevick A, Miller SM, et al. Communicating genetic test results to the family: a six-step skills-building strategy. Fam Community Health 2001; 24(3):13–26.

77. American Society of Human Genetics Board of Directors, American College of Medical Genetics Board of Directors. Points to consider: ethical, legal, and psychosocial implications of genetic testing in children and adolescents. Am J Hum Genet 1995; 57(5):1233–1241.

78. Nelson RM, Botkin JR, Kodish ED, et al. Ethical issues with genetic testing in pediatrics. Pediatrics 2001; 107(6):1451–1455.

79. Strahm B, Malkin D. Hereditary cancer predisposition in children: genetic basis and clinical implications. Int J Cancer 2006; 119(9):2001–2006.

80. Collins F. Commentary on the ASCO statement on genetic testing for cancer susceptibility. J Clin Oncol 1996; 14(5):1738–1740.

81. Tercyak KP, Peshkin BN, DeMarco TA, et al. Parent-child factors and their effect on communicating *BRCA1/2* test results to children. Patient Educ Couns 2002; 47(2):145–153.

82. Campbell E, Ross LF. Professional and personal attitudes about access and confidentiality in the genetic testing of children: a pilot study. Genet Testing 2003; 7(2):123–130.

83. Campbell E, Ross LF. Parental attitudes and beliefs regarding the genetic testing in children. Community Genet 2005; 8(2):94–102.

84. Hamann HA, Croyle RT, Venne VL, et al. Attitudes toward the genetic testing of children among adults in a Utah-based kindred tested for a *BRCA1* mutation. Am J Med Genet 2000; 92(1):25–32.

85. Duncan RE, Delatycki MB. Predictive testing in young people for adult-onset conditions: where is the empirical evidence? Clin Genet 2006; 69(1):8–16.

86. Elger BS, Harding TW. Testing adolescents for a hereditary breast cancer gene (*BRCA1*). Respecting their autonomy is in their best interest. Arch Pediatr Adolesc Med 2000; 154(2): 113–119.

87. Sharpe NF, Carter RF. Susceptibility testing. In: Sharpe NF, Carter RF, eds. Genetic Testing: Care, Consent, and Liability. New Jersey: John Wiley & Sons, Inc., 2006:268–291.

88. McConkie-Rosell A, Spiridigliozzi GA. "Family matters": a conceptual framework for genetic testing in children. J Genet Couns 2004; 13(10):9–29.

89. Simpson JL, Carson SA, Cisneros P. Preimplantation genetic diagnosis (PGD) for heritable neoplasia. J Natl Cancer Inst Monogr 2005; 34:87–90.

90. Offit K, Kohut K, Clagett B, et al. Cancer genetic testing and assisted reproduction. J Clin Oncol 2006; 24(29):4775–4782.

91. Dyer C. HFEA widens its criteria for preimplantation diagnosis. BMJ 2006; 332(7551):1174.

92. Offit K, Levran O, Mullaney B, et al. Shared genetic susceptibility to breast cancer, brain tumors, and Fanconi anemia. J Natl Cancer Inst 2003; 95(20):1548–1551.

4

Cancer Risks in *BRCA1* and *BRCA2* Mutation Carriers

Kenneth Offit and Peter Thom
Clinical Genetics Service, Department of Medicine, Memorial Sloan-Kettering Cancer Center, New York, New York, U.S.A.

INTRODUCTION

More than a decade after the discovery of the *BRCA1* and *BRCA2* genes, there remains scholarly debate regarding the precise magnitude and spectrum of cancer risks to individuals carrying mutations of these genes (1–9). The ranges of risk estimates derived have emerged from different types of studies performed over the past decade, and thus the ranges of risks reported may reflect the biases of the ascertainment methodologies employed. Alternatively, or additionally, environmental or other modifying genetic factors may impact on kindreds, segregating *BRCA* mutations. Modifying genetic factors may include those intrinsic to the mutation itself, i.e., genotype–phenotype correlations, as well as extrinsic modifiers due to coinheritance of mutations in other genes. A significant variance in penetrance estimates conveyed to women at the time of genetic counseling may pose vexing challenges as they consider the intricacies of treatment options, including preventive surgeries. This chapter will provide an overview of the various methods that have been utilized to estimate risk associated with *BRCA* mutations, will highlight the genotype/phenotype associations that have been observed, and will review the risk for tumors other than breast and ovarian cancer in carriers of *BRCA1/2* mutations. The conclusion that will emerge is that clinicians can draw on a large literature providing relatively stable estimations of risks tailored to individuals in families affected by multiple cases of breast or related cancers, or individuals in the general population lacking evidence of a family history of syndromic cancers.

DEFINITION OF RISKS

Before analyzing studies that have derived *BRCA*-associated cancer risks it is important to review the nomenclature utilized herein. This nomenclature includes the concepts of relative risks (RRs) and odds ratios (ORs) drawn from epidemiological studies, and the concept of penetrance rooted in genetics.

RR is derived from cohort studies, which compare subjects exposed versus unexposed to a risk factor (environmental or genetic). RR is calculated by dividing the number of subjects exposed to the risk factor who develop a disease by the number of unexposed subjects who develop the disease per unit time (10,11). *Penetrance* is the proportion of those with a specific genotype who develop the expected phenotype (10). It is generally expressed as age-specific penetrance, the percentage of individuals affected by the disease by a specific age, or within an age group. *Retrospective* studies measure the association between exposures and disease looking backward in time. Retrospective analyses may be *cohort studies* or *case–control studies*. These differ based on how the subjects are chosen. Cohort studies generally select two groups of individuals on the basis of exposure versus nonexposure to a risk factor. The outcome that is measured is the disease incidence in each group; incidence of disease in the exposed group divided by that in the unexposed group, expressed as an RR. Most cohort studies are prospective, starting at a point in time with individuals free of a disease and following them forward. However, a cohort can also be identified retrospectively and followed up to the present. There can be bias in studies that appear to be retrospective cohort studies, but which in fact are not. This is particularly true when cohorts are assembled according to, for example, their ability to come for a genetic test because of the ascertainment bias from prior interventions (e.g., surgeries) that may impact their cancer risk (12). In some studies, the RR of an event, for example the occurrence of breast cancer over time, is derived as a *hazard ratio*, calculated from a proportional hazards regression model. Case–control studies are retrospective studies and use outcome as the starting point: two groups are selected on the basis of differing outcomes, one with and another without disease. Exposures to risk factors are then determined. The relative proportion of those with the disease who are exposed to a risk factor (in this case a *BRCA* mutation) is compared to the proportion without the disease exposed to the risk factor, resulting in an OR. The OR is an approximation of the RR (10).

Genetic linkage studies have been effective at discovering highly penetrant genes that cause breast and ovarian cancer (13–16). As will be discussed, penetrance rates derived from these highly selected kindreds would be assumed, by definition, to be overestimates, since the criterion for ascertainment was biased toward multiplex (multiply affected) kindreds (17–24).

MUTATION LOCUS: GENOTYPE/PHENOTYPE CORRELATIONS

The *BRCA1* gene consists of 24 exons encoding 1863 amino acids (25). To date, more than 1000 deleterious mutations have been found in *BRCA1*. The earliest suggestion that variable breast and ovarian cancer risks are associated with mutation position appeared in the initial analysis of clinical testing for *BRCA1* mutations by one laboratory in the United States (26). Subsequently, Gayther et al. (27) found a significant relationship between the 5' and 3' locations of the *BRCA1* mutation loci and the RR for breast versus ovarian cancer, but this was not confirmed by Struewing et al. (28), and subsequent studies have weakened the case for phenotype/genotype correlations in *BRCA1* (29,30).

BRCA2 is also a large gene (27 exons, 3418 amino acids). Over 500 mutations in *BRCA2* have been described. The existence of phenotype/genotype correlations with respect to *BRCA2* mutations has been more strongly supported than those initially reported for *BRCA1*. A study by Gayther et al. (31) described a pattern of phenotype/genotype correlations. Families with a high incidence of ovarian cancer tended to have mutations clustered in a 3.3 kb region of exon 11 bounded by nucleotides 3035 and 6629, which was termed the ovarian cancer cluster region (OCCR). The authors speculated that this clustering of ovarian cancer could result from mutations with higher ovarian cancer penetrance, lower breast cancer penetrance, or a combination of both. Additional support

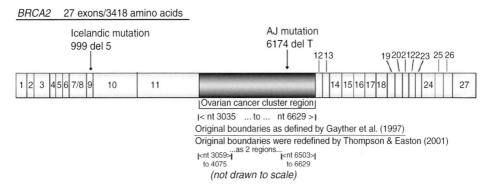

Figure 1 The ovarian cancer cluster region in *BRCA2*. The region bounded by nucleotides 3059 to 4075 and 6503 to 6629 were associated with a decreased RR of breast cancer (0.63) and an increased RR of ovarian cancer (1.88) (Thompson and Easton, 2001). *Abbreviations*: AJ, Ashkenazi Jewish founder mutation position; RR, relative risk. *Source*: From Refs. 31–34.

for the phenotype/genotype correlations being associated with the OCCR has come from studies of Ashkenazi Jews involving the *6174delT* founder mutation, which lies inside the *BRCA2* OCCR. This mutation is found in ovarian cancer patients about four times as often as in those with breast cancer (29,32). Further, the Icelandic *BRCA2* founder mutation *999delT*, which is outside the OCCR, is found with a similar frequency in both breast and ovarian cancer cases (33).

As shown in Figure 1, the OCCR was further elucidated by Thompson and Easton (34), who refined the boundaries of the region. The kindreds for this study were gathered by the Breast Cancer Linkage Consortium (BCLC) (36) from 20 centers in Western Europe, the United States, and Canada and consisted of 164 kindreds with 92 distinct mutations. Using a larger dataset and more sophisticated statistical analyses than the earlier studies, this group optimally defined the OCCR as bounded by nucleotides 3059 to 4075 and 6503 to 6629. Individuals in this study with mutations in the OCCR had a decreased RR of breast cancer (0.63) and an increased RR of ovarian cancer (1.88).

PENETRANCE AS A REFLECTION OF THE BIOLOGY OF *BRCA*, AND HETEROGENEITY OF MUTATION TYPES

In the United States, breast and ovarian cancers together have a significant incidence in the general population: birth to death incidence for breast cancer is 12.67%, and for ovarian cancer, it is 1.44% (37). The frequency of all *BRCA1/2* mutations has been estimated as 0.0008 (~1/1250) in the general U.S. population and 0.0129 for Ashkenazi Jews (~1/77) (38). *BRCA1/2* mutation carriers are likely to be subject to the same risk factors that influence the general population, though the manner in which these factors operate in *BRCA1/2* mutation carriers may differ (38–43). Penetrance estimates for *BRCA1/2* mutation–positive individuals represent the sum of genetic and nongenetic influences. Thus, for *BRCA1/2* mutation–positive individuals, penetrance represents the incidence of the disease due to the specific mutation plus the incidence of the disease in the general population.

A metapopulation, for example the United States, is a mix of subpopulations. In addition to the founder mutations observed in Ashkenazi Jews, significant frequency differences have been described between subpopulations represented within the U.S.

metapopulation (44–47). One study noted substantial differences in hazard ratios between *BRCA1* and *BRCA2* mutations—11 versus 23, respectively—and between protein-truncating mutations versus missense and splice-site mutations—13, 30, and 30, respectively (48). Large genomic rearrangements, including deletions, also exist, further contributing to the heterogeneity, and the frequency of these deletions also varies among genetic subpopulations. In one study, a 12% rate of such rearrangements was noted in 269 U.S. kindreds, but this was 0% among a subset of 31 Ashkenazi kindreds (49). However, this study probably overestimated the frequency of large rearrangements because of oversampling of multiplex kindreds. Similarly, Petrij-Bosch et al. (50) studied 170 multiplex Dutch kindreds who had been tested negative for *BRCA1* by methods that did not search for large-scale deletions and demonstrated a 36% rate of large-scale rearrangements. If, as appears to be the case, *BRCA1/2* mutation types and frequencies have different distributions in different subpopulations, and different types of mutations convey different risks, then penetrance calculations in a mixed metapopulation will vary according to the mix of subpopulations represented.

PENETRANCE ESTIMATES FROM LINKAGE STUDIES

In the process of assembling large kindreds for mapping, and ultimately the positional cloning of *BRCA1* and *BRCA2*, it was possible to make early estimates of penetrance for these genes. The subjects had been selected for linkage studies from kindreds with multiple, multigenerational cases of breast and/or ovarian cancer. These studies yielded penetrance estimates of 83% to 87% and 44% to 63%, respectively, for breast and ovarian cancer by the age of 70 years (18,23,51). A maximum-likelihood statistical approach to deriving penetrance estimates for *BRCA2* based on two large breast/ovarian cancer families linked to *BRCA2* yielded estimates of risk of breast cancer by the age of 70 years of 79.5% in females and 6.3% in males (52).

PENETRANCE ESTIMATES FROM SERIES BASED ON DIRECT
BRCA GENOTYPING

Following the identification of *BRCA1* and *BRCA2*, it became possible to directly genotype individuals and to derive penetrance by examining the family structure of these probands. These series, in which the index case or proband was selected on the basis of having breast cancer and then being genotyped, have been referred to as "case proband" studies or "genotyped affected proband" series (1,53). In case proband series, there may be significant bias, depending on how the cases were ascertained. In true "population-based" case proband studies, the index cases are selected without regard to family history or other factors (54). Cases ideally are collected from population-based registries, ideally by a random selection. However, in practice, because active participation in the study is required, only a fraction of eligible participants may take part; thus, even such "population-based" series may reflect ascertainment bias. Another means to gather case probands is the hospital-based series using, preferably, incident and not prevalent cases so as to avoid survival bias. Finally, there are "volunteer" case proband series, one of which, performed in New York, generated considerable discussion because of the potential biases in selection. In contrast to case proband series are the control proband series, in which the index case is not selected because of the phenotype under study (breast cancer), but is unaffected. Such an approach avoids the pitfalls of "size-biased sampling," in which case probands may share many nongenetic risk factors associated with breast cancer, whereas the control probands may not (1). Because of the relative rarity of *BRCA* mutations, there have been comparatively few control proband series.

The major case proband series that derived penetrance rates and confidence intervals are shown in Figure 2 which displays a range of risk estimates corresponding to various studies. These studies have been divided into three general groups: the first group consisting of "multiple case" ascertainments including linkage-based families and clinic-based ascertainments; the second group consisting of hospital-based and volunteer ascertainments, all of "affected proband" type with the exception of the Washington, DC, area "control proband" volunteer study; and the third group of true population-based studies in which breast or ovarian cancer cases were ascertained from registries, and were not subject to bias due to ascertainment according to family history, or other biases associated with hospital-based or volunteer cases. As seen in Figure 2, the ranges of risk are generally highest for the first group, intermediate for the second, and lowest for the third. One exception is an Italian clinic-based series in which the authors noted that their clinic population had remarkably weak family histories of cancer and indicated that their ascertainment should be "considered intermediate ... between a multiple-case ... and population-based ... study" (56).

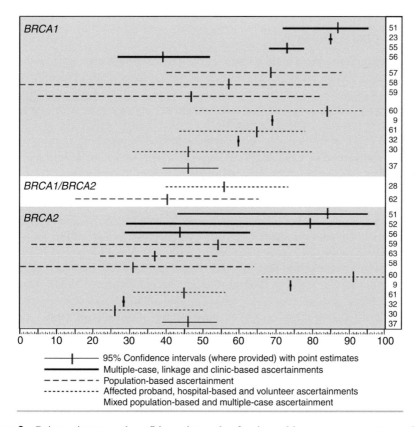

Figure 2 Point estimates and confidence intervals of estimated breast cancer penetrance by the age of 70 years in various categories of studies, including multiple case, linkage and linkage ascertainments, population-based ascertainments, and "affected proband" hospital-based and volunteer ascertainments (see text).

A key potential bias in all "genotyped affected proband" studies is that the formula used to calculate penetrance in the kin-cohort method assumes a steady mutation frequency. It is anticipated that because *BRCA1/2* mutations significantly affect mortality, these mutation frequencies decrease with increasing age cohorts. In the Washington, DC, area study (28,53,64), for example, the carrier frequency in females 20 to 29 years of age was 2.7%, whereas the frequency in females over 60 was 0.7%. In male subjects, the corresponding figures were 2.3% and 1.5%, respectively. It is also assumed in the methods to calculate penetrance that mutations are in a "steady state"; i.e., that mutations do not appear de novo. Thus, in the kin-cohort model devised to calculate penetrance, it is assumed that 50% of the parents (the kin-cohort) will have inherited the same mutation. However, it is biologically possible that neither parent inherited the mutation seen in the proband. De novo mutations in *BRCA* have been reported (65,66). While it is assumed that the frequency of *BRCA* de novo mutations is not as high as the 30% to 50% reported for some genes (e.g., *NF1*, *APC*), the exact frequency has not been determined systematically. Indeed, in the course of cosegregation studies of *BRCA* missense variants of unknown significance, we have observed cases of de novo missense variants (Offit, unpublished observation). A relatively low rate of de novo *BRCA* mutations would have an impact on kin-cohort derived penetrance estimates. In addition, underreporting of relatives affected with breast cancer can also serve to underestimate penetrance estimates derived using this approach (2).

Control Proband Series

Control proband series are limited by the relative rarity of *BRCA* mutations, as well as the complexity and cost of genotyping thousands of control individuals to identify a handful of *BRCA* mutation–carrying kindreds. A crucial factor in the feasibility of this type of study design was the discovery of "founder" mutations among a genetic isolate amenable to research participation. The discovery of three "Ashkenazi" mutations, two in *BRCA1* and one in *BRCA2*, is detailed elsewhere in this volume. The frequency of these mutations was directly measured in a number of studies involving Ashkenazi Jewish participants. We and others found that about 2.5% of Ashkenazi Jews carried one of these founder mutations (28, 67–71). For the Washington, DC, area control proband study (28,53,67), the subjects were recruited via posters in Jewish community centers, and through radio and newspaper ads in both Jewish and general media outlets in the Washington, DC, area. This cross-sectional study included 5318 self-identified Ashkenazi individuals >20 years old, in the Washington, DC, area, all of whom were subsequently genotyped for the two *BRCA1* founder mutations and 5087 of whom were genotyped for the Ashkenazi *BRCA2* founder mutation. After genetic testing, the researchers compared family histories of mutation carriers and noncarriers. Using the kin-cohort design, cancer risks were compared in first-degree relatives of probands with *BRCA* mutations ("carrier kins") and without *BRCA* mutations ("noncarrier kins"), assuming that 50% of the time, these first-degree relatives would carry the same mutation. It should be noted that the mutation-carrying probands in such a cross-sectional model may or may not have had the cancer phenotype; the authors allowed the use of affected individuals as probands for reasons of convenience in obtaining family history information. Penetrance calculations were based on weighted-average probabilities. Using this approach, the estimated penetrance at the age of 70 years for either breast or ovarian cancer was calculated to be 63%, considerably lower than the estimates derived from linkage studies.

Despite this study design, the Washington area study and the kin-cohort method present a number of potentially confounding issues. Most importantly, the family history of cancer may be a significant factor in the decision to volunteer for such a study (72). In the Washington area study, the combined incidence of breast and ovarian cancer among noncarriers at 70 years of age was found to be 13% to 14%, somewhat higher than the 9% rate in the general population. When compared with the Surveillance, Epidemiology, and End Results (SEER) (37) registry, noncarriers in this study group had a 68% increased incidence of breast cancer and a 48% increase in ovarian cancer. One explanation for the selection bias in volunteers was the observation that "participants were highly educated, with over 57% reporting a postgraduate degree" (28), compared to about 9% with postgraduate degrees in the general population (73). Level of education has been positively correlated with later prima-gravida and having less children, both factors associated with higher breast cancer risks (74). According to the National Jewish Population Survey 2000–2001 (75), almost half the number of Jewish women aged 35 to 39 are nulliparous, compared to a fifth of all U.S. women. In the Washington study, these selection biases may have contributed to overestimating the penetrance of *BRCA* compared to a true metapopulation-based approach.

Case Proband Studies

In case proband studies, breast (or ovarian) cancer cases are identified from population-based registries, incident hospital series, or clinical ascertainments; family histories are then documented. Using a variety of statistical models, including the kin-cohort model, the age-specific rates of breast cancer are calculated. In most studies, cancer rates in mutation carriers were compared with those in noncarriers, although in some studies, a variety of sources for controls were used, including published data on expected cancer rates from SEER or other population registries.

The major case proband series that derived penetrance rates and confidence intervals are shown in Figure 2. The Anglian Breast Cancer Study Group (59) included 1435 breast cancer index cases diagnosed at <55 years of age who were then genotyped, resulting in the identification of 24 *BRCA1/2* mutation carriers. The rate of expected cancer, using population statistics from England and Wales, was compared to the observed rate in both carrier relatives and noncarrier relatives. Thorlacius et al. (63) studied 541 female and 34 male breast cancer cases unselected for family history. These subjects were genotyped for the Icelandic founder mutation in *BRCA2*, and 69 such cases were identified. Data from the Icelandic Cancer Registry were then used to compare the history of cancer in first-degree relatives of carriers and noncarriers. Warner et al. (32) ascertained 457 Ashkenazi female breast cancer cases unselected for either age or family history, of whom 412 were tested for the three Ashkenazi founder mutations; 48 carriers were identified. Control groups consisted of 360 non-Ashkenazi female breast cancer cases and 380 Ashkenazi Jewish females with no history of cancer. Based on reported family histories, the RR for breast cancer (and prostate cancer) in first-degree relatives of carriers and noncarriers was estimated using the kin-cohort model.

Three studies have used ovarian cancer cases as case probands. One study analyzed mothers and sisters of 922 women with incident ovarian cancer (cases) and 922 women with no history of ovarian cancer (controls) (57). The estimated risk of breast cancer by the age of 80 years was 73.5% in mutation carriers and 6.8% in noncarriers, with an ovarian cancer risk of 27.8% in carriers and 1.8% in noncarriers. Antoniou et al. (76) used one dataset consisting of 112 kindreds having two or more cases of epithelial ovarian cancer who were then tested for *BRCA1/2* mutations, and a second set including 374 ovarian cancer cases, unselected for family history, who were then typed for *BRCA1* mutations. Twelve mutation carriers were identified and the family history of cancer was analyzed in the extended pedigrees of these kindreds. A third study selected subjects from 649 incident cases of ovarian cancer in Ontario (77). These women were tested for the 11 most common mutations in *BRCA1/2*, resulting in the identification of 60 case probands. Risks of various cancers were compared in first-degree relatives of carriers and noncarriers using a proportional hazards regression model. As noted by these authors, one advantage of using ovarian cancer case probands is that they do not reflect shared underlying risk factors for breast cancer (3).

Using a completely different approach, the group at Memorial Hospital identified Ashkenazi subjects from a series of primary breast cancer incident cases at three hospitals without reference to familial aggregation of cancer (30). The important distinction in this method is that no family data—neither history nor genotyping of relatives—were utilized. The control group was the same as the Washington study: 3434 Ashkenazi women without a previous history of breast cancer. All subjects were genotyped for the three Ashkenazi founder mutations. This study relied only on the comparison of mutation frequencies in the cases versus controls and the age-specific rates of breast cancer in the general population. In this study, the penetrance was derived from three factors: the population incidence rate from SEER data, the gene mutation prevalence, and the age-specific RR of breast cancer in carriers. This methodology extended that of an earlier study by Fodor et al. (70) by using age-specific incidence to improve accuracy. In the Fodor et al. (70) study, *BRCA* mutation frequencies were determined in 1715 cancer-free individuals at the time of prenatal screening and in 268 breast cancer patients, yielding 18 mutation carriers. ORs were estimated from a standard Mantel–Haentzel test. It is worth noting that the penetrance for *BRCA1* mutation carriers of breast cancer by the age of 70 years for these two studies mark the lower bounds shown in Figure 2: 46% for *BRCA1* and 26% for *BRCA2* in the Satagopan series. This method assumes that the general population incidence (SEER data) and the control group incidence of breast cancer (3434 Ashkenazi Jewish) are equivalent. As previously discussed with respect to the Washington, DC, kin-cohort study, and as will be examined in more detail shortly, this assumption is questionable. The controls (noncarriers) had a breast/ovarian cancer incidence of 13% to 14% at the age of 70 years compared to 9% per the SEER data. The authors pointed out, however, that overall breast cancer incidence in Israel is no higher than in the United States, suggesting no overall increase in rates of breast cancer in those of Ashkenazi or other Jewish backgrounds. However, in view of the differences found in control rates of breast cancer, the authors performed a sensitivity analysis, assuming that breast cancer in Ashkenazi women was 10% or 20% higher than U.S. rates. The effect on penetrance derived was minimal (30).

In 2003, Antoniou et al. (61) performed a meta-analysis of 22 previous studies estimating *BRCA1/2* penetrance using over 8000 index cases unselected for family history comprised of females (86%) or males (2%) with breast cancer and females with epithelial ovarian cancer (12%). Calculations of penetrance were estimated using a modified segregation analysis based on disease occurrence in relatives of mutation-positive individuals. Variations in penetrance were examined using the following variables: type of mutation (genotype/phenotype correlation will be discussed later in this chapter), type of cancer, age at diagnosis, birth cohorts, and location of each study. The goal of this methodology was to better reflect the risks for mutation carriers in both low-risk and high-risk families. The average risk of breast cancer for *BRCA1* carriers was estimated to be 65% by the age of 70 years, and the corresponding estimate for *BRCA2* carriers was 45%. For those ascertained through early onset index cases (<35 years old), the breast cancer risk to *BRCA1* carriers was appreciably higher, 87%. For *BRCA1* carriers identified through breast cancer cases, the breast cancer risk was higher than when identification was through ovarian cancer cases. Ovarian cancer risk did not differ by type of ascertainment case for *BRCA1*. The authors found no age of onset effect for *BRCA2* carriers when cases had breast cancer. And for *BRCA2* mutation carriers, breast cancer risk was higher if identified through breast cancer index cases, and ovarian cancer risk was higher if identified through ovarian cancer index cases.

The kindreds in most of the studies included in this meta-analysis were selected on the basis of an affected index case. Other genetic and/or environmental risk factors are likely to be over-represented in these cases, thus leading to overestimates of penetrance. However, the authors argue that in real-life clinical practice, a minimum of one affected relative would be required to initiate genetic testing; so the penetrance estimates derived in this study are appropriate for clinical purposes. The statistical model used is dependent on RR measurements, and all study locations included in the meta-analysis were presumed to have general population breast cancer incidences equivalent to England and Wales. Population incidence measurements are highly dependent on breast cancer screening programs as was illustrated by the ~25% increase in breast cancer incidence in the United Kingdom during the half decade after the implementation of a nationwide program (78). This study did not control for this factor.

Just as a general consensus to the issue of *BRCA* penetrance was suggested by the meta-analysis of Antoniou et al. (61), in 2003, the "New York Breast Cancer Study" (NYBCS) appeared (9). This study attempted to ascertain 1008 Ashkenazi Jewish incident cases with invasive breast cancer without regard to family history or age of onset. Penetrance estimates in this study were slightly higher for both *BRCA1* and, in particular, for *BRCA2* than other population-based analyses; the cumulative risk of breast cancer at 70 years of age was 69% for *BRCA1* and 74% for *BRCA2*. These results were generally confirmatory of previous studies providing clinical testing as an incentive for study participation. The researchers confirmed a birth-cohort effect (described later in this chapter), as well as two significant lifestyle modifiers, both associated with a later age of onset: physical activity during teenage years; and lighter weight at menarche. The ensuing scholarly response and authors' reply serves as a useful summary of the limitations and challenges in the study design reviewed in this chapter (7–9). Wacholder et al. (8) noted several potential ascertainment biases in the NYBCS which would have led to an overestimate of penetrance estimates. In general, these concerns included a reliance on "case probands" (enriching in all breast and ovarian cancer risk factors in these individuals), the possible bias toward including probands from multiplex families, including deceased relatives only with cancer diagnoses, and a number of other potential signs of bias resulting from absence of a number of technical details of methodology in the original report. Although several of the technical questions raised by Wacholder et al. (8) were to some extent addressed by the NYBCS authors, the fundamental limitations of this type of study remain (1). For example, the observation that over half of probands included in the NYBCS reported a family history of a first- or a second-degree relative affected with breast cancer, compared to less than a third of probands with a similar family history in a true "population based" study by Hopper et al. (54), supports the view that, however well intentioned the efforts, the "volunteer" and "referral" mechanism of ascertainment in the NYBCS and similar studies results in a skewed study population. Easton et al. (7) questioned the ratio of observed mutation carriers to expected carriers in the NYBCS. Although a good part of this discrepancy in the frequency of carriers was due to the failure to use SEER age-specific breast cancer rates, even with this adjustment, there appeared to be risk factor differentials between the Ashkenazi Jewish population and the metapopulation from which SEER tables are derived.

Subsequent to the New York Ashkenazi penetrance study, there have been additional studies on the penetrance of *BRCA* mutations in large series using sophisticated methods of statistical analysis. In a retrospective study by the Cancer Genetics Network (38), 676 Ashkenazi families and 1272 families of other ethnicities, including 282 population-based cases, were analyzed utilizing a novel retrospective likelihood approach to correct for bias induced by oversampling of participants with a positive family history. The estimated cumulative breast cancer risk at the age of 70 years was consistent with previous population-based studies: 46% in *BRCA1* carriers and 43% in *BRCA2* carriers, with ovarian cancer risks of 39% and 22%, respectively (38).

Prospective Studies

As mentioned at the outset, the most robust estimates of cancer risks associated with *BRCA* mutations will come from prospective cohort studies. Many of these studies are now coming to a point in time and a threshold in size as to provide stable estimates of true RR of cancer.

A study in Holland followed 139 women with pathogenic *BRCA1* or *BRCA2* mutations (79). At the point of enrollment, none of the women had cancer histories. During the course of the study, 76 women underwent prophylactic mastectomies, and none of these women developed subsequent breast cancer. The remaining 63 women remained under regular surveillance. The median age of the women in the surveillance group was 39.5 years. Using a model assuming a constant hazard ratio for the surveillance group, the authors concluded that the annual incidence of breast cancer for *BRCA1* mutation–positive individuals is 2.5%. Using a similar approach, another group prospectively compared the effect of surveillance versus prophylactic salpingo-oophorectomy on subsequent breast and ovarian cancer incidence (80). This group prospectively documented an incidence among the surveillance-only group that exceeded even that of the early linkage studies; the incidence of breast cancer and *BRCA*-related gynecologic cancer was observed to be 53 cases per 1000 woman-years, higher than the 21 to 42 cases per 1000 woman-years that would be predicted on the basis of linkage studies (23,36). However, when eight patients in whom cancer was diagnosed during the first year of follow-up (prevalent cases) were excluded from the analysis, the incidence of cancer in our cohort was 25 per 1000 woman-years, within the range derived from linkage studies, and the same as estimated in the Dutch prospective series.

BREAST CANCER RISK IN MALES

Familial clustering of female breast cancer was demonstrated as early as 1926 (81), and epidemiological studies have shown that although both men and women with breast cancer are more likely to have family histories in first-degree relatives than unaffected individuals, men with breast cancer were even more likely to have a first-degree relative with ovarian cancer than affected women (82,83). It is noteworthy that initial linkage studies of *BRCA1* did not reveal an association with male breast cancer (14,84). Linkage studies for *BRCA2*, on the other hand, did contain male breast cancer cases (16). Germline analyses of 50 men affected with breast cancer unselected for family history revealed that 14% of these men carried a *BRCA2* mutation (85). Easton et al. (52), in a study of two large kindreds linked to *BRCA2*, estimated the cumulative risk of breast cancer in male carriers to be 6.3% by the age of 70 years. In an analysis of 164 *BRCA2* kindreds, a similar estimate for cumulative risk emerged: 6.9% for male breast cancer by the age of 80 years, 80 to 100 times the general population risk (34). Thorlacius et al. (63) studied 34 male and 541 female breast cancer cases in Iceland, unselected for family history. Thirteen of these 34 men (38%) had the Icelandic *BRCA2* founder mutation compared to a 10.4% carrier rate among the 541 women. This suggests a high index of suspicion for *BRCA2* mutations in kindreds with male breast cancer, a fact that has been incorporated into predictive models of *BRCA1/2* prevalence (86). A German study of breast and ovarian cancer patients found that 23% harbored mutations in *BRCA2* if there was at least one case of male breast cancer in the family (87). Although the risk of breast cancer in male *BRCA1* carriers is less than for *BRCA2*, it is not inconsiderable. The frequency of the *BRCA1* mutations among Ashkenazi male breast cancer patients in Israel was three to four times the expected rate (88). Brose et al. (55) estimated a 58-fold increase in risk of breast cancer among 483 males carrying *BRCA1* mutations. Finally, although the risk of breast cancer for men with *BRCA1/2* mutations is a fraction of that for women, at least one study has estimated the overall lifetime risk of any cancer for male relatives of *BRCA2* mutation carriers is higher than that for female relatives (77). If true, *BRCA2* testing criteria, currently almost exclusively based on the clinical discovery of breast and ovarian cancer cases, may need to be more inclusive.

MODIFIERS OF PENETRANCE AND BREAST CANCER GENES OTHER THAN *BRCA*

Several studies have noted an increased penetrance for *BRCA1/2* in more recent birth cohorts. The NYBCS (9) confirmed Narod's earlier observation of a significant increase in breast cancer risk by the age of 50 years in birth cohorts after 1940 (67% after 1940, 24% before 1940) (39). Ovarian cancer risk did not differ by birth cohort. This increase in incidence for *BRCA1/2* mutation carriers parallels an increase in breast cancer in the general U.S. population over that period (37). Antoniou et al. (61) analyzed the results of 22 studies in which cases were unselected for family history. The RR for breast cancer among *BRCA1/2* mutation carriers in the post-1960 birth cohorts was two to three times the RR in the preceding four decades. A study of Austrian *BRCA1* mutation–positive women found that those from birth cohorts after 1958 had a significantly higher incidence of breast cancer by 40 years of age than those from earlier birth cohorts: 46% versus 27%, respectively (89). Finally, Tryggvadottir et al. (90) quantified the increase in breast cancer risk in the Icelandic population between 1921 and 2002. During this period in Iceland, the overall cumulative incidence of breast cancer by the age of 70 years increased from 2.3% to 7.4%. Among carriers of a common Icelandic *BRCA2* mutation, the increase over the same period was from 17.9% to 65.5%, roughly the equivalent multiple.

Environmental factors and reproductive lifestyle changes have certainly contributed to the gradual, long-term increase in cumulative incidence of breast cancer, but more recent age-related changes in diagnostic screening have led to more abrupt increases in detection of breast cancer. For example, after the implementation of a nationwide breast-screening program in the United Kingdom, breast cancer incidence between 50 to 64 years of age increased by ~25% in the half decade from 1987 to 1992 (78).

Disaggregating the relative effects of screening and etiologic events is a daunting endeavor. Because the baseline incidence of breast cancer is higher for mutation carriers, small changes in either of these factors may have large multiplier effects on penetrance estimates for mutation carriers. This may account for some of the variance in penetrance estimates seen in both population-based and case-based studies. Figure 2, showing the penetrance estimates for *BRCA1/2* mutation carriers, illustrates just how widely varied these estimates are. For example, some studies have estimated a higher cumulative risk for *BRCA2* mutation carriers compared to *BRCA1* mutation carriers (59,91), while others have estimated the opposite (61). In addition to the sources of analytic and ascertainment biases mentioned earlier in this chapter, the differences in penetrance found in the specific populations in these studies may have resulted from population-specific mutations.

The incidence of breast cancer varies significantly by geographical location. Although these differences may be diminishing over time, those who live in developed countries currently have up to five times the RR of those who live in developing nations (92,93). Neither susceptibility genes, such as *BRCA1/2*, nor familial clustering can account for this degree of geographical variability. Furthermore, studies of migrants who have moved from low- to high-incidence areas have shown that within one decade, their breast cancer rates approached the local rates, and within one to two generations, their offspring adopted local breast cancer incidence rates (94–96). Thus, it is clear that one's environment, and sociocultural influences, are significant contributors to overall breast cancer incidence along with genetic variation.

The combined frequency of *BRCA1/2* mutations is relatively low in most populations, from 0.1% to 0.4 % (91,97). Do other known heritable causes account for the residual risk of familial breast cancer? To date, as covered in other chapters of this volume, major genes associated with breast cancer susceptibility include *MSH2/MLH1* (Muir–Torre syndrome), *TP53* (Li–Fraumeni syndrome), *PTEN* (Cowden syndrome), *STK11* (Peutz–Jeghers syndrome), and the low-penetrance mutations of *CHEK2*. However, these gene mutations are all relatively rare and cannot explain the residual risk of familial breast cancer beyond that attributable to *BRCA1/2*. Despite intensive investigation, other major breast cancer genes are yet to be identified, and it is believed that a number of low-penetrance genes with high population frequencies represent the majority of the residual familial risk (98). Whether these other putative genes modify the effects of *BRCA1/2* or represent independent etiologies is a matter of ongoing research (Chapter 8). However, their impact on penetrance is relevant to this discussion. As established earlier in this discussion, when penetrance estimates for *BRCA1/2* are derived from case probands, particularly if those probands are members of high-risk families, all breast and ovarian cancer risk factors, including putative genetic modifiers, will likely be over-represented in these individuals. Penetrance estimates based on the assumption that the susceptibility gene under investigation, e.g., *BRCA1*, is the sole cause of the disease may incur significant error, and the bias in these estimates is a direct function of all other risk factors present in mutation carriers (1).

TYPES OF CANCER ASSOCIATED WITH *BRCA1/2* MUTATIONS

Ovarian Cancer

The most significant cancer, other than breast cancer, in individuals with *BRCA1/2* mutations is ovarian cancer, as reflected in the nomenclature, hereditary breast ovarian cancer (HBOC) syndrome. As with breast cancer, early linkage studies probably overestimated the penetrance of ovarian cancer for *BRCA1/2* mutation carriers with estimates by the age of 70 years of 44% for *BRCA1* carriers (51) and 27% for *BRCA2* carriers (97). In contrast, later studies, utilizing nonlinkage-based ascertainments, derived lower penetrances. Struewing et al. (28) estimated the penetrance for ovarian cancer in those who harbored one of the three Ashkenazi Jewish *BRCA1/2* founder mutations to be

16% by the age of 70 years. The Anglian Breast Cancer Study Group (59) estimated the combined penetrance of *BRCA1/2* for ovarian cancer by the age of 80 years at 22%. In 2002, Antoniou et al. (91) estimated the penetrance of *BRCA1* for ovarian cancer by the age of 70 years to be 25.9% and the corresponding estimate for *BRCA2* was 9.1%. A meta-analysis of 22 studies with a total of over 8000 index cases of breast and/or ovarian cancer patients unselected for family history, 500 of whom carried *BRCA1/2* mutations, was performed by Antoniou et al. (61). The average cumulative risk of ovarian cancer by the age of 70 years for *BRCA1* was 39% and for *BRCA2* was 11%. The corresponding figures were higher in families with early-onset index cases: 51% for *BRCA1*; 32% for *BRCA2*. In this analysis, for *BRCA1*, the ovarian cancer risk was highest when a breast cancer index case was <35 years of age. For *BRCA2*, the cumulative risks were higher when based on ovarian cancer index cases. In an Italian study by Marroni et al. (56), ovarian cancer penetrances were 43% at the age of 70 years in *BRCA1* carriers and 15% at the age of 70 years in *BRCA2* carriers. A paper by Chen et al. (38) estimated the cumulative ovarian cancer risk at the age of 70 years to be 39% in *BRCA1* carriers and 22% in *BRCA2* carriers. The study by Chen et al. included 676 Ashkenazi kindreds and 1272 non-Ashkenazi kindreds with greater than three diagnoses of breast or ovarian cancer in each family. Thus, as was the case for estimates of breast cancer penetrance when broken down by *BRCA1* versus *BRCA2* subtypes, ovarian cancer penetrance estimates are generally higher in *BRCA1* mutation carriers, ranging from 16% to 44%, compared to 9.1% to 27% for *BRCA2* mutation carriers.

Fallopian tube (FT) cancers are generally grouped with ovarian cancer because of the clinico–pathologic similarities of the two. Somatic loss of wild-type *BRCA* alleles in FT tumor tissue supports a link to HBOC (99). The BCLC (36) estimated a 500-fold excess of FT cancer among known and suspected *BRCA2* mutation carriers when compared with the general population rate calculated from the East Anglian Cancer Registry in England. A number of studies have found associations between FT cancer and *BRCA1* (100,101); a systematic study of the frequency of *BRCA* mutations in 44 unselected FT index cases from the Ontario Cancer Registry in Canada revealed five with a *BRCA1* mutation (11.4%) and two with a *BRCA2* mutation (4.5%) (102). The authors also found a roughly twofold excess risk of ovarian and breast cancers among first-degree relatives of mutation carriers. A subsequent study of 381 *BRCA1* mutation–positive women calculated a 120-fold excess risk of FT cancers in this group compared to the estimated general population risk (55). Levine et al. (103) examined all Ashkenazi cases of both FT cancer and primary peritoneal cancer at two New York City medical centers during the period 1981–2001. Of 29 FT cancer cases thus ascertained, five (17%) had mutations; all five had *BRCA1* mutations and one patient had an additional *BRCA2* mutation. The estimated RR of FT cancer for *BRCA* mutation carriers was 11.3.

Cancers Other Than Breast and Ovarian Cancer

Table 1 groups studies, by type, that have examined the association of cancers other than breast and ovarian/FT cancers with *BRCA1/2* mutations, or in families with breast and/or ovarian cancer. Inclusion in the table was restricted to claims of statistically significant findings.

Colorectal Cancer

Early linkage studies and family-based studies in which there was no genotyping of colorectal cancer cases observed significant associations between *BRCA1/2* mutations

Table 1 Genotype/Phenotype Correlation Studies. Listed by Type (see text). Associating *BRCA1/2* Mutations with Cancer Risks

Studies (by type)	Gene type	Actual or actual/ potential carriers	No. of families	Colon/ rectal	Stomach	Kidney/ bladder	Pancreas	Liver	Gall bladder bile duct	Uterine	Pertonium	Fallopian tube	Cervix	Prostate	Lymphoma	Squamous cell skin	Leukemia	Melanoma	Other cancers combined
Linkage																			
	BRCA1																		
Ford, 1994 (51)		464	33	4.1	NS	NS	NS	NS	NS	NS			NS	3.3	NS		NS	NS	4.2
	BRCA2																		
The Breast Cancer Linkage Consortium, 1999 (36)		3728	173	NS	2.6	NS	3.5	4.2	5.0	NS			NS	4.6	NS		NS	2.6	2.5
Inferred genotype																			
	BRCA1																		
Johannsson, 1999 (104)		29/596 ♀		4.1R	5.2	X	NS		X					X		NS	X		5.3
Johannsson, 1999 (104)		29/549 ♂		NS	NS	NS	NS		NS					NS		6.0	NS		NS
Risch, 2001 (77)		291 CR/ 4,378 n		NS	6.2	NS	NS			NS				NS			2.6		♂NS/♀3.6
	BRCA2																		
Sigurdsson, 1997 (105)		53 ♂	16											4.6					
Johannsson, 1999 (104)		20/383 ♂	20	NS	NS	NS								2.4	NS		NS	NS	2.0
Risch, 2001 (77)		160 CR/ 4,378 n		2.5	NS	NS	NS			NS				NS			NS		♂1.7/♀NS
	BRCA1/2																		
Moslehi, 2000 (29)		1,222 CR/ 2,213 n		NS	NS		3.1			NS				3.5				NS	♂1.6/♀1.9

Genotyped proband																
Brose, 2002 (55)	*BRCA1*	381♀/102♂	147								120					NS
Thompson, 2002 (106)		2245	699	2.0	6.9	NS	2.8	4.1	2.6		3.7	NS	NS	NS	NS	NS
Struewing, 1997 (28)	*BRCA1/2*	120/5218 AJ	NS	2.0	NS	NS	2.3	NS	NS			4.2	NS	NS	NS	NS
Association	*BRCA1*															
Kirchhoff, 2004B (107)		6/586 AJ										NS				
Edwards, 2003 (108)	*BRCA2*	5/263										23.0				
Ozcelik, 1997 (109)		4/39 AJ					8.3									
Kirchhoff, 2004A (112)		8/251 AJ										4.8				
Hubert, 1999 (110)	*BRCA1/2*	3/87										NS				
Vazina, 2000 (111)		5/174										NS				
Levine, 2003 (103)		AJ 22 PPC/ 29 FT	NS							37.7	11.3					
Kirchhoff, 2004A (112)		6/586 AJ														♂NS/♀2.3

Note: Inclusion in the table was restricted to studies showing statistically significant findings, or significant null results.

Abbreviations: AJ, Ashkenazi Jews; BC, breast cancer; CR, carriers' relatives; FT, fallopian tube; n, noncarriers' relatives; NS, not significant; PPC, primary peritoneal carcinoma; R, rectal only; X, not reported.

and colorectal cancers. Using linkage kindreds, Ford et al. (51) estimated the RR for colon cancer in *BRCA1* carriers as 4.1. Johannsson et al. (104) used the Swedish Cancer Registry to derive an RR based on cancer in family members of mutation carriers (29 *BRCA1* index cases and 20 *BRCA2* index cases). Among female relatives of *BRCA1* mutation carriers, they estimated the RR of colon cancer to be 4.1, but there was no excess risk found among male relatives. Based on kindreds derived from 649 unselected ovarian cancer index cases, Risch et al. (77) observed an elevated risk of colon cancer for *BRCA2* mutation carriers with an RR of 2.5; no significant increase in risk was found for *BRCA1* mutation carriers. Studies by Brose et al. (55), with subjects drawn from risk evaluation clinics, and by Thompson and Easton (106), with participants drawn from 699 kindreds across 30 centers in Western Europe and North America, both estimated a twofold RR for colon cancer among carriers of *BRCA1* mutations. These family-based studies were "indirect" in that genotyping was not performed on colon cancer cases themselves, and histologic confirmation of reported family history information was also generally not provided. This leaves open the possibility for reporting bias in cases compared to controls. Chen-Shtoyerman et al. (113), in a study of 225 unselected Ashkenazi Jewish colorectal cancer patients, found the frequency of *BRCA1/2* founder mutations in this group to be close to the average for the general Ashkenazi population, suggesting no increase in the risk of colorectal cancer to mutation carriers. Kirchhoff et al. (112) found no increased RR for colon cancer in *BRCA1/2* mutation carriers, based on the frequency of the founder mutations in 586 Ashkenazi colon cancer patients unselected for family history, with an unaffected Ashkenazi control group of 5012 individuals. Similarly, Niell et al. (114) found no association between *BRCA* mutations and colorectal cancer in 1002 case patients compared to 1038 control subjects. These later studies suggest that if there is a risk for colorectal neoplasia in *BRCA* mutation carriers, it is very modest at best.

Stomach (Gastric) Cancer

A study by Brose et al. (55) estimated a significantly increased risk of gastric cancer among *BRCA1* mutation carriers (RR = 6.9), although no increase was noted in the Thompson and Easton Study (106). Risch et al. (77) derived a similar RR of stomach cancer for *BRCA1* mutation–positive individuals, but a nonsignificant risk for *BRCA2* mutation carriers. Johannsson et al. (104) stratified their study by gender, as well as by gene mutation, and found a significantly elevated risk of stomach cancer in female *BRCA1* carriers (RR = 5.2) but not in male carriers. They noted that classification of some of the stomach cancers may have been erroneous. The BCLC study (36) estimated an RR of stomach cancer of 2.6 based on a comparison of the observed incidence in the cohort with SEER and International Agency for Research on Cancer (IARC) data. Histologic confirmation of history of cancer was attempted only in probands and first-degree relatives, and was successful in only 48% of such cases. Because direct genotyping association studies of gastric cancer in Ashkenazi Jews have not yet been performed to confirm this association, and because the unconfirmed diagnosis of gastric and ovarian cancers may be confounding variables, the association of *BRCA* mutations and gastric cancer remains speculative.

Pancreatic Cancer

Several studies have claimed an increased risk of pancreatic cancer largely with *BRCA2* mutation carriers; indeed *BRCA2* somatic mutations were first identified in a pancreatic tumor (16). Thompson and Easton observed an elevated risk of pancreatic cancer, RR = 2.3, in *BRCA1* mutation carriers (106), a finding that was confirmed in a smaller, highly selected series (55), but in only one of two larger, unselected series of *BRCA*-mutated ovarian cancer probands (29,77). The BCLC study (36) also found a significant excess risk of pancreatic cancer in *BRCA2* mutation carriers in the study group and estimated the RR of pancreatic cancer to be 3.5. A study by Hahn et al. (115) included 26 European, non-Ashkenazi families with two or more histologically confirmed cases of pancreatic cancer and found 12% of these families to be positive for *BRCA2* mutations. Murphy et al. (116) ascertained 29 U.S. kindreds with three or more cases of pancreatic cancer where two were first-degree relatives. Five families (17%) were found to harbor *BRCA2* mutations. A higher than expected number of Ashkenazi individuals with pancreatic cancer harbored *BRCA2* mutations in a large association study (109); and two previous studies noted that a family history of pancreatic cancer was a predictor of an increased frequency of *BRCA2* mutations (117,118). Finally, a study by Lal et al. (119) ascertained 102 subjects from among newly diagnosed, histologically verified pancreatic cancer patients. Of these individuals, 14 were Ashkenazi, three of whom had a *BRCA2* and one had a *BRCA1* mutation. Thus, while the risk of pancreatic cancer is clearly associated with *BRCA2* mutations, its association with *BRCA1* mutations is still under study.

Prostate Cancer

Early linkage studies suggested an RR of prostate cancer of 3.3 among the 33 multiplex kindreds studied (51). When broken down by *BRCA1* versus *BRCA2*, the linkage consortium found no increased risk in *BRCA1*-linked kindreds (106), but in *BRCA2* mutation carriers, a statistically significant increase in the risk for prostate cancer was noted (RR = 4.6) (36). The RR was higher for prostate cancer before the age of 65 years (RR = 7.3). Sigurdsson et al. (105) ascertained 53 mutation-positive first-degree male relatives of breast cancer probands in known Icelandic *BRCA2* kindreds. Among these men, the estimated RR of prostate cancer was 4.6. Among mutation-positive second-degree male relatives, the corresponding RR was 2.5. The 383 men in another study by Johannsson et al. (104) were all from known Icelandic *BRCA2*-linked kindreds and had been diagnosed with cancer. Standardized morbidity rates estimated for prostate cancer were 2.4 after male breast cancer index cases were excluded. Struewing et al. (28) compared prostate cancer incidence among first-degree relatives of carriers versus noncarriers of *BRCA1/2* Ashkenazi founder mutations. The RR of prostate cancer for relatives of carriers was 4.2. However, Risch et al. (77) found no significant differences in RR for prostate cancer in *BRCA1* or *BRCA2* carriers compared to noncarriers, a finding similar to that of Moslehi et al. (29). Association studies have not been in agreement about the excess risk of prostate cancer attributable to *BRCA1/2*. Hubert et al. (110) found no excess frequency of *BRCA1/2* mutations among 83 Ashkenazi with prostate cancer, unselected for family history or age; however, Kirchhoff et al. (107) noted an increased risk of prostate cancer in a larger number of cases studied. The risk was not associated with an earlier age at onset, and was seen only in Ashkenazi *BRCA2* but not *BRCA1* mutation carriers. Thus, prostate cancer risk is increased in *BRCA2* mutation carriers, but because of the absence of earlier onset, preventive health implications are modest.

Uterine Cancer

Recent large studies have not shown an increased risk of uterine cancer in women with *BRCA* mutations who do not take tamoxifen (120). However, a rare subtype of uterine serous papillary cancer (USPC), resembling serous papillary carcinoma of the ovary or the peritoneum, may be associated with *BRCA* mutations. USPC is more aggressive than endometrial uterine cancer, is generally diagnosed in late stages, usually has a poor prognosis, and responds to treatment modalities employed in ovarian cancer (121). A study by Biron-Shental et al. (122) found that 6 of 22 patients (27%) with USPC had *BRCA1* or *BRCA2* mutations; four of the six had prior histories of breast or ovarian cancer. The authors of these three studies have suggested, based on these data, that USPC may be part of the spectrum of HBOC syndrome.

No increase in uterine cancers was noted in the linkage consortium analysis of *BRCA2* mutation–carrying kindreds (36). Moslehi et al. (29) estimated that for first-degree relatives of ovarian cancer cases with *BRCA* mutations, the RR for uterine cancer was 6.5 at the age of 75 years; however, this was based only on four cases of reported cancer in relatives of *BRCA1* mutation carriers. Risch et al. (77), based on a population-based series of 649 ovarian cancer cases, estimated the RR of uterine cancer to first-degree relatives of carriers to be not significantly elevated when compared to the relatives of noncarriers. Thompson and Easton (106) in a study of 699 kindreds and 2245 *BRCA1* mutation carriers, estimated the RR of uterine cancer to carriers of *BRCA1* mutations to be 2.65. However, in this study, as well as the previous studies, the *BRCA* genotype was inferred in relatives and/or the reported family histories of uterine cancers were not confirmed. Indeed, Thompson et al. indicate that some of the reported cases of uterine cancer may have been ovarian cancers. In a consecutive series of 199 Ashkenazi patients with endometrial carcinoma tested for the presence of *BRCA1/2* mutations, only three (1.5%) were found to have *BRCA1/2* mutations, which is below the ~2.5% frequency in the Ashkenazi population at large (123). None of these were of serous papillary subtype. The issue of uterine cancer risk in *BRCA* mutation carriers takes on significance because of the question regarding whether hysterectomy (removal of the uterus) as well as oophorectomy (removal of ovaries and FTs) represents the optimal risk-reducing surgical intervention in *BRCA* mutation carriers. Since large series have thus far not demonstrated an increased risk for uterine cancer in *BRCA* mutation carriers (120), oophorectomy and removal of the FTs remains an acceptable option to hysterectomy and oophorectomy. A separate issue in this clinical decision relates to possible risks associated with residual FT-derived tissue. Such foci, along with the larger amount of peritoneal tissue, remain potential sources for hereditary gynecologic malignancies in patients following risk-reducing surgeries.

Malignant Melanoma

An increased risk of cutaneous malignant melanoma associated with having an affected family member was quantified (OR = 2.69) in a study by Holman and Armstrong (124). It has been estimated that 8% to 12% of cases are attributable to inherited factors (11). There is a known association of malignant melanoma with a mutation in *CDKN2* on chromosome 9 that codes for p16, another important regulator of the cell division cycle (125). Several studies have demonstrated an association of *BRCA* mutations and malignant melanoma. In 3728 individuals in 173 breast–ovarian cancer families with *BRCA2* mutations, the BCLC (36) estimated a statistically significant RR for malignant melanoma of 2.58. However, a study by van Asperen et al. (126) noted no significant excess risk of malignant melanoma associated with *BRCA* mutations in first-degree relatives of mutation carriers in 139 *BRCA2* families; and Johannesdottir et al. (33) concluded that *BRCA2* accounts for a significant fraction of breast and ovarian cancer, but only a small proportion of other cancers, including malignant melanoma.

Risk of Contralateral Breast Cancer

The 10-year risks of contralateral breast cancer following the diagnosis of breast cancer in women who did not have an oophorectomy or take tamoxifen were 43.4% for *BRCA1* carriers and 34.6% for *BRCA2* carriers, confirming the estimates made from linkage studies (127). This risk can be reduced substantially by hormonal chemoprevention and/ or oophorectomy. Indeed, the widespread clinical acceptance of these procedures will impact on future prospective estimates of contralateral breast cancer risk in *BRCA* mutation carriers.

CONCLUSIONS

Although the major risks associated with inherited mutations of *BRCA1* and *BRCA2* are now well described, there remains debate about the precise magnitude and spectrum of risks due to syndromic cancers. The ranges of risks reported to date may reflect the inherent biases in the ascertainment methodologies employed, and more recent studies may provide more stable estimates of these risks (128). In addition, environmental and other genetic modifying factors impact on kindreds, segregating *BRCA* mutations. These modifying genetic factors include those intrinsic to the mutation itself, i.e., mutation-specific genotype–phenotype correlations, as well as extrinsic modifiers, which are still under study. Although the unraveling of this myriad of genetic and epigenetic modifiers will pose a daunting challenge in the laboratory, the translation of this information in the clinic can be facilitated by adopting a relatively simple framework. In counseling individuals with *BRCA* mutations, the range of penetrance estimates need not pose a barrier to responsible clinical intervention. For ovarian cancer risk, even assuming the lowest penetrance figures published to date, with risks on the order of one in five (28), this must be compared to the "baseline" risk of "sporadic" ovarian cancer of one in 70. This gradient is more than enough to justify risk-reducing interventions, including oophorectomy after childbearing in the absence of a reliable means for screening or chemoprevention (79). In the case of breast cancer, risks on the order of 50% to 80% have not been high enough to justify preventive surgery for most women in North America (129); the availability of magnetic resonance imaging and emerging new screening methodologies provides a reasonable first approach to high-risk screening for many women (130), with risk-reducing surgery a more acceptable option for others. For individuals who desire more precise penetrance estimates, "kinship-specific" penetrance can further refine the estimate based on data from his or her kinship, e.g. the age of onset of mutation-positive relatives. For the individual with a single instance of breast cancer in the absence of a family history, risks derived from population-based studies can be cited, taking into account the potential biases of these methodologies (2,5). For an individual in multiplex kindred, risks more in line with linkage-derived data can be provided (4). Importantly, for cancer risks other than breast and ovarian, it is prudent to rely on studies in which the pathology of tumor types has been confirmed and direct genotyping performed.

Ultimately, the concept of penetrance is of molecular genetic as well as clinical significance in breast cancer clinical risk management. Important insights will emerge from the further study of genetic epidemiologic risk factors associated with the penetrance of inherited *BRCA* mutations. The eventual elucidation of genetic and environmental "protective factors" and "risk modifiers" in unaffected elderly individuals with *BRCA* mutations may prove as useful and important biologically as the discovery of the *BRCA* genes themselves.

ACKNOWLEDGMENTS

This work was partially supported through the Lomangino family genetics fund and the Truettner family research fund.

REFERENCES

1. Begg CB. On the use of familial aggregation in population-based case probands for calculating penetrance. J Natl Cancer Inst 2002; 94(6):1221–1226.
2. Amos CR. On the use of familial aggregation in population based case probands for calculating penetrance. J Natl Cancer Inst 2003; 95:74–75.
3. Risch H, Narod S. On the use of familial aggregation in population based case probands for calculating penetrance. J Natl Cancer Inst 2003; 95(1):73–74.
4. Pharoah PP, Antoniou A, Hopper J, et al. On the use of familial aggregation in population based case probands for calculating penetrance. J Natl Cancer Inst 2003; 95(1):75–76.
5. Whittemore AS, Gong G. On the use of familial aggregation in population based case probands for calculating penetrance. J Natl Cancer Inst 2003; 95(1):76–77.
6. Burke W, Austin MA. On the use of familial aggregation in population based case probands for calculating penetrance. J Natl Cancer Inst 2003; 95(1):78–79.
7. Easton DF, Hopper JL, Thomas DC, et al. Breast cancer risks for *BRCA1/2* carriers. Science 2004; 306:2187–2191; author reply 2187–2191.
8. Wacholder S, Struewing JP, Hartge P, et al. Breast cancer risks for *BRCA1/2* carriers. Science 2004; 306:2187–2191; author reply 2187–2191.
9. King MC, Marks JH, Mandell JB. Breast and ovarian cancer risks due to inherited mutations in *BRCA1* and *BRCA2*. Science 2003; 302(5645):643–646. author reply 2004; 306: 2187–2191.
10. Offit K. Clinical cancer genetics: risk counseling and management. New York: Wiley-Liss, 1998.
11. Offit K, Brown K. Quantitating familial cancer risk: a resource for clinical oncologists. J Clin Oncol 1994; 12(8):1724–1736.
12. Offit K, Kauff N. Reducing the risk of gynecologic cancer in the Lynch syndrome. N Engl J Med 2006; 354(3):293–295.
13. Hall JM, Lee MK, Newman B, et al. Linkage of early-onset familial breast cancer to chromosome 17q21. Science 1990; 250(4988):1684–1689.
14. Miki Y, Swensen J, Shattuck-Eidens D, et al. A strong candidate for the breast and ovarian cancer susceptibility gene *BRCA1*. Science 1994; 266(5182):66–71.
15. Wooster R, Neuhausen SL, Mangion J, et al. Localization of a breast cancer susceptibility gene, *BRCA2*, to chromosome 13q12-13. Science 1994; 265(5181):2088–2090.
16. Wooster R, Bignell G, Lancaster J, et al. Identification of the breast cancer susceptibility gene *BRCA2*. Nature 1995; 378(6559):789–792.
17. Claus EB, Risch N, Thompson WD. Genetic analysis of breast cancer in the cancer and steroid hormone study. Am J Hum Genet 1991; 48(2):232–242.
18. Easton DF, Bishop DT, Ford D, et al. Genetic linkage analysis in familial breast and ovarian cancer: results from 214 families. The Breast Cancer Linkage Consortium. Am J Hum Genet 1993; 52(4):678–701.
19. King MC, Rowell S, Love SM. Inherited breast and ovarian cancer. What are the risks? What are the choices? JAMA 1993; 269(15):1975–1980.
20. Claus EB, Risch N, Thompson WD. Autosomal dominant inheritance of early-onset breast cancer. Implications for risk prediction. Cancer 1994; 73(3):643–651.
21. Goldgar DE, Fields P, Lewis CM, et al. A large kindred with 17q-linked breast and ovarian cancer: genetic, phenotypic, and genealogical analysis. J Natl Cancer Inst 1994; 86(3): 200–209.

22. Porter DE, Cohen BB, Wallace MR, et al. Breast cancer incidence, penetrance and survival in probable carriers of *BRCA1* gene mutation in families linked to *BRCA1* on chromosome 17q12-21. Br J Surg 1994; 81(10):1512–1515.

23. Easton DF, Ford D, Bishop DT. Breast and ovarian cancer incidence in *BRCA1*-mutation carriers Breast Cancer Linkage Consortium. Am J Hum Genet 1995; 56(1):265–271.

24. Rebbeck TR, Couch FJ, Kant J, et al. Genetic heterogeneity in hereditary breast cancer: role of *BRCA1* and *BRCA2*. Am J Hum Genet 1996; 59(3):547–553.

25. Schuyer M, Berns EM. Is TP53 dysfunction required for *BRCA1*-associated carcinogenesis? Mol Cell Endocrinol 1999; 155(1–2):143–152.

26. Shattuck-Eidens D, McClure M, Simard J, et al. A collaborative survey of 80 mutations in the *BRCA1* breast and ovarian cancer susceptibility gene. Implications for presymptomatic testing and screening. JAMA 1995; 273(7):535–541.

27. Gayther SA, Warren W, Mazoyer S, et al. Germline mutations of the *BRCA1* gene in breast and ovarian cancer families provide evidence for a genotype-phenotype correlation. Nat Genet 1995; 11(4):428–433.

28. Struewing JP, Hartge P, Wacholder S, et al. The risk of cancer associated with specific mutations of *BRCA1* and *BRCA2* among Ashkenazi Jews. N Engl J Med 1997; 336(20): 1401–1408.

29. Moslehi R, Chu W, Karlan B, et al. *BRCA1* and *BRCA2* mutation analysis of 208 Ashkenazi Jewish women with ovarian cancer. Am J Hum Genet 2000; 66(4):1259–1272.

30. Satagopan JM, Offit K, Foulkes W, et al. The lifetime risks of breast cancer in Ashkenazi Jewish carriers of *BRCA1* and *BRCA2* mutations. Cancer Epidemiol Biomarkers Prev 2001; 10(5):467–473.

31. Gayther SA, Mangion J, Russell P, et al. Variation of risks of breast and ovarian cancer associated with different germline mutations of the *BRCA2* gene. Nat Genet 1997; 15(1): 103–105.

32. Warner E, Foulkes W, Goodwin P, et al. Prevalence and penetrance of *BRCA1* and *BRCA2* gene mutations in unselected Ashkenazi Jewish women with breast cancer. J Natl Cancer Inst 1999; 91(14):1241–1247.

33. Johannesdottir G, Gudmundsson J, Bergthorsson JT, et al. High prevalence of the 999del5 mutation in Icelandic breast and ovarian cancer patients. Cancer Res 1996; 56(16): 3663–3665.

34. Thompson D, Easton D. Variation in cancer risks, by mutation position, in *BRCA2* mutation carriers. Am J Hum Genet 2001; 68(2):410–419.

35. Cancer risks in *BRCA2* mutation carriers. The Breast Cancer Linkage Consortium. J Natl Cancer Inst 1999; 91:1310–1316.

36. National Cancer Institute: Surveillance, Epidemiology and End Results (SEER) Program. http://seer.cancer.gov/cgi-bin/csr/1975_2003/search.pl#results (accessed May 2006).

37. Chen S, Iversen ES, Friebel T, et al. Characterization of *BRCA1* and *BRCA2* mutations in a large United States sample. J Clin Oncol 2006; 24(6):863–871.

38. Narod SA, Goldgar D, Cannon-Albright L, et al. Risk modifiers in carriers of *BRCA1* mutations. Int J Cancer 1995; 64(6):394–398.

39. Chang-Claude J, Becher H, Eby N, et al. Modifying effect of reproductive risk factors on the age at onset of breast cancer for German *BRCA1* mutation carriers. J Cancer Res Clin Oncol 1997; 123(5):272–279.

40. Jernstrom H, Lerman C, Ghadirian P, et al. Pregnancy and risk of early breast cancer in carriers of *BRCA1* and *BRCA2*. Lancet 1999; 354(9193):1846–1850.

41. Rebbeck TR, Kantoff PW, Krithivas K, et al. Modification of *BRCA1*-associated breast cancer risk by the polymorphic androgen-receptor CAG repeat. Am J Hum Genet 1999; 64(5):1371–1377.

42. Hartge P, Chatterjee N, Wacholder S, et al. Breast cancer risk in Ashkenazi *BRCA1/2* mutation carriers: effects of reproductive history. Epidemiology 2002; 13(3):255–261.

43. Narod SA. Modifiers of risk of hereditary breast and ovarian cancer. Nat Rev Cancer 2002; 2(2):113–123.

44. Thorlacius S, Sigurdsson S, Bjarnadottir, et al. Study of a single *BRCA2* mutation with high carrier frequency in a small population. Am J Hum Genet 1997; 60(5):1079–1084.

45. Gorski B, Jakubowska A, Huzarski T, et al. A high proportion of founder *BRCA1* mutations in Polish breast cancer families. Int J Cancer 2004; 110(5):683–686.

46. Pal T, Permuth-Wey J, Holtje T, et al. *BRCA1* and *BRCA2* mutations in a study of African American breast cancer patients. Cancer Epidemiol Biomarkers Prev 2004; 13(11): 1794–1799.

47. Weitzel JN, Lagos V, Blazer KR, et al. Prevalence of *BRCA* mutations and founder effect in high-risk Hispanic families. Cancer Epidemiol Biomarkers Prev 2005; 14(7):1666–1671.

48. Scott CL, Jenkins MA, Southey MC, et al. Average age-specific cumulative risk of breast cancer according to type and site of germline mutations in *BRCA1* and *BRCA2* estimated from multiple-case breast cancer families attending Australian family cancer clinics. Hum Genet 2003; 112(5–6):542–551.

49. Walsh T, Casadei S, Coats KH, et al. Spectrum of mutations in *BRCA1*, *BRCA2*, CHEK2, and TP53 in families at high risk of breast cancer. JAMA 2006; 295(12):1379–1388.

50. Petrij-Bosch A, Peelen T, van Vliet M, et al. *BRCA1* genomic deletions are major founder mutations in Dutch breast cancer patients. Nat Genet 1997; 17(3):341–345.

51. Ford D, Easton DF, Bishop DT, et al. Risks of cancer in *BRCA1*-mutation carriers. Breast Cancer Linkage Consortium. Lancet 1994; 343(8899):692–695.

52. Easton DF, Steele L, Fields P, et al. Cancer risks in two large breast cancer families linked to *BRCA2* on chromosome 13q12-13. Am J Hum Genet 1997; 61(1):120–128.

53. Wacholder S, Hartge P, Struewing JP, et al. The kin-cohort study for estimating penetrance. Am J Epidemiol 1998; 148(7):623–630.

54. Hopper JL, Bishop DT, Easton DF. Population-based family studies in genetic epidemiology. Lancet 2005; 366(9494):1397–1406.

55. Brose MS, Rebbeck TR, Calzone KA, et al. Cancer risk estimates for *BRCA1* mutation carriers identified in a risk evaluation program. J Natl Cancer Inst 2002; 94(18):1365–1372.

56. Marroni F, Aretini P, D'Andrea E, et al. Penetrances of breast and ovarian cancer in a large series of families tested for *BRCA1/2* mutations. Eur J Hum Genet 2004; 12(11):899–906.

57. Whittemore AS, Gong G, Itnyre J. Prevalence and contribution of *BRCA1* mutations in breast cancer and ovarian cancer: results from three U.S. population-based case-control studies of ovarian cancer. Am J Hum Genet 1997; 60(3):496–504.

58. Bonadona V, Sinilnikova OM, Chopin S, et al. Contribution of *BRCA1* and *BRCA2* germ-line mutations to the incidence of breast cancer in young women: results from a prospective population-based study in France. Genes Chromosomes Cancer 2005; 43(4):404–413.

59. Prevalence and penetrance of *BRCA1* and *BRCA2* mutations in a population-based series of breast cancer cases. Anglian Breast Cancer Study Group. Br J Cancer 2000; 83:1301–1308.

60. Lalloo F, Varley J, Ellis D, et al. Prediction of pathogenic mutations in patients with early-onset breast cancer by family history. Lancet 2003; 361(9363):1101–1102.

61. Antoniou A, Pharoah PD, Narod S, et al. Average risks of breast and ovarian cancer associated with *BRCA1* or *BRCA2* mutations detected in case Series unselected for family history: a combined analysis of 22 studies. Am J Hum Genet 2003; 72(5):1117–1130.

62. Hopper JL, Southey MC, Dite GS, et al. Population-based estimate of the average age-specific cumulative risk of breast cancer for a defined set of protein-truncating mutations in *BRCA1* and *BRCA2*. Australian Breast Cancer Family Study. Cancer Epidemiol Biomarkers Prev 1999; 8(9):741–747.

63. Thorlacius S, Struewing JP, Hartge P, et al. Population-based study of risk of breast cancer in carriers of *BRCA2* mutation. Lancet 1998; 352(9137):1337–1339.

64. Struewing JP, Hartge P, Wacholder S, et al. The risk of cancer associated with specific mutations of BRCA1 and BRCA2 among Ashkenazi Jews. N Engl J Med 1997; 336(20): 1401–1408.

65. Tesoriero A, Andersen C, Southey M, et al. De novo *BRCA1* mutation in a patient with breast cancer and an inherited *BRCA2* mutation. Am J Hum Genet 1999; 65(2):567–569.

66. Robson M, Scheuer L, Nafa K, et al. Unique de novo mutation of *BRCA2* in a woman with early onset breast cancer. J Med Genet 2002; 39(2):126–128.
67. Struewing JP, Abeliovich D, Peretz T, et al. The carrier frequency of the *BRCA1* 185delAG mutation is approximately 1 percent in Ashkenazi Jewish individuals. Nat Genet 1995; 11(2):198–200.
68. Oddoux C, Struewing JP, Clayton CM, et al. The carrier frequency of the *BRCA2* 6174delT mutation among Ashkenazi Jewish individuals is approximately 1%. Nat Genet 1996; 14(2): 188–190.
69. Roa BB, Boyd AA, Volcik K, et al. Ashkenazi Jewish population frequencies for common mutations in *BRCA1* and *BRCA2*. Nat Genet 1996; 14(2):185–187.
70. Fodor FH, Weston A, Bleiweiss IJ, et al. Frequency and carrier risk associated with common *BRCA1* and *BRCA2* mutations in Ashkenazi Jewish breast cancer patients. Am J Hum Genet 1998; 63(1):45–51.
71. Hartge P, Struewing JP, Wacholder S, et al. The prevalence of common *BRCA1* and *BRCA2* mutations among Ashkenazi Jews. Am J Hum Genet 1999; 64(4):963–970.
72. Gail MH, Pee D, Benichou J, et al. Designing studies to estimate the penetrance of an identified autosomal dominant mutation: cohort, case-control, and genotyped-proband designs. Genet Epidemiol 1999; 16(1):15–39.
73. U.S. Census Bureau. Educational Attainment 2000. http://www.census.gov/prod/2003pubs/c2kbr-24.pdf (accessed May 2006).
74. Braaten T, Weiderpass E, Kumle M, et al. Explaining the socioeconomic variation in cancer risk in the Norwegian Women and Cancer Study. Cancer Epidemiol Biomarkers Prev 2005; 14(1):2591–2597.
75. The National Jewish Population Survey 2000–2001: Strength, Challenge and Diversity in the American Jewish Population. Sept. 2003. http://www.census.gov/prod/cen2000/index.html (accessed May 2006).
76. Antoniou AC, Gayther SA, Stratton JF, et al. Risk models for familial ovarian and breast cancer. Genet Epidemiol 2000; 18(2):173–190.
77. Risch HA, McLaughlin JR, Cole DE, et al. Prevalence and penetrance of germline *BRCA1* and *BRCA2* mutations in a population series of 649 women with ovarian cancer. Am J Hum Genet 2001; 68(3):700–710.
78. Quinn M, Allen E. Changes in incidence of and mortality from breast cancer in England and Wales since introduction of screening. United Kingdom Association of Cancer Registries. BMJ 1995; 311(7017):1391–1395.
79. Meijers-Heijboer H, van Geel B, van Putten WL, et al. Breast cancer after prophylactic bilateral mastectomy in women with a *BRCA1* or *BRCA2* mutation. N Engl J Med 2001; 345(3):159–164.
80. Kauff ND, Satagopan JM, Robson ME, et al. Risk-reducing salpingo-oophorectomy in women with a *BRCA1* or *BRCA2* mutation. N Engl J Med 2002; 346(21):1609–1615.
81. Lane-Claypon JE. A further report on cancer of the breasts, with special reference to its associated antecedent conditions. Report on Public Health and Medical Subjects, no. 32. London, England: Ministry of Health, 1926.
82. Rosenblatt KA, Thomas DB, McTiernan A, et al. Breast cancer in men: aspects of familial aggregation. J Natl Cancer Inst 1991; 83(12):849–854.
83. Amos CI, Struewing JP. Genetic epidemiology of epithelial ovarian cancer. Cancer 1993; 71: 566–572.
84. Narod SA, Ford D, Devilee P, et al. An evaluation of genetic heterogeneity in 145 breast-ovarian cancer families. Breast Cancer Linkage Consortium. Am J Hum Genet 1995; 56(1): 254–264.
85. Couch FJ, Farid LM, DeShano ML, et al. *BRCA2* germline mutations in male breast cancer cases and breast cancer families. Nat Genet 1996; 13(1):123–125.
86. Marroni F, Aretini P, D'Andrea E, et al. Evaluation of widely used models for predicting *BRCA1* and *BRCA2* mutations. J Med Genet 2004; 41(4):278–285.

87. Meindl A. Comprehensive analysis of 989 patients with breast or ovarian cancer provides *BRCA1* and *BRCA2* mutation profiles and frequencies for the German population. Int J Cancer 2002; 97(4):472–480.

88. Struewing JP, Coriaty ZM, Ron E, et al. Founder *BRCA1/2* mutations among male patients with breast cancer in Israel. Am J Hum Genet 1999; 65(6):1800–1802.

89. Kroiss R, Winkler V, Bikas, et al. Younger birth cohort correlates with higher breast and ovarian cancer risk in European *BRCA1* mutation carriers. Hum Mutat 2005; 26(6):583–589.

90. Tryggvadottir L, Sigvaldason H, Olafsdottir GH, et al. Population-based study of changing breast cancer risk in Icelandic *BRCA2* mutation carriers, 1920–2000. J Natl Cancer Inst 2006; 98(2):116–122.

91. Antoniou AC, Pharoah PD, McMullan G, et al. A comprehensive model for familial breast cancer incorporating *BRCA1*, *BRCA2* and other genes. Br J Cancer 2002; 86(1):76–83.

92. McPherson K, Steel CM, Dixon JM. ABC of breast diseases. Breast cancer-epidemiology, risk factors, and genetics. BMJ 2000; 321(7261):624–628.

93. Parkin DM. International variation. Oncogene 2004; 23(38):6329–6340.

94. Ziegler RG, Hoover RN, Pike MC, et al. Migration patterns and breast cancer risk in Asian-American women. J Natl Cancer Inst 1993; 85(22):1819–1827.

95. Tyczynski J, Tarkowski W, Parkin DM, et al. Cancer mortality among Polish migrants to Australia. Eur J Cancer 1994; 30A(4):478–484.

96. Parkin DM, Khlat M. Studies of cancer in migrants: rationale and methodology. Eur J Cancer 1996; 32A(5):761–771.

97. Ford D, Easton DF, Stratton M, et al. Genetic heterogeneity and penetrance analysis of the *BRCA1* and *BRCA2* genes in breast cancer families. The Breast Cancer Linkage Consortium. Am J Hum Genet 1998; 62(3):676–689.

98. Balmain A, Gray J, Ponder B. The genetics and genomics of cancer. Nat Genet 2003; 33:238–244.

99. Zweemer RP, van Diest PJ, Verheijen RH, et al. Molecular evidence linking primary cancer of the fallopian tube to *BRCA1* germline mutations. Gynecol Oncol 2000; 76(1):45–50.

100. Friedman LS, Szabo CI, Ostermeyer EA, et al. Novel inherited mutations and variable expressivity of *BRCA1* alleles, including the founder mutation 185delAG in Ashkenazi Jewish families. Am J Hum Genet 1995; 57(6):1284–1297.

101. Tonin P, Moslehi R, Green R, et al. Linkage analysis of 26 Canadian breast and breast-ovarian cancer families. Hum Genet 1995; 95(5):545–550.

102. Aziz S, Kuperstein G, Rosen B, et al. A genetic epidemiological study of carcinoma of the fallopian tube. Gynecol Oncol 2001; 80(3):341–345.

103. Levine DA, Argenta PA, Yee CJ, et al. Fallopian tube and primary peritoneal carcinomas associated with *BRCA* mutations. J Clin Oncol 2003; 21(22):4222–4227.

104. Johannsson O, Loman N, Moller T, et al. Incidence of malignant tumours in relatives of *BRCA1* and *BRCA2* germline mutation carriers. Eur J Cancer 1999; 35(8):1248–1257.

105. Sigurdsson S, Thorlacius S, Tomasson J, et al. *BRCA2* mutation in Icelandic prostate cancer patients. J Mol Med 1997; 75(10):758–761.

106. Thompson D, Easton DF. Cancer Incidence in *BRCA1* mutation carriers. Breast Cancer Linkage Consortium. J Natl Cancer Inst 2002; 94(18):1358–1365.

107. Kirchhoff T, Kauff ND, Mitra N, et al. *BRCA* mutations and risk of prostate cancer in Ashkenazi Jews. Clin Cancer Res 2004B; 10(9): 2918–2921.

108. Edwards SM, Kote-Jarai Z, Meitz J, et al. Two percent of men with early-onset prostate cancer harbor germline mutations in the *BRCA2* gene. Am J Hum Genet 2003; 72(1):1–12.

109. Ozcelik H, Schmocker B, Di Nicola N, et al. Germline *BRCA2* 6174delT mutations in Ashkenazi Jewish pancreatic cancer patients. Nat Genet 1997; 16(1):17–18.

110. Hubert A, Peretz T, Manor O, et al. The Jewish Ashkenazi founder mutations in the *BRCA1/BRCA2* genes are not found at an increased frequency in Ashkenazi patients with prostate cancer. Am J Hum Genet 1999; 65(3):921–924.

111. Vazina A, Baniel J, Yaacobi Y, et al. The rate of the founder Jewish mutations in *BRCA1* and *BRCA2* in prostate cancer patients in Israel. Br J Cancer 2000; 83(4):463–466.

112. Kirchhoff T, Satagopan JM, Kauff ND, et al. Frequency of *BRCA1* and *BRCA2* mutations in unselected Ashkenazi Jewish patients with colorectal cancer. J Natl Cancer Inst 2004A; 96(1): 2–3.

113. Chen-Shtoyerman R, Figer A, Fidder HH, et al. The frequency of the predominant Jewish mutations in *BRCA1* and BRCA2 in unselected Ashkenazi colorectal cancer patients. Br J Cancer 2001; 84(4):475–477.

114. Niell BL, Rennert G, Bonner JD, et al. *BRCA1* and *BRCA2* founder mutations and the risk of colorectal cancer. J Natl Cancer Inst 2004; 96(1):15–21.

115. Hahn SA, Greenhalf B, Ellis I, et al. *BRCA2* germline mutations in familial pancreatic carcinoma. J Natl Cancer Inst 2003; 95(3):214–221.

116. Murphy KM, Brune KA, Griffin C, et al. Evaluation of candidate genes *MAP2K4*, *MADH4*, *ACVR1B*, and *BRCA2* in familial pancreatic cancer: deleterious *BRCA2* mutations in 17%. Cancer Res 2002; 62(13):3789–3793.

117. Phelan CM, Lancaster JM, Tonin P, et al. Mutation analysis of the *BRCA2* gene in 49 site-specific breast cancer families. Nat Genet 1996; 13(1):120–122.

118. Tonin P, Weber B, Offit K, et al. Frequency of recurrent *BRCA1* and *BRCA2* mutations in Ashkenazi Jewish breast cancer families. Nat Med 1996; 2(11):1179–1183.

119. Lal G, Liu G, Schmocker B, et al. Inherited predisposition to pancreatic adenocarcinoma: role of family history and germ-line p16, *BRCA1*, and *BRCA2* mutations. Cancer Res 2000; 60(2):409–416.

120. Beiner ME, Finch A, Rosen B, et al. Hereditary Ovarian Cancer Clinical Study Group. The risk of endometrial cancer in women with BRCA1 and BRCA2 mutations. A prospective study. Gynecol Oncol 2007; 104(1):7–10.

121. Lavie O, Ben-Arie A, Pilip A, et al. *BRCA2* germline mutation in a woman with uterine serous papillary carcinoma—case report. Gynecol Oncol 2005; 99(2):486–488.

122. Biron-Shental T, Drucker L, Altaras M, et al. High incidence of *BRCA1-2* germline mutations, previous breast cancer and familial cancer history in Jewish patients with uterine serous papillary carcinoma. Eur J Surg Oncol 2006; 32(10):1097–1100.

123. Levine DA, Lin O, Barakat RR, et al. Risk of endometrial carcinoma associated with *BRCA* mutation. Gynecol Oncol 2001; 80(3):395–398.

124. Holman CD, Armstrong BK. Pigmentary traits, ethnic origin, benign nevi, and family history as risk factors for cutaneous malignant melanoma. J Natl Cancer Inst 1984; 72:257–266.

125. Borg A, Sandberg T, Nilsson K, et al. High frequency of multiple melanomas and breast and pancreas carcinomas in *CDKN2A* mutation-positive melanoma families. J Natl Cancer Inst 2000; 92:1260–1266.

126. van Asperen CJ, Brohet RM, Meijers-Heijboer EJ, et al. Cancer risks in *BRCA2* families: estimates for sites other than breast and ovary. J Med Genet 2005; 42:711–719.

127. Metcalfe K, Lynch HT, Ghadirian P, et al. Contralateral breast cancer in BRCA1 and BRCA2 mutation carriers. J Clin Oncol 2004; 22(12):2328–2335.

128. Offit K. *BRCA* mutation frequency and penetrance: new data, old debate. J Natl Cancer Inst 2006; 98:1675–1677.

129. Scheuer L, Kauff N, Robson M, et al. Outcome of preventive surgery and screening for breast and ovarian cancer in *BRCA* mutation carriers. J Clin Oncol 2001; 20(5):1260–1268.

130. Robson ME, Offit K. Breast MRI for women with hereditary cancer risk. J Am Med Assoc 2004; 292(11):1368–1370.

5
PTEN and Cowden Syndrome

Kevin M. Zbuk and Jennifer Stein
Genomic Medicine Institute, Lerner Research Institute, Cleveland Clinic Foundation, Cleveland, Ohio, U.S.A.

Charis Eng
Genomic Medicine Institute, Lerner Research Institute and Taussig Cancer Center, Cleveland Clinic Foundation, and Department of Genetics and Case Comprehensive Cancer Center, Case Western Reserve University School of Medicine, Cleveland, Ohio, U.S.A.

INTRODUCTION

The *PTEN* hamartoma tumor syndrome (PHTS) includes not only the entity Cowden syndrome (CS, MIM 158350) which is the focus of this chapter, but also Bannayan-Riley-Ruvalcaba syndrome (BRRS, MIM 153480), Proteus syndrome (PS, MIM 176920), and Proteus-like syndrome (PSL) (1). Disorders in this heterogeneous group are all, to varying degrees, associated with germline mutations of the *PTEN* tumor suppressor, localized to 10q23.2 (2,3). PTEN is a dual-specificity phosphatase, having both phospholipid and protein phosphatase activities (4–6). PTEN plays a crucial role in controlling cell growth, cell spreading, and mediating apoptosis and cell cycle arrest.

CS is an underrecognized, underdiagnosed, autosomal dominant disorder. Patients with CS are at increased risk of developing breast, thyroid, and endometrial cancers in addition to benign neoplasias of these same organs and characteristic mucocutaneous manifestations including papillomatous papules and trichilemmomas (7). BRRS is characterized by macrocephaly, lipomas, hemangiomas, and speckled penis (8). PS and PSL are complex disorders characterized by hemihypertrophy, subcutaneous tumors and various bone, and cutaneous and vascular anomalies (9). Although BRRS, PS, and PSL have not historically been associated with increased cancer risk, current expert opinion is that all patients with germline *PTEN* mutations, irrespective of phenotypic classification, follow the cancer surveillance recommendations suggested for CS, emphasizing the importance of recognizing all facets of the PHTS (1).

CLINICAL DESCRIPTION OF CS

CS, named after Rachel Cowden, the first reported patient with the disorder (10), is characterized by multiple hamartomas which can affect any organ from all three germ cell layers, including the characteristic mucocutaneous manifestations and benign and malignant neoplasms of the breast, thyroid, and endometrium (7). Underscoring the fulminant nature of the malignancies, Rachel Cowden died at the age of 31 of metastatic breast cancer (11).

Published estimates of CS incidence are 1/200,000 (12). However, because many of the signs are common in the general population (e.g., fibrocystic breast disease and uterine leiomyomas), and there is considerable variability in presentation, the disorder is underrecognized, and the true incidence is likely much higher (1). The proportion of isolated and familial cases is not precisely known but it appears 40% to 60% of cases may be sporadic (13). Although an increased female:male prevalence of CS is described, this is likely in part related to ascertainment bias since benign and malignant breast and endometrial neoplasms are features of the operational criteria for diagnosis. A similar phenomenon is seen with BRRS, and it's increased male:female prevalence, which is discussed below.

Diagnostic Criteria

Diagnostic criteria were initially developed by the International Cowden Consortium to systemically study CS in the context of localizing the susceptibility gene (2). While these original criteria are robust, with >80% of patients strictly meeting these criteria harboring a germline *PTEN* mutation (14), they are also complex and likely too stringent for routine clinical care. In addition, clinicians not familiar with the disorder may fail to recognize certain pathognomonic features such as papillomatous papules and trichilemmomas. Thus, a major goal of current research is to determine the most parsimonious criteria for referral to a cancer genetics clinic for consideration of *PTEN* mutation testing. The working criteria established by the National Comprehensive Cancer Network Genetics/High Risk Panel (Table 1) (15) have recently been updated and are designed to aid the clinician in the identification of patients appropriate for referral to a cancer genetics specialist. These guidelines additionally offer recommendations on the management of patients who test either positive or negative for germline *PTEN* mutations, and these are outlined in the section entitled Clinical Management of CS.

Component Malignancies

Breast Cancer in CS

Component malignancies in CS include breast, thyroid (16), and endometrial carcinomas (Table 2) (17). The most common malignancy seen in CS is adenocarcinoma of the breast, with lifetime risks in female CS patients estimated to be 25% to 50% compared with the lifetime risk of 12% to 13% in the general population (18,19). As commonly described in other hereditary breast cancer predisposition syndromes, the average age of breast cancer diagnosis is lower in patients with CS compared with that in sporadic cases. In CS, the average age of diagnosis is between 38 and 46 years while the average age of diagnosis is 55 to 65 years in sporadic cases (19). There has only been a single systematic study looking at histologies in CS-related breast carcinomas, but without knowing the germline *PTEN* status (20). In this study of 59 breast neoplasias belonging to 19 unrelated CS cases, 35 (59%) had some malignant pathology. All cases of invasive breast cancer were ductal histology, with the exception of a single case of tubular carcinoma. The distribution of tumor grades was similar to that seen in sporadic breast cancer. No data on the estrogen or progesterone receptor status of the carcinomas was described. There also seems to be an increased risk of in situ carcinomas at an earlier age than in sporadic cases, and there was a higher frequency of sclerosis and fibrotic hamartomatous tissue present in the breast pathologic samples from individuals with CS. The hamartomatous tissue was often bilateral and extensive and led to frequent biopsies. Interestingly, in over 50% of

Table 1 Current Operational Diagnostic Criteria for the Diagnosis of CS—2006

Pathognomonic criteria	Operational diagnosis in an individual
Adult LDD	Mucocutaneous lesions alone if
Mucocutaneous lesions	Six or more facial papules, of which three or more
Trichilemmomas, facial	must be trichilemmomas, or
Acral keratoses	Cutaneous facial papules and oral mucosal
Papillomatous papules	papillomatosis, or
Mucosal lesions	Oral mucosal papillomatosis and acral keratoses, or
	Palmoplantar keratoses, six or more
	Two or more major criteria or
	One major and ≥3 minor or ≥four minor
Major criteria	Operational diagnosis in a family where one individual
Breast cancer	is diagnostic for CS
Thyroid cancer (especially follicular)	The pathognomonic criteria
Macrocephaly (megalencephaly)	Any one major criteria with or without minor criteria
(i.e., ≥97th percentile)	Two minor criteria
Endometrial cancer	History of BRRS
Minor criteria	
Other thyroid lesions (e.g., multinodular goiter, adenoma)	
Mental retardation (i.e., IQ ≤ 75)	
GI hamartomas	
Fibrocystic breast disease	
Lipomas	
Fibromas	
GU tumors (especially renal cell carcinoma)	
GU abnormalities (eg. horseshoe kidney)	
Uterine fibroids	

Abbreviations: BRRS, Bannayan-Riley-Ruvalcaba syndrome; CS, Cowden syndrome; GI, gastrointestinal; GU, gastrourinary; LDD, Lhermitte-Duclos disease.

malignant specimens examined, the carcinoma appeared to occur within these areas of hamartomatous tissue. It was hypothesized that the malignancy may have developed from within a mammary hamartoma, although the etiologic relationship between the two remains unclear. Breast cancer risk may be increased in male CS patients, although its frequency is currently unknown (14,21). Bilateral breast cancer has been described in patients with CS (20,22), but it is unclear whether its occurrence is more common in CS than in apparently sporadic cases. Similarly, there is no literature confirming that patients with CS have an increased risk of developing a second breast malignancy after initial resection, although the "field defect" present secondary to a germline *PTEN* mutation would suggest this is likely the case, and such evidence exists for other heritable breast cancer syndromes, especially *BRCA1/2* (23).

Additional Malignancies Seen in CS

The lifetime risk of epithelial thyroid cancer in CS is approximately 10% (1). Follicular thyroid cancer is felt to be the most common histology seen but papillary thyroid cancer has also been observed (16). However, it is suspected that some cases described as

Table 2 Common Manifestations of CS

Mucocutaneous manifestations	99%
Trichilemmomas	
Papillomatous papules	
Acral keratosis	
Breast lesions	
Fibrocystic breasts/fibroadenomas adenocarcinoma	76% of affected females
	30–50% of affected females
Macrocephaly	30–40%
Thyroid abnormalities	50–67%
Multinodular goiter	
Adenomas	
Follicular thyroid carcinoma	3–10%
Gastrointestinal lesions	
Hamartomatous polyps	40%
Esophageal glycogenic acanthosis	
Genitourinary abnormalities	
Multiple uterine leiomyomas (fibroids)	44% of affected females
Bicornuate uterus	

Abbreviation: CS, Cowden syndrome.

papillary thyroid cancer may in fact represent the papillary variant of follicular thyroid cancer. Medullary thyroid cancer is not a component of CS. The frequency of endometrial cancer in patients with CS is not yet clearly defined, but may be as high as 5% to 10% (7,24). There is an increased risk of clear cell renal cell carcinoma, but the frequency of this component malignancy is currently unknown (17). In addition, melanomas and glial tumors may occur more commonly in patients with CS, but current evidence is not strong enough to warrant their addition to the diagnostic criteria given their frequency in the general population.

Mucocutaneous Manifestations

The mucocutaneous manifestations of CS are the most common, yet the most difficult to recognize, with an estimated penetrance of 99% by the end of the third decade (17). The characteristic skin lesions of CS are trichilemmomas and papillomatous papules (25). Trichilemmomas are hamartomas of the infundibulum of the hair follicle and are characteristically found at or near the hairline while papillomatous papules are condyloma-like lesions occurring frequently on the face, hands, feet, or oral mucosa. It is not uncommon to see papillomatous papules proliferate at pressure points particularly on the palmar and plantar surfaces. Additional cutaneous manifestations include acral keratoses, small punctate lesions commonly seen on the palmar surface of the hands, which are often associated with a central depression or "pit." Lipomas are a feature, but are seen more commonly in BRRS (14). Patients appear predisposed to excessive scarring, even cheloid formation, at the site of traumatic or iatrogenic scars.

Nonmalignant Solid Organ Involvement

At least 50% of patients with CS exhibit benign breast disease (26). In a series of specimens from CS patients who had undergone breast biopsies or resections, 98% had evidence of benign breast lesions (20). The spectrum of lesions includes ductal hyperplasia, intraductal papillomas, sclerosing adenosis, lobular atrophy and fibroadenomas, dense stromal fibrosis, and fibrocystic changes (20,26). These benign manifestations, in addition to the breast hamartomas described previously, are often bilateral and extensive (20), making surveillance in patients with CS considerably more difficult.

Benign thyroid lesions including adenomas, hamartomas, and multinodular goiter occur in 50% to 67% of all affected patients (16). It is suspected that Hashimoto thyroiditis occurs at an increased frequency in CS, especially in patients who are of non-Asian ancestry; this belief is supported by early literature describing Hashimoto thyroiditis as a component of BRRS (8). Currently, functional disorders of the thyroid resulting in hyperthyroidism or hypothyroidism in the absence of adenomas or goiter are not considered components of CS.

Nearly 50% of female patients with CS develop uterine leiomyomas (26), which, although common in the general population, occur at an early age (often in the third decade) in CS and are often multiple and large (1). Genitourinary malformations such as horseshoe kidney and bicornuate uterus occur at an increased frequency (1). Hamartomatous gastrointestinal (GI) polyps occur, but symptomatic polyps are felt to occur less frequently than in BRRS. Esophageal glycogenic acanthosis has been described, which has the appearance of elevated gray-white plaques in the distal mucosa of the esophagus. It has been suggested that the presence of both glycogenic acanthosis and colonic polyps in an individual is quite specific to CS (27). In a series of 11 individuals with CS (10 with germline *PTEN* mutations), all had diminutive, asymptomatic hamartomatous or lipomatous polyps in both the upper and lower GI tracts, and all with the exception of the *PTEN* mutation negative patient also had esophageal glycogenic acanthosis (28). A recent study additionally found unexpected germline *PTEN* mutations in 9% of patients with unclassified hyperplastic/adenomatous polyposis syndromes (29).

Central Nervous System Manifestations

Macrocephaly, often quite pronounced, is common, with head circumference >2 SD above the mean in greater than 40% of patients (26). More specifically, the increased head circumference is due to megalencephaly, an increase in brain volume. In addition, the head is often dolichocephalic even when head circumference is normal. Developmental delay is described but is less common in CS than in BRRS. Adult onset Lhermitte-Duclos disease (LDD) has recently been moved to the pathognomonic criteria (previously a major criteria) for the diagnosis of CS (Table 1) (15). LDD is characterized by cerebellar enlargement secondary to granule cell and Purkinje cell hypertrophy (30). Resulting signs and symptoms include those of increased intracranial pressure (e.g., headache, vomiting, and altered level of consciousness) and ataxia from cerebellar dysfunction. Thus, even though LDD is not a malignancy, the morbidity and the mortality of this disorder are very significant. Patients with LDD demonstrate significant variability in the course of disease. Some have progressive disease, which is eventually fatal despite recurrent surgical excisions, while others have stable disease that does not require surgical excisions.

CLINICAL DESCRIPTION OF BRRS

BRRS is a developmental disorder whose most commonly recognized features are macrocephaly, hemangiomas, lipomas, speckled penis, and mental retardation (8).

Macrocephaly occurs in the vast majority of patients, and developmental delay is seen in 25% to 50% (8). Symptomatic intestinal hamartomas are reported more often in BRRS (occurring in up to 40% of patients) compared with CS. Such hamartomas can lead to GI bleeding, bowel obstruction, anemia and chronic diarrhea (31,32). The rarity of the syndrome precludes accurate estimates of the penetrance of these features. Pigmented macules on the penis ("speckled penis") appear to be the most specific finding, but can be subtle, and not initially present at birth (33). This feature may lead to ascertainment bias, with BRRS more frequently reported in males.

Cancer Predisposition in BRRS

The risk of malignancy in BRRS is not well defined. Historically, there is no mention of cancer predisposition in early BRRS literature (8,31), as follow up of cases into adulthood is virtually never reported. However, once it was realized that CS and BRRS are allelic (34) (discussed later), this opinion has changed. In addition, the single largest study of genotype–phenotype correlation in patients with BRRS demonstrated a strong correlation between germline *PTEN* mutations and both benign (fibroadenomas) and malignant breast diseases in families with BRRS or CS/BRRS overlap (families consisting of individuals who meet CS criteria in addition to individuals felt to have BRRS) (35). This finding solidified the recommendation that all patients with *PTEN* mutations, irrespective of phenotypic presentation, be screened for cancer in the same manner as a patient with CS, and led to the evolution of the concept of PHTS.

PTEN, A DUAL-SPECIFICITY PHOSPHATASE

The clinical syndrome of CS was first described in 1963 (10); however the locus for CS was not mapped to 10q23 until 1996 (2) and *PTEN* itself was not identified until 1997, where its somatic role in sporadic cancer cell lines was noted (36,37). Sequence analysis showed a large region of homology to chicken tensin, bovine auxilin, and a protein tyrosine-phosphatase domain, from which the name "PTEN" was coined [for *p*hosphatase and *ten*sin homolog, deleted on chromosome 10 (*ten*)]. A third group identified *PTEN* by searching for novel human protein tyrosine phosphatases (38). They identified *TEP1* [transforming growth factor (TGF)–regulated and epithelial cell-enriched phosphatase], which was subsequently shown to be identical to *PTEN*.

PTEN spans nine exons and encodes a 403 amino acid protein. Functionally, PTEN can be regarded as a dual-specificity phosphatase on several levels (1). PTEN has been shown to dephosphorylate both serine/threonine and tyrosine residues (4). Thus, PTEN is a dual-specificity protein phosphatase. In this role, PTEN dephosphorylates focal adhesion kinase to inhibit cell migration and cell spreading (39). In addition, PTEN appears to regulate cyclin D1 and the cell survival pathway mitogen-activated protein kinase (MAPK) through its protein phosphatase activity (40). However, PTEN is also a phospholipid phosphatase whose major substrate is phosphoinositol-3,4,5-triphosphate, a major lipid second messenger that is required for Akt recruitment to the plasma membrane and its subsequent activation (41). Through this action, PTEN opposes the action of phosphoinositol-3-kinase and negatively regulates the Akt pathway by inhibiting the phosphorylation of Akt (Fig. 1). Through this inhibition, it mediates cell cycle arrest at G1 and/or apoptosis (42), through the action of downstream effectors such as BAD (43). BAD, BCl-xL/BCl-2 Associated Death Promoter and FAS. FAS, TNF receptor superfamily, member 6.

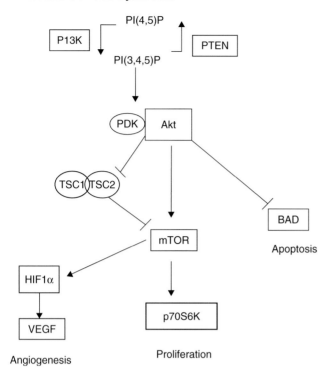

Figure 1   *PTEN* as a regulator of the Akt pathway. PI3K activation leads to increased levels of PIP3 and subsequent activation of Akt through the action of PDK. Akt subsequently regulates a variety of processes including angiogenesis, cellular proliferation, and apoptosis. By dephosphorylating PIP3, PTEN downregulates the Akt pathway. *Abbreviations*: BAD, Bcl-xL/Bcl-2-Associated Death Promoter; FAS, TNF receptor superfamily member 6; HIF1α, hypoxia inducible factor 1 alpha; mTOR, mammalian target of rapamycin; PDKI, 3-phosphoinositide-dependent protein kinase 1; PIP3, phosphoinositol-3,4,5-triphosphate; PI3K, phosphoinositol-3-kinase; TSC, tuberous sclerosis protein; VEGF, vascular endothelial growth factor.

PTEN has nuclear localization sequence–like sequences that are required for transport of PTEN into the nucleus (44). Although traditionally felt to exert its effect solely in the cytoplasm, it now appears that nuclear PTEN is required for cell cycle arrest, while cytoplasmic PTEN is required for apoptosis. Cytoplasmic PTEN downregulates phosphorylation of Akt and upregulates p27 whereas nuclear PTEN downregulates cyclin D1 and prevents the phosphorylation of MAPK. Thus nuclear-cytoplasmic partitioning differentially regulates cell cycle control and apoptosis (45). Abnormalities of this partitioning may play an important role in PTEN dysfunction, and this hypothesis has become a major focus of ongoing research.

PTEN MUTATIONS IN CS

The International Cowden Consortium mapped the susceptibility locus for CS to 10q22-q23 (2) and subsequently demonstrated that germline mutations of *PTEN* cause CS (46). Utilizing strict operational criteria, >80% of individuals with CS harbor a germline *PTEN* mutation (14) (Table 3). Initial studies of families meeting strict operational criteria for CS demonstrate no genetic heterogeneity (2). To date, no additional disease susceptibility loci have been confirmed for CS. It is thus believed that CS is a monoallelic disorder.

Table 3 *PTEN* Hamartoma Tumor Syndromes

Syndrome	*PTEN* mutation frequency	Clinical features
CS	85%	Benign and malignant breast, thyroid, and endometrial neoplasias, trichilemmomas, papillomatous papules, macrocephaly
BRRS	60%	Macrocephaly, developmental delay, hemangiomas, lipomas, speckled penis
PS	10–20%	Congenital malformations, hemihypertrophy, hamartomatous overgrowths, epidermal nevi, and hyperostosis
PSL	60%	Features suggestive but not meeting diagnostic criteria of PS
ASD with macrocephaly	~10–20% (exact figure unknown)	*PTEN* mutations associated with extreme macrocephaly (>4 SD above mean)
Macrocephaly and VATER association	Unknown (confirmatory studies needed)	VATER

Abbreviations: ASD, autism spectrum disorder; BRRS, Bannayan-Riley-Ruvalcaba syndrome; CS, Cowden syndrome; PHTS, PTEN hamartoma tumor syndromes; PS, Proteus syndrome; PSL, Proteus syndrome like; SD, standard deviation; VATER, vertebral malformations, anal malformations, trachea-esophageal atresia, radial/renal malformations.

Therefore, to additionally characterize patients with CS who are mutation negative, novel mechanisms leading to *PTEN* dysfunction including nuclear-cytoplasmic PTEN trafficking and splice site variation are being actively studied.

Genotype–Phenotype Correlation in CS

Approximately two-thirds of germline *PTEN* mutations are found in exons 5, 7, and 8, and approximately 40% of all CS mutations are located in exon 5, although this exon represents only 20% of the coding sequence (1,14). This reflects the biological significance of this domain, which encodes the phosphatase core motif. There is a correlation between the presence of germline *PTEN* mutations and breast carcinoma in probands meeting operational criteria for CS (14). In other words, the risk of breast cancer may be higher in those patients and families with a clinical diagnosis of CS who harbor germline *PTEN* mutations. Additionally, mutations within the phosphatase core motif and 5' of it appear to be associated with involvement of five or more organs, suggesting a correlation between mutations in this region of *PTEN* and disease severity (14). A recent study has demonstrated that promoter mutations are present in 10% of mutation negative patients with CS (47). Importantly, the functional significance of these mutations was confirmed by biochemical studies that demonstrate increased phosphorylated Akt levels, confirming PTEN dysfunction in these patients. This study demonstrated a very strong cancer phenotype associated with the identified *PTEN* promoter mutations. Breast cancer was diagnosed in six out of nine and thyroid cancer was diagnosed in three out of nine (thyroid cancer and breast cancer occurred simultaneously in two out of nine). In all, seven out of nine (78%) promoter mutation positive families demonstrated a component malignancy. *PTEN* promoter mutations were not seen in patients with BRRS in this study.

In a pivotal study, Zhou et al. performed mutational analysis on tissue blocks from 18 unselected, unrelated patients with adult onset LDD and demonstrated that 15 (83%) of 18 samples were found to carry a *PTEN* mutation (48). All individuals with mutations were adult-onset patients, while the three without mutations were diagnosed in infancy or childhood. Immunohistochemistry revealed that 75% of the LDD samples had complete or partial loss of PTEN expression accompanied by elevated phosphorylated Akt, which occurred specifically in the dysplastic gangliocytoma cells. Thus, germline mutations in *PTEN* are associated with adult onset LDD, but not LDD diagnosed in infancy or childhood. Subsequently, germline *PTEN* mutations in patients with LDD have been documented in several additional series (49–51).

Early data suggest that certain naturally occurring *PTEN* splice variants occur more frequently in patients with CS than in normal controls and that these splice variants have differential effects on the ability of PTEN to regulate downstream molecular targets, thus suggesting that splice variants may play a role in the pathogenesis of CS (52,53). Intriguingly, there appears to exist splice variant genotype–phenotype correlation, with patients with CS and BRRS showing differential expression of splice variants compared to each other and compared with normal controls (52).

PTEN MUTATIONS IN BRRS

Approximately 60% of patients with BRRS harbor germline *PTEN* mutations, both in isolated and familial cases, and the frequency of germline *PTEN* mutations appears to be similar in both familial and apparently sporadic BRRSs (35). Therefore, at least a subset of BRRS and CS are allelic. In addition, the mutational spectra of CS and BRRS overlap (1), lending further proof that CS and BRRS are allelic as does the existence of CS/BRRS overlap families, in which cases of CS and BRRS are both present in the family (35). Approximately 65% of all distinct *PTEN* mutations found in CS occurred in the first five exons or in the promoter region, while 60% of all distinct *PTEN* mutations found in BRRS occurred within exons 6 to 9 (1,35). Thus, CS mutations appear to cluster in the 5' region while BRRS mutations cluster in the 3' region of *PTEN*. Further exploration of mechanisms of PTEN dysfunction has revealed that 10% of patients with classic BRRS harbor large deletions encompassing *PTEN* that would not be detectable by traditional polymerase chain reaction (PCR)–based mutation analysis (47). Such deletions occured exclusively in patients or families with BRRS, but not in individuals or families with CS only.

Genotype–Phenotype Correlation in BRRS

The presence of germline *PTEN* mutations in BRRS probands correlates with the presence of benign and malignant breast lesions in BRRS and additionally correlates with the presence of lipomas, compared with BRRS probands without mutations (35). CS/BRRS clinical overlap families have a >90% germline *PTEN* mutation frequency (35). CS/BRRS overlap families tend to have germline *R130X* and *R335X* mutations, occurring in slightly under half of such families.

OTHER *PTEN* MUTATION–RELATED DISORDERS

Germline *PTEN* mutations have been documented in 10% to 20% of patients with PS and 60% of patients with PSL (54–56). Additionally germline *PTEN* mutations were documented in 17% of patients with autism spectrum disorder associated with extreme macrocephaly (57) and a patient with macrocephaly and *v*ertebral malformations, *a*nal malformations, *t*rachea-*e*sophageal atresia, *r*adial/*r*enal malformations (VATER) association (58).

CLINICAL MANAGEMENT OF CS

Managing the Cutaneous Manifestations of CS

The mucocutaneous manifestations of CS are not life threatening and if asymptomatic, observation alone is prudent. When symptomatic, topical agents, curettage, cryosurgery, or laser ablation may provide only temporary relief. A single case reported documented successful treatment of cutaneous lesions with acitretin (59). Surgical excision is sometimes complicated by cheloid formation and, commonly, recurrence of the lesions.

Management of Malignancy in CS

The treatment of the malignant manifestations of PHTS is generally the same as for their sporadic counterparts. Several caveats deserve mention however. Like other hereditary breast cancer syndromes, the risk of second primaries, not only within the breasts but also in other affected organs, is increased in CS, although no data exists on the frequency of their occurrence. In addition, some women with CS have extensive fibrocystic changes and/or fibroadenomas that make surveillance difficult. For these reasons, the clinician and patient need to consider on an individualized basis of the appropriateness of mastectomy versus lumpectomy, in addition to giving consideration to performing prophylactic mastectomy of the contralateral breast (see section entitled Prevention of Breast Cancer in CS).

Thyroid cancer should be treated with total thyroidectomy. Additionally, it is expert opinion that patients with thyroid adenomas, in whom surgery is deemed necessary, also be treated with complete thyroidectomy given the very high prevalence of benign thyroid neoplasias in CS that may make surveillance after hemithyroidectomy extremely difficult. In addition, the risk of developing a malignancy in the remaining thyroid tissue and the difficulty of repeated thyroid resection support this opinion.

Potential Use of Targeted Therapies in CS

Agents such as rapamycin, which are mammalian targets of rapamycin (mTOR) inhibitors, are often suggested as rational choices for utilizing targeted therapy in CS given the effect of PTEN on modulating this downstream molecule (Fig. 1). Given the toxicity associated with these agents, limiting treatment to patients with malignancy when considering mTOR inhibitors and pAkt inhibitors (when clinically available) appears rational at this juncture. Mechanistically, an additional limitation of mTOR inhibitors in CS is that mTOR lies downstream of the lipid phosphatase activity of PTEN but has no interaction downstream of its protein phosphatase. As such, mTOR inhibitors would leave pathways such as the MAPK pathway unchecked, a potentially harmful proposition. Additionally, the Akt pathway plays a crucial role in normal development and homeostasis, and literature is emerging that documents serious adverse effects from iatrogenically blocking the Akt pathway (60–62).

PREVENTION OF BREAST CANCER IN CS

Some women with CS consider prophylactic mastectomy, especially if breast tissue is dense, making surveillance difficult, or if repeated breast biopsies have been necessary. Prophylactic mastectomy reduces the risk of breast cancer by 90% in women at high risk (63), although no studies have specifically addressed this intervention in patients with CS. There is no direct evidence to support the routine use of agents such as tamoxifen or raloxifene in individuals with CS to reduce the risk of developing breast cancer. Physicians should discuss the limitations of the evidence and the risks and benefits of chemoprophylaxis with each individual. In addition, the clinician must discuss the increased risk of endometrial cancer associated with tamoxifen use in this population that is already at increased risk for this malignancy.

CANCER SURVEILLANCE IN CS

The most important aspect of management of "any" individual with a *PTEN* mutation is increased cancer surveillance. Cancer surveillance recommendations are updated annually by the National Comprehensive Cancer Network (NCCN) (15) as part of the Genetic/Familial High-Risk Assessment: Breast and Ovarian guideline. The 2006 guidelines recommend the following interventions:

General

- Annual comprehensive physical examination starting at age 18 years (or five years before the youngest component cancer diagnosis in the family), with attention paid to skin changes and the neck region
- Consider annual dermatologic examination
- Annual urinalysis. Consider annual cytology and renal ultrasound examination if the family history is positive for renal cell carcinoma.

Breast Cancer

Women

- Monthly breast self-examination beginning at age 18 years
- Annual clinical breast examinations beginning at age 25 years or 5 to 10 years earlier than the earliest known breast cancer diagnosis in the family (whichever is earlier)
- Annual mammography and breast magnetic resonance imaging (MRI) beginning at age 30 to 35 years or 5 to 10 years before the earliest known breast cancer diagnosis in the family (whichever is earlier)

Men should perform monthly breast self-examination.

Thyroid Cancer

- Baseline thyroid ultrasound examination at age 18 years
- Consider annual thyroid ultrasound examination thereafter

Endometrial Cancer

- "*Premenopausal women*": Annual blind repel (suction) biopsies beginning at age 35 to 40 years (or five years before the youngest endometrial cancer diagnosis in the family).
- "*Postmenopausal women*": Annual transvaginal ultrasound examination with biopsy of suspicious areas.

MANAGEMENT OF BRRS

Given the arguments described earlier in this chapter, it is recommended that individuals with BRRS harboring a germline *PTEN* mutation undergo the same surveillance as individuals with CS. In addition it has been suggested that individuals with BRRS should also be monitored for complications related to GI hamartomatous polyposis. Reasonable interventions include annual measurement of serum hemoglobin levels and prompt endoscopic evaluation of concerning GI symptoms such as lower GI bleeding, altered bowel habits, or persistent abdominal pain (32). Management of hemangiomas and arteriovenous malformations can be problematic. Chemoembolization and excision are often ineffective, with lesions recurring rapidly (64). Recently, there has been anecdotal success with the use of antiangiogenic agents. The rationale for the use of these agents is demonstrated by the modulation of angiogenesis by *PTEN* (Fig. 1).

GENETIC COUNSELING

It is suspected that up to 50% of all patients with CS or BRRS do not have a family history of either syndrome, either because their disease is the result of a de novo mutation or because the condition has gone undiagnosed in previous generations (35). Because this disorder is underdiagnosed, the de novo mutation rate is difficult to determine. Once a clinical diagnosis is established or suspected, *PTEN* mutation analysis is indicated in the setting of genetic counseling. If a *PTEN* mutation is identified in the proband, the most straightforward approach is to offer genetic testing to the parents of the individual carrying the mutation. If a parent of the proband has CS or BRRS (either meets diagnostic criteria or has a *PTEN* mutation), the probability that other siblings could inherit the family-specific mutation is 50%. Conversely, if the parents of an affected proband have a negative clinical examination and no germline *PTEN* mutation, the risk to the proband's siblings is negligible, since germline mosaicism has not been reported in CS or BRRS, to date. Molecular diagnostic testing of *PTEN* is appropriate for at-risk individuals younger than 18 years given the possible early presentation of symptoms in those with BRRS and PS. A patient has been recently described with a clinical diagnosis of CS in whom follicular thyroid cancer developed at six years of age (65). The earliest diagnosis of breast cancer is at 14 years of age (16,19).

For probands who meet diagnostic criteria but do not have an identifiable *PTEN* mutation, both parents should undergo thorough clinical examination to help determine if either parent has features that have gone previously undiagnosed. If a mutation is not identified in a pedigree, the diagnosis of CS/BRRS in family members must be excluded on clinical grounds with the caveat that a negative exam in a young child does not rule out the diagnosis. Such families should be offered enrollment in ongoing research exploring novel mechanisms of PTEN dysfunction. Management of patients with a clinical diagnosis of CS but no identifiable *PTEN* mutation should be individualized based on personal and family history (15).

An additional challenge facing the cancer geneticist is the fact that many features of CS are common in the general population and can run in families as isolated conditions due to other genetic or nongenetic reasons. As discussed previously, CS can be difficult to diagnose, given the common nature of many of the clinical features and variable penetrance. Thus a major barrier to genetic counseling is that many patients remain unrecognized and are not referred for counseling in the first place. Ongoing education of the medical community with respect to CS remains an important goal. This will be more readily achieved once the most parsimonious criteria for referral to a cancer genetics specialist are determined as a result of ongoing clinical research.

CONCLUSION

It has been less than a decade since the discovery that germline *PTEN* mutations cause CS; however much has already been learned about this unique tumor suppressor and its evolving spectrum of associated disorders. The discovery of promoter mutations and large genomic deletions of *PTEN* has increased the probability of identifying a *PTEN* mutation in a patient with a clinical diagnosis of CS or BRRS. Considerable headway has also been made toward understanding novel mechanisms of PTEN dysfunction including differential expression of naturally occurring *PTEN* splice variants and nuclear-cytoplasmic compartmentalization of PTEN, which may offer important insight into the mechanism of phenotypic manifestation in mutation negative patients. Finally, the complex signaling pathways involving PTEN are becoming better understood, and the use of targeted therapy, even in the setting of cancer prevention, may soon become a reality.

ACKNOWLEDGMENTS

The authors dedicate this chapter to all our patients and their families who have participated in our research and/or who have informally taught us valuable clinical lessons. CE thanks her many collaborators and genetic counselors nationally and internationally who have participated, in one way or another, in PHTS research. The *PTEN* work in the Eng lab has been partially funded by the American Cancer Society, the Department of Defense Breast Cancer Research Program, and the Susan G. Komen Breast Cancer Foundation (to CE). CE is a recipient of the Doris Duke Distinguished Clinical Scientist Award. KMZ is a Crile Fellow of the Cleveland Clinic Foundation.

REFERENCES

1. Eng C. *PTEN*: one gene, many syndromes. Hum Mutat 2003; 22:183–198.
2. Nelen MR, et al. Localization of the gene for Cowden disease to 10q22-23. Nature Genet 1996; 13:114–116.
3. Waite KA, Eng C. Protean PTEN: form and function. Am J Hum Genet 2002; 70: B29–B44.
4. Myers MP, et al. *PTEN*, the tumor suppressor from human chromosome 10q23, is a dual specificity phosphatase. Proc Natl Acad Sci U S A 1997; 94:9052–9057.

5. Stambolic V, et al. Negative regulation of PKB/Akt-dependent cell survival by the tumor suppressor PTEN. Cell 1998; 95:1–20.

6. Maehama T, Dixon JE. The tumor suppressor, PTEN/MMAC1, dephosphorylates the lipid second messenger, phosphatidylinositol 3,4,5-trisphosphate. J Biol Chem 1998; 273: 13375–13378.

7. Pilarski R, Eng C. Will the real Cowden syndrome please stand up (again)? Expanding mutational and clinical spectra of the PTEN hamartoma tumour syndrome. J Med Genet 2004; 41:323–326.

8. Gorlin RJ, Cohen MM, Condon LM, Burke BA. Banayan-Riley-Rvalcabe syndrome. Am J Med Genet 1992; 44:307–314.

9. Biesecker LG, et al. Proteus syndrome: diagnostic criteria, differential diagnosis and patient evaluation. Am J Med Genet 1999; 84:389–395.

10. Lloyd KM, Denis M. Cowden's disease: a possible new symptom complex with multiple system involvement. Ann Intern Med 1963; 58:136–142.

11. Brownstein MH, Wolf M, Bilowski JB. Cowden's disease: a cutaneous marker of breast cancer. Cancer 1978; 41:2393–2398.

12. Nelen MR, et al. Novel PTEN mutations in patients with Cowden disease: absence of clear genotype-phenotype correlations. Eur J Hum Genet 1999; 7:267–273.

13. Eng C, Parsons R. Cowden syndrome. In: Vogelstein B, Kinzler KW, eds. The Genetic Basis of Human Cancer. New York: McGraw-Hill, 1998:519–526.

14. Marsh DJ, et al. Mutation spectrum and genotype-phenotype analyses in Cowden disease and Bannayan-Zonana syndrome, two hamartoma syndromes with germline PTEN mutation. Hum Mol Genet 1998; 7:507–515.

15. The NCCN Genetic/Familial High-Risk Assessment: Breast and Ovarian Guideline (V.1.2007) © 2006 National Comprehensive Cancer Network, Inc. Available at: http:// www.nccn.org. Accessed January 1, 2007. To view the most recent and complete version of the guideline, go online to www.nccn.org.

16. Starink TM, et al. The Cowden syndrome: a clinical and genetic study in 21 patients. Clin Genet 1986; 29:222–233.

17. Eng C. Will the real Cowden syndrome please stand up: revised diagnostic criteria. J Med Genet 2000; 37:828–830.

18. Eng C. Cowden syndrome. J Genet Counsel 1997; 6:181–191.

19. Longy M, Lacombe D. Cowden disease. Report of a family and review. Ann Génet 1996; 39: 35–42.

20. Schrager CA, Schneider D, Gruener AC, Tsou HC, Peacocke M. Clinical and pathological features of breast disease in Cowden's syndrome: an underrecognised syndrome with an increased risk of breast cancer. Hum Pathol 1997; 29:47–53.

21. Fackenthal JD, et al. Male breast cancer in Cowden syndrome patients with germline PTEN mutations. J Med Genet 2001; 38:159–164.

22. Reifenberger J, et al. Cowden's disease: clinical and molecular genetic findings in a patient with a novel PTEN germline mutation. Br J Dermatol 2003; 148:1040–1046.

23. Metcalfe K, et al. Contralateral breast cancer in BRCA1 and BRCA2 mutation carriers. J Clin Oncol 2004; 22:2328–2335.

24. Marsh DJ, et al. Germline PTEN mutations in Cowden syndrome-like families. J Med Genet 1998; 35:881–885.

25. Mallory SB. Cowden syndrome (multiple hamartoma syndrome). Dermatol Clin 1995; 13: 27–31.

26. Hanssen AMN, Fryns JP. Cowden syndrome. J Med Genet 1995; 32:117–119.

27. Kay PS, Soetikno RM, Mindelzun R, Young HS. Diffuse esophageal glycogenic acanthosis: an endoscopic marker of Cowden's disease. Am J Gastroenterol 1997; 92: 1038–1040.

28. Weber HC, Marsh D, Lubensky I, Lin A, Eng C. Germline PTEN/MMAC1/TEP1 mutations and association with gastrointestinal manifestations in Cowden disease. Gastroenterology 1998; 114S:G2902.

29. Sweet K, et al. Molecular classification of patients with unexplained hamartomatous and hyperplastic polyposis. JAMA 2005; 294:2465–2473.

30. Ambler M, Pogacar S, Sidman R. Lhermitte-Duclos disease (granule cell hypertrophy of the cerebellum). Pathologic analysis of the first familial cases. J Neuropathol Exp Neurol 1969; 28:622–647.

31. Ruvalcaba RHA, Myhre S, Smith DW. Sotos syndrome with intestinal polyposis and pigmentary changes of the genitalia. Clin Genet 1980; 18:413–416.

32. Hendriks YM, et al. Bannayan-Riley-Ruvalcaba syndrome: further delineation of the phenotype and management of *PTEN* mutation-positive cases. Fam Cancer 2003; 2: 79–85.

33. Parisi M, et al. The spectrum and evolution of phenotypic findings in *PTEN* mutation positive cases of Bannayan-Riley-Ruvalcaba syndrome. J Med Genet 2001; 38:52–57.

34. Marsh DJ, et al. Germline mutations in *PTEN* are present in Bannayan-Zonana syndrome. Nat Genet 1997; 16:333–334.

35. Marsh DJ, et al. *PTEN* mutation spectrum and genotype-phenotype correlations in Bannayan-Riley-Ruvalcaba syndrome suggest a single entity with Cowden syndrome. Hum Mol Genet 1999; 8:1461–1472.

36. Li J, et al. *PTEN*, a putative protein tyrosine phosphatase gene mutated in human brain, breast and prostate cancer. Science 1997; 275:1943–1947.

37. Steck PA, et al. Identification of a candidate tumour suppressor gene, *MMAC1*, at chromosome 10q23.3 that is mutated in multiple advanced cancers. Nat Genet 1997; 15:356–362.

38. Li DM, Sun H. TEP1, encoded by a candidate tumor suppressor locus, is a novel protein tyrosine phosphatase regulated by transforming growth factor beta. Cancer Res 1997; 57: 2124–2129.

39. Tamura M, et al. PTEN interactions with focal adhesion kinase and suppression of the extracellular matrix-dependent phosphotidyinositol 3-kinase/Akt cell survival pathway. J Biol Chem 1999; 274:20693–20703.

40. Weng LP, Brown JL, Eng C. PTEN coordinates G1 arrest by down regulating cyclin D1 via its protein phosphatase activity and up regulating p27 via its lipid phosphatase activity. Hum Mol Genet 2001; 10:599–604.

41. Stambolic V, et al. Negative regulation of PKB/Akt-dependent cell survival by the tumor suppressor PTEN. Cell 1998; 95:29–39.

42. Li DM, Sun H. PTEN/MMAC1/TEP1 suppresses the tumorigenecity and induces G1 cell cycle arrest in human glioblastoma cells. Proc Natl Acad Sci U S A 1998; 95: 15406–15411.

43. Di Cristofano A, et al. Impaired Fas response and autoimmunity in *PTEN*+/− mice. Science 1999; 285:2122–2125.

44. Chung JH, Ginn-Pease ME, Eng C. Phosphatase and tensin homologue deleted on chromosome 10 (*PTEN*) has nuclear localization signal-like sequences for nuclear import mediated by major vault protein. Cancer Res 2005; 65:4108–4116.

45. Chung JH, Eng C. Nuclear-cytoplasmic partitioning of phosphatase and tensin homologue deleted on chromosome 10 (*PTEN*) differentially regulates the cell cycle and apoptosis. Cancer Res 2005; 65:8096–8100.

46. Liaw D, et al. Germline mutations of the *PTEN* gene in Cowden disease, an inherited breast and thyroid cancer syndrome. Nat Genet 1997; 16:64–67.

47. Zhou XP, et al. Germline *PTEN* promoter mutations and deletions in Cowden/Bannayan-Riley-Ruvalcaba syndrome result in aberrant PTEN protein and dysregulation of the phosphoinositol-3-kinase/Akt pathway. Am J Hum Genet 2003; 73:404–411.

48. Zhou XP, et al. Germline inactivation of *PTEN* and dysregulation of the phosphoinositol-3-kinase/Akt pathway cause human Lhermitte-Duclos disease in adults. Am J Hum Genet 2003; 73:1191–1198.

49. Perez-Nunez A, et al. Lhermitte-Duclos disease and Cowden disease: clinical and genetic study in five patients with Lhermitte-Duclos disease and literature review. Acta Neurochir (Wien) 2004; 146:679–690.

50. Derrey S, et al. Association between Cowden syndrome and Lhermitte-Duclos disease: report of two cases and review of the literature. Surg Neurol 2004; 61:447–454; discussion 454.

51. Sutphen R, et al. Severe Lhermitte-Duclos disease with unique germline mutation of *PTEN*. Am J Med Genet 1999; 82:290–293.

52. Sarquis MS, et al. Distinct expression profiles for PTEN transcript and its splice variants in Cowden syndrome and Bannayan-Riley-Ruvalcaba syndrome. Am J Hum Genet 2006; 79: 23–30.

53. Agrawal S, Eng C. Differential expression of novel naturally occurring splice variants of PTEN and their functional consequences in Cowden syndrome and sporadic breast cancer. Hum Mol Genet 2006; 15:777–787.

54. Zhou XP, et al. Association of germline mutation in the *PTEN* tumour suppressor gene and a subet of Proteus and Proteus-like syndromes. Lancet 2001; 358:210–211.

55. Loffeld A, et al. Epidermal naevus in Proteus syndrome showing loss of heterozygosity for an inherited *PTEN* mutation. Br J Dermatol 2006; 154:1194–1198.

56. Smith JM, et al. Germline mutation of the tumour suppressor *PTEN* in Proteus syndrome. J Med Genet 2002; 39:937–940.

57. Butler MG, et al. Subset of individuals with autism spectrum disorders and extreme macrocephaly associated with germline *PTEN* tumour suppressor gene mutations. J Med Genet 2005; 42:318–321.

58. Reardon W, Zhou XP, Eng C. A novel germline mutation of the *PTEN* gene in a patient with macrocephaly, ventricular dilatation and features of VATER association. J Med Genet 2001; 38:820–823.

59. Cnudde F, Boulard F, Muller P, Chevallier J, Teron-Abou B. Cowden disease: treatment with acitretine. Ann Dermatol Venereol 1996; 123:739–741.

60. Fujio Y, Nguyen T, Wencker D, Kitsis RN, Walsh K. Akt promotes survival of cardiomyocytes in vitro and protects against ischemia-reperfusion injury in mouse heart. Circulation 2000; 101:660–667.

61. Zdychova J, Komers R. Emerging role of Akt kinase/protein kinase B signaling in pathophysiology of diabetes and its complications. Physiol Res 2005; 54:1–16.

62. Sausville EA, et al. Phase I trial of 72-hour continuous infusion UCN-01 in patients with refractory neoplasms. J Clin Oncol 2001; 19:2319–2333.

63. Rebbeck TR, et al. Bilateral prophylactic mastectomy reduces breast cancer risk in *BRCA1* and *BRCA2* mutation carriers: the PROSE Study Group. J Clin Oncol 2004; 22:1055–1062.

64. Turnbull MM, Humeniuk V, Stein B, Suthers GK. Arteriovenous malformations in Cowden syndrome. J Med Genet 2005; 42:e50.

65. Hachicha M, et al. Cowden's disease: a new paediatric observation. Arch Pediatr 2006; 13: 459–462.

6

Li–Fraumeni Syndrome

Louise C. Strong

University of Texas M.D. Anderson Cancer Center, Houston, Texas, U.S.A.

HISTORICAL PERSPECTIVE

In 1969, Li and Fraumeni published a paper that led to the identification of a new hereditary cancer syndrome known as Li–Fraumeni Syndrome (LFS) (1). They reported four families with an unusual clustering of childhood soft tissue sarcomas, young onset breast cancer, and a variety of other tumors, and suggested this might represent a new familial syndrome; they followed those findings with a systematic survey of the cancer family history of over 600 U.S. children with rhabdomyosarcoma (2) that revealed additional components of the syndrome including adrenal cortical carcinoma and brain tumors. The syndrome was distinctly different from most familial cancer aggregates in the diversity of tumor types and young ages of cancer diagnosis.

Other investigators in other populations as well confirmed the occurrence of LFS, largely by ascertainment through childhood sarcoma patients (3,4), and provided statistical evidence for a genetic etiology (5).

Li and Fraumeni prospectively followed their original families and accrued additional cases, and in 1988 described clinical criteria for the syndrome (Table 1) (6). These criteria included a proband with a sarcoma diagnosed before age 45 years, a first degree relative with any cancer before age 45 and an additional close relative in the same lineage with any cancer before age 45 or sarcoma at any age. Their work demonstrated the continuing increased cancer risk in the original families over time, with new cancers in individuals previously affected, and cancer in new generations. New cancers arose both spontaneously and in areas of previous radiation therapy. Breast cancer and sarcomas continued to be the most common cancers, accounting for the majority of first and subsequent tumors.

In 1990, Malkin et al. (7) and Srivastava et al. (8) identified a germ line mutation in the tumor suppressor gene p53 in 5/5 and 1/1 LFS families, identifying mutations known to be deleterious based on the substantial data on tumor-specific p53 mutations. The mutations as well segregated in the families. Given the knowledge of p53 as the most commonly mutated gene in human cancer (9), and its established role in many different cancers, it seemed that p53 represented the major gene responsible for LFS.

WHAT IS LFS?

LFS is a clinical, descriptive diagnosis. Not all kindreds that fit the clinical criteria have a p53 germ line mutation, and certainly some individuals have a p53 germ line

Table 1 Diagnostic Criteria for Li–Fraumeni Syndrome and Li–Fraumeni-Like Syndrome

Li–Fraumeni syndrome (6)	Li–Fraumeni-like syndrome (11)
Proband <45 years with a sarcoma	Proband with any childhood tumor, or sarcoma, brain tumor, or adrenocortical tumor <45 years
Plus first degree relative <45 years with any cancer	Plus first or second degree relative in the same lineage with typical LFS tumor at any age or any cancer <45 years
Plus additional first and second degree relative in the same lineage aged <45 years with any cancer or sarcoma at any age	Plus another first or second degree relative in the same lineage with any cancer <60 years

mutation without meeting the full clinical criteria. The classic familial criteria fail to account for de novo mutations, which are not rare (10). As genetic testing has become available and other tumor types have been identified in p53 mutation carriers, Birch et al. (11) developed less rigorous clinical criteria referred to as Li–Fraumeni-like syndrome (LFL) (Table 1). LFL included a wider range of proband diagnoses and of ages of relatives at cancer diagnosis. As might be expected, the "classic" LFS families have a higher frequency of a p53 germ line mutation of some 77%, while the LFL families have a frequency of 40% (12). Other criteria have differed modestly from LFL, varying the proband tumor type or range of cancer age of onset (13,14). Specific tumors that seem to have a relatively high probability of a germ line p53 mutation include childhood adrenal cortical carcinoma (15,16), choroid plexus tumors (17), and childhood rhabdomyosarcoma occurring before age 3 years (18). Birch et al. (19) suggested that malignant phylloides tumors are associated with LFS; given standard coding they would probably be included in the overall breast cancer figures and the distinction missed. These conflicting definitions have raised important questions: What is the true phenotype of a p53 mutation carrier? Is there genetic heterogeneity in LFS? The semantic question becomes, should LFS remain a clinical entity as originally described, or should the definition include the phenotypes associated with a p53 germ line mutation? The more practical question is, what are the indications for p53 mutation testing?

As noted above, not all LFS kindreds have a p53 germ line mutation (14). While some mutations may be missed due to lack of sensitivity of the mutation testing used, rearrangements seem to be relatively rare (20), and the high frequency of mutations identified in classic LFS families imply that few mutations are missed (12). Further, p53 can be ruled out by linkage analysis in some kindreds (21,22). Bell et al. (23) reported a germ line mutation in the hCHK2 gene in some LFS kindreds, but it now appears to be a low-penetrant gene modifying breast cancer risk by about twofold (24,25). Bachinski et al. (26) recently reported a region of chromosome 1q showing linkage in two LFS families. However to date most LFS appears attributable to p53 germ line mutations, and our further discussion of breast cancer in LFS will focus on p53 mutation carriers.

THE P53 TUMOR SUPPRESSOR GENE

P53 was originally identified in 1979 in a study to identify gene products that bound to the large T antigen of SV40 (27,28). It was not until 1989 that it became clear that p53 was a tumor suppressor gene and not an oncogene (29). P53 is the gene most commonly mutated in human cancer (9), and many believe that in those tumors with wild-type p53, the p53 pathway is otherwise abrogated (30). While p53 is not necessary for normal development (31), it plays a major role in the DNA damage response pathway. The protein functions as a transcription activator or repressor. On DNA damage, p53 is activated and can induce cell cycle arrest, permitting DNA repair before the cell progresses through S phase, or apoptosis. Thus p53 is involved in eliminating those cells with damaged DNA that could not faithfully reproduce daughter cells with intact DNA, those cells with damaged DNA that might give rise to cancer. P53 was dubbed "guardian of the genome" by David Lane in 1992 (32). In addition p53 has been found to play an important role in angiogenesis, differentiation, and senescence.

P53 has been shown to function in part as a transcription activator or repressor in response to DNA damage. Loss of p53 function is associated with loss of the cell cycle arrest and apoptotic functions, and hence permissive for accumulation of DNA damage. Some 75% of germ line mutations in LFS or somatic mutations in tumors are missense mutations (unlike most cancer susceptibility genes) and most affect the transcriptional activity of p53. The missense mutations are clustered in five conserved domains, primarily the DNA-binding domains, with certain distinct "hotspots" that account for some 30% of germ line p53 mutations (codons 175, 213, 245, 248, 273, and 282). Common mutations involve the DNA contact sites (codons 248 and 273), or sites that stabilize the p53 structure as codon 175. However a wide range of frameshift, nonsense, and splice mutations are observed as well, with large deletions or rearrangements extremely rare (14).

TUMOR-SPECIFIC LOSS OF HETEROZYGOSITY VS. HAPLOINSUFFICIENCY

Tumor development associated with a p53 germ line mutation was initially thought to occur via the classic Knudson two hit model, with tumor-specific loss of heterozygosity (LOH), showing loss of the wild-type allele (7). However in a systematic study of tumors from p53 mutation carriers, Varley et al. (33) noted that less than half of the tumors showed loss of wild-type p53. Further, over half of the tumors from p53 heterozygous knockout mice were found to retain the wild-type allele, and the wild-type allele was functional; the tumors expressed wild-type protein on exposure to gamma radiation and activated or repressed the appropriate wild-type p53 downstream targets (34). These data supported a haplo-insufficiency model for p53 in tumorigenesis. This model has been further elucidated by the demonstration that in p53 heterozygous knockout cells the p53 basal and stress response levels of mRNA and protein are reduced to 25% of the wild-type levels, leaving the cell with a reduced p53 stress response and aberrant p53-dependent cell cycle regulation, perhaps leading to genomic instability and increased tumor development (35).

ANIMAL MODELS

Much of our current knowledge of the role of p53 in tumor development has come from mouse models, including the studies of LOH cited above. There are excellent reviews of the history of the p53 null and heterozygous mice (36–38) and of the mice with p53 missense mutations that are more analogous to those occurring in LFS (39). These findings have greatly influenced current thinking in LFS research, notably in the search for risk modifiers and future therapeutics, as discussed below.

FREQUENCY OF GERM LINE P53 MUTATIONS IN BREAST CANCER

The earliest publications on LFS focused on childhood soft tissue sarcoma and breast cancer (1,2), with most ascertainment through the less common childhood sarcomas. However, with the opportunity to test for a specific gene, focus shifted to the far more common, and often familial, breast cancer. The question was, what fraction of breast cancer, young, familial, bilateral, or associated with other cancers, might be attributable to germ line p53 mutations? A flurry of papers appeared in the literature from the early 1990s, studying different clinical groups of breast cancer and using various techniques to identify mutations. However, few p53 germ line mutations were observed using criteria of familial breast cancer (40–46), bilateral breast cancer (47), age at breast cancer diagnosis less than 31, 35, or 40 years (48–50), breast cancer associated with a personal or family history of multiple primary tumors (51), or breast cancer associated with no more than one sarcoma in the index case or relative and not meeting LFS criteria (12,52). In all of the above studies the frequency of p53 germ line mutations failed to reach the 10% level recommended by American Society of Clinical Oncology (ASCO) for initiating genetic testing. Indeed, given the high frequency of breast cancer in the general population, neither the definition of classic LFS (6), LFL (11,14) nor the French LFS group criteria for p53 mutation testing (13) specify breast cancer as part of the classification scheme!

The above cited studies indicate that the only good predictor of a p53 germ line mutation is a cancer family history of LFS or LFL. However for health-care providers to apply those criteria family members must accurately report the family history. Lalloo et al. (48,53) conducted a population-based study of 100 patients with breast cancer diagnosed before age 31 years, with testing for *BRCA1, 2*, and p53. A three-generation pedigree was collected at diagnosis, with hospital records, cancer registry or death certificate documentation; of the 31 familial cases with hospital notes available, only 14 were found to have reported an accurate family history. In the series four p53 mutation carriers were identified, none of whom had an LFS cancer family history identified at diagnosis. Two mutations were in patients later found to have LFS or LFL family histories but not reported at diagnosis, and two were in sporadic patients, including one confirmed de novo mutation. Schneider et al. (54) also noted that fewer than half of the respondents recruited because of a known familial p53 mutation were able to report a cancer family history that would have led to p53 mutation testing. This was significantly below the accuracy level of *BRCA* mutation kindred respondents.

There may be other limitations to identifying p53 mutation carriers based on LFS/ LFL cancer family history. Anticipation, an earlier age at diagnosis in successive generations, has been reported from the overall Database of Germ line p53 Mutations (55) and from a series of p53 mutation kindreds identified by systematic study of childhood sarcoma probands (56). None of the seven p53 mutation kindreds from the latter study would have been selected for mutation testing at the time of the proband diagnosis had LFS/ LFL criteria been applied. Thus anticipation may potentially mask the LFS/LFL phenotype.

In summary, there are no guidelines that offer both high predictive value and high sensitivity for breast cancer cases. All the criteria based on family history fail to detect new mutations; however, selection based on young age alone does not meet ASCO or other satisfactory guidelines of 10% probability of a mutation.

The lack of a consistent algorithm to identify those at high risk for LFS is particularly concerning given the estimates of Lalloo et al. (48,53) from their population-based study of women with breast cancer before the age of 31 years; they estimated the birth prevalence of p53 germ line mutation carriers to be 1 in 5000, a high figure that will need to be confirmed.

PENETRANCE FOR BREAST CANCER IN P53 MUTATION CARRIERS

Overall data from the IARC TP53 Database (14) confirm findings of smaller series that breast cancer is the most common cancer in LFS, accounting for about 25% to 30% of all cancers. For p53 mutation carriers the median age of breast cancer onset is 33 years, significantly earlier than for non-p53 LFS at 42.5 years. To date no genotype–phenotype correlation, that is, no association of specific p53 mutations by structural or functional domain, or by mutation type, has been observed for breast cancer overall; however, breast cancer median age of onset was significantly younger in those with mutations in the DNA-binding domain (average age 32 years) as compared with missense mutations not in the DNA-binding domain (average age 42 years); age of onset for those with inactivating or likely null mutations was similar to that for mutations in the DNA-binding domain (median age 33 years) (14). This is in contrast to previous findings (57) of a higher incidence and earlier onset of breast cancer in those with mutations in the core DNA-binding domain compared to those with protein truncating or other inactivating mutations.

Overall data demonstrate a very high risk of breast cancer in female p53 mutation carriers (this author is not aware of any reported male breast cancer in p53 germ line mutation carriers). Breast cancer accounts for about 50% of the female cancers (14). While penetrance data specifically on breast cancer are not available, penetrance for cancer for women overall has been estimated. Chompret et al. (10) studied 13 germ line p53 mutation kindreds ascertained through childhood cancer patients with cancer family history before age 46 or multiple primary tumors, and noted an earlier onset for cancer in carrier women as compared to carrier men. They estimated the lifetime cancer risk for women carriers to be nearly 100%, with the risk greatest between ages 16 and 45, with a probability 84% of being affected by age 45, and with breast cancer accounting for 80% of the cancers in that age group. The findings of Hwang et al. (58) were similar, with a much higher risk of cancer in female carriers as compared to male carriers; however that excess risk was not entirely attributable to breast cancer. The period of highest risk for women was from age 20 to 45 years. Cumulative cancer risk estimates were 18% at age 20, 77% by age 40, and 93% by age 50, with breast cancer the most common cancer. Segregation analysis demonstrated an incredibly high relative risk of 1000-fold for female mutation carriers to noncarriers, and a sevenfold increased risk for female carriers as compared to male carriers (59). The data as well-provided statistical evidence for a modifier locus that greatly increases cancer risk for female as compared to male carriers.

RISK OF MULTIPLE PRIMARY CANCERS IN MUTATION CARRIERS

In the initial LFS report (1), some family members had multiple primary cancers. Many case reports and series have noted the association of LFS, p53 germ line mutations, and multiple primary tumors (60–69). The increased risk of subsequent neoplasms was clearly demonstrated in the follow-up studies of the 24 LFS kindreds (6,70), citing the high risk for those with young age of first cancer diagnosis, the occurrence not only of second but of third malignant neoplasms, the spectrum of multiple primary tumors that was primarily composed of the same component tumors observed as initial tumors, and the high frequency of tumors arising in radiation-treated areas. The analysis was not based on p53 mutation status but classic LFS, and included 8 p53 mutation kindreds, 8 non-p53 LFS, and 8 unknown genotype LFS. With an additional 10 to 30 years follow-up the cumulative risk of a second malignant neoplasm was 57% (±10%) SE at 30 years after the first cancer diagnosis, and for a third malignant neoplasm was 38% (±12%) at 10 years after second tumor diagnosis. The highest cumulative risk was observed for those with soft tissue sarcoma as the first cancer (64% (±16%) at 20 years, 100% at 30 years), and the highest relative risk was in those with first cancer diagnosis before age 19 years. Interestingly the risk for multiple primary cancers was similar for p53 and non-p53 LFS. Hwang et al. (58) reported only on p53 mutation carriers with a systematic ascertainment not based on family history or multiple primary tumors, and noted a relative risk of a second cancer of 12 (95% CI 7–20), with a cumulative risk of more than 50% over 20 years. Lalloo et al. (48,53) noted that p53 mutation carriers accounted for most of the second cancers in their series of young (diagnosis before age 31 years) breast cancer patients.

BREAST CANCER AS A FIRST OR SUBSEQUENT CANCER IN LFS

Not only is breast cancer the most common cancer observed in LFS, it plays a major role in subsequent cancers. In the Hisada et al. (71) series, 200 LFS patients had at least one cancer, including 104 females and 96 males; among 30 patients who developed one or more additional cancers, 19 (63%) were in females. The 19 females who had multiple primary tumors experienced a total of 46 cancers (original plus subsequent), with breast cancer accounting for 26.

Forty-five of the original tumors were female breast, and 10 of those patients developed at least one additional tumor, including eight with an additional breast cancer. Breast cancer also accounted for 5/6 (83%) of second cancers in those with an initial sarcoma (the other common original tumor). These data overall suggest an extremely high probability of breast cancer in LFS females, most of which occur before age 45, with a remarkably high probability of a second breast cancer. In Hwang et al. (58), the cumulative risk of female breast cancer in a p53 mutation carrier was over 60% by age 40 years (Strong et al., unpublished data).

RADIATION AND CHEMOTHERAPY RISKS

Most series of LFS families, as well as case reports, have noted not only the high risk of multiple primary tumors but the frequent occurrence of new cancers in radiation-treated sites (48,53,58,60,71–73). Hisada et al. (71) observed only one of 14 subsequent breast cancers arising in a previously irradiated area; however most of the subsequent sarcomas arose in previously irradiated areas, and studies of childhood cancer survivors, especially young soft tissue patients (67,74), have noted a significant excess of female breast cancer, both within and in the absence of radiation therapy.

It seems clear that there is an extremely high risk of multiple primary tumors in LFS patients, occurring both spontaneously and in irradiated sites. This is consistent with observations in heterozygous p53 knockout mice in which radiation significantly accelerates tumor development (75). Many authors have suggested that radiation not be used for cancer treatment in p53 mutation carriers if feasible, and have recommended that the young p53 mutation carrier with breast cancer be treated with a mastectomy instead of conservative surgery with radiotherapy (48,53,76). With this potential impact on treatment, the need to identify the LFS patient becomes more critical, and the need to obtain accurate cancer family history in young breast cancer patients more urgent. Given the second cancer risk in non-p53 LFS kindreds, even testing for p53 may not provide an adequate discriminant (71).

More limited data are available on the role of chemotherapy in the occurrence of multiple primary neoplasms in LFS patients. However the small number of case reports of apparent therapy-related leukemia or myelodysplasia in pediatric (64) and adult (68,69) LFS patients suggest that systematic studies of the risks should be undertaken.

RISK MODIFIERS

The diversity of tumor types and ages within LFS families has been noted since the original report and confirmed with mutation testing (1,14,58), suggesting that additional factors influence tumor development. Early studies of p53 heterozygous knockout mice demonstrated that the tumor types observed were in part dependent on the genetic background of the mice (77). More recently Wu et al. (59) provided statistical evidence for the presence of risk modifiers in p53 mutation kindreds, with a differential effect on female and male carriers. Thus there is reason to try to identify risk modifiers in p53 mutation carriers. Bond et al. (78) investigated variants in the negative regulator of p53, MDM2, a gene that encodes a protein that binds directly to p53 and inhibits its activity. In mice, variation in MDM2 levels significantly affects tumorigenesis, and in human tumors, overexpression of MDM2 is thought to substitute for p53 mutation (79). Bond et al. (78) identified a relatively common variant in the MDM2 promoter (SNP309, with the variant G allele frequency 33–40%) that enhances binding to Sp1 and leads to increased levels of MDM2 mRNA and protein, with reduced stability of p53 in response to cellular stress. In p53 mutation carriers, a significantly earlier age of cancer onset (7–10 years) has been observed in the carriers of at least one SNP309 G allele (78,80–82). Further, those with the SNP309 G allele had a higher frequency of multiple primary tumors (78). More recent work (83) has demonstrated that the SNP309 G allele effect is sex-specific and affects cancer risk exclusively in females, presumably related to the increased affinity for the Sp1 cotranscriptional activator for multiple hormone receptors including the estrogen receptor. It remains to be determined how much this allele accounts for the excess cancer risk in female mutation carriers.

Bougeard et al. (80) have studied the p53 Arg72Pro polymorphism, the hypothesis being that the Arg72 allele, shown to have a greater effect in inducing apoptosis (84), would modify risk. They showed that compared to the Pro72 allele, the Arg72 allele has an effect of reducing the age at cancer onset in p53 mutation carriers. The combined effect of the G allele at SNP309 and one Arg allele at TP53 72 was to reduce the mean age of first tumor onset by 25 years. While numbers of patients studied to date are small, these data strongly support the notion of risk modifiers of p53, and suggest that, given the number of positive and negative regulators of p53 (39), there may be many others yet to be identified.

Anticipation, or the increased cancer risk or earlier age of cancer onset in successive generations, may also serve as a risk modifier in p53 mutation kindreds (55,56). This phenomenon could easily mask the classic signs of LFS, such that mutation carriers with childhood cancer may not present with an LFS/LFL cancer family history. In the longitudinal series of Strong et al. (4,5,58,85), none of the seven proven p53 mutation kindreds would have been identified as LFS at the proband presentation, yet 25 years later all but one, probably a new mutation, fulfill classic LFS. A possible biological mechanism for this effect may involve the shortening of telomeres in p53 mutation carriers (82).

BREAST CANCER PROGNOSIS IN LFS

Many studies have indicated that a p53 somatic mutation is an independent poor prognostic indicator for breast cancer (86), with some data suggesting that the prognosis may be influenced by the nature of the mutation (87). Miller et al. (30) have shown that an expression signature for p53 functional status in breast cancer is more predictive of outcome than p53 sequence analysis, and suggest that p53 may be functionally attenuated in the absence of DNA sequence variants. From those data one might assume that the breast cancer in germ line p53 mutation carriers would also carry a poor prognosis; surprisingly little data are available to support that expectation, and the absence of data perhaps speaks loudly. Given that there are no published survival data for breast cancer in p53 mutation carriers, the frequent reports of multiple primary tumors occurring over 10 to 30 years (71) suggest that many of these patients do not succumb to their breast cancer. Unlike *BRCA1,2* mutation carriers (88), no distinct pathology or prognosis has been associated with the breast cancer in p53 mutation carriers. In the Hwang et al. (58) series, the overall cancer survival for p53 germ line mutation carriers and controls were not different (Strong et al., unpublished data), suggesting that there is not a uniquely poor prognosis. The relative rarity of p53 germ line mutation carriers will make any distinct positive or negative response to specific agents difficult to determine. Despite the increased radiation sensitivity with respect to increased cancer risk associated with p53 mutations in mouse and human (71,75), no unusual acute toxicities have been described in response to radiation or cytotoxic agents.

CANCER SURVEILLANCE AND PREVENTION

Recently the American Cancer Society issued new guidelines for breast screening based on level of risk (89). These recommendations include annual screening with MRI as an adjunct to mammography for women with a 20% to 25% lifetime breast cancer risk, based on evidence accumulated from prospective trials of *BRCA* mutation carriers, and Expert Consensus Opinion for LFS. The *BRCA* studies indicated an increased sensitivity, but reduced specificity, for MRI as compared with mammography. Importantly, fewer interval cancers occurred in the annual MRI screening groups. The recommended age to begin MRI and mammography screening was 30 years, although it was noted that consideration should be given to individual factors such as age of breast cancer diagnosis in the family. The use of MRI is particularly appealing for LFS patients, given the previously cited concerns regarding radiation exposure.

Moule et al. (76) have suggested consideration of long-term tamoxifen treatment for chemoprevention of breast cancer in LFS, given animal data (90) suggesting it could be effective. However it might not be feasible for the young LFS population at risk. Prophylactic mastectomy may also be a viable option for some patients.

Unfortunately there are no defined guidelines for screening or prevention for most LFS cancers. The most frequent tumors would be soft tissue sarcoma, osteosarcoma and brain tumors, none of which lend themselves to presymptomatic screening. New imaging techniques or serum proteomic discriminants are clearly needed. Given the lack of specificity for a distinct cancer type within a family, with the possible exception of adrenal cortical tumors, it is difficult to recommend aggressive screening. Patient education regarding symptoms, regular physical examinations with a physician aware of LFS risk and tumor spectrum, and application of noninvasive screening for melanoma and perhaps colon cancer (91) at an early age seem reasonable.

PSYCHOSOCIAL AND ETHICAL IMPLICATIONS OF GERM LINE P53 MUTATION TESTING

Genetic counseling and testing for p53 germ line mutations has been available since the mid-1990s, but even in kindreds with known mutations the uptake has been below 40% (92).

As genetic counseling and testing for cancer susceptibility has become more common, guidelines for testing have been updated. Current ASCO guidelines support genetic testing in the setting of pre- and posttest counseling if the individual has a personal or family history suggestive of a cancer susceptibility syndrome, the test can be adequately interpreted, and results will affect medical management (93). The increasing integration of p53 mutation status into medical management as evidenced by the recommendation for breast MRI screening and for relative avoidance of radiation therapy provides a more compelling rationale for genetic testing than previously available. As new therapies are developed that target specific lesions in the p53 pathway, additional benefits from knowledge of the p53 status may accrue. Others benefits of knowing one's genotype may come from the opportunity to make informative reproductive choices (94). For those at risk, the benefits also lie in the relief of anxiety for those who test negative for a known familial mutation.

Barriers to effective p53 testing include the previously cited difficulty in defining the guidelines for testing with adequate sensitivity and positive predictive value, the difficulty in eliciting an accurate LFS family history, concerns about insurance and employment discrimination, and concerns about psychological stress of knowing carrier status with the lack of validated risk reduction strategies. Dorval et al. (95) have shown that in the pretest counseling session unaffected at risk individuals from LFS kindreds could reasonably predict their emotional response to positive and negative results disclosure; for those testing positive for the mutation the actual distress responses were less than those estimated. Thus both carriers and noncarriers were able to complete the process without adverse psychological outcomes. While these findings may be in part due to the self-selected nature of the participants, genetic testing is always an option, so that those who may be less confident of their ability to cope may not elect to be tested. Peterson et al. (96) reported use of a video format decision aid for at risk individuals in families with known p53 mutations. The families were dispersed and knowledge of the cancer family history was generally limited. The decision aid provided an opportunity to facilitate awareness of hereditary cancer risks within families. Compared with baseline date, the intervention was associated with significantly increased knowledge about LFS and genetic testing, decreased decisional conflict regarding testing, and decreased cancer worries. This tool provided an opportunity to reach out to those in genetically underserved areas, and provide them with information to determine whether to seek genetic counseling.

In summary, there are likely to be increasing benefits to testing at risk individuals, as well as additional tools to provide support for individuals facing the choice of genetic testing for cancer susceptibility. Fear of discrimination should not have to enter into the decision process.

FUTURE DIRECTIONS

Although LFS is rare, p53 somatic mutations in tumors are not, so there is much interest in identifying new approaches to tumor treatment based on the tumor p53 genotype or functional status. Several groups have developed gene therapy approaches to tumor treatment, with the simple idea that replacing the wild-type p53 would resolve the problem. There has been some success in local control with this approach in various tumors, using an adenoviral p53 delivery system (97,98). Could this approach help patients with germ line p53 mutations? There is now at least "proof of principle," an example of p53 therapy in a LFS patient, with evidence of treated tumor regression (99).

In this case an LFS patient had multiple lesions of an aggressive embryonal carcinoma refractory to treatment. One lesion was responsible for the symptoms, and was treated with experimental advexin p53 therapy. The treated tumor showed significant, well-documented regression, while the untreated lesions progressed. While this approach may not be practical for many patients as tumor has to be accessible for injection, it represents a new example of "molecular cancer therapeutics," and some hope for "personalized medicine" for LFS patients (100).

In mouse models additional new treatments that target the p53 pathway have been shown to cause significant tumor regression. As most human tumors include mutation or functional inactivation of the p53 pathway, one approach is to reactivate the p53 pathway to initiate apoptosis or senescence. Several papers have recently surprisingly demonstrated that established mouse tumors were sensitive to p53 reactivation (101–103). For these strategies to be helpful in LFS tumors, presumably the wild-type allele or some other p53 family member would have to be activated. Other approaches include developing small molecule inhibitors of the p53 negative regulator MDM2, such as the nutlins (104,105), thus freeing up more p53. An additional approach that might be more relevant to LFS patients focuses on genes and proteins that are downstream of p53, including the p53 family member p73 (106). This creative study targeted another negative regulator of p53 (and family members p63 and p73) iASPP, a protein that is often overexpressed in breast cancer. The investigators used a minimal p53-derived apoptotic peptide to bind iASPP and derepress p73, subsequently activating p73-mediated cell death. While tumors have returned in all of these model systems, the initial regression has been impressive, and there is expectation that further combined therapies may be even more effective.

CONCLUSIONS

Breast cancer is the most common cancer in LFS, and occurs at an extremely early age. There are recommended modalities to screen (MRI and mammography) and manage (mastectomy without radiation therapy) the breast cancer successfully in many cases. However, successful screening and management require early recognition of LFS to initiate screening, a problem given the limited knowledge of LFS cancer family history, the frequency of de novo mutations, and the lack of a highly sensitive and highly predictive algorithm to identify LFS patients. Further, management of a young onset breast cancer in LFS may be only the beginning; the patient will be at continuing cancer risk throughout life. Optimal patient management could require multidisciplinary teams of oncologists, geneticists, genetic counselors, diagnostic radiologists, "alert clinicians," chemoprevention specialists, biomarker laboratories, etc., teams and resources rarely available. Patient advocacy groups have been difficult to maintain for the rare cancer-prone LFS; however as more at risk individuals are seeking counseling and the LFS knowledge base expanding, there may be a new opportunities to develop needed support groups. With the research focus on mechanisms to maintain or reactivate the p53 pathway, new approaches to prevention and treatment will hopefully emerge.

REFERENCES

1. Li FP, Fraumeni JF Jr. Soft-tissue sarcomas, breast cancer, and other neoplasms. A familial syndrome? Ann Intern Med 1969a; 71:747–52.

2. Li FP, Fraumeni JF Jr. Rhabdomyosarcoma in children: epidemiologic study and identification of a familial cancer syndrome. J Natl Cancer Inst 1969b; 43:1365–73.
3. Birch JM, Hartley AL, Marsden HB, et al. Excess risk of breast cancer in the mothers of children with soft tissue sarcomas. Br J Cancer 1984; 49:325–31.
4. Strong LC, Stine M, Norsted TL. Cancer in survivors of childhood soft tissue sarcoma and their relatives. J Natl Cancer Inst 1987; 79:1213–20.
5. Williams WR, Strong LC. Genetic epidemiology of soft tissue sarcomas in children. In: Muller H, Weber W, editors. Familial Cancer, First International Research Conference, Basel: Karger, 1985:151–3.
6. Li FP, Fraumeni JF Jr, Mulvihill JJ, et al. A cancer family syndrome in twenty-four kindreds. Cancer Res 1988; 48:5358–62.
7. Malkin D, Li FP, Strong LC, et al. Germ line p53 mutations in a familial syndrome of breast cancer, sarcomas, and other neoplasms. Science 1990; 250:1233–8.
8. Srivastava S, Zou ZQ, Pirollo K, et al. Germ-line transmission of a mutated p53 gene in a cancer-prone family with Li–Fraumeni syndrome. Nature 1990; 348:747–9.
9. Hollstein M, Sidransky D, Vogelstein B, et al. p53 Mutations in human cancers. Science 1991; 253:49–53.
10. Chompret A, Brugieres L, Ronsin M, et al. p53 Germline mutations in childhood cancers and cancer risk for carrier individuals. Br J Cancer 2000; 82:1932–7.
11. Birch JM, Hartley AL, Tricker KJ, et al. Prevalence and diversity of constitutional mutations in the p53 gene among 21 Li–Fraumeni families. Cancer Res 1994a; 54:1298–304.
12. Evans DG, Birch JM, Thorneycroft M, et al. Low rate of TP53 germline mutations in breast cancer/sarcoma families not fulfilling classical criteria for Li–Fraumeni syndrome. J Med Genet 2002; 39:941–4.
13. Chompret A, Abel A, Stoppa-Lyonnet D, et al. Sensitivity and predictive value of criteria for p53 germline mutation screening. J Med Genet 2001; 38:43–7.
14. Olivier M, Goldgar DE, Sodha N, et al. Li–Fraumeni and related syndromes: correlation between tumor type, family structure, and TP53 genotype. Cancer Res 2003; 63:6643–50.
15. Wagner J, Portwine C, Rabin K, et al. High frequency of germline p53 mutations in childhood adrenocortical cancer. J Natl Cancer Inst 1994; 86:1707–10.
16. Varley JM, McGown G, Thorncroft M, et al. Are there low-penetrance TP53 Alleles? Evidence from childhood adrenocortical tumors. Am J Hum Genet 1999; 65:995–1006.
17. Krutilkova V, Trkova M, Fleitz J, et al. Identification of five new families strengthens the link between childhood choroid plexus carcinoma and germline TP53 mutations. Eur J Cancer 2005; 41(11):1597–603.
18. Diller L, Sexsmith E, Gottlieb A, et al. Germline p53 mutations are frequently detected in young children with rhabdomyosarcoma. J Clin Invest 1995; 95:1606–11.
19. Birch JM, Alston RD, McNally RJ, et al. Relative frequency and morphology of cancers in carriers of germline TP53 mutations. Oncogene 2001; 20:4621–8.
20. Bougeard G, Brugieres L, Chompret A, et al. Screening for TP53 rearrangements in families with the Li–Fraumeni syndrome reveals a complete deletion of the TP53 gene. Oncogene 2003; 22:840–6.
21. Evans SC, Mims B, McMasters KM, et al. Exclusion of a p53 germline mutation in a classic Li–Fraumeni syndrome family. Hum Genet 1998; 102:681–6.
22. Birch JM, Heighway J, Teare MD, et al. Linkage studies in a Li–Fraumeni family with increased expression of p53 protein but no germline mutation in p53. Br J Cancer 1994b; 70: 1176–81.
23. Bell DW, Varley JM, Szydlo TE, et al. Heterozygous germ line hCHK2 mutations in Li–Fraumeni syndrome. Science 1999; 286:2528–31.
24. Sodha N, Houlston RS, Bullock S, et al. Increasing evidence that germline mutations in CHEK2 do not cause Li–Fraumeni syndrome. Hum Mutat 2002; 20:460–2.
25. Siddiqui R, Onel K, Facio F, et al. The TP53 mutational spectrum and frequency of CHEK2*1100delC in Li–Fraumeni-like kindreds. Fam Cancer 2005; 4:177–81.

26. Bachinski LL, Olufemi S-E, Zhou X, et al. Genetic mapping of a third Li–Fraumeni syndrome (LFS) predisposition locus to human chromosome 1q23. Cancer Res 2005; 65:427–9.

27. Lane DP, Crawford LV. T antigen is bound to a host protein in SV40 transformed cells. Nature 1979; 278:261–3.

28. Linzer DIH, Levine AJ. Characterisations of a 54,000 MW cellular SV40 tumor antigen present in SV40-transformed cells and uninfected embryonal carcinoma cells. Cell 1979; 17: 43–52.

29. Finlay CA, Hinds PW, Levine AJ. The p53 proto-oncogene can act as a suppressor of transformation. Cell 1989; 57:1083–93.

30. Miller LD, Smeds J, George J, et al. An expression signature for p53 status in human breast cancer predicts mutation status, transcriptional effects, and patient survival. Proc Natl Acad Sci 2005; 102:13550–5.

31. Donehower LA, Harvey M, Slagle BL, et al. Mice deficient for p53 are developmentally normal but susceptible to spontaneous tumours. Nature 1992; 356:215–21.

32. Lane DP. p53 Guardian of the genome. Nature 1992; 358:15–6.

33. Varley JM, Thorncroft M, McGown G, et al. A detailed study of loss of heterozygosity on chromosome 17 in tumours from Li–Fraumeni patients carrying a mutation to the TP53 gene. Oncogene 1997; 14:865–71.

34. Venkatachalam S, Shi YP, Jones SN, et al. Retention of wild-type p53 in tumors from p53 heterozygous mice: reduction of p53 dosage can promote cancer formation. EMBO J 1998; 17:4657–67.

35. Lynch CJ, Milner J. Loss of one p53 allele results in four-fold reduction of p53 mRNA and protein: a basis for p53 haplo-insufficiency. Oncogene 2006; 25:3463–70.

36. Attardi LD, Jacks T. The role of p53 in tumour suppression: lessons from mouse models [review]. Cell Mol Life Sci 1999; 55:48–63.

37. Donehower LA. The p53-deficient mouse: a model for basic and applied cancer studies [review]. Semin Cancer Biol 1996; 7:269–78.

38. Lozano G, Liu G. Mouse models dissect the role of p53 in cancer and development. Semin Cancer Biol 1998; 8:337–44.

39. Lozano G, Zambetti GP. What have animal models taught us about the p53 pathway? [review] J Pathol 2005; 205:206–20.

40. Prosser J, Elder PA, Condie A, et al. Mutations in p53 do not account for heritable breast cancer: a study in five affected families. Br J Cancer 1991; 63:181–4.

41. Warren W, Eeles RA, Ponder BA, et al. No evidence for germline mutations in exons 5-9 of the p53 gene in 25 breast cancer families. Oncogene 1992; 7:1043–6.

42. Patel UA, Perry M, Crane-Robinson C. Screening for germline mutations of the p53 gene in familial breast cancer patients. Eur J Clin Invest 1995; 25:132–7.

43. Zelada-Hedman M, Borresen-Dale AL, Claro A, et al. Screening for TP53 mutations in patients and tumours from 109 Swedish breast cancer families. Br J Cancer 1997; 75:1201–4.

44. Rapakko K, Allinen M, Syrjakoski K, et al. Germline TP53 alterations in Finnish breast cancer families are rare and occur at conserved mutation-prone sites. Br J Cancer 2001; 84: 116–9.

45. Balz V, Prisack HB, Bier H, et al. Analysis of BRCA1, TP53, and TSG101 germline mutations in German breast and/or ovarian cancer families. Cancer Genet Cytogenet 2002; 138:120–7.

46. Walsh T, Casadei S, Coats KH, et al. Spectrum of mutations in BRCA1, BRCA2, CHEK2, and TP53 in families at high risk of breast cancer. JAMA 2006; 295:1379–88.

47. Lidereau R, Soussi T. Absence of p53 germ-line mutations in bilateral breast cancer patients. Hum Genet 1992; 89:250–2.

48. Lalloo F, Varley J, Moran A, et al. BRCA1, BRCA2 and TP53 mutations in very early-onset breast cancer with associated risks to relatives. Eur J Cancer 2006; 42:1143–50.

49. Sidransky D, Tokino T, Helzlsouer K, et al. Inherited p53 gene mutations in breast cancer. Cancer Res 1992; 52:2984–6.

50. Borresen AL, Andersen TI, Garber J, et al. Screening for germ line TP53 mutations in breast cancer patients. Cancer Res 1992; 52:3234–6.

51. Martin AM, Kanetsky PA, Amirimani B, et al. Germline TP53 mutations in breast cancer families with multiple primary cancers: is TP53 a modifier of BRCA1? J Med Genet 2003; 40:e34.

52. Manoukian S, Peissel B, Pensotti V, et al. Germline mutations of TP53 and BRCA2 genes in breast cancer/sarcoma families. Eur J Cancer 2007; 43:6.

53. Lalloo F, Varley J, Ellis D, Early Onset Breast Cancer Study Group et al. Prediction of pathogenic mutations in patients with early-onset breast cancer by family history. Lancet 2003; 361:1101–2.

54. Schneider KA, DiGianni LM, Patenaude AF, et al. Accuracy of cancer family histories: comparison of two breast cancer syndromes. Genet Test 2004; 8:222–8.

55. Trkova M, Hladikova M, Kasal P, et al. Is there anticipation in the age at onset of cancer in families with Li–Fraumeni syndrome? J Hum Genet 2002; 47:381–6.

56. Brown BW, Costello TJ, Hwang S-J, et al. Generation or birth cohort effect in Li–Fraumeni syndrome. Hum Genet 2005; 118:489–98.

57. Birch JM, Blair V, Kelsey AM, et al. Cancer phenotype correlates with constitutional TP53 genotype in families with the Li–Fraumeni syndrome. Oncogene 1998; 17:1061–8.

58. Hwang S-J, Lozano G, Amos CI, et al. Germline p53 mutations in a cohort with childhood sarcoma: sex differences in cancer risk. Am J Hum Genet 2003; 72:975–83.

59. Wu C-C, Shete S, Amos CI, et al. Joint effects of germ-line p53 mutation and sex on cancer risk in Li–Fraumeni syndrome. Cancer Res 2006; 66:8287–92.

60. Malkin D, Jolly KW, Barbier N, et al. Germline mutations of the p53 tumor-suppressor gene in children and young adults with second malignant neoplasms. N Engl J Med 1992; 326: 1309–15.

61. Felix CA, Strauss EA, D'Amico D, et al. A novel germline p53 splicing mutation in a pediatric patient with a second malignant neoplasm. Oncogene 1993; 8:1203–10.

62. King P, Craft AW, Malcolm AJ. p53 Expression in three separate tumours from a patient with Li–Fraumeni's syndrome. J Clin Pathol 1993; 46:676–7.

63. Russo CL, McIntyre J, Goorin AM, et al. Secondary breast cancer in patients presenting with osteosarcoma: possible involvement of germline p53 mutations. Med Pediatr Oncol 1994; 23:354–8.

64. Felix CA, Hosler MR, Provisor D, et al. The p53 gene in pediatric therapy-related leukemia and myelodysplasia. Blood 1996; 87:4376–81.

65. Nadav Y, Pastorino U, Nicholson AG. Multiple synchronous lung cancers and atypical adenomatous hyperplasia in Li–Fraumeni syndrome. Histopathology 1998; 33:52–4.

66. Potzsch C, Voigtlander T, Lubbert M. p53 Germline mutation in a patient with Li–Fraumeni syndrome and three metachronous malignancies. J Cancer Res Clin Oncol 2002; 128: 456–60.

67. Cohen RJ, Curtis RE, Inskip PD, et al. The risk of developing second cancers among survivors of childhood soft tissue sarcoma. Cancer 2005; 103:2391–6.

68. Kuribayashi K, Matsunaga T, Sakai T, et al. A patient with TP53 germline mutation developed Bowen's disease and myelodysplastic syndrome with myelofibrosis after chemotherapy against ovarian cancer. Intern Med 2005; 44:490–5.

69. Anensen N, Skavland J, Stapnes C, et al. Acute myelogenous leukemia in a patient with Li–Fraumeni syndrome treated with valproic acid, theophyllamine and all-trans retinoic acid: a case report. Leukemia 2006; 20:734–6.

70. Li FP, Fraumeni JF Jr. Prospective study of a family cancer syndrome. JAMA 1982; 47: 2692–4.

71. Hisada M, Garber JE, Fung CY, et al. Multiple primary cancers in families with Li–Fraumeni syndrome. J Natl Cancer Inst 1998; 90:606–11.

72. Limacher JM, Frebourg T, Natarajan-Ame S, et al. Two metachronous tumors in the radiotherapy fields of a patient with Li–Fraumeni syndrome. Int J Cancer 2001; 96:238–42.

73. Evans DG, Birch JM, Ramsden RT, et al. Malignant transformation and new primary tumours after therapeutic radiation for benign disease: substantial risks in certain tumour prone syndromes. J Med Genet 2006; 43:289–94.

74. Heyn R, Haeberlen V, Newton WA, et al. Second malignant neoplasms in children treated for rhabdomyosarcoma. Intergroup Rhabdomyosarcoma Study Committee. J Clin Oncol 1993; 11:262–70.

75. Kemp CJ, Wheldon T, Balmain A. p53-Deficient mice are extremely susceptible to radiation-induced tumorigenesis. Nature Genet 1994; 8:66–9.

76. Moule RN, Jhavar SG, Eeles RA. Genotype phenotype correlation in Li–Fraumeni syndrome kindreds and its implications for management. Fam Cancer 2006; 5:129–33.

77. Harvey M, McArthur MJ, Montgomery CA Jr, et al. Genetic background alters the spectrum of tumors that develop in p53-deficient mice. FASEB J 1993; 7:938–43.

78. Bond GL, Hu W, Bond EE, et al. A single nucleotide polymorphism in the Mdm2 promoter attenuates the p53 tumor suppressor pathway and accelerates tumor formation in humans. Cell 2004; 119:591–602.

79. Bond GL, Levine AJ. A single nucleotide polymorphism in the p53 pathway interacts with gender, environmental stresses and tumor genetics to influence cancer in humans [review]. Oncogene 2007; 26:1317–23.

80. Bougeard G, Baert-Desurmont S, Tournier I, et al. Impact of the MDM2 SNP309 and TP53 Arg72Pro polymorphism on age of tumour onset in Li–Fraumeni syndrome. J Med Genet 2006; 43:531–3.

81. Ruijs MW, Schmidt MK, Nevanlinna H, et al. The single-nucleotide polymorphism 309 in the MDM2 gene contributes to the Li–Fraumeni syndrome and related phenotypes. Eur J Hum Genet 2007; 15:110–4.

82. Tabori U, Nanda S, Druker H, et al. Younger age of cancer initiation is associated with shorter telomere length in Li–Fraumeni Syndrome. Cancer Res 2007; 67:1415–8.

83. Bond GL, Hirshfield KM, Kirchhoff T, et al. MDM2 SNP309 accelerates tumor formation in a gender-specific and hormone-dependent manner. Cancer Res 2006; 66(10):5104–10.

84. Dumont P, Leu JI, Della PA III, et al. The codon 72 polymorphic variants of p53 have markedly different apoptotic potential. Nat Genet 2003; 33:357–65.

85. Lustbader ED, Williams WR, Bondy ML, et al. Segregation analysis of cancer in families of childhood soft-tissue sarcoma patients. Am J Hum Genet 1992; 51:344–56.

86. Petitjean A, Achatz MI, Borresen-Dale AL, et al. TP53 mutations in human cancers: functional selection and impact on cancer prognosis and outcomes [review]. Oncogene 2007; 26:2157–65.

87. Lai H, Ma F, Trapido E, et al. Spectrum of p53 tumor suppressor gene mutations and breast cancer survival. Breast Cancer Res Treat 2004; 83:57–66.

88. Honrado E, Benitez J, Palacios J. Histopathology of BRCA1- and BRCA2-associated breast cancer. Crit Rev Oncol Hematol 2006; 59:27–39.

89. Saslow D, Boetes C, Burke W, et al. American Cancer Society guidelines for breast screening with MRI as an adjunct to mammography. Cancer J Clin 2007; 57:75–89.

90. Hursting SD, Perkins SN, Haines DC, et al. Chemoprevention of spontaneous tumorigenesis in p53-knockout mice. Cancer Res 1995; 55:3949–53.

91. Wong P, Verselis SJ, Garber JE, et al. Prevalence of early onset colorectal cancer in 397 patients with classic Li–Fraumeni syndrome. Gastroenterology 2006; 130:73–9.

92. Patenaude AF, Schneider K, Kieffer SA, et al. Acceptance of invitations for p53 and BRCA1 predisposition testing: factors influencing potential utilization of cancer genetic testing. Psycho Oncol 1996; 5:241–50.

93. American Society of Clinical Oncology Policy Statement Update: Genetic Testing for Cancer Susceptibility. J Clin Oncol 2003; 21:2397–406.

94. Rechitsky S, Verlinsky O, Chistokhina A, et al. Preimplantation genetic diagnosis for cancer predisposition. Reprod Biomed 2002; 5:148–55.

95. Dorval M, Patenaude AF, Schneider KA, et al. Anticipated versus actual emotional reactions to disclosure of results of genetic tests for cancer susceptibility: findings from p53 and BRCA1 testing programs. J Clin Oncol 2000; 18:2135–42.

96. Peterson SK, Pentz RD, Blanco AM, et al. Evaluation of a decision aid for families considering p53 genetic counseling and testing. Genet Med 2006; 8:226–33.

97. Swisher SG, Roth JA, Komaki R, et al. Induction of p53-regulated genes and tumor regression in lung cancer patients after intratumoral delivery of adenoviral p53 (INGN 201) and radiation therapy. Clin Cancer Res 2003; 9:93–101.

98. Reid TR, Freeman S, Post L, et al. Effects of Onyx-015 among metastatic colorectal cancer patients that have failed prior treatment with 5-FU/leucovorin. Cancer Gene Ther 2005; 12: 673–81.

99. Senzer N, Nemunaitis J, Nemunaitis M, et al. p53 Therapy in a patient with Li–Fraumeni syndrome. Mol Cancer Ther 2007; 6:1478–82.

100. Kurzrock R. Studies in target-based treatment. Mol Cancer Ther 2007; 6:1477.

101. Martins CP, Brown-Swigart L, Evan GI. Modeling the therapeutic efficacy of p53 restoration in tumors. Cell 2006; 127:1323–34.

102. Ventura A, Kirsch DG, McLaughlin ME, et al. Restoration of p53 function leads to tumour regression in vivo. Nature 2007; 445:661–5.

103. Xue W, Zender L, Miething C, et al. Senescence and tumour clearance is triggered by p53 restoration in murine liver carcinomas. Nature 2007; 445:656–60.

104. Vassilev LT. MDM2 inhibitors for cancer therapy. Trends Mol Med 2007; 13:23–31.

105. Sarek G, Kurki S, Enback J, et al. Reactivation of the p53 pathway as a treatment modality for KSHV-induced lymphomas. J Clin Invest 2007; 117:1019–28.

106. Bell HS, Dufes C, O'Prey J, et al. A p53-derived apoptotic peptide derepresses p73 to cause tumor regression in vivo. J Clin Invest 2007; 117:1008–18.

7

Rare Causes of Inherited Breast Cancer Susceptibility

Katherine L. Nathanson
University of Pennsylvania School of Medicine, Philadelphia, Pennsylvania, U.S.A.

INTRODUCTION

The major genes associated with inherited susceptibility to breast cancer are *BRCA1* and *BRCA2*. However, breast cancer is a component of other cancer susceptibility syndromes, including Li-Fraumeni syndrome (LFS), Cowden syndrome, Peutz-Jeghers syndrome (PJS), and hereditary gastric cancer. LFS and Cowden disease, caused by mutations in *TP53* and *PTEN*, respectively, are discussed in Chapters 6 and 5. This chapter is divided into two major parts: (*i*) other rare familial cancer syndromes with breast cancer as a component and (*ii*) mutations in DNA damage response genes associated with an increased risk of breast cancer, notably in families with multiple breast cancer cases.

RARE FAMILIAL CANCER SYNDROMES WITH BREAST CANCER AS A COMPONENT

Peutz-Jeghers Syndrome

PJS is characterized by hamartomatous polyps in the small bowel and pigmented macules of the buccal mucosa, lips, fingers, and toes (1). Mutations in *STK11/LKB1*, a serine-threonine kinase located on chromosome 19q13.3, have been identified in 50% to 80% of patients with PJS (2–8). *STK11/LKB1* is the only kinase identified as leading to cancer predisposition when inactivated in the germline. Loss of the wild type allele in hamartomas and adenocarcinomas in patients with PJS is consistent with its role as tumor suppressor gene (9). Of note, despite the increased risk of breast cancer associated with PJS, mutations in *STK11/LKB1* do not appear to play an important role in sporadic breast cancers (10). As mutations cannot be identified in all patients with PJS, it has been postulated that there is a second gene, which is suggested to be located at 19q13.4 (11,12).

Several studies have examined the cancer risk in Peutz-Jeghers patients. PJS patients are at greatly increased risk of gastrointestinal cancers and gynecological cancers (13–15). Prior to the identification of *LKB1* as the causative gene in PJS, it had been suggested that the risk of breast cancer was increased in PJS patients based on case reports of early onset and bilateral breast cancer. The first retrospective study looking at cancer risk in Peutz-Jeghers families described an increased relative risk in affected women for breast and gynecological tumors together of 20.3 (13). In that study, the mean age of breast cancer diagnosis was 39. However, only 16 women were included in the study. A follow-up study by Giardiello et al. using a PJS registry also showed a 15-fold increased risk of breast cancer (16). However, as the study was registry based, it may not have contained systematic follow-up of all patients, thus risk could be inflated.

Two more recent studies have evaluated breast cancer risk in patients with PJS, with disparate results. The larger study by Hearle et al. incorporates data from eight centers seeing patients with PJS, which includes data from several earlier papers—the two cited above as well as a study of 240 patients with PJS reported on by Lim et al. in 2004 (8,13,14,16). Hearle et al. included PJS patients both with and without identified mutations in *LKB1*. Seventy percent of 226 women with PJS had mutations. Sixteen of the women developed breast cancer (and one male) in an age range of 35 to 61. The risk of breast cancer did not differ between those with and without identified mutations. The risk for developing breast cancer was 8% [95% confidence interval (CI) 4–17], 13% (95% CI 7–24), 31% (95% CI 18–50), and 45% (95% CI 27–68) at ages 40, 50, 60, and 70, respectively. The authors estimate that this translates into a six-fold increased relative risk. Of note, this relative risk is lower than that previously published in the studies incorporated into this series of PJS patients. In contrast, a study by Mehenni et al. comprising only patients with identified *LKB1* mutations did not find an increased risk of breast cancer (15). The study included 73 women, only one of which developed breast cancer. However, the risks for gastrointestinal cancers (63% 95% CI 23–82) were similar to those reported by Hearle et al. (57% 95% CI 39–76), suggesting that the populations are not substantially different with respect to other cancer risks. It is possible that the differences are due to inclusion of patients without identified mutations in the study by Hearle et al., but the risk is not significantly different in patients with and without detectable mutations in *LKB1* (14). As the patients come from different populations, it is possible that other factors modify the penetrance and, thus, breast cancer risk associated with PJS, such as age of menarche and menopause, parity, and genetic variants in other genes. However, modifiers likely would not explain such a large difference in risk. Based on the papers with higher risk, screening for breast cancer in PJS patients is recommended starting at age 20, with mammography every two years and breast exam by a physician yearly (1). In addition, these patients may be eligible for research screening studies that include women at high risk of breast cancer and breast magnetic resonance imaging (MRI) should be considered.

Hereditary Diffuse Gastric Cancer

Hereditary gastric cancer is a rare autosomal dominant cancer susceptibility syndrome in which patients have a greatly increased risk of diffuse gastric cancer—67% (95% CI 39–99) for men and 83% for women (95% CI 58–99) by age 80 (17). Germline mutations have been identified in E-cadherin (*CDH1*) (18) located at 16p22.1. Huntsman et al. have suggested six criteria for the clinical diagnosis of hereditary diffuse gastric cancer (HDGC), however only 30% of families meeting these criteria have identified *CHD1* mutations (19). In families with a documented case of diffuse gastric cancer at or before age 50 and a family history of gastric cancer, 50% have identified mutations in *CDH1*. Several studies have supported the importance of prophylactic gastrectomy in families with *CDH1* mutations, as 17 of 18 asymptomatic carriers with prophylactic gastrectomy demonstrated early (intramucosal) gastric cancers (20–23).

Multiple studies have supported an increased risk for lobular breast cancer in HDGC families (17,19,23–25). In sporadic lobular breast cancers, there commonly is loss of E-cadherin expression usually resulting from the somatic mutation of one allele and loss of heterozygosity of *CDH1* (26,27). The initial observation was made by Keller et al. who reported a woman with a germline mutation in *CDH1* with metachronous development of diffuse gastric cancer and lobular breast cancer (24). Subsequently, after review of the breast cancer pathology in HDGC families it was found for those that could be located, lobular breast cancer was diagnosed (17). Lobular breast cancer is observed in HDGC families with and without *CDH1* mutations (19). Recently, the criteria for genetic testing for *CDH1* mutations have been expanded to include any family with both gastric cancer and lobular breast cancer based on mutation positive families that meet this criterion (23).

The penetrance for lobular breast cancer is estimated to be 39% by age 80 (95% CI 12–84) in women with germline *CDH1* mutations in the absence of other causes of cancer/mortality. Thus, this estimate is based on women who are unaffected with gastric cancer, and as the prevalence of gastric cancer is so high, a woman is much more likely to develop gastric cancer before breast cancer. When the two cancer risks are combined, the risk of gastric cancer is 72% and of breast cancer is 18% (17). Screening for lobular breast cancer in families with HDGC is recommended starting at age 35 or five years earlier than the earliest age of diagnosis. Importantly, in addition to routine screening with physician exam and mammography, MRI is recommended due to the increased difficulty of detecting lobular breast cancers using traditional methods, such as mammography (28).

VARIANTS IN DNA DAMAGE RESPONSE GENES ASSOCIATED WITH AN INCREASED RISK OF BREAST CANCER, NOTABLY IN FAMILIES WITH MULTIPLE BREAST CANCER CASES

Ataxia Telangiectasia Mutated

Individuals homozygous for germline mutations in ataxia telangiectasia mutated (*ATM*) have ataxia telangiectasia (AT), an autosomal recessive disorder characterized by cerebellar ataxia, oculocutaneous telangiectasias, radiation hypersensitivity, and an increased incidence of malignancy (29). AT homozygotes have cancer risks 60 to 180 times greater than the general population including non-Hodgkins lymphoma (nearly 100% lifetime risk) and breast and ovarian cancer (30). Heterozygosity for germline mutations in *ATM* was initially hypothesized by Swift et al. to confer an increased breast cancer risk and that screening mammography, a source of ionizing radiation, could theoretically increase the penetrance of such mutations (31). An initial study supporting the hypothesis was criticized due to the exceptionally low rate of breast cancer among the controls. In addition, subsequent studies did not consistently support a link between *ATM* mutation heterozygosity and breast cancer susceptibility, thus the association remained controversial for many years.

Two major approaches have been used to address the issue of whether females with heterozygous mutations in *ATM* are at increased risk of breast cancer. The first approach is the study of families ascertained through the identification of a proband affected with AT, and comparison of breast cancer risk female family members to the general population or married-in family members. Unaffected family members of AT patients consistently have an increased risk of breast cancer, with relative risks ranging from 1.5 to 9 (32–41). Later studies, which include more families, have reported relative risks between 2.4 and 3.4, with higher risks among younger women. Many of the earlier studies also suggested a higher risk of breast cancer among younger women. Two recent studies from the Nordic countries and United Kingdom are the largest to date of heterozygous *ATM* mutation carriers ascertained through families with members with AT. In the study from the Nordic countries, 1445 blood relatives of 75 AT patients were evaluated (42). Olsen et al. found a standardized incidence ratio (SIR) of 1.7 (95% CI 1.2–2.4), which was increased to 2.9 among those under age 55 (95% CI 1.8–4.5). The risk was most pronounced among mothers of the AT proband (SIR 8.1, 95% CI 3.3–17). When these women were excluded, there was no increased risk of breast cancer among female carriers of the *ATM* mutation. Given that risk was limited to mothers of probands, the authors question a direct relationship between *ATM* heterozygosity and breast cancer risk and postulate rather an in utero effect. In the study from the United Kingdom, cancer incidence and mortality data was obtained for 1160 relatives of 169 AT patients, including 247 obligate heterozygotes (43). As genotype was unknown, Thompson et al. factored in the probability of the family member being a heterozygote into their calculations when comparing the rate of cancers in *ATM* heterozygotes to those expected to the general population. They found a relative risk of 2.23 (95% CI 1.16–4.28) for *ATM* heterozygotes as compared to the general population; the risk increased to 4.94 (95% CI 1.9–12.9) in those under 50 years of age. Unlike the study by Olsen et al., they did not find a risk restricted to mothers of AT patients; in fact, the highest risk was seen in aunts of AT carriers—2.6 (95% CI 1.33–5.5). However, mothers and aunts were the groups with the highest SIRs. Together, these results support a moderate increase in breast cancer risk in female heterozygous carriers of *ATM* mutations.

A second approach has been to use mutational analysis in early onset breast cancer cases to define the contribution of *ATM* to breast cancer risk. In the first such study of 401 women diagnosed with breast cancer under the age 40, *ATM* mutation frequency did not differ from that of controls (44). However, protein truncation testing (PTT) was used for mutation screening, which may have missed some mutations. Null results also were reported by Izatt et al. in 100 breast cancer cases under the age of 40 and by Chen et al. in 100 breast cancer patients with a family history, as well as several smaller studies (45–49). In a study of 483 unselected Norwegian breast cancer cases, 150 under age 55, screened for the Norwegian founder *ATM* mutations, no increase in prevalence over controls was found (50). However, Broeks et al. did find an increased rate of *ATM* mutations in 82 patients diagnosed with breast cancer before age 45, 40% of whom had contralateral disease and all of whom had been exposed to low-dose radiation at a young age (51). This study suggested that exposure to even low-dose radiation at a young age may be an important component of breast cancer risk in the presence of an *ATM* mutation. The most recent, and most definitive study, examined the full sequence of *ATM* (63 exons) in 443 familial breast cancer cases (*BRCA1/2* negative, at least three breast cancer cases) and 521 controls (52). Using familial based cases gives an estimated four-fold increase in power over sporadic cases. Twelve deleterious mutations were identified in cases and two in controls ($p = 0.0043$). These results demonstrate that heterozygous *ATM* mutations are associated with breast cancer with a relative risk of 2.37 (95% CI 1.5–3.8). Unlike the family-based studies, there was no difference in relative risk in breast cancer cases under age 50, although the estimated risk under age 50 (2.5, 95% CI 1.41–4.17) is within the range predicted by those studies. The proband phenotype and family history were not significantly different in the breast cancer case probands with identified *ATM* mutations as compared with those without such mutations.

The type of mutation in *ATM* (missense vs. truncating) has been postulated to be associated with differing risks of breast cancer (53), with missense mutations carrying a higher risk of breast cancer. The model initially was suggested based on the apparent differences in risk identified using the two methods outlined above—family-based studies of AT patients and case–control studies of breast cancer patients. Gatti et al. suggested that missense mutations would have a dominant negative phenotype, resulting in a more striking phenotype than simple-loss of protein. While this hypothesis would have explained the lack of identified *ATM* mutation carriers in studies of breast cancer patients, there did not appear to be a difference in breast cancer risk in families of AT patients with truncating and missense mutations. While some initial studies appeared to support this hypothesis (54,55), more recent studies have not supported a correlation between missense mutations and higher breast cancer risk. In a more recent study, missense mutations were associated with a decreased risk of breast cancer (43). In a study by Rahman et al. of 433 breast cancer cases and 521 controls, 37 nonsynonymous variants were identified, 12 in both cases and controls, 13 only in cases and 10 only in controls (52). Two of the variants present only in cases previously had been demonstrated to be associated with AT. None of the remaining nonsynonymous variants were associated with either case or control status nor did they cluster in any region of the protein. These studies do not support any difference in risk between missense and protein truncating mutations in *ATM*.

In summary, the risk associated with a heterozygous *ATM* mutation, based on studies of AT families and breast cancer probands, has converged on an approximately two-fold increase in risk. The estimate of breast cancer population attributable risk due to *ATM* mutations is 0.86% (95% CI 0.32–1.72). Although recent studies have clarified the association of *ATM* heterozygous mutations with breast cancer risk, there are a number of unanswered questions which need to be addressed by larger studies (or pooled resources). Such questions include why some studies show a much greater association in the mothers of AT patients than in more distant relatives and whether there are mutation specific differences in breast cancer risk. In addition, important clinical questions remain to be answered: whether exposure to radiation, both diagnostic and therapeutic, is associated with increased sensitivity in carriers of *ATM* mutations and how and if clinical testing for *ATM* mutations should be implemented. Currently clinical testing for *ATM* mutations is not recommended.

Checkpoint Kinase 2

Checkpoint kinase 2 (CHEK2), encoded by the gene *CHEK2* located on chromosome 22q12.1, is a protein involved in cell-cycle control. CHEK2 plays an important role in mediating cell-cycle progression in response to DNA damage (56). In response to DNA damage, it is quickly activated by *ATM*-mediated phosphorylation (57–59). When activated, the encoded protein is known to inhibit CDC25C phosphatase, preventing entry into mitosis, and has been shown to stabilize the tumor suppressor protein p53, leading to cell-cycle arrest in G1. Data suggest that the interaction between *CHEK2* and *BRCA1* may affect whether homologous recombination or nonhomologous end joining is used for repair of double-stranded breaks rather than the specific process of repair (60,61).

An initial study of LFS kindreds suggested that *CHEK2* was a potential LFS gene (62). While it is no longer thought that *CHEK2* plays a role in LFS, two variants in *CHEK2* were identified in the initial study, 1100delC and I157T, which subsequently have been studied as breast cancer susceptibility alleles. *CHEK2* 1100delC, which abolishes the kinase activity, has found in multiple studies to confer a two-fold increased risk of breast cancer across different populations (63–72). The mutation has been found at varying frequencies across populations with the highest frequency in the Netherlands, 3.7% in women with breast cancer diagnosed under age 50 (73). The initial study by

Stratton et al. found the 1100delC mutation at a frequency of 1.1% in healthy controls and 5.1% in 718 probands from breast cancer families from Europe and America ($p = 0.00000003$) (64). The increase in risk associated with the variant in families without *BRCA1* or *BRCA2* mutations was 1.70 (95% CI 1.32–2.20). Closely following up on this was the study from Finland by Nevanlinna and colleagues who also found the variant at increased frequency in 506 familial breast cancer cases [5.5% vs. 1.4%, odds ratio (OR) 4.2; 95% CI 2.4–7.2; $p = 0.0002$] (65). The largest study was done by the *CHEK2* Breast Cancer Case-control Consortium of 10,860 breast cancer cases and 9065 controls; they found the 1100delC mutation in 1.9% of cases and 0.7% of controls (OR 2.34; 95% CI 1.72–3.20) (66). Various studies have confirmed an association with bilateral breast cancer, earlier age of diagnosis, and having a first degree relative with breast cancer (64–66,68). Two studies have examined an association between ionizing radiation and the 1100delC mutation. In patients with bilateral breast cancer, Broeks et al. found the highest percentage of variants in those who had received radiation therapy for their first primary breast cancer, 7.7%, as compared with 3% in those who had not received radiation therapy (67). In 2311 female breast cancer cases and 496 controls from the Ontario and Northern California Breast Cancer Family Registries, a great number of *CHEK2* variants were found in women over age 45 who were exposed more than 15 years prior to their diagnosis (OR 4.28; 95% CI 1.5–12.2) (74). As *CHEK2* plays a role in DNA damage response to ionizing radiation, it is not unexpected that women carrying the variant, which leads to lower protein levels, would be more sensitive and more likely to develop breast cancer after exposure to radiation.

The cumulative risk of breast cancer has been estimated to be 13.7% by age 70 for carriers of the 1100delC mutation, as compared with 6.1% for noncarriers (66). The *CHEK2* Consortium estimated that 0.7% of breast cancer and 0.5% of the excess familial risk is due to this variant in the UK. Using a population-based series of 469 bilateral breast cancer cases, Peto et al. estimate a cumulative risk of 23.8% of breast cancer for first degree relatives of women with bilateral breast cancer and the 1100delC mutation whom also carry the mutation (SIR 12.11; 95% CI 5.23–23.88) (75). Of note, first degree relatives who did not carry the mutation also have an increased risk of breast cancer (SIR 3.48; 95% CI 2.96–4.09). The higher cumulative risk estimated in the latter study for carriers of the 1100delC mutation likely is due to the influence of other shared factors, either environmental or genetic, that contribute to the increased breast cancer risk in families with bilateral breast cancer cases. The *CHEK2* mutation also has been suggested to be associated with a poor prognosis. In 1479 women from the Netherlands with a median follow-up of 10 years, the 1100delC variant was observed in 54 women (3.7%). These women had a higher risk of second primary breast cancer (HR 2.1; 95% CI 1.0–4.3), decreased recurrence-free survival (HR 1.7; 95% CI 1.2–2.4), and breast cancer-specific survival (HR 1.4; 95% CI 1.0–2.1) compared with noncarriers (73). The authors argue that the worsened prognosis should prompt clinical screening for the *CHEK2* mutation at the time of diagnosis so that more intensive therapy or follow-up could be done. However, the rarity of the variant in most populations and borderline significant findings argue against such screening. Narod and Lynch suggest that based on the incident rates reported by Weischer et al. (74), 2000 *CHEK2* positive Danish women would have to be followed for five years to find 40 new cancers (and 400,000 women would have to be screened to identify those 2000 women), making a prospective study logistically and monetarily improbable (76). At this time, clinical testing is not recommended for the *CHEK2* 1100delC mutation. There are several studies underway examining its use in the clinic, which may serve to clarify if mutation testing can and should be used in a clinical scenario.

Interestingly, the 1100delC mutation was not found at increased frequency in *BRCA1/2* mutation carriers. It is possible that the low frequency of the *CHEK2 1100delC* in *BRCA1/2* mutation carriers is due to the fact that *CHEK2*, *BRCA1*, and *BRCA2* lie in the same pathway, and that this pathway is subverted in the mutation carriers, and thus there is little additive effect of the *CHEK2* mutation (64). However, both *CHEK2* and *BRCA1/2* mutations are rare, so it is possible that they coexist, but at such rarity that together they remain unidentified.

Additional mutations have been identified in *CHEK2*. Most relevant to female breast cancer is *I157T* (470 T > C), the frequency of which also is population dependant. The variant does not appear to contribute to breast cancer susceptibility in the United Kingdom, North America, and the Netherlands (77). However, it does appear to contribute to breast cancer susceptibility in Finland, Poland, Germany, and Byelorussia with an increased frequency of breast cancer cases as compared with controls (78–80), albeit associated with lower risk of breast cancer (OR 1.4 in two studies) than the 1100delC mutation. In the latter populations, the estimated breast cancer attributable risk is similar at ~2%, and in Finland, the estimated cumulative risk of breast cancer is 8.1% in carriers (as compared with 5.5% for noncarriers).

BARD1-BRCA1-Associated RING Domain

BRCA1-associated really-interesting-new-gene (RING) domain protein (*BARD1*) was identified in a yeast two-hybrid screen as a binding partner of *BRCA1* (81). Like *BRCA1*, BARD1 has a RING-finger domain; *BRCA1* and BARD1 form a functional heterodimer through the interaction of those domains (82). The interaction of BRCA1 and BARD1 serves to stabilize the two proteins. Mutations in *BRCA1* in the RING domain abrogate the interaction between BRCA1 and BARD1 and are associated with susceptibility to breast and ovarian cancers (83). The heterodimer appears to act as a ubiquitin ligase that targets cell-cycle regular and DNA repair proteins for degradation (84). Similar to *BRCA1*, knockout of *BARD1* leads to early embryonic lethality (85).

As mutations in *BRCA1* and *BRCA2* account for only 30% to 40% of familial breast cancer, *BARD1* was an excellent candidate as an additional breast cancer susceptibility gene based on its interaction with *BRCA1*, because as well as their functional similarity, both have a RING finger domain. Several studies screened high risk breast and breast/ovarian cancer families without mutations in *BRCA1* and *BRCA2* for mutations in *BARD1*. These studies did not find any evidence that *BARD1* was a breast cancer susceptibility gene. Ghimenti et al. screened 40 families by single-strand conformation polymorphism and identified five mutations including *1139del21* and *Cys557Ser* (86). None of the mutations were associated with allelic loss of *BARD1* and so did not support a role as *BARD1* as a tumor suppressor associated with cancer susceptibility. In a similar manner, Ishitobi et al. screened 60 families and found several missense mutations, most of which had been previously observed and the same in-frame deletion *1139del21* (87). The authors investigated *Val507Met* as a low penetrance susceptibility allele for breast cancer in a small association study of 142 population-based breast cancers and 155 healthy controls; they suggest that it is associated with an increased risk of breast cancer in 69 postmenopausal women with an OR of 2.05 (95% CI 1.01–4.16). Nevanlinna et al. resequenced *BARD1* in 45 Finnish familial breast cancer kindreds and seven patients with breast and ovarian cancer, again finding only known missense mutations (88). The largest study screened 126 Finnish families and found four missense and three synonymous amino acid changes (89). They suggest that six of these amino acid changes are neutral, as their frequency in the familial cases was not different from that in control populations. However, they suggest that the Cys557Ser variant is a low penetrance breast cancer susceptibility allele, which they find in 5.6% of 126 familial breast cancer cases, 2.7% of 188 unselected cases, and 1.4% of 1018 controls, $p = 0.005$ for the comparison of familial cases and controls. The most significant finding was in 94 familial probands with a family history of breast cancer only (7.4% vs. 1.4%, $p = 0.001$). Based on this study, three larger studies of the Cys557Ser variant as a low penetrance breast cancer susceptibility allele have been done, all done in Nordic countries, two of which show a positive association. The negative study was done in Finland by Vahteristo et al. in 1811 familial breast cancer probands (577Ser frequency 1.4%), 1565 unselected breast cancer cases (2.2%), and 1083 controls (2.5%). Using 1090 cases with breast cancer and 703 from Iceland, Stacey et al. found an association with breast cancer (OR 1.28; 95% CI 1.11–3.01), which was pronounced in family history positive cases (OR 2.41; 95% CI 1.22–4.75, $p = 0.015$) (90). In carriers of the Iceland founder *BRCA2* mutation, 999del5 and the Cys557Ser allele, the OR was 3.11 (95% CI 1.16–8.4). The authors also note that the 577Ser allele is associated with an increased risk of second primary breast cancer and specific subtypes of breast cancer, lobular and medullary. The largest study by the Nordic consortium included 2906 breast and ovarian cancer cases and 3591 controls from Finland, Iceland, Denmark, Sweden, and Norway (91). In this study, 557Ser was found at increased frequency in probands from breast and/or ovarian cancer families with and without *BRCA1* or *BRCA2* mutations as compared with controls for ORs of 2.6 (95% CI 1.7–4.0) and 3.2 (95% CI 1.2–38), respectively. While the consortium included prostate and colorectal cancer cases, the association with disease only was found with breast cancer cases. The 557Ser allele appears to have arisen from a common ancestor of Northern European origin (90). In Iceland, it clusters in one geographic area; Icelandic and Utah CEPH carriers of the variant have the same haplotype. The *BARD1* 557Ser allele is found at a higher frequency in Northern Europe and in two large case–control studies is associated with breast cancer, particularly in those with a positive family history. However, the increase in risk is small and likely only to play a significant role in those whom already have a *BRCA2* 999del5 mutation. Mutation testing is not in use on a clinical basis.

Fanconi Anemia Genes

Fanconi anemia (FA) is a rare autosomal recessive disease, clinically characterized in most patients by growth retardation, radial aplasia (malformation of the thumb and forearms), hyperpigmentation of the skin, kidney malformation, developmental delay, as well as other congenital malformations (92). However, some patients do not have any dysmorphic features or congenital malformations. Aplastic anemia presenting in the first decade of life frequently occurs. The rate of bone marrow failure is estimated to be 90% by age 40 (93). The estimated risks of developing hematological and nonhematological malignancies are 33% and 28%, respectively by age 40 (93). Of interest, *FANCD1* and, more recently, *FANCN* are associated with an increased cancer prone phenotype as compared with other complementation groups. In *FANCD1*, the average of leukemia is 2.2 years of age as compared with 13.4 years for other complementation groups (94). For *FANCD1* patients, the cumulative probability of malignancy is 97% by age five (95). In both *FANCD1* and *FANCN*, patients are prone to Wilms tumor and medulloblastoma as opposed to the hematological malignancies common in other complementation groups (96,97). The cells of patients with FA are characterized by hypersensitivity to interstrand DNA crosslinking agents (Mitomycin C, diepoxybutane) and the formation of aberrant chromosomal structures in response to them (98). FA is an excellent example of genetic heterogeneity, with the syndrome caused by 13 complementation groups that are clinical recognized (Table 1).

Swift et al. had first hypothesized that heterozygotes would be at increased risk for cancer in 1971; however, this was not supported by his study in 1980 of extended families of 25 heterozygotes (99). Additional studies also did not support an increased cancer risk for heterozygotes (100). However, FA is caused by multiple genes, unlike AT, and it remained a possibility that mutations in some of the genes could be associated with breast cancer susceptibility, which would not be identified in the heterogeneous group, particularly as the majority of cases are associated with mutations in one gene—*FANCA*. FA clearly was linked to breast cancer susceptibility when *BRCA2* was identified as the causative gene for the complementation group *FANCD1* (101). Based on the identification of *BRCA2* in *FANCD1* patients, other FA genes were candidates for breast cancer susceptibility genes. A survey of mutations in *FANCA*, *FANCC*, *FANCD2*, *FANCE*, *FANCF*, and *FANCG* in 88 familial breast cancer cases negative for mutations in *BRCA1* and *BRCA2* identified two missense mutations (in *FANCA* and *FANCE*) in the genes (102). In addition, *FANCD2* has been screened for mutations in 30 Australian *BRCA1/2* negative families without identification of pathogenic mutations (103). These studies suggested that these FA genes were not associated with breast cancer susceptibility.

Studies of other FA genes, however, have suggested an association with breast cancer susceptibility. The gene implicated in *FANCJ*, *BRIP1* (*BRCA1 interacting protein* C-terminal helicase *1*), has been extensively studied in association with breast cancer families without *BRCA1* or *BRCA2* mutations, resulting in the detection of one frameshift and several missense mutations, all of which did not cosegregate with breast cancer in the families (103–108). The conclusion was that mutations in *BRIP1* did not play a

Table 1 Fanconi Anemia Genes and Their Association with *FANCD2* Monoubiquitination and Breast Cancer Susceptibility

Subtype	Gene	Chromosomal location	Required for *FANCD2* monoubiquitination	Implicated in breast cancer susceptibility
A	*FANCA*	16q24.3	Yes	No
B	*FANCB*	Xp22.31	Yes	No
C	*FANCC*	9q22.3	Yes	No
D1	*BRCA2*	13q12.3	No	Yes
D2	*FANCD2*	3p25.3	–	No
E	*FANCE*	6p22-21	Yes	No
F	*FANCF*	11p15	Yes	No
G	*FANCG/ XRCC9*	9p13	Yes	No
I	Unknown	–	Yes	–
J	*BACH1/ BRIP1*	17q22-24	No	Yes
L	*FANCL/ PHF9/ POG*	2p16.1	Yes	–
M	*FANCM/ Hef*	14q21.3	Yes	–
N	*PalB2*	16p12.1	No	Yes

significant role in familial breast cancer. However, in 1212 women with breast cancer (*BRCA1/2* mutation negative), all of which had at least one first degree relative with breast cancer and/or ovarian cancer, Rahman et al. identified nine with mutations as compared with two in 2081 controls ($p = 0.003$) (109). They estimated the relative risk for breast cancer associated with mutations in *BRIP1* as 2.0 (95% CI 1.2–3.2), which was increased in those less than 50 years old to 3.5 (95% CI 1.7–5.7). There was no difference in frequency of missense mutations between cases and controls. These data implicate *BRIP1* as a low penetrance gene conferring susceptibility to breast cancer. In addition, Rahman et al. suggested that heterozygous mutations within the genes of the FA core complex (*FANCA, FANCB, FANCC, FACE, FANCG, FANCL, FANCM*), which mediate the monoubiquinination of *FANCD2* may not contribute to breast cancer susceptibility. In contrast, mutations in genes downstream of *FANCD2*, such as *BRCA2* and *BRIP1*, may contribute to breast cancer susceptibility.

Most recently, *PalB2* (*p*artner *a*nd *l*ocalizer of *B*RCA2) has been implicated as a causative gene for FA and low penetrance gene for breast cancer. *PalB2* was identified through coimmunoprecipitation with *BRCA2* (110). *PalB2* binds with *BRCA2* with up to 50% complexed and colocalizes with *BRCA2* in nuclear foci after DNA damage. Mutations in *PalB2* were identified in 10 of 923 familial breast cancer cases, in this case defined as at least one breast cancer at any age and two relatives also affected with breast cancer, as compared with none in 1084 controls ($p = 0.0004$) (111). Nine mutations were identified in families with female breast cancer only, one in a family that also contained male breast cancer. The relative risk was estimated at 2.3 (95% CI 1.4–3.9; $p = 0.0025$), which increased to 3.0 for women under the age of 50 (95% CI 1.4–3.9). However, the median age of diagnosis was 46, not significantly different from that of all families, with a mean age of diagnosis of 49. Not unexpectedly, mutations in *PalB2* did not completely cosegregate with cancer in families. *PalB2* also functions downstream of FANCD2 monoubiquinination, suggesting that a common pathway for FA genes which contribute to breast cancer susceptibility.

DNA Data Repair Genes and Breast Cancer Susceptibility

The data presented above show an emerging picture of mutations in DNA damage repair genes and breast cancer susceptibility. In regards to FA genes, the data suggest that mutations in DNA damage repair genes that function in homologous recombination downstream of FANCD2 monoubiquinination are likely to be associated with breast cancer susceptibility. However, many questions remain unanswered. Mutations in *BRCA1*, *BRCA2*, and *TP53* confirm a high risk of breast cancer (approximately 10-fold) and contribute to 15% to 20% of familial breast cancer. Mutations in *ATM*, *CHEK2*, *BRIP1*, and *PalB2*, despite interacting with and functioning in the same pathway as *BRCA1*, *BRCA2*, and/or *TP53*, confirm a lower risk of breast cancer. Even taken together mutations in *ATM*, *CHEK2*, *BRIP1*, and *PalB2* are very rare accounting for an estimated 2.3% of breast cancer risk (111). What accounts for the differences in risk, and also do other genes in this pathway play yet unidentified roles in breast cancer susceptibility? Also do all of these genes function independently of each other with nonoverlapping mutations? While the link between *BRCA1*, *BRCA2*, and *TP53* and breast cancer susceptibility has been known for many years, the reason why mutations in these genes are associated with a higher risk of breast cancer rather than other cancers remains unknown. Similarly, the reason why mutations in *ATM*, *CHEK2*, *BRIP1*, and *PalB2* also appear to be associated with breast cancer is unknown, except for an association with *CHEK2* mutations and prostate cancer (112,113). In part the bias toward breast cancer may be because similar large-scale studies of mutational analysis in familial cancer probands of other cancers have not been completed and so they may be associated with other cancers in the future. Nonetheless, the link between mutations in DNA damage repair genes that function in homologous recombination and breast cancer is well documented and future studies will explore it further.

REFERENCES

1. McGarrity TJ, Amos C. Peutz-Jeghers syndrome: clinicopathology and molecular alterations. Cell Mol Life Sci 2006; 63:2135–2144.
2. Hemminki A, Markie D, Tomlinson I, et al. A serine/threonine kinase gene defective in Peutz-Jeghers syndrome. Nature 1998; 391:184–187.
3. Mehenni H, Gehrig C, Nezu J, et al. Loss of LKB1 kinase activity in Peutz-Jeghers syndrome, and evidence for allelic and locus heterogeneity. Am J Hum Genet 1998; 63: 1641–1650.
4. Olschwang S, Markie D, Seal S, et al. Peutz-Jeghers disease: most, but not all, families are compatible with linkage to 19p13.3. J Med Genet 1998; 35:42–44.
5. Ylikorkala A, Avizienyte E, Tomlinson IP, et al. Mutations and impaired function of LKB1 in familial and non-familial Peutz-Jeghers syndrome and a sporadic testicular cancer. Hum Mol Genet 1999; 8:45–51.
6. Wang ZJ, Churchman M, Avizienyte E, et al. Germline mutations of the LKB1 (STK11) gene in Peutz-Jeghers patients. J Med Genet 36:365–368.
7. Boardman LA, Couch FJ, Burgart LJ, et al. Genetic heterogeneity in Peutz-Jeghers syndrome. Hum Mutat 2000; 16:23–30.
8. Lim W, Olschwang S, Keller JJ, et al. Relative frequency and morphology of cancers in STK11 mutation carriers. Gastroenterology 2004; 126:1788–1794.
9. Wang ZJ, Ellis I, Zauber P, et al. Allelic imbalance at the LKB1 (STK11) locus in tumours from patients with Peutz-Jeghers' syndrome provides evidence for a hamartoma-(adenoma)-carcinoma sequence. J Pathol 1999; 188:9–13.
10. Bignell GR, Barfoot R, Seal S, Collins N, Warren W, Stratton MR. Low frequency of somatic mutations in the LKB1/Peutz-Jeghers syndrome gene in sporadic breast cancer. Cancer Res 1998; 58:1384–1386.
11. Mehenni H, Blouin JL, Radhakrishna U, et al. Peutz-Jeghers syndrome: confirmation of linkage to chromosome 19p13.3 and identification of a potential second locus, on 19q13.4. Am J Hum Genet 1997; 61:1327–1334.
12. Hearle N, Lucassen A, Wang R, et al. Mapping of a translocation breakpoint in a Peutz-Jeghers hamartoma to the putative PJS locus at 19q13.4 and mutation analysis of candidate genes in polyp and STK11-negative PJS cases. Genes Chromosomes Cancer 2004; 41: 163–169.
13. Boardman LA, Thibodeau SN, Schaid DJ, et al. Increased risk for cancer in patients with the Peutz-Jeghers syndrome. Ann Intern Med 1998; 128:896–899.
14. Hearle N, Schumacher V, Menko FH, et al. Frequency and spectrum of cancers in the Peutz-Jeghers syndrome. Clin Cancer Res 2006; 12:3209–3215.
15. Mehenni H, Resta N, Park JG, Miyaki M, Guanti G, Costanza MC. Cancer risks in LKB1 germline mutation carriers. Gut 2006; 55:984–990.
16. Giardiello FM, Brensinger JD, Tersmette AC, et al. Very high risk of cancer in familial Peutz-Jeghers syndrome. Gastroenterology 2000; 119:1447–1453.
17. Pharoah PD, Guilford P, Caldas C. Incidence of gastric cancer and breast cancer in CDH1 (E-cadherin) mutation carriers from hereditary diffuse gastric cancer families. Gastroenterology 2001; 121:1348–1353.
18. Guilford P, Hopkins J, Harraway J, et al. E-cadherin germline mutations in familial gastric cancer. 1998; 392:402–405.

19. Brooks-Wilson AR, Kaurah P, Suriano G, et al. Germline E-cadherin mutations in hereditary diffuse gastric cancer: assessment of 42 new families and review of genetic screening criteria. J Med Genet 2004; 41:508–517.

20. Huntsman DG, Carneiro F, Lewis FR, et al. Early gastric cancer in young, asymptomatic carriers of germ-line E-cadherin mutations. N Engl J Med 2001; 344:1904–1909.

21. Chun YS, Lindor NM, Smyrk TC, et al. Germline E-cadherin gene mutations: is prophylactic total gastrectomy indicated? Cancer 2001; 92:181–187.

22. Charlton A, Blair V, Shaw D, Parry S, Guilford P, Martin IG. Hereditary diffuse gastric cancer: predominance of multiple foci of signet ring cell carcinoma in distal stomach and transitional zone. Gut 2004; 53:814–820.

23. Suriano G, Yew S, Ferreira P, et al. Characterization of a recurrent germ line mutation of the E-cadherin gene: implications for genetic testing and clinical management. Clin Cancer Res 2005; 11:5401–5409.

24. Keller G, Vogelsang H, Becker I, et al. Diffuse type gastric and lobular breast carcinoma in a familial gastric cancer patient with an E-cadherin germline mutation. Am J Pathol 1999; 155: 337–342.

25. Zhu ZG, Yu YY, Zhang Y, et al. Germline mutational analysis of CDH1 and pathologic features in familial cancer syndrome with diffuse gastric cancer/breast cancer proband in a Chinese family. Eur J Surg Oncol 2004; 30:531–535.

26. Berx G, Cleton-Jansen A-M, Nollet F, et al. E-cadherin is a tumour/invasion suppressor gene mutated in human lobular breast cancers. EMBO J 1995; 14:6107–6116.

27. Berx G, Becker KF, Hofler H, van Roy F. Mutations of the human E-cadherin (CDH1) gene. Hum Mutat 1998; 12:226–237.

28. Schelfout K, Van Goethem M, Kersschot E, et al. Preoperative breast MRI in patients with invasive lobular breast cancer. Eur Radiol 2004; 14:1209–1216.

29. Wright J, Teraoka S, Onengut S, et al. A high frequency of distinct ATM gene mutations in ataxia-telangiectasia. Am J Hum Genet 1996; 59:839–846.

30. Morrell D, Cromartie E, Swift M. Mortality and cancer incidence in 263 patients with ataxia-telangiectasia. J Natl Cancer Inst 1986; 77:89–92.

31. Swift M, Morrell D, Cromartie E, Chamberlin AR, Skolnick MH, Bishop DT. The incidence and gene frequency of ataxia-telangiectasia in the United States. Am J Hum Genet 1986; 39: 573–583.

32. Swift M, Reitnauer PJ, Morrell D, Chase CL. Breast and other cancers in families with ataxia-telangiectasia. N Engl J Med 1987; 316:1289–1294.

33. Swift M, Morrell D, Massey RB, Chase CL. Incidence of cancer in 161 families affected by ataxia-telangiectasia [see comments]. N Engl J Med 1991; 325:1831–1836.

34. Easton DF. Cancer risks in A-T heterozygotes. Int J Radiat Biol 1994; 66:S177–S182.

35. Inskip HM, Kinlen LJ, Taylor AM, Woods CG, Arlett CF. Risk of breast cancer and other cancers in heterozygotes for ataxia-telangiectasia. Br J Cancer 1999; 79:1304–1307.

36. Janin N, Andrieu N, Ossian K, et al. Breast cancer risk in ataxia telangiectasia (AT) heterozygotes: haplotype study in French AT families. Br J Cancer 1999; 80:1042–1045.

37. Su Y, Swift M. Mortality rates among carriers of ataxia-telangiectasia mutant alleles. Ann Intern Med 2000; 133:770–778.

38. Olsen JH, Hanemann JM, Borresen-Dale AL, et al. Cancer in patients with Ataxia-Telangiectasia and in their relatives in the Nordic countries. J Natl Cancer Inst 2001; 93.

39. d'Almeida AK, Cavaciuti E, Dondon MG, et al. Increased risk of breast cancer among female relatives of patients with ataxia-telangiectasia: a causal relationship? Br J Cancer 2005; 93:730–732; author reply; 732.

40. Andrieu N, Cavaciuti E, Lauge A, et al. Ataxia-telangiectasia genes and breast cancer risk in a French family study. J Dairy Res 2005; 72 Spec No: 73–80.

41. Cavaciuti E, Lauge A, Janin N, et al. Cancer risk according to type and location of ATM mutation in ataxia-telangiectasia families. Genes Chromosomes Cancer 2005; 42:1–9.

42. Olsen JH, Hahnemann JM, Borresen-Dale AL, et al. Breast and other cancers in 1445 blood relatives of 75 Nordic patients with ataxia telangiectasia. Br J Cancer 2005; 93:260–265.

43. Thompson D, Duedal S, Kirner J, et al. Cancer risks and mortality in heterozygous ATM mutation carriers. J Natl Cancer Inst 2005; 97:813–822.

44. FitzGerald MG, Bean JM, Hegde SR, et al. Heterozygous ATM mutations do not contribute to early onset of breast cancer [see comments]. Nat Genet 1997; 15: 307–310.

45. Izatt L, Greenman J, Hodgson S, et al. Identification of germline missense mutations and rare allelic variants in the ATM gene in early-onset breast cancer. Genes, Chromosomes Cancer 1999; 26:286–294.

46. Chen J, Birkholtz GG, Lindblom P, Rubio C, Lindblom A. The role of ataxia-telangiectasia heterozygotes in familial breast cancer. Cancer Res 1998; 58:1376–1379.

47. Vorechovsky I, Luo L, Lindblom A, et al. ATM mutations in cancer families. Cancer Res 1996; 56:4130–4133.

48. Shayeghi M, Seal S, Regan J, et al. Heterozygosity for mutations in the ataxia telangiectasia gene is not a major cause of radiotherapy complications in breast cancer patients. Br J Cancer 1998; 78:922–927.

49. Bebb G, Glickman B, Gelmon K, Gatti R. "AT risk" for breast cancer [see comments]. Lancet 1997; 349:1784–1785.

50. Laake K, Vu P, Andersen TI, et al. Screening breast cancer patients for Norwegian ATM mutations. Br J Cancer 2000; 83:1650–1653.

51. Broeks A, Urbanus JH, Floore AN, et al. ATM-heterozygous germline mutations contribute to breast cancer-susceptibility. Am J Hum Genet 2000; 66:494–500.

52. Renwick A, Thompson D, Seal S, et al. ATM mutations that cause ataxia-telangiectasia are breast cancer susceptibility alleles. Nat Genet 2006; 38:873–875.

53. Gatti RA, Tward A, Concannon P. Cancer risk in ATM heterozygotes: a model of phenotypic and mechanistic differences between missense and truncating mutations. Mol Genet Metab 1999; 68:419–423.

54. Stankovic T, Kidd AM, Sutcliffe A, et al. ATM mutations and phenotypes in ataxia-telangiectasia families in the British Isles: expression of mutant ATM and the risk of leukemia, lymphoma, and breast cancer. Am J Hum Genet 1998; 62:334–345.

55. Chenevix-Trench G, Spurdle AB, Gatei M, et al. Dominant negative ATM mutations in breast cancer families. J Natl Cancer Inst 2002; 94:205–215.

56. Bartek J, Lukas J. Chk1 and Chk2 kinases in checkpoint control and cancer. Cancer Cell 2003; 3:421–429.

57. Ahn JY, Schwarz JK, Piwnica-Worms H, Canman CE. Threonine 68 phosphorylation by ataxia telangiectasia mutated is required for efficient activation of Chk2 in response to ionizing radiation. Cancer Res 2000; 60:5934–5936.

58. Matsuoka S, Rotman G, Ogawa A, Shiloh Y, Tamai K, Elledge SJ. Ataxia telangiectasia-mutated phosphorylates Chk2 in vivo and in vitro. Proc Natl Acad Sci U S A 2000; 97: 10389–10394.

59. Matsuoka S, Huang M, Elledge SJ. Linkage of ATM to cell cycle regulation by the Chk2 protein kinase. Science 1998; 282:1893–1897.

60. Zhang J, Willers H, Feng Z, et al. Chk2 phosphorylation of BRCA1 regulates DNA double-strand break repair. Mol Cell Biol 2004; 24:708–718.

61. McPherson JP, Lemmers B, Hirao A, et al. Collaboration of Brca1 and Chk2 in tumorigenesis. Genes Dev 2004; 18:1144–1153.

62. Bell DW, Varley JM, Szydlo TE, et al. Heterozygous germ line hCHK2 mutations in Li-Fraumeni syndrome. Science 1999; 286:2528–2531.

63. Lee SB, Kim SH, Bell DW, et al. Destabilization of CHK2 by a missense mutation associated with Li-Fraumeni Syndrome. Cancer Res 2001; 61:8062–8067.

64. Meijers-Heijboer H, van den Ouweland A, Klijn J, et al. Low-penetrance susceptibility to breast cancer due to CHEK2(*)1100delC in noncarriers of BRCA1 or BRCA2 mutations. Nat Genet 2002; 31:55–59.

65. Vahteristo P, Bartkova J, Eerola H, et al. A CHEK2 genetic variant contributing to a substantial fraction of familial breast cancer. Am J Hum Genet 2002; 71:432–438.

66. Consortium CBCC-C. CHEK2*1100delC and susceptibility to breast cancer: a collaborative analysis involving 10,860 breast cancer cases and 9,065 controls from 10 studies. Am J Hum Genet 2004; 74:1175–1182.

67. Broeks A, de Witte L, Nooijen A, et al. Excess risk for contralateral breast cancer in CHEK2*1100delC germline mutation carriers. Breast Cancer Res Treat 2004; 83:91–93.

68. Oldenburg RA, Kroeze-Jansema K, Kraan J, et al. The CHEK2*1100delC variant acts as a breast cancer risk modifier in non-BRCA1/BRCA2 multiple-case families. Cancer Res 2003; 63:8153–8157.

69. Osorio A, Rodriguez-Lopez R, Diez O, et al. The breast cancer low-penetrance allele 1100delC in the CHEK2 gene is not present in Spanish familial breast cancer population. Int J Cancer 2004; 108:54–56.

70. Rajkumar T, Soumittra N, Nancy NK, et al. BRCA1, BRCA2 and CHEK2 (1100 del C) germline mutations in hereditary breast and ovarian cancer families in South India. Asian Pac J Cancer Prev: APJCP 2003; 4:203–208.

71. Offit K, Pierce H, Kirchhoff T, et al. Frequency of CHEK2*1100delC in New York breast cancer cases and controls. BMC Med Genet 2003; 4:1.

72. Sodha N, Bullock S, Taylor R, et al. CHEK2 variants in susceptibility to breast cancer and evidence of retention of the wild type allele in tumours. Br J Cancer 2002; 87:1445–1448.

73. Schmidt MK, Tollenaar RA, de Kemp SR, et al. Breast cancer survival and tumor characteristics in premenopausal women carrying the CHEK2*1100delC germline mutation. J Clin Oncol 2007; 25:64–69.

74. Bernstein JL, Teraoka SN, John EM, et al. The CHEK2*1100delC allelic variant and risk of breast cancer: screening results from the Breast Cancer Family Registry. Cancer Epidemiol Biomarkers Prev 2006; 15:348–352.

75. Johnson N, Fletcher O, Naceur-Lombardelli C, dos Santos Silva I, Ashworth A, Peto J. Interaction between CHEK2*1100delC and other low-penetrance breast-cancer susceptibility genes: a familial study. Lancet 2005; 366:1554–1557.

76. Narod SA, Lynch HT. CHEK2 mutation and hereditary breast cancer. J Clin Oncol 2007; 25: 6–7.

77. Schutte M, Seal S, Barfoot R, et al. Variants in CHEK2 other than 1100delC do not make a major contribution to breast cancer susceptibility. Am J Hum Genet 2003; 72: 1023–1028.

78. Kilpivaara O, Vahteristo P, Falck J, et al. CHEK2 variant I157T may be associated with increased breast cancer risk. Int J Cancer 2004; 111:543–547.

79. Cybulski C, Gorski B, Huzarski T, et al. CHEK2 is a multiorgan cancer susceptibility gene. Am J Hum Genet 2004; 75:1131–1135.

80. Bogdanova N, Enssen-Dubrowinskaja N, Feshchenko S, et al. Association of two mutations in the CHEK2 gene with breast cancer. Int J Cancer 2005; 116:263–266.

81. Wu LC, Wang ZW, Tsan JT, et al. Identification of a RING protein that can interact in vivo with the BRCA1 gene product. Nat Genet 1996; 14:430–440.

82. Meza JE, Brzovic PS, King MC, Klevit RE. Mapping the functional domains of BRCA1. Interaction of the ring finger domains of BRCA1 and BARD1. J Biol Chem 1999; 274: 5659–5665.

83. Brzovic PS, Meza J, King MC, Klevit RE. The cancer-predisposing mutation C61G disrupts homodimer formation in the NH2-terminal BRCA1 RING finger domain. J Biol Chem 1998; 273:7795–7799.

84. Irminger-Finger I, Jefford CE. Is there more to BARD1 than BRCA1? Nat Rev Cancer 2006; 6:382–391.

85. McCarthy EE, Celebi JT, Baer R, Ludwig T. Loss of Bard1, the heterodimeric partner of the Brca1 tumor suppressor, results in early embryonic lethality and chromosomal instability. Mol Cell Biol 2003; 23:5056–5063.

86. Ghimenti C, Sensi E, Presciuttini S, et al. Germline mutations of the BRCA1-associated ring domain (BARD1) gene in breast and breast/ovarian families negative for BRCA1 and BRCA2 alterations. Genes Chromosomes Cancer 2002; 33:235–242.

87. Ishitobi M, Miyoshi Y, Hasegawa S, et al. Mutational analysis of BARD1 in familial breast cancer patients in Japan. Cancer Lett 2003; 200:1–7.

88. Vahteristo P, Syrjakoski K, Heikkinen T, et al. BARD1 variants Cys557Ser and Val507Met in breast cancer predisposition. Eur J Hum Genet 2006; 14:167–172.

89. Karppinen SM, Heikkinen K, Rapakko K, Winqvist R. Mutation screening of the BARD1 gene: evidence for involvement of the Cys557Ser allele in hereditary susceptibility to breast cancer. J Med Genet 2004; 41:e114.

90. Stacey SN, Sulem P, Johannsson OT, et al. The BARD1 Cys557Ser variant and breast cancer risk in Iceland. PLoS Med 2006; 3:e217.

91. Karppinen SM, Barkardottir RB, Backenhorn K, et al. Nordic collaborative study of the BARD1 Cys557Ser allele in 3956 patients with cancer: enrichment in familial BRCA1/ BRCA2 mutation-negative breast cancer but not in other malignancies. J Med Genet 2006; 43:856–862.

92. www.genetests.org.

93. Kutler DI, Singh B, Satagopan J, et al. A 20-year perspective on the International Fanconi Anemia Registry (IFAR). Blood 2003; 101:1249–1256.

94. Wagner JE, Tolar J, Levran O, et al. Germline mutations in BRCA2: shared genetic susceptibility to breast cancer, early onset leukemia, and Fanconi anemia. Blood 2004; 103: 3226–3229.

95. Alter BP, Rosenberg PS, Brody LC. Clinical and molecular features associated with biallelic mutations in FANCD1/BRCA2. J Med Genet 2006.

96. Reid S, Renwick A, Seal S, et al. Biallelic BRCA2 mutations are associated with multiple malignancies in childhood including familial Wilms tumour. J Med Genet 2005; 42:147–151.

97. Reid S, Schindler D, Hanenberg H, et al. Biallelic mutations in PALB2 cause Fanconi anemia subtype FA-N and predispose to childhood cancer. Nat Genet 2006.

98. Taniguchi T, D'Andrea AD. Molecular pathogenesis of Fanconi anemia: recent progress. Blood 2006; 107:4223–4233.

99. Swift M, Caldwell RJ, Chase C. Reassessment of cancer predisposition of Fanconi anemia heterozygotes. J Natl Cancer Inst 1980; 65:863–867.

100. Potter NU, Sarmousakis C, Li FP. Cancer in relatives of patients with aplastic anemia. Cancer Genet Cytogenet 1983; 9:61–65.

101. Howlett NG, Taniguchi T, Olson S, et al. Biallelic inactivation of BRCA2 in Fanconi anemia [see comments]. Science 2002; 297:606–609.

102. Seal S, Barfoot R, Jayatilake H, Stratton MR, Rahman N. Breast Cancer Susceptibility Collaboration. Evaluation of Fanconi anemia genes in familial breast cancer predisposition. Cancer Res 2003; 63:8596–8599.

103. Lewis AG, Flanagan J, Marsh A, et al. Mutation analysis of FANCD2, BRIP1/BACH1, LMO4 and SFN in familial breast cancer. Breast Cancer Res 2005; 7:R1005–R1016.

104. Luo L, Lei H, Du Q, et al. No mutations in the BACH1 gene in BRCA1 and BRCA2 negative breast-cancer families linked to 17q22. Int J Cancer 2002; 98:638–639.

105. Rutter JL, Smith AM, Davila MR, et al. Mutational analysis of the BRCA1-interacting genes ZNF350/ZBRK1 and BRIP1/BACH1 among BRCA1 and BRCA2-negative probands from breast-ovarian cancer families and among early-onset breast cancer cases and reference individuals. Hum Mutat 2003; 22:121–128.

106. Karppinen SM, Vuosku J, Heikkinen K, Allinen M, Winqvist R. No evidence of involvement of germline BACH1 mutations in Finnish breast and ovarian cancer families. Eur J Cancer 2003; 39:366–371.

107. Levran O, Attwooll C, Henry RT, et al. The BRCA1-interacting helicase BRIP1 is deficient in Fanconi anemia. Nat Genet 2005; 37:931–933.

108. Litman R, Peng M, Jin Z, et al. BACH1 is critical for homologous recombination and appears to be the Fanconi anemia gene product FANCJ. Cancer Cell 2005; 8:255–265.

109. Seal S, Thompson D, Renwick A, et al. Truncating mutations in the Fanconi anemia J gene BRIP1 are low-penetrance breast cancer susceptibility alleles. Nat Genet 2006; 38: 1239–1241.

110. Xia B, Sheng Q, Nakanishi K, et al. Control of BRCA2 cellular and clinical functions by a nuclear partner, PALB2. Mol Cell 2006; 22:719–729.

111. Rahman N, Seal S, Thompson D, et al. PALB2, which encodes a BRCA2-interacting protein, is a breast cancer susceptibility gene. Nat Genet 2006.

112. Cybulski C, Wokolorczyk D, Huzarski T, et al. A large germline deletion in the Chek2 kinase gene is associated with an increased risk of prostate cancer. J Med Genet 2006; 43: 863–866.

113. Dong X, Wang L, Taniguchi K, et al. Mutations in CHEK2 associated with prostate cancer risk. Am J Hum Genet 2003; 72:270–280.

8

Low-Penetrance Genes in Breast Cancer

Paul D. P. Pharoah
Department of Oncology, University of Cambridge, Cambridge, U.K.

INTRODUCTION

For many years the main focus of the research effort into the inherited basis of breast cancer was the search for single, strong, but rarely mutated predisposing genes that cause a subset of the disease with Mendelian inheritance. More recently, attention has switched to the systematic study of common genetic variation in complex disease susceptibility with the promise of a "polygenic" approach to the prevention and treatment of common diseases. This change of focus has been enabled by the completion of the human genome sequence and the subsequent generation of detailed information about the range of genetic differences between individuals. Some have claimed that the greater under-standing of genetic risk factors and their interactions with the environment will allow diseases to be predicted and to be prevented at both individual and population levels, by directing interventions at individuals shown to be at high risk (1,2). Others are less sure (3–5): in particular, they question whether molecular testing for common genetic variants can have sufficient predictive power to be of practical use either for the individual or for defining risk groups in the population at large. In this chapter, I will review the evidence for the polygenic model of breast cancer susceptibility, discuss progress toward identifying low-penetrance alleles, and comment on the clinical utility and public health relevance of these alleles.

THE EVIDENCE FOR LOW-PENETRANCE GENES

Breast cancer, like other common cancers, exhibit some degree of familial clustering, with disease being approximately two-fold more common in first-degree relatives of cases (6,7). The higher rate of most cancers in the monozygotic twins of cases than in dizygotic twins or siblings suggests that most of the familial clustering is the result of genetic variation rather than lifestyle or environmental factors (8,9). Further evidence for the relative importance of genetic factors comes from the observation that more distant relatives of a case (i.e., those beyond the nuclear family) are also at increased risk of disease even though they would be expected to share environmental or lifestyle factors to a lesser degree (6). Furthermore, the magnitude of the risks in distant relatives is close to those predicted by simple genetic models such as a dominant model or an additive polygenic model.

Some of the familial clustering of breast cancer occur as part of specific inherited breast cancer syndromes, where disease results from single genes conferring a high risk. Several genes associated with these syndromes have been identified including *BRCA1*, *BRCA2*, *PTEN*, and *TP53*. However, the susceptibility alleles in these genes are rare in the population and they account for a small minority of the inherited component of cancer. Highly penetrant variants in the breast cancer susceptibility genes *BRCA1* and *BRCA2* account for less than 20% of the genetic risk of breast cancer with other rarer high-penetrance genes such as *TP53*, ataxia telangiectasia–mutated (*ATM*), and *PTEN* counting for less than 5% (10). Other *BRCA1/2*-like genes are unlikely to exist as the majority of multiple case families can be accounted for by *BRCA1* or *BRCA2* (11) and, despite extensive research efforts, attempts to identify similar highly penetrant cancer susceptibility genes, using family based linkage studies, have failed.

Mathematical modeling of the familial aggregation of breast cancer in the population can provide important clues about the range of genetic models that best account for the familial aggregation of breast cancer not due to the high penetrance *BRCA* genes. Two such studies have been published. The first study used data from a series of 856 breast cancer cases from Australia that were diagnosed under the age of 40 and had been tested for mutations in *BRCA1* and *BRCA2* (12). The model that fit these data the best was that of a single recessive allele that conferred a high disease risk. Another study analyzed the occurrence of breast cancer in the relatives of patients in the Anglian Breast Cancer Study, a population-based series of ~1500 cases, all of whom were screened for mutations in *BRCA1* and *BRCA2* (13). Two models were found to fit the data well. The model best describing the data was a polygenic model, in which susceptibility to breast cancer is conferred by a large number of alleles. The risk associated with any individual allele is small; but the effects are multiplicative so that a woman with several susceptibility alleles is at high risk. The second model was that of a single common recessive allele (frequency 0.24). This recessive allele was estimated to confer a relative risk (RR) of 21 for rare homozygotes compared with common homozygotes and heterozygotes, corresponding to a moderately high lifetime penetrance of 42%.

The polygenic and recessive models were also applied to a series of multiple case families not due to *BRCA* mutations (14). The polygenic model fitted these data well, but the fit of the recessive model was not so good. Furthermore, a large meta-analysis of observational epidemiological studies found that the familial breast cancer risk to siblings is similar to that to mothers, suggesting that any recessive component for the excess familial risk is at best small (7). These observations, together with the failure of genetic linkage studies to identify further breast cancer susceptibility genes, suggest that a single gene recessive model is less plausible than a polygenic model of inheritance.

Thus, the evidence for the polygenic model of breast cancer susceptibility is persuasive and it is likely to be an appropriate model for many common cancers and other diseases. However, the number of risk alleles and their properties (allele frequencies and risks conferred) are not known. Indeed, a wide variety of possibilities are consistent with a polygenic model for cancer susceptibility, ranging from a handful of alleles of moderate risk to a large number of alleles each conferring a slight increase in risk across a wide range of allele frequencies, or a combination of the two.

PROGRESS TOWARD IDENTIFYING COMMON LOW-PENETRANCE ALLELES

The main alternative to linkage studies for disease gene mapping is the association study, in which the frequency of a genetic variant in diseased individuals (cases) and individuals without the disease (controls) are compared (15,16). Allelic association is present when the distribution of genotypes differs in cases and controls. Such an association provides evidence that the locus under study, or a neighboring locus, is related to disease susceptibility. Association studies for disease genes depend on the "common variant: common disease" hypothesis (17). Genetic variants that arose many generations ago may, for a variety of reasons, have become common in the present population at frequencies ranging from a few percent upward. Some of these variants may predispose to common diseases of late onset, and combinations of these variants are proposed to underlie differences in disease susceptibility. Association mapping will be a powerful tool for mapping such loci with moderate effects. However, it is not clear how much of the genetic predisposition to cancer is due to alleles with moderate effects or how many such alleles exist.

The genetic association study has been used as a method to map cancer susceptibility alleles for over four decades, but the advent of modern molecular genetics has seen a dramatic increase in the use of this type of study in the past five years (18). These efforts have, perhaps, been most notable for their few successes. However, most studies carried out so far have been based on the candidate gene/candidate polymorphism approach. Candidate genes are those that encode proteins thought to be involved in carcinogenesis, such as those involved in apoptosis, cell-cycle control, carcinogen metabolism, or DNA repair, or those known to be somatically altered in cancer. The rationale for the candidate gene approach is that by maximizing the biological plausibility, the chances of success are increased. However, the approach is limited by its reliance on existing knowledge to identify candidate genes based on function.

Perhaps the only confirmed low-penetrance breast cancer susceptibility allele identified to date is the *1100delc* variant in *CHEK2*. *CHEK2* encodes a G2 checkpoint kinase that plays a critical role in DNA damage repair. It is the human ortholog of the yeast *Cds1* and *Rad53* G2 checkpoint kinases (19). Activation of these proteins in response to DNA damage prevents cellular entry into mitosis. In mammalian cells, activation of *CHEK2* in response to ionizing radiation is regulated through phosphorylation by *ATM* (20). Activated *CHEK2* phosphorylates critical cell-cycle proteins, including p53, Cdc25C, Cdc25A, and *BRCA1*, promoting cell-cycle arrest and activation of DNA repair (21–24).

The protein truncating variant in *CHEK2*, *1100delc*, was originally identified by Bell et al. in a woman with breast cancer who had a family history compatible with Li-Fraumeni syndrome (25). The same variant was subsequently identified in affected women in a large multiple-case family with breast cancer from the Netherlands that did not show linkage to *BRCA1* or *BRCA2* (26). Further analyses demonstrated that this variant was present in 18/1620 (1.1%) of controls from England, the Netherlands, and the United States, but it was present in 55/1071 (5.1%) of breast cancer cases from multiple-case families that did not segregate *BRCA1* or *BRCA2* mutations, a frequency difference that was highly statistically significant. Haplotype analysis confirmed that all *CHEK2*1100delC* mutations derived from a common founder. A similar association was found in another study based on 1035 unselected breast cancer cases, 507 breast cancer cases with a positive family history, and 1885 controls from Finland (27). The frequencies in familial breast cancer cases and controls were very similar to that observed by Meijers-Heijboer et al. (4.5% in cases vs. 1.4% in controls) (26). Meijers-Heijboer et al. found an even higher frequency in cases with a family history of male breast cancer, suggesting an association between *CHEK2*1100delc* and male breast cancer, but this association was not replicated in a series of male patients with breast cancer unselected for family history (28). The association was subsequently confirmed in an analysis of 10 case–control studies from five countries comprising 10,860 cases unselected for family history and 9065 controls. The *1100delc* variant was found in 1.9% of cases and 0.7% of controls [odds ratio = 2.3; 95% confidence interval (CI) 1.7–3.2]. There was some evidence for a higher prevalence of *1100delc* among cases with a family history and at younger ages of diagnosis, a pattern of risk consistent with the polygenic model. Assuming a constant RR with age, and a carrier frequency of 0.5%, the estimated absolute risk of breast cancer would be 14% by age 70 compared with 6% in noncarriers. However, *CHEK2*1100delc* only makes a small contribution to the overall burden of breast cancer as it accounts for just 0.5% of the excess familial risk.

There have been many reports of other low-penetrance alleles for breast cancer, but few initial reports of "significant" associations have been replicated by independent studies and no allele has been confirmed with the stringent levels of statistical significance required for genetic association studies. There has been some debate about the major reasons for nonreplication (29,30), but the most likely explanation is that most initial reports are false positives, and the most common reason for this is simply chance (type I error), exacerbated by publication bias. Where the prior probability of association is low, stringent levels of significance are required to reduce the chance of a false positive to acceptable levels (31,32). This can be illustrated as follows: A dominant breast cancer susceptibility allele with a population frequency of 30% that confers a modest increase in risk of disease of 30% (RR = 1.3) would account for approximately 1% of the excess familial RR. Therefore, under a log additive model, the maximum number of such disease alleles is 80 (20% of the excess risk explained by known genes). Assuming there are 10^7 polymorphic loci across the genome, the probability that a random candidate variant will be associated with disease is no more than 1 in 100,000 (prior probability). If any of these loci are tested for association with 90% statistical power to detect a true association at the 0.01 level of significance, the probability that a statistically significant association is a true positive is just 0.08%. This is analogous to the false positive report probability described by Wacholder et al. (31). Even if the significance level is made more stringent at 10^{-4} the positive predictive value improves to only 8%. The prior may be improved by judicious selection of candidate genes or polymorphisms based on underlying biology, although the results of genome-wide association (GWA) studies in other diseases suggest that any weighting of the evidence based on what we know of molecular biology should, at best, be small (33). Of course, in reality, the expected number of loci, their allele frequencies and risk, or the number of variant loci in the genome are not known. Nevertheless, adoption of stringent significance levels, perhaps 10^{-5} for candidate gene studies and 10^{-7} for whole-genome studies, would avoid most of the problems of nonreplication (34). Nonreplication may also occur because the replication studies are too small to detect low-to-moderate risk alleles with sufficient power. The major lesson to be derived from these observations is that large sample sizes are needed to detect and confirm, at appropriate levels of statistical significance, genetic variants that confer modest risks (35,36).

FUTURE DIRECTIONS

Despite the lack of success so far, it seems likely that the next 5 to 10 years will see rapid developments in our understanding of the polygenic basis of breast cancer. The reasons for this optimism lie in the potential of empirical, GWA studies, which, until recently have not been feasible. A new era of GWA association has been made possible by two major advances. Firstly our knowledge of human genomic architecture has been advanced dramatically by projects such as the International Hap Map project which seeks to identify and catalog common genetic variation in human population (37). Secondly, new genotyping technologies now enable hundreds of thousands of markers to be assayed in large numbers of samples, at a reasonable cost. It is estimated that there are approximately 11 million single nucleotide polymorphisms (SNPs) in the genome with a minor allele frequency of 1% or greater, of which approximately seven million have a frequency of 5% or greater (38,39). Currently available genotyping platforms provide marker sets which, although not yet perfect, should provide a high degree of coverage of the common variants in the genome (40). The potential of GWA studies is exemplified by the identification of a common polymorphic variant in *CFH* that confers an increased risk of age-related macular degeneration (41). Two GWA studies of breast cancer have been recently published.

Further reason for optimism comes from the establishment of multicenter collaborations that enable much larger sample sizes and the confirmation of results at genome-wide levels of significance. The *CHEK2* consortium has developed into the Breast Cancer Association Consortium (BCAC) with over 20 participating case–control studies. Initial analyses of 20 candidate polymorphisms have confirmed *CASP8* D302N as a low-penetrance breast cancer polymorphism, with the common D-allele associated with an increase in risk [odds ratio = 1.13 (95% CI 1.08–1.18)] (unpublished data). Similarly the Consortium of Cohorts was formed by National Cancer Institute (NCI) to address the need for large-scale collaborations for study of gene–gene and gene–environment interactions in the etiology of breast and prostate cancer (42).

The association studies' design relies on the "common disease: common variant" hypothesis. It is, however, equally possible that much of the variation in cancer risk is due to rarer alleles. Indeed, virtually all susceptibility alleles identified to date have frequencies of less than 1%. These include both high-penetrance mutations and low-penetrance variants in *ATM* and *CHEK2* that predispose to breast cancer. The identification of rare variants that confer modest risks is possible, but the problems are formidable. Firstly, very large sample sizes are required: the *CHEK2 1100delc* variant was initially identified in a family based study and only confirmed with a total sample size of almost 20,000. And second, much less is known about the occurrence of rare variants across the genome, as current efforts to identify genetic variation have concentrated on common polymorphisms identifiable by resequencing small numbers of individuals. Identifying rare variants will require resequencing much larger numbers of individuals, perhaps concentrating on individuals from high risk families where the frequencies may be higher. Furthermore, because the numbers of rare variants will be much larger, the problems of multiple testing (lower prior probability of association) will be much greater. Finally, the frequencies of such alleles are likely to vary between populations.

The relative importance of common and rare variants in cancer susceptibility cannot be inferred from existing data and remains a major uncertainty overhanging future studies. Nevertheless, the identification of common alleles is more tractable and, because they would explain a greater fraction of disease burden, is of more direct public health relevance. Therefore it is logical to concentrate on these. However, alleles are likely to be rare if there is any degree of selection against the variant, for example if homozygotes are nonviable. If most cancer susceptibility is related to fundamental processes of cellular control, rare alleles may turn out to be the more important component.

CLINICAL RELEVANCE OF INDIVIDUAL LOW-PENETRANCE ALLELES

What then, might be the impact of the identification of genetic risk factors for disease, in terms of disease prevention at the level of the population? Several authors have pointed out that individual susceptibility genes are unlikely to contribute much to disease prevention (5). For example, consider a highly penetrant allele that is rare in the population (allele frequency = 0.001 or carrier frequency = 0.002). Note that deleterious alleles of *BRCA1* and *BRCA2* occur in the population with a combined frequency of about 0.003 in populations where there are no common founder mutations (43). Suppose that the mutation confers a 10-fold increase in risk in carriers with a corresponding lifetime risk of disease in a carrier of 50%. Such an allele would be present in 2% of all cases. If we have an intervention, e.g., chemoprevention, that reduces disease risk by 40% the absolute risk reduction in carriers is 20% (40% of 50%). Thus, for every five (100/20) carriers treated we would prevent one case. This is the numbers needed to treat. However, if we identified carriers by testing (or "screening") the population, we would need to screen 2500 individuals (5/0.002) to prevent one case. This is the number needed to screen (NNS). A population screening program to detect and treat carriers would reduce total disease burden by 0.8% if uptake of testing and treatment were complete. The *CHEK2 1100delc* is only slightly more common than this (carrier frequency = 0.005), but confers a substantially smaller risk. Again assuming we have an intervention that reduces risk by 40%, the absolute risk reduction is just 5.6%, and so for every 18 carriers treated 1 case would be prevented. The NNS is 3570. A population screening program to detect and treat carriers would also reduce total disease burden by 0.8% if uptake of testing and treatment were complete.

Let us now consider a more common, low-penetrance genetic variant, which carries a two-fold increase in disease risk, a lifetime risk of disease of 10%, and is present in 5% of the population. The variant would be present in 9.5% of all cases. An intervention that reduces risk by 40% (absolute risk reduction 4%) will have an NNS of 500, and, at best, could reduce total disease burden by 3.8%. Common alleles with risk of this magnitude are likely to be the exception and it is much more likely that the alleles identified by the new generation of GWA studies will confer risk of 1.1 to 1.3. The clinical utility of testing for these alleles will be extremely limited.

DISEASE PREVENTION UNDER THE POLYGENIC MODEL

The possibility that genetic susceptibility to breast cancer is due to several loci, each conferring a modest independent risk, seems reasonable. In practice, the number of loci involved will be finite, but once there are more than four to five loci the distribution of risk will be similar to the polygenic model except at the extreme tails. A key aspect of the model is the standard deviation of the polygenic risk distribution, because this determines the power of the distribution to discriminate high and low risk individuals (44). The estimate of the standard deviation obtained by Antoniou et al. is a property of the segregation analysis model (13) and it is also close to that predicted by other studies of familial risk. The RRs of disease in monozygotic twins ($\lambda_{monozygotic}$) and siblings ($\lambda_{sibling}$) are related to each other and to the predicted standard deviation of the polygenic log-normal risk distribution by the equation

$$\lambda_{monozygotic} = \lambda_{sibling}^2 = e^{\sigma^2}$$

Assuming $\lambda_{sibling}$ to be equal to 2, as estimated by many observational epidemiologic studies, this equation solves to predict a standard deviation of 1.2. The familial RRs for many other common cancers are also around 2 to 3 (6,45), which suggests that the distribution of risk for these cancers will be similar to that we have observed for breast cancer. Thus, the potential benefits of a targeted high risk approach to disease prevention are also likely to be similar.

The practical use of risk information should be considered in two contexts: that of the individual and that of the population as defined by Rose (46). In both cases, our analysis suggests that a "risk profile" that is based on the combination of known genotype and other risk factors is likely to provide risk discrimination which will be of practical value in health care terms. Whether genetic testing in whole populations would be socially or economically acceptable remains unknown and is likely to depend on whether useful action can be seen to result. But it does seem clear that the use of combinations of risk factors is potentially able to overcome many of the limitations of single risk factors, which have been the cause of skepticism about the practical utility of molecular genotyping for common, low risk genes (4,5). For example, in respect of individual risk, a single gene which conferred a RR of breast cancer of 1.5-fold would increase the risk of breast cancer to an individual from the U.K. population average of 5.7% by age 70 to around 8.5%. On the other hand, a full polygenic genotypic risk profile might identify one woman in 30 who has a risk by age 70 of 20% or more (44). Little is known about how individuals will perceive and respond to such risks; but the discriminatory power of the polygenic risk profile is clear.

At the population level, the effects are even more striking. In Figure 1 the predicted polygenic risk distribution in the population and the prior risk distribution in cases (44) are shown. According to the polygenic model, 12% of the population have a risk of breast cancer of 1 in 10 or more by age 70; and half the total breast cancer incidence falls within that 12% of the population. Different cut-offs can be chosen to give the best combination of high risk and proportion of total breast cancer incidence that is included within the high risk group, to suit the purpose in hand. An important feature of the high risk groups

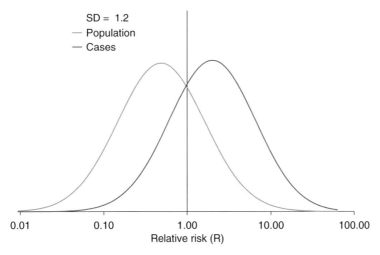

Figure 1   Log–normal distribution of genetic risk in population. Relative risks are shown on a log scale, while the arithmetical average risk for the entire population has been set at 1.0. The risk distribution in individuals who will develop breast cancer (cases) is shifted to the right. The SD describes the spread of risk between high and low values within the population, and thus the potential to discriminate different levels in different individuals. *Abbreviation*: SD, standard deviation.

defined by the model is that most of the individuals within them will be at risk because of the combined effect of several predisposing alleles. This implies that interventions that are based on specific mechanisms of predisposition will individually deal with only a proportion of the excess cancer risk; and that except for predisposing genes with major effects, generic interventions are more likely to be appropriate.

Risk profiles may also be used to define low risk groups. Thus, only 12% of breast cancer incidence falls within the 50% of women at lowest risk. Exclusion of the low risk groups from interventions, if it were socially acceptable, might be very cost effective. For example, screening of the whole population by mammography should reduce breast cancer mortality by approximately 30% (47). If mammography were offered only to the half of the population in the highest risk group by the genetic profile, total breast cancer mortality would still be reduced by 26%, a "loss" of only 4%. There would be additional benefits, since the benefit:harm ratio is likely to be improved by targeting the high risk group. These arguments assume that the efficacy of any intervention is independent of genotype: if that is not the case, the dividend from genotyping may be greater or smaller depending on whether the cancers in high risk individuals are more or less responsive to the intervention.

These arguments and examples also assume that all of the genetic factors that contribute to the estimated risk distribution can be identified and typed. In practice, this goal is some way off (18). Nevertheless, it seems plausible that GWA studies currently in progress will identify a reasonable number of susceptibility alleles in the next two years. Assume 10 risk alleles are identified, each with an allele frequency of 0.3, and each

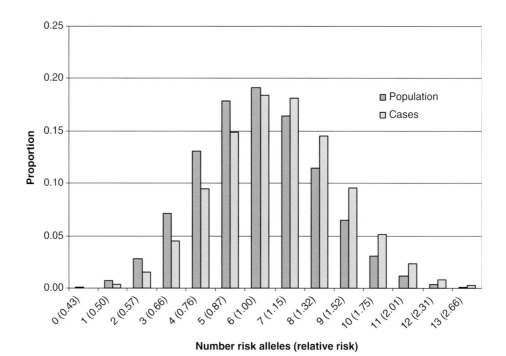

Figure 2 Distribution of risk groups in population for 10 putative risk alleles each with a minor allele frequency of 0.3 and each conferring a relative risk of 1.15. Proportion of population carrying >13 risk alleles extremely small.

conferring a RR of 1.15 with a multiplicative mode of action. In total, these alleles would account for approximately 5% of the excess familial risk of breast cancer. It would be possible to identify 21 risk groups in the population (individuals carrying 0–20 risk alleles). The RR between the lowest risk group and the highest would be 16.4, being 0.43 for the low risk group and 7.1 for the high risk group with the average RR set at 1. In Figure 2, the distribution of the different risk groups in the population and the proportion of all cases that these groups would account for are shown. It can be seen that even if current research efforts identify 10 low penetrance alleles, their clinical utility will be limited. Approximately 23% of the population will carry eight risk alleles or more. This high risk group will have a risk of disease 1.7-fold higher than the low risk group and will account for 33% of cases. Even with 20 susceptibility alleles, the clinical utility is limited, with the 19% of the population that carry 15 risk alleles or more being at 2.08 times the risk compared with those who carry 14 risk alleles or less, and 33% of cases occur in the high risk group.

CONCLUSION

There is good evidence to support the polygenic model for breast cancer susceptibility. Single common low penetrance genes will be of limited clinical utility, but if all the disease-associated alleles that contribute to breast cancer susceptibility were known the potential benefits of targeted preventive interventions are clear at both the level of the individual and when considering disease burdens in populations. A major challenge for molecular genetics and genetic epidemiology is to identify some or all of these alleles.

REFERENCES

1. Bell J. The new genetics in clinical practice. Br Med J 1998; 316:618–620.
2. Beaudet AL. 1998 ASHG presidential address. Making genomic medicine a reality. Am J Hum Genet 1999; 64:1–13.
3. Friend SH. Breast cancer susceptibility testing: realities in the post-genomic era [news; comment]. Nat Genet 1996; 13:16–17.
4. Holtzman NA, Marteau TM. Will genetics revolutionize medicine? N Engl J Med 2000; 343: 141–144.
5. Vineis P, Schulte P, McMichael AJ. Misconceptions about the use of genetic tests in populations. Lancet 2001; 357:709–712.
6. Amundadottir LT, Thorvaldsson S, Gudbjartsson DF, et al. Cancer as a complex phenotype: pattern of cancer distribution within and beyond the nuclear family. PLoS Med 2004; 1:e65.
7. Collaborative group on hormonal factors in breast cancer. Familial breast cancer: collaborative reanalysis of individual data from 52 epidemiological studies including 58,209 women with breast cancer and 101,986 women without the disease. Lancet 2001; 358:1389–1399.
8. Lichtenstein P, Holm NV, Verkasalo PK, et al. Environmental and heritable factors in the causation of cancer—analyses of cohorts of twins from Sweden, Denmark and Finland. N Engl J Med 2000; 343:78–85.
9. Peto J, Mack TM. High constant incidence in twins and other relatives of women with breast cancer. Nat Genet 2000; 26:411–414.
10. Easton DF. How many more breast cancer predisposition genes are there? Breast Cancer Res 1999; 1:14–17.
11. Ford D, Easton DF, Stratton M, et al. Genetic heterogeneity and penetrance analysis of the BRCA1 and BRCA2 genes in breast cancer families. Am J Hum Genet 1998; 62:676–689.

12. Cui J, Antoniou AC, Dite GS, et al. After BRCA1 and BRCA2-what next? Multifactorial segregation analyses of three-generation, population-based Australian families affected by female breast cancer. Am J Hum Genet 2001; 68:420–431.

13. Antoniou AC, Pharoah PDP, McMullen G, Day NE, Ponder BAJ, Easton DF. Evidence for further breast cancer susceptibility genes in addition to *BRCA1* and *BRCA2* in a population based study. Genetic Epidemiol 2001; 21:1–18.

14. Antoniou AC, Pharoah PDP, McMullen G, et al. A comprehensive model for familial breast cancer incorporating *BRCA1*, *BRCA2* and other genes. Br J Cancer 2002; 86:76–83.

15. Risch N. Searching for genetic determinants in the new millennium. Nature 2000; 405: 847–856.

16. Cardon LR, Bell JI. Association study designs for complex diseases. Nat Rev Genet 2001; 2: 91–99.

17. Chakravarti A. Population genetics—making sense out of sequence. Nat Genet 1999; 21: 56–60.

18. Pharoah PDP, Dunning AM, Ponder BAJ, Easton DF. Association studies for finding cancer-susceptibility genetic variants. Nat Rev Cancer 2004; 4:850–860.

19. Matsuoka S, Huang M, Elledge SJ. Linkage of ATM to cell cycle regulation by the Chk2 protein kinase. Science 1998; 282:1893–1897.

20. Matsuoka S, Rotman G, Ogawa A, Shiloh Y, Tamai K, Elledge SJ. Ataxia telangiectasia-mutated phosphorylates Chk2 in vivo and in vitro. Proc Natl Acad Sci U S A 2000; 97: 10389–10394.

21. Zeng Y, Forbes KC, Wu Z, Moreno S, Piwnica-Worms H, Enoch T. Replication checkpoint requires phosphorylation of the phosphatase Cdc25 by Cds1 or Chk1. Nature 1998; 395: 507–510.

22. Chehab NH, Malikzay A, Appel M, Halazonetis TD. Chk2/hCds1 functions as a DNA damage checkpoint in G(1) by stabilizing p53. Genes Dev 2000; 14:278–288.

23. Lee JS, Collins KM, Brown AL, Lee CH, Chung JH. hCds1-mediated phosphorylation of BRCA1 regulates the DNA damage response. Nature 2000; 404:201–204.

24. Falck J, Mailand N, Syljuasen RG, Bartek J, Lukas J. The ATM-Chk2-Cdc25A checkpoint pathway guards against radioresistant DNA synthesis. Nature 2001; 410:842–847.

25. Bell DW, Varley JM, Szydlo TE, et al. Heterozygous germ line hCHK2 mutations in Li-Fraumeni syndrome. Science 1999; 286:2528–2531.

26. Meijers-Heijboer H, van den Ouweland A, Klijn J, et al. Low-penetrance susceptibility to breast cancer due to CHEK2(*)1100delC in noncarriers of BRCA1 or BRCA2 mutations. Nat Genet 2002; 31:55–59.

27. Vahteristo P, Bartkova J, Eerola H, et al. A CHEK2 genetic variant contributing to a substantial fraction of familial breast cancer. Am J Hum Genet 2002; 71:432–438.

28. Neuhausen S, Dunning A, Steele L, et al. Role of CHEK2*1100del*c* in unselected series of non-BRCA1/2 male breast cancers. Int J Cancer 2004; 108:477–478.

29. Ioannidis JP, Ntzani EE, Trikalinos TA, Contopoulos-Ioannidis DG. Replication validity of genetic association studies. Nat Genet 2001; 29:306–309.

30. Lohmueller KE, Pearce CL, Pike M, Lander ES, Hirschhorn JN. Meta-analysis of genetic association studies supports a contribution of common variants to susceptibility to common disease. Nat Genet 2003; 33:177–182.

31. Wacholder S, Chanock S, Garcia-Closas M, El Ghormli L, Rothman N. Assessing the probability that a positive report is false: an approach for molecular epidemiology studies. J Natl Cancer Inst 2004; 96:434–442.

32. Ioannidis JP. Why most published research findings are false? PLoS Med 2005; 2:e124.

33. Todd JA. Statistical false positive or true disease pathway? Nat Genet 2006; 38:731–733.

34. Risch N, Merikangas K. The future of genetic studies of complex diseases. Science 1996; 273: 1516–1517.

35. Dahlman I, Eaves IA, Kosoy R, et al. Parameters for reliable results in genetic association studies in common disease. Nat Genet 2002; 30:149–150.

36. Colhoun HM, McKeigue PM, Davey Smith G. Problems of reporting genetic associations with complex outcomes. Lancet 2003; 361:865–872.
37. International HapMap Consortium. The International HapMap Project. Nature 2003; 426: 789–796.
38. Kruglyak L, Nickerson DA. Variation is the spice of life. Nat Genet 2001; 27:234–236.
39. Livingston RJ, von Niederhausern A, Jegga AG, et al. Pattern of sequence variation across 213 environmental response genes. Genome Res 2004; 14:1821–1831.
40. Barrett JC, Cardon LR. Evaluating coverage of genome-wide association studies. Nat Genet 2006; 38:659–662.
41. Klein RJ, Zeiss C, Chew EY, et al. Complement factor H polymorphism in age-related macular degeneration. Science 2005; 308:385–389.
42. Hunter DJ, Riboli E, Haiman CA, et al. A candidate gene approach to searching for low-penetrance breast and prostate cancer genes. Nat Rev Cancer 2005; 5:977–985.
43. Antoniou AC, Durocher F, Smith P, Simard J, Easton DF. BRCA1 and BRCA2 mutation predictions using the BOADICEA and BRCAPRO models and penetrance estimation in high-risk French-Canadian families. Breast Cancer Res 2006; 8:R3.
44. Pharoah PDP, Antoniou A, Bobrow M, et al. Polygenic susceptibility to breast cancer: implications for prevention. Nat Genet 2002; 31:33–36.
45. Goldgar DE, Easton DF, Cannon-Albright LA, Skolnick MH. A systematic population based assessment of cancer risk in first degree relatives of cancer probands. J Natl Cancer Instit 1994; 86:1600–1608.
46. Rose G. Sick individuals and sick populations. Int J Epidemiol 1985; 14:32–38.
47. Kerlikowske K, Grady D, Rubin SM, Sandrock C, Ernster VL. Efficacy of screening mammography: a meta-analysis. J Am Med Assoc 1995; 273:149–154.

SECTION 3: ASSESSMENT AND DISSEMINATION OF CLINICAL RISKS FOR *BRCA1/2* MUTATION CARRIERS

9

Biology of *BRCA1-* and *BRCA2*-Associated Carcinogenesis

Jenny Llamas and Lawrence C. Brody
Molecular Pathogenesis Section, Genome Technology Branch, National Human Genome Research Institute, Bethesda, Maryland, U.S.A.

INTRODUCTION

In the decade since the discovery of the *BRCA1* and *BRCA2* genes, our understanding of their function has grown tremendously, albeit, slowly. We have advanced from knowing virtually nothing about these genes (other than they were cancer risk factors) to a point where new classes of anti-tumor drugs are being tested based on knowledge of the *BRCA1* and *BRCA2* "pathway." The cloning of these genes was heralded as a great breakthrough in breast cancer research. In retrospect, identifying the genes was the simple part. It took 10 years because the technology and infrastructure that support positional cloning were not yet mature. Why did it require another decade to develop an understanding of the function of these genes? Much of the explanation can be placed on our difficulty is fleshing out new aspects of biology when handed genes of unknown function that lack sequence similarity to known genes. Such was the case for *BRCA1* and *BRCA2*. Their amino acid sequence bore little resemblance to any previously cloned genes. Prior to their cloning, data from tumors suggested that both *BRCA1* and *BRCA2* are tumor suppressor genes. Having the genes in hand has allowed those in the field to investigate all aspects of *BRCA1* and *BRCA2* biology. This chapter is not intended to be an exhaustive review of the field; rather, our intent was to focus on those advances most directly relevant to the clinician.

We now know that in addition to being tumor suppressor genes, *BRCA1* and *BRCA2* are involved in the signaling and repair of DNA. *BRCA1* has also been shown to play a role in cell cycle regulation and transcription. Mutations in either gene lead to a compromise of DNA repair (1), resulting in DNA replication errors. In the current working model, this extra mutational load ultimately leads to the development of breast or ovarian cancer. Like those with "sporadic cancers," the increased risk of breast or ovarian cancer in mutation carriers is affected by age and hormone-related factors. The influence of hormones is shown by the increased incidence of breast cancer among women with a late age at menarche, late age at menopause, and late age at first full-term pregnancy—each of these estimated to increase the probability of developing breast cancer by 1.5- to 3-fold (2). A positive family history, however, is the strongest risk factor for developing breast cancer. It has been shown that the risk of breast cancer increases with the number of family members affected, the closeness of kinship, and the earlier in age that family members are affected (2). Precise risk estimates on how these factors interact with different mutations have not been determined. However, the existence of these factors has provided a context for biological research.

BRCA1 AND *BRCA2*—COMMON FEATURES

Large Proteins

BRCA1 and *BRCA2* are both large proteins (Fig. 1). *BRCA1* is a 1863–amino acid protein with a predicted mass of 207 kDa (3). Its 5592 nucleotides are distributed in 24 exons spread over 81 kilobases (kb) of genomic DNA (4). *BRCA2* is an even larger 3418–amino acid polypeptide with a mass of 384 kDa (3). It consists of 11,385 protein-coding nucleotides in 27 exons spread over 70 kb of Chromosome 13 (4). The sequence of *BRCA2* is not related to that of *BRCA1* but does contains eight versions of a sequence of 20 to 30 amino acids, BRC repeats, separated by varying intervals, all encoded by exon 11 (4).

Evolutionary Divergence

The amino acid sequences of *BRCA1* and *BRCA2* are poorly conserved across mammalian species. For example, the sequence identity of human *BRCA1* with mouse Brca1 is 56% (5) and human *BRCA2* with mouse Brca2 is 59% (6). This is far below the average (>80% identity) for human/mouse gene comparisons. Yet, *BRCA1* can rescue

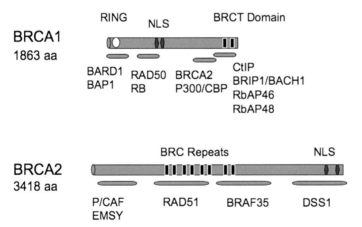

Figure 1 Functional domains and interacting proteins of *BRCA1* and *BRCA2*. Schematic diagrams of *BRCA1* (*top panel*) and *BRCA2* (*bottom panel*) proteins. Specific functional domains are indicated above the protein. Interacting proteins and the approximate location of their binding are indicated below the protein. Domains in *BRCA1* include RING domain in the amino terminus. This domain includes the ubiquitin ligase activity and binding site for BARD1. The central portion of the protein contains two NLS. The carboxy terminus of the protein includes two conserved BRCT repeats. Proteins that directly interact with *BRCA1* are shown. Gray oval indicates the region of *BRCA1* to which they bind. In the illustration of *BRCA2*, the location of the eight BRC repeats sequences are indicated. Two NLS sequences are present near the carboxyl terminus. Select proteins that interact with *BRCA2* are shown. *Abbreviations*: BARD1, *BRCA1*-associated ring domain; BRCT, *BRCA1* C-terminal; NLS, nuclear localization signals; RING, really interesting new gene.

embryonic lethality of Brca1-mutant mice and *BRCA2* can rescue DNA damage sensitivities of a hamster Brca2-mutant cell line (5), implying functional conservation of the protein. In contrast, other tumor suppressor genes such as *MSH2* or *XPA* show sequence conservation across mammalian species with identity between human and mouse of 92% and 86%, respectively (5).

Although *BRCA1* and *BRCA2* have overall poor sequence conservation, they are characterized by regions of higher sequence conservation. *BRCA1* has a conserved N-terminal really interesting new gene (RING) finger domain and a C-terminal *BRCA1* C-terminal (BRCT) domain capable of mediating transcriptional activation when linked to a suitable DNA-binding domain (7). The C-terminal region and BRC repeats in the central portion of *BRCA2* are also somewhat well conserved (5).

Gene Expression

While it is natural to focus of breast and ovarian tissues, *BRCA1* and *BRCA2* are expressed in all tissues. This expression pattern underscores the fact that these genes play a general role in all cells. Expression levels vary from tissue to tissue and *BRCA1* mRNA is highly expressed in several tissues, especially in rapidly proliferating cells undergoing differentiation. In mouse (and presumably humans), this includes mammary epithelial cells during puberty, pregnancy, and lactation (8). *BRCA1* is highly expressed during S phase and *BRCA1* protein is distributed diffusely throughout the nucleoplasm of resting cells and G1 cells (9). At the start of DNA synthesis, *BRCA1* proteins appear to accumulate in discrete nuclear bodies or foci that also contain *BRCA1*-associated ring domain (BARD1), *BRCA2*, and Rad51 (9). The pattern of expression of *BRCA2* is generally similar to *BRCA1* but differential expression is observed in endocrine tissues, including the testis during spermatogenesis and the breast during pregnancy (7).

Control of DNA Before Cell Cycle

Hormone Regulation

Evidence suggests that *BRCA1* functions as a coregulator for steroid hormone receptors and alters steroid hormone action, contributing to the tissue-specific pattern of tumorigenesis in *BRCA1* mutation carriers (10). The cancer specificity seems to be contributed by the interplay between *BRCA1* and the estrogen-signaling pathway, as *BRCA1* has been known as a negative regulator of estrogen receptor (ER)-α signals (11). *BRCA1* repression of ER-α activity is noticeable by the inhibition of estrogen-stimulated expression of *pS2*, cathepsin D, and a number of other estrogen-responsive genes (12). This inhibition of ER-α could be a result of both a direct interaction of the *BRCA1* and ER-α proteins and a *BRCA1*-mediated downregulation of the expression of *p300*, a transcriptional coactivator of ER-α (12).

Data suggest a possible model for *BRCA1* carcinogenesis in which genomic instability leads to the initiation of cancerous cells, while the loss of normal restraint on hormonal stimulation of mammary epithelial cell proliferation allows amplification of these preexisting cancerous cells (7). Findings from a study testing the effect of exogenous hormones in mice with a mammary-targeted deletion of the full length *BRCA1* isoform (Brca1Co/CoMMTV-Cre) (10) suggest that *BRCA1* deficiency abolishes the homeostatic mechanisms that limit the proliferative response to estrogen or progesterone alone and enhances the response to the combination of estrogen plus progesterone. Also, a study of 11,847 individuals from 699 *BRCA1*-mutant breast cancer families (7) suggests that in addition to breast and ovarian cancers, *BRCA1* mutation carriers have an increased risk of pancreatic, endometrial, and cervical cancers and prostate cancers in men younger than 65 years of age. However, *BRCA2* mutations have not been linked to cervical and endometrial cancers, suggesting that endocrine factors may contribute to *BRCA1*-dependent cancer development (7).

BRCA1 PROTEIN

Knockout Studies

Animal models are powerful tools for understanding the mechanisms of human diseases, their prevention, and therapy. In the laboratory mouse, homologous recombination can be used to alter the genome at specific locations (13,14). Strains of mice in which a gene of interest has been made nonfunctional or "knocked-out" are now commonly created to study an unknown or incompletely known gene function, as was done with *BRCA1* (15). *BRCA1* homozygous knockout mice (two null alleles) die at embryonic day 7.5 or 10.5 (3). Death appears to result from an overall lack of cell proliferation, not through alterations of programmed cell death (apoptosis) as might be expected of a tumor suppressor gene (3). Thus, these studies suggest that expression of *BRCA1* is directly involved in cell growth. Further support for cell growth regulation by *BRCA1* is found when looking at mice with targeted deletion of exon 11 of *BRCA1* (2), which results in centrosome amplification, defective G2-M checkpoint control, and genetic instability.

Domains

The *BRCA1* protein comprises a distinctive approximately 100–amino acid RING (named for the prototype gene containing this domain, really interesting new gene) domain at its *N*-terminus, and a pair of approximately 90–amino acid BRCT repeats at its *C*-terminus (Fig. 1) (16). The importance of these two functional domains in the tumor suppressor function of *BRCA1* is highlighted by the finding that most of the missense mutations, unambiguously shown to be cancer-predisposing mutations, map to either RING or BRCT domain. However, these domains appear to be functionally distinct.

RING Domain

The functional importance of the RING domain lies in its role as an E3 ubiquitin ligase in the ubiquitin–proteasome pathway (Fig. 2). The ubiquitin–proteasome pathway is responsible for targeting proteins for degradation and thus maintains appropriate levels of intracellular proteins. The "signal" component of this pathway is ubiquitin—an abundant and essential 76–amino acid cellular protein. In the classical pathway, this protein is used by cells as a covalent modifier of other proteins to target them for degradation via translocation to the proteasome—the organelle of protein degradation (17). More recently, it has been appreciated that ubiquitin can also be used as a signal to activate or repress a target protein's function without leading to its destruction.

Ubiquitination is carried out by a three-enzyme complex (E1–E3). The pathway proceeds through an enzymatic cascade where the product of the first reaction becomes the substrate for the next. Any given cell has one E1, several "E2"s and many "E3"s (see below). Substrate specificity is determined by the E3 component. First the E1, ubiquitin-activating enzyme, charges the carboxy-terminal glycine on the ubiquitin peptide in an ATP-dependent step (17). Ubiquitin is then transferred to E2, a ubiquitin-conjugating enzyme, via a thioester linkage. The charged E2 next interacts with E3 ubiquitin ligase,

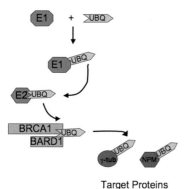

Target Proteins

Figure 2 *BRCA1* has ubiquitin ligase activity. UBQ (*gray arrow*) is first linked to the E1 ubiquitin-activating enzyme. The E1 enzyme transfers the ubiquitin to the ubiquitin-conjugating enzyme, E2. Heterodimers containing BARD1 and *BRCA1* have ubiquitin ligases activity. Substrate specificity is determined by the E3 member of the enzyme cascade. In the case of *BRCA1*–BARD1, this dimer brings the E2 conjugating enzyme to the target. Two targets of *BRCA1*–BARD1 are shown, gamma tublin (γ-tub) and nucleolar phosphoprotein nucleophosmin (NPM, see text). *Abbreviations*: BARD1, *BRCA1* associated ring domain; NPM, nucleolar phosphoprotein nucleophosmin; UBQ, ubiquitin.

whereby E3 mediates the transfer of ubiquitin to the target protein. This first conjugated ubiquitin is the site where additional ubiquitin proteins add to form a polyubiquitin chain, which serves as the protein degradation signal. Lastly, the polyubiquitinated target protein undergoes proteolytic cleavage by the proteasome. However, some protein substrates are not polyubiquitinated and are modified by a single ubiquitin. Monoubiquitination plays an important role as a signal in protein trafficking and extracellular receptor internalization (18).

The total number of E3 ligases is not yet known. The human genome contains approximately 17 E2 enzymes and a single E1 enzyme (18). Thus, the E3 ligases are critical in providing for the substrate specificity of the ubiquitination reaction. These RING-containing E3 ligases such as *BRCA1* and its stabilizing binding partner BARD1 (19) are thought to function by bringing the E2 into proximity with the target protein and then catalyzing the transfer of the ubiquitin from the E2 to the substrate (18). Loss of the *BRCA1* E3 ubiquitin ligase activity would prevent proteasome degradation of its target proteins or disrupt *BRCA1*-mediated signaling. This could alter intracellular activity or levels of critical proteins and thereby alter the regulation of cellular processes that may lead to tumor development. Cancer-predisposing missense mutations within the RING domain of *BRCA1* have been shown to eliminate the ubiquitin ligase activity of *BRCA1* (20). Thus, it appears that the RING domain plays a critical role in *BRCA1* function and that this role can be directly related to the manner in which normal *BRCA1* activity prevents tumor formation.

BRCT Domain

While mutations in the RING domain result in a loss of ubiquitin ligase activity, cancer-associated mutations in the carboxy terminal BRCT domain of *BRCA1* lead to a loss of its transcriptional activation function and loss of binding to RNA polymerase II and can also prevent *BRCA1* from being transported to the nucleus for DNA damage repair (20). The BRCT repeats are believed to fold back and pack together in order to form a highly structured carboxy-terminal domain, and several cancer mutations with single amino acid substitutions or premature stop sites within that region can have a broad impact on the overall conformation of *BRCA1* (21). A change in conformation has the potential to affect *BRCA1* localization and it is possible that the reduced efficiency of nuclear import contributes to the loss of some of these nuclear activities.

Interacting Proteins

Inferred Function

BRCA1 has been defined as being a predominantly nuclear-localized protein. Its nuclear expression and phosphorylation status increase as cells enter S-phase of the cell cycle and remain high during mitosis (21). About four hours after mitosis is complete, and cells enter G1 resting phase, *BRCA1* expression decreases through ubiquitination and proteasome-dependent degradation (21). The nuclear staining pattern of *BRCA1* is consistent with its nuclear functions in different types of transcriptional activation, cell cycle control, and DNA repair pathways.

Transcriptional Activation

Many of *BRCA1*'s biologic actions may be mediated through regulation of transcription. Although *BRCA1* is not a DNA-binding transcription factor, it can interact with a variety of transcription factors to either promote or inhibit their activity. For example, *BRCA1* has been shown to be a coactivator of transcription by bringing together enhancer-binding proteins such as p53, STAT1 (18), C-Myc, JunB, ATF1, and others (7). *BRCA1* can also interact with components of the basal transcriptional machinery (RNA Helicase A, RNA polymerase II), transcriptional coregulators, and chromatin-modifying proteins such as p300/CBP, the retinoblastoma protein (RB1), histone deacetylases (HDACs), and other transcriptional regulatory proteins (Fig. 1) (7). The role that this transcriptional activity plays in tumor formation remains unclear.

Cell-Cycle Arrest

The *BRCA1*–BARD1 dimer with E3 ubiquitin ligase function has been linked to cell cycle checkpoint functions. The centrosome component, γ-tubulin, is ubiquitylated by *BRCA1*–BARD1 heterodimer in vitro, specifically at lysine residues at position 48 and 344 in γ-tubulin (2). Expression of a γ-tubulin mutated at lysine 48 caused a pronounced amplification of the centrosomes.

 In addition, *BRCA1*–BARD1 has also been shown to ubiquitinate the nucleolar phosphoprotein nucleophosmin (NPM, also known as B23) (22). NPM interacts with *BRCA1*–BARD1 and colocalizes with BARD1 and *BRCA1* in mitotic cells (23). Located mainly in the nucleolus, NPM's primary function is thought to be ribosomal biogenesis (24), although other functions such as upregulation by genotoxic stress (25,26), an apoptosis inhibitor, histone chaperone activity in chromatin remodeling, and centrosome duplication (22) have been ascribed to NPM. Importantly, most NPM functions overlap with or implicate *BRCA1*, providing an understanding of how *BRCA1* may play a critical role in cell cycle regulation.

DNA Damage Repair

A large amount of evidence suggests that *BRCA1* plays a role in DNA repair (Fig. 3). *BRCA1*-deficient cells have defects in DNA repair pathways, including the repair of

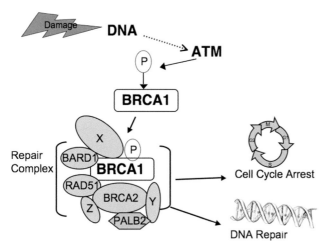

Figure 3 *BRCA1*- and *BRCA2*-mediated DNA damage response. Damage to DNA is sensed by the ATM protein. ATM signals to a variety of proteins, thereby initiating the cellular response to damage. The kinase portion of ATM phosphorylates *BRCA1* ("P" in oval) on specific serine residues. Upon phosphorylation, *BRCA1* enters into a large protein complex that translocates to sites of DNA damage. Some members of this complex are shown (gray ovals). Ovals XYZ represent a large number of additional proteins in this complex. Proteins in the complex carry out specific functions in DNA repair. Other members of the complex signal to cell cycle checkpoint proteins, causing the cell to arrest. Depending on the nature of the DNA damage, the cell will either complete DNA repair or enter into the apoptosis pathway. *Abbreviation*: BARD1, *BRCA1*-associated ring domain.

double strand breaks by homologous recombination, nonhomologous end-joining, and nucleotide excision repair (11). Cellular DNA repair factors are known to aggregate in the nucleus in discrete "foci." *BRCA1* colocalizes to these DNA damage–induced nuclear foci and in nuclear dots during S-phase (21). Additionally, an amino terminal fragment of *BRCA1*, when coexpressed with BARD1, monoubiquitylates the histone protein Histone 2AX (H2AX) in vivo and in vitro (23), implying *BRCA1*–BARD1 activity is involved in chromatin modification. H2AX and *BRCA1* colocalize in discrete foci at sites of DNA damage (27). And, although the exact function of H2AX is not well understood, mice lacking H2AX exhibit sensitivity to DNA damage and chromosomal instability (23). In general, histone proteins are responsible for condensing nuclear DNA into chromatin and their modification perhaps leads to the loosening of this compaction. Thus, it is possible that ubiquitylation of the specialized histone, H2AX by *BRCA1*–BARD1 at DNA breaks, facilitates the action of DNA repair enzymes.

Two possible mechanisms through which *BRCA1* may play a role in DNA damage repair have been proposed. One focuses on the findings that *BRCA1* interacts with proteins of the DNA damage repair machinery either directly or indirectly. For instance, Rad51 and Rad50 are *BRCA1*-interacting proteins, which function in homologous recombination and DNA damage repair (11). Also, a group of proteins associate with *BRCA1* to form a large complex called *BRCA1*-associated genome surveillance complex (BASC), which includes tumor suppressors and DNA damage repair proteins, MSH2, MSH6, MLH1, ATM, BLM, and the RAG50-MRE11-NBS1 protein complex (11). The second possible mechanism centers on the finding that *BRCA1* regulates the transcription of genes involved in DNA damage repair. Three genes, *Gadd45* (a DNA damage repair and response gene), *DDB2* (a gene defective in Xeroderma Pigmentosum group E cells and encoding the p48-damaged DNA-binding protein), and *XPC*—all involved in nucleotide excision repair, have been found to be regulated by *BRCA1* (11). In general, the "transcription" model is less well supported than the "interaction" model.

BRCA2 PROTEIN

Compared to *BRCA1*, fewer investigators have focused their efforts on *BRCA2*. *BRCA2* was cloned after *BRCA1* and is much larger, resulting in complications in manipulating the cloned gene and performing functional analyses. For instance, more than 1800 distinct mutations have been reported in the Breast Cancer Information Core (BIC) Database in *BRCA2*, with most mutations being small deletions of insertions, leading to frame shifts and premature termination of the protein (28). This is consistent with the loss of function that is expected with clinically significant mutations in tumor suppressor genes.

However, few functional tests have been reported and they only cover a limited part of the gene. Moreover, 97% of the more 1000 missense mutations in BIC have been classified as variants with unknown significance (28).

The extreme size of *BRCA2* appears to provide a large number of binding sites for proteins partners (Figs. 1 and 3). These protein partners include Rad51, *BRCA1*, P/CAF, DSS1, BRAF35, USP11, FANCD2 and G, androgen receptor (AR), BCCIPα/β, and the recently identified proposed oncoprotein EMSY and also partner and localizer of *BRCA2* (PALB2) (Figs. 1 and 3) (29). PALB2 colocalizes with *BRCA2* in nuclear foci and promotes its localization and stability in nuclear structures (chromatin, nuclear matrix). These structures function in recombination-based DNA repair and cell cycle checkpoints (29). *BRCA2*'s association with multiple proteins, therefore, makes it likely that *BRCA2* functions at least partly as a scaffold protein aiding in the formation of high-order, multiprotein complexes of biological importance.

Knockout Studies

To study the function of *BRCA2*, homozygous knockout mice have been created. In most cases, the complete loss of function of *BRCA2* from mice carrying homozygous truncation mutations in the 5' region of exon 11 die at day 8.5 of embryogenesis (2). However, mice with heterozygous mutations (BRCA+/–) are phenotypically normal (2). If *BRCA2* knockout mice are crossed to mice lacking *p53*, the offspring live until day 11.5, suggesting that the loss of *BRCA2* results in apoptosis unless the *p53* pathway has also been mutated (2). This suggests that *BRCA2* interacts with the *p53*-mediated DNA damage checkpoint. Therefore, the available evidence indicates that *BRCA2* is a "caretaker," like *p53*, which serves to maintain genomic integrity (30). When this function is lost, genetic defects accumulate. Somatic defects in specific genes are directly responsible for cancer formation.

BRC Repeats

The central binding domain of multiple BRC repeats (Fig. 1) is highly conserved in several mammalian species, suggesting a biological function. For instance, the BRC repeats play a major role in the control, localization, and function of Rad51. There are eight repeats in *BRCA2* designated as BRC1 to BRC8. BRC1, BRC2, BRC3, BRC4, BRC7, and BRC8, are highly conserved, and bind to Rad51 (29,31)—a key protein that covers the processed single-stranded DNA overhangs of double-stranded breaks (DSBs) and promotes homologous recombination, which suggests a role in DNA damage repair. However, BRC5 and BRC6 are less well conserved and do not bind to Rad51 (31). Moreover, mutations within these repeats are associated with cancer predisposition. The deletions of several BRC repeats in mice lead to cancer (32), and the somatic mutations in BRC repeats have been found to be associated with breast cancer (33).

BRCA2 and Fanconi Anemia

The notion that *BRCA2* is solely involved in breast and ovarian cancer was challenged recently. Investigators working on a rare inherited disorder, Fanconi Anemia (FA), discovered that mutations in *BRCA2* cause certain subtypes of FA (34). FA is characterized by developmental defects, bone marrow failure, and susceptibility to certain types of cancer, most notably, acute myelogenous leukemia. Cells from FA patients exhibit chromosome fragility and are hypersensitive to DNA-damaging agents. FA is genetically heterogeneous; mutations in 12 different genes cause FA. One of these genes, FANCD1 was found to be *BRCA2*. Most forms of FA are inherited as a recessive trait. Patients with FANCD1-associated FA have mutations in both copies of *BRCA2* (biallelic mutation). In contrast, in *BRCA2*-related breast cancer, only one copy of the gene is mutated (heterozygous mutation). While this is a rapidly evolving field, it is now clear that the majority of the proteins implicated in FA reside in one of two multiprotein complexes. These complexes are responsible for resolving cross-links in DNA. While the exact mechanics of the DNA repair process has yet to be worked out, it is clear *BRCA1*, *BRCA2* and *FA* genes are functionally connected. This connection has given rise to the term FA/BRCA pathway. This connection was reinforced by the finding that mutations in one member of the FA complex, FANCJ/BRIP1 (a DNA helicase), have been associated with early onset breast cancer (35).

FROM FUNCTION TO PATHOLOGY

In the future, mutation screening and specific treatments may be guided by the specific pathological and molecular features found in tumors arising in those carrying *BRCA1* and *BRCA2* mutations. A detailed description of the histopathological features of *BRCA1* and *BRCA2* tumors are covered elsewhere in this volume. The functional bases for these differences are not yet understood. *BRCA1*-associated carcinomas are more likely to have the basal cell phenotype, a subtype of high histological grade, highly proliferating, ER- and HER2-negative breast carcinoma, and are frequently aneuploid (36–38). This phenotype is rarely found in *BRCA2* carcinomas, which are of higher histological grade than sporadic age-matched controls but tend to be ER and progesterone receptor positive (36). Instead, there has been a strong suggestion that *BRCA2*-linked carcinomas display a "tubular-lobular" phenotype (38). If loss of either *BRCA1* or *BRCA2* results in a disruption of DNA repair, why would the *BRCA1* and *BRCA2* tumors have different phenotypes? The answer may lie in subtle gene-specific differences.

Apart from variation in histophenotype, other molecular pathological features distinguish *BRCA1* from *BRCA2*. The expression of cell cycle proteins differs in *BRCA1*-compared to *BRCA2*-associated tumors. The expression of the cell cycle proteins cyclins A, B1, and E and SKP2 are associated with *BRCA1* phenotype, whereas cyclin D1 and p27 expression are associated with *BRCA2* carcinomas (36). In addition, *BRCA2*-associated tumors resemble sporadic cancers in steroid receptor expression, but *BRCA2* tumors show a higher frequency of *p53* mutations and poor tubule formation, without the other features of *BRCA1* tumors (39). *BRCA2* is also able to directly bind to Rad51 by its BRC repeats and alter its activity while *BRCA1*, although in complex with Rad51, does not directly bind to it (40). Thus, investigating the possible effects or contribution these various proteins exert in tumor development may lead to potential therapeutic targets.

TREATMENT IMPLICATIONS

Ionizing Radiation

Exposure to ionizing radiation (IR) results in DNA damage, most significantly DSBs. In normal cells, DNA damage induces cell cycle arrest to prevent the spread of deleterious cells and activates repair pathways to correct genomic defects. IR as the basis of radiotherapy is a standard treatment used against cancer and is indicated for approximately 60% of cancer patients (41). Yet, even though it is an important cancer therapy, improving outcomes after radiation therapy remains an important clinical goal. To date, certain biologically targeted therapies have been shown to enhance radiation response. However, currently available agents are targeted to specific gene mutations and benefit only a small subset of patients with solid tumors (41). The ideal radiosensitizer then should be relatively nontoxic and enhance the clinical effectiveness of IR in a broad range of tumors. Are there aspects of *BRCA1* and *BRCA2* function that might impact radiation treatment?

Recent work suggests that phosphorylated H2AX (γ-H2AX) plays an important role in the recruitment and/or retention of DNA repair and checkpoint proteins such as *BRCA1*, MRE11/Rad50/NBS1 complex MDC1, and 53BP1 (41). Cells treated with peptide inhibitors of γ-H2AX demonstrate increased radiosensitivity following radiation compared with untreated irradiated cells (41). Therefore, therapies that either block γ-H2AX foci formation by inhibiting upstream kinase activity or directly inhibit H2AX function, interfering with DNA damage repair processes, should be investigated for use as potential radiosensitizing agents.

The involvement of *BRCA1* and *BRCA2* in DSB DNA repair has led to questioning whether *BRCA1* and *BRCA2* patients would respond favorably to IR. Such a treatment kills *BRCA*-deficient tumor cells more efficiently than sporadic tumor cells by creating damage that would not be repaired, resulting in cell death. A problem with this approach is that this treatment is nonselective and neighboring cells would also be subject to the detrimental effects of IR. However, in a large clinical study, no significant differences in the incidence of local reactions to radiation were reported in *BRCA1* and *BRCA2* carriers versus noncarriers (40).

Hormonal Treatment

The benefits of hormonal therapy remain controversial. From a therapeutic point of view, hormone therapy will not be indicated for most *BRCA1* tumors, as they are frequently ER and progesterone receptor negative but can be used in most *BRCA2* and non-*BRCA1* and *BRCA2* carcinomas (36). From a preventative standpoint, tamoxifen, a commonly used antihormonal therapy, has been observed to have a protective effect on women with moderate risk factors (36) and reduce the incidence of breast cancers that were ER positive. Yet, the data specific for *BRCA1* mutations remains unclear. In addition, tamoxifen has been shown to have adverse effects on the endometrium. A study showed that women, predominantly over 50 years, who had been treated with tamoxifen had a threefold greater risk of developing invasive endometrial cancer with a rate of approximately 1% over five years (42). Despite data (see above) directly connecting *BRCA1* to estrogen, it is difficult to estimate the benefit of tamoxifen without specifically testing the effect in a large series of women with *BRCA1* or *BRCA2* cancer-predisposing mutations.

Inhibitors

Tangible evidence that research into the basic biology of *BRCA1* and *BRCA2* can have a direct impact on cancer treatment comes in the form of emerging new drug targets. Two of these, PARP1 and HDACs, have a direct connection to *BRCA1* and *BRCA2* biology.

PARP1

Cells suffer (and can tolerate) thousands of single-stranded breaks (SSBs) in a 24-hour period. Normally, these types of breaks are efficiently repaired. SSBs left unrepaired in dividing cells are converted to DSBs, during DNA replication. In contrast to SSBs, unrepaired DSBs are poorly tolerated by the cell. Accumulation of more than a few DSBs triggers cell death (43). Therefore, a potentially tumor cell–specific treatment would take advantage of the prediction that *BRCA1*- and *BRCA2*-deficient cells are DSB repair deficient. Such cells would be sensitive to increases in the "load" of DSBs. In mammals, the main SSB repair enzyme is poly(ADP-ribose) polymerase 1 (PARP1). In normal cells, drugs that specifically inhibit PARP1 are relatively nontoxic. It is predicted that in *BRCA1*- and *BRCA2*-deficient cells, inhibition of PARP1 would flood the cell with unrepaired DSBs. Thus, inhibition of PARP1 would result in tumor cell death. Normal surrounding tissue containing a wild-type allele of *BRCA1–BRCA2* would not be affected. This approach has been successful in model systems (44,45). Additional cell types and different PARP1 inhibitors are currently being tested (46).

Histone Deacetylases

The ability of *BRCA1* to bind to chromatin-modifying enzymes such as HDAC has led to the development of two models (40) by which *BRCA1* might regulate transcription. In the first model, *BRCA1* may recruit HDAC complexes to specific promoters and thereby repress transcription of a particular gene. In the second model, *BRCA1* may activate transcription by displacing HDAC complexes from specific promoters. Inhibitors of HDACs may then possibly serve as anticancer agents as their inhibition would result in an increase in histone acetylation, leading to the transcriptional activation of a few genes, the expression of which causes inhibition of tumor growth. Thus, HDAC inhibitors can potentially be used as treatment/prevention options for *BRCA1* tumors by compensating for the lack of *BRCA1* expression.

CLINICAL SIGNIFICANCE AND CONCLUSIONS

While considerable work will be required before either of the inhibitor approaches discussed above move from the research laboratory to the clinic, they represent novel strategies and new drug targets. The rationale for these approaches is a direct outgrowth of research into the biology of *BRCA1* and *BRCA2*. Such work serves as an example how new and unanticipated directions can spring from basic investigations.

Since their identification, extensive research has been carried out to elucidate the function of *BRCA1* and *BRCA2* in breast and ovarian cancer. Efforts have been directed toward identifying the biochemical pathways that rely on *BRCA1* and *BRCA2* as a way to develop targeted therapies and potentially benefit mutation carriers. Research has revealed that *BRCA1* and *BRCA2* play significant role in various basic cellular processes such as transcriptional activation, cell cycle control, and DNA repair. This knowledge has the potential to expand and enhance our ability to detect and treat *BRCA1*- and *BRCA2*-associated cancers.

REFERENCES

1. Welcsh PL, King MC. BRCA1 and BRCA2 and the genetics of breast and ovarian cancer. Hum Mol Genet 2001; 10(7):705–713.
2. Arnold MA, Goggins M. BRCA2 and predisposition to pancreatic and other cancers. Expert Rev Mol Med 2001; 3:1–10.
3. Brody LC, Biesecker BB. Breast cancer susceptibility genes. BRCA1 and BRCA2. Medicine (Baltimore) 1998; 77(3):208–226.
4. Brody LC, Biesecker BB. Breast cancer: the high-risk mutations. Hosp Pract (Minneap) 1997; 32(10):59–63,67–68,70–72 passim.
5. Jasin M. Homologous repair of DNA damage and tumorigenesis: the BRCA connection. Oncogene 2002; 21(58):8981–8993.
6. Warren M, et al. Structural analysis of the chicken BRCA2 gene facilitates identification of functional domains and disease causing mutations. Hum Mol Genet 2002; 11(7):841–851.
7. Rosen EM, Fan S, Isaacs C. BRCA1 in hormonal carcinogenesis: basic and clinical research. Endocr Relat Cancer 2005; 12(3):533–548.
8. Marquis ST, et al. The developmental pattern of Brca1 expression implies a role in differentiation of the breast and other tissues. Nat Genet 1995; 11(1):17–26.
9. Baer R, Ludwig T. The BRCA1/BARD1 heterodimer, a tumor suppressor complex with ubiquitin E3 ligase activity. Curr Opin Genet Dev 2002; 12(1):86–91.
10. Katiyar P, et al. Regulation of progesterone receptor signaling by BRCA1 in mammary cancer. Nucl Recept Signal 2006; 4:e006.
11. Deng CX, Wang RH. Roles of BRCA1 in DNA damage repair: a link between development and cancer. Hum Mol Genet 2003; 12 Spec No 1:R113–R123.
12. Ma Y, et al. The breast cancer susceptibility gene BRCA1 regulates progesterone receptor signaling in mammary epithelial cells. Mol Endocrinol 2006; 20(1):14–34.
13. Austin CP, et al. The knockout mouse project. Nat Genet 2004; 36(9):921–924.
14. Evers B, Jonkers J. Mouse models of BRCA1 and BRCA2 deficiency: past lessons, current understanding and future prospects. Oncogene 2006; 25(43):5885–5897.
15. Hakem R, de la Pompa JL, Mak TW. Developmental studies of Brca1 and Brca2 knock-out mice. J Mammary Gland Biol Neoplasia 1998; 3(4):431–445.
16. Glover JN. Insights into the molecular basis of human hereditary breast cancer from studies of the BRCA1 BRCT domain. Fam Cancer 2006; 5(1):89–93.
17. Mani A, Gelmann EP. The ubiquitin-proteasome pathway and its role in cancer. J Clin Oncol 2005; 23(21):4776–4789.
18. Starita LM, Parvin JD. Substrates of the BRCA1-dependent ubiquitin ligase. Cancer Biol Ther 2006; 5(2):137–141.
19. Mallery DL, Vandenberg CJ, Hiom K. Activation of the E3 ligase function of the BRCA1/BARD1 complex by polyubiquitin chains. Embo J 2002; 21(24):6755–6762.
20. Sankaran S, et al. Identification of domains of BRCA1 critical for the ubiquitin-dependent inhibition of centrosome function. Cancer Res 2006; 66(8):4100–4107.
21. Henderson BR. Regulation of BRCA1, BRCA2 and BARD1 intracellular trafficking. Bioessays 2005; 27(9):884–893.

22. Sato K, et al. Nucleophosmin/B23 is a candidate substrate for the BRCA1-BARD1 ubiquitin ligase. J Biol Chem 2004; 279(30):30919–30922.

23. Irminger-Finger I, Jefford CE. Is there more to BARD1 than BRCA1? Nat Rev Cancer 2006; 6(5):382–391.

24. Savkur RS, Olson MO. Preferential cleavage in pre-ribosomal RNA byprotein B23 endoribonuclease. Nucleic Acids Res 1998; 26(19):4508–4515.

25. Yang C, Maiguel DA, Carrier F. Identification of nucleolin and nucleophosmin as genotoxic stress-responsive RNA-binding proteins. Nucleic Acids Res 2002; 30(10): 2251–2260.

26. Wu MH, Yung BY. UV stimulation of nucleophosmin/B23 expression is an immediate-early gene response induced by damaged DNA. J Biol Chem 2002; 277(50):48234–48240.

27. Ward IM, Chen J. Histone H2AX is phosphorylated in an ATR-dependent manner in response to replicational stress. J Biol Chem 2001; 276(51):47759–47762.

28. Thomassen M, et al. A missense mutation in exon 13 in BRCA2, c.7235G>A, results in skipping of exon 13. Genet Test 2006; 10(2):116–120.

29. Xia B, et al. Control of BRCA2 cellular and clinical functions by a nuclear partner, PALB2. Mol Cell 2006; 22(6):719–729.

30. Zhang H, Tombline G, Weber BL. BRCA1, BRCA2, and DNA damage response: collision or collusion? Cell 1998; 92(4):433–436.

31. Chen CF, et al. Expression of BRC repeats in breast cancer cells disrupts the BRCA2-Rad51 complex and leads to radiation hypersensitivity and loss of G(2)/M checkpoint control. J Biol Chem 1999; 274(46):32931–32935.

32. Donoho G, et al. Deletion of Brca2 exon 27 causes hypersensitivity to DNA crosslinks, chromosomal instability, and reduced life span in mice. Genes Chromosomes Cancer 2003; 36(4):317–331.

33. Galkin VE, et al. BRCA2 BRC motifs bind RAD51-DNA filaments. Proc Natl Acad Sci USA 2005; 102(24):8537–8542.

34. Howlett NG, et al. Biallelic inactivation of BRCA2 in Fanconi anemia. Science 2002; 297(5581):606–609.

35. Kennedy RD, D'Andrea AD. The Fanconi Anemia/BRCA pathway: new faces in the crowd. Genes Dev 2005; 19(24):2925–2940.

36. Honrado E, Benitez J, Palacios J. The molecular pathology of hereditary breast cancer: genetic testing and therapeutic implications. Mod Pathol 2005; 18(10):1305–1320.

37. Lalloo F, Evans DG. The pathology of familial breast cancer: clinical and genetic counselling implications of breast cancer pathology. Breast Cancer Res 1999; 1(1):48–51.

38. Marcus JN, et al. Hereditary breast cancer: pathobiology, prognosis, and BRCA1 and BRCA2 gene linkage. Cancer 1996; 77(4):697–709.

39. Hodgson SV, Morrison PJ, Irving M. Breast cancer genetics: unsolved questions and open perspectives in an expanding clinical practice. Am J Med Genet C Semin Med Genet 2004; 129(1):56–64.

40. Yarden RI, Papa MZ. BRCA1 at the crossroad of multiple cellular pathways: approaches for therapeutic interventions. Mol Cancer Ther 2006; 5(6):1396–1404.

41. Kao J, et al. Gamma-H2AX as a therapeutic target for improving the efficacy of radiation therapy. Curr Cancer Drug Targets 2006; 6(3):197–205.

42. Eeles RA, Powles TJ. Chemoprevention options for BRCA1 and BRCA2 mutation carriers. J Clin Oncol 2000; 18(21 suppl):93S–99S.

43. Roos WP, Kaina B. DNA damage-induced cell death by apoptosis. Trends Mol Med 2006; 12(9):440–450.

44. Bryant HE, et al. Specific killing of BRCA2-deficient tumours with inhibitors of poly(ADP-ribose) polymerase. Nature 2005; 434(7035):913–917.

45. Farmer H, et al. Targeting the DNA repair defect in BRCA mutant cells as a therapeutic strategy. Nature 2005; 434(7035):917–921.

46. De Soto JA, Deng CX. PARP-1 inhibitors: are they the long-sought genetically specific drugs for BRCA1/2-associated breast cancers? Int J Med Sci 2006; 3(4):117–123.

10
Genetic Testing and Counseling Issues

Jill Stopfer
*Abramson Cancer Center, University of Pennsylvania, Philadelphia,
Pennsylvania, U.S.A.*

Vickie Venne
Huntsman Cancer Center, University of Utah, Salt Lake City, Utah, U.S.A.

Katherine Schneider
Dana Farber Cancer Institute, Boston, Massachusetts, U.S.A.

INTRODUCTION

Major advances in the understanding of the molecular basis of cancer have made it possible to identify families where breast cancer risk has a strong inherited basis. Individuals who perceive themselves to be at high cancer risk are increasingly seeking out clinical genetics services that assess their cancer risk and provide management recommendations. Physicians are also increasingly referring patients for genetic testing, since identification of genetic risk may influence certain patient treatment choices both around the time of diagnosis, such as whether to have prophylactic surgery as part of their definitive treatment, and during long-term management. Comprehensive cancer genetics clinics, often involving oncology and genetics professionals, offer these services to individuals largely concerned about the implications of their family history of cancer. In addition, clinicians in many specialties are being called upon by their patients to provide information about genetics and cancer risk.

Genetic counseling is a key component of the cancer risk assessment process (1,2), and includes education regarding the genetics of cancer, the likelihood of developing cancer as well as the likelihood of carrying a genetic susceptibility mutation, the benefits and limitations of genetic susceptibility testing, and appropriate cancer screening and prevention strategies. The goal is to empower patients to make informed decisions regarding screening, prevention, and genetic testing by providing him or her with the necessary genetic, medical, and psychosocial information. Attention to psychosocial issues is critical for effective genetic counseling (3). This chapter will focus on the process of providing genetic counseling and testing for individuals at risk for hereditary forms of breast cancer. A thorough review of cancer risks associated with various hereditary breast cancer syndromes and risk assessment models is included in other chapters in this volume.

IDENTIFICATION OF HEREDITARY CANCER RISK

Eliciting an accurate family history is a core activity when assessing risk for cancer and remains the single most cost-effective approach to identifying individuals for genetic counseling and testing and for implementation of cancer risk management strategies (4). Clinicians sometimes rely on answers to the inquiry, "tell me, who in the family has had cancer," as the sole method for obtaining this type of information. Unfortunately, this approach may or may not reveal enough information to perform an accurate risk assessment. Patients may not know the details of their family history without first checking with other relatives and asking pointed questions. In other cases, patients may not have the correct understanding of a relative's diagnosis, and without medical records, the appropriate diagnosis may be missed. Clinicians may put the onus of obtaining medical records, preferably a pathology report, on the patient. Often, comprehensive cancer genetics programs will provide assistance to the patient in obtaining these records. Although histories of breast cancer in close relatives have been shown to be accurate (5), attempts should be made to confirm other tumor types critical to the diagnosis of a hereditary cancer syndrome. Histories of ovarian cancer, especially in relatives removed by more than one generation, are less accurate than histories of breast cancer (6,7). Confirmation of ovarian cancer histology is also helpful since nonepithelial ovarian cancers, such as germ-cell tumors, are not associated with inherited risk due to *BRCA1* or *BRCA2*. Since the presence of an epithelial ovarian or fallopian tube cancer in the family may significantly affect the likelihood of a *BRCA1/2* mutation and thus impact subsequent management recommendations, attempts should always be made to confirm this diagnosis. Records on deceased individuals can be obtained with the signature on a medical release form from the next of kin, although sometimes proof of executorship is also required to obtain private health information.

Failure to obtain an appropriate family history could result in a missed diagnosis of a hereditary cancer syndrome, and subsequently, this in turn may lead to lost opportunities for cancer risk management and risk reduction. In addition, missing the diagnosis of a hereditary cancer syndrome has led to a series of "failure to diagnose" lawsuits or liability cases (8). This section will outline strategies for the cancer genetics specialist as well as generalist for obtaining accurate family history information.

Obtaining Family History Information

Many individuals can be identified as candidates for genetic counseling and testing in either a primary-care setting or an oncology setting. Surgeons, family practice providers, internists, obstetrician/gynecologists, and oncologists should all inquire about a minimum of three generations of family history of all cancers. Genetic counselors typically employ a pedigree with standard symbols, which include females drawn as circles and males as squares (9). The proband refers to the individual who has presented for genetic counseling and is indicated on the pedigree with an arrow. The three-generation family history must include at a minimum information on the proband's siblings, children, parents, grand-parents, maternal and paternal aunts and uncles, and maternal and paternal grandparents. The pedigree should be extended to include cousins as well as nieces and nephews. Family history information can be documented on even more distant relatives if the proband can identify additional relatives affected by cancer. The cancer pedigree should include all the individuals from each generation, whether affected with cancer or not, so that the ratio of affected to unaffected family members can be appreciated. Recording the family history of cancers in this manner also assists with the recognition of the mode of transmission of risk. Additionally, the pedigree should include information on all surgical procedures in affected and unaffected family members such as bilateral oophorectomy performed either for prophylaxis or for a benign condition or removal of skin lesions. Such surgeries may impact that individuals risk for cancer (as would be the case with oophorectomy) or may indicate another possible unsuspected cancer in the pedigree, such as a melanoma. An example of a cancer pedigree is presented in Figure 1 and important details of the family history are listed in Figure 2.

When reviewing a family history questionnaire with a patient, it is helpful to clarify primary versus metastatic cancer sites and to ask about precursor lesions. Typically, ductal carcinoma in situ is counted in the risk assessment with the same weight as an invasive cancer whereas lobular carcinoma in situ is not (10,11). In addition, it is essential to inquire about both maternal and paternal histories of cancer, since mutations in dominant cancer susceptibility genes can be inherited from either a mother or father.

Recording ethnicity is important for breast cancer risk assessment. For example, mutations in *BRCA1/2* are found much more commonly among those of Eastern European Jewish ancestry (Ashkenazis), with an incidence of 1 in 40 (12,13), as opposed to 1 in 500 in non-Ashkenazis (14,15). Clinicians are advised to inquire about any known Jewish ancestry rather than to ask the proband if she is Jewish. An individual may not self-identify as Jewish but have Ashkenazi ancestry in the affected cancer lineage. Such information will impact the likelihood of having a *BRCA1/2* mutation as well as the testing strategy. Founder mutations have also been detected in a number of other groups including those of Dutch, French Canadian, Icelandic, and Swedish ancestry among others (15–18).

Taking a detailed family history can be a time-consuming endeavor. A useful strategy is to provide a family history screening questionnaire that can be mailed out in advance or completed in a waiting room. This allows the proband time to contact other family members if necessary and provides direction regarding the type of information needed. An example showing the structure of a family history questionnaire is provided in Figure 3.

Once the pedigree is recorded in the medical record, it can be updated at each subsequent encounter with the patient, since family histories change over time.

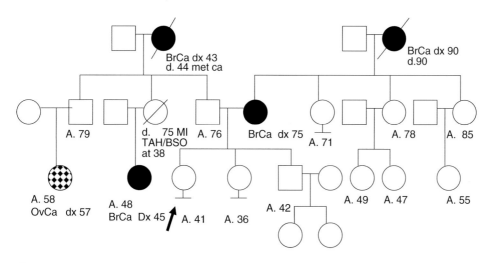

Figure 1 A cancer-focused pedigree.

For each family member with cancer, record the following information:
- What was the primary type of cancer?
- What was the age at diagnosis, current age or age at death?
- What was the cause of death?
- Was the cancer unilateral or bilateral (for paired organs)?
- Possible environmental exposure that might have influenced cancer risk, such as smoking, alcohol, radiation therapy and asbestos

Additional information to record on all women with breast cancer (if possible)
- Type of treatment, including surgery, chemotherapy, hormonal therapy, radiation therapy and reconstruction
- Estrogen and progesterone receptor status (positive or negative)
- Her-2 neu status
- Recurrence information
- Treatment location(s)

For all family members without a cancer diagnosis:
- What are their current ages?
- If deceased, what was their age and cause of death?
- Did they have any prophylactic surgeries, such as hysterectomy, oophorectomy or mastectomy?

Ethnic Background
- For both maternal and paternal side, record countries of origin of ancestors
- Record history of Eastern European Jewish (Ashkenazi ancestry)

Figure 2 Information to include in cancer pedigree.

Sometimes hereditary risk only reveals itself with the passing of years, so patients should also be encouraged to keep their providers abreast of new cancer diagnoses in the family. Reassessment of the significance of the pedigree may lead to changes in recommendations for cancer risk management as well as a possible diagnosis of a hereditary cancer syndrome. The generalist who is not going to be performing an in depth risk family history assessment may also find some of the National Comprehensive Cancer Network's (NCCN's) referral criteria for Hereditary Breast/ Ovarian Syndrome (Table 1), Li–Fraumeni Syndrome (Table 2), and Cowden Syndrome (Table 3) helpful.

DIAGNOSING A HEREDITARY BREAST CANCER SYNDROME

Armed with the cancer pedigree, the clinician can now examine the history for clues about the presence of a hereditary cancer syndrome. These syndromes in general confer very significant lifetime cancer risks due to a mutation in a single germline cancer susceptibility gene inherited in an autosomal-dominant manner. Typical families demonstrate multiple affected family members in several generations, often with early ages of onset. There may be skipped generations however, since these conditions are not 100% penetrant—even those who carry a mutation in a cancer susceptibility gene may live their lives at increased risk but never develop cancer. In addition, histories of female cancers such as breast cancer may be masked due to generations with a high ratio of males to females or small sibships.

NAME First, Last and Maiden Name	DATE OF BIRTH	DATE OF DEATH (If applicable)	AFFECTED WITH CANCER? Yes or No	LOCATION OF CANCER (Eg. Breast, Colon, Pancreas, etc.)	YEAR OF CANCER DIAGNOSIS	HOSPITAL WHERE CANCER DIAGNOSED
You Mary Smith	12/2/1964		Yes	Breast	2000	Hospital of the University of Pennsylvania
Your Mother						
Your Father						
Your Mother's Mother						
Your Mother's Father						
Your Father's Mother						
Your Father's Father						
Your Children						
Your Mother's Brothers and Sisters						
Your Father's Brothers and Sisters						
Your Maternal First Cousins						
Your Paternal First Cousins						
Your Nieces and Nephews						
Other Relatives with Cancer						

Figure 3 Example of a family history questionnaire.

Only about 5% to 10% of breast cancer is due to strong inherited risk conferred by a dominant gene mutation (19). Inherited risk due to mutations in the *BRCA1* and *BRCA2* genes are the most commonly identified type of genetic risk for breast cancer. Currently, the bulk of clinical genetic testing for breast cancer risk is focused on identifying mutations in the *BRCA1/2* genes. However, it is critical that both clinicians and patients are aware that these are not the only genes that can increase breast cancer risk. Care must be taken to communicate the possibility of a different hereditary cancer syndrome raising breast cancer risk or the possibility of inherited risk due to an unidentified gene or set of genes. As clinical testing opportunities broaden to include additional low-penetrant genes, and possibly panels of these genes, it is likely that more families with the concerning patterns of breast cancer will have the source of their risk identified.

GENETIC COUNSELING AND TESTING PROCESS

Cancer genetic counseling is a communication process dealing with an individual's risks of developing specific inherited forms of cancer. The process of genetic counseling helps individuals understand and adapt to the medical, psychological, and familial implications of genetic contributions to cancer risk. Genetic counseling typically includes interpretation of family and medical histories to assess risk, education about inheritance, discussions about options for managing risk, prevention, and research participation (20).

Genetic counseling can, but does not always, lead to genetic testing. Genetic counseling is, however, a critical part of any genetic testing and should be provided by a

Table 1   Referral Criteria for Testing for Hereditary Breast/Ovarian Cancer (*BRCA1* and *BRCA2*)

Patient meets one or more of the following criteria:
  Member of a family with a known *BRCA1/2* mutation
  Personal history of breast cancer and one or more of the following:
    Diagnosed at or below age 40, with or without additional family history
    Diagnosed at or below age 50 or two breast primaries, with one or more close blood relative
    with breast cancer diagnosed at or below age 50
    One or more close relative with epithelial ovarian cancer
  Personal history of breast cancer and one or more of the following:
    Two or more close relatives with breast cancer and/or epithelial ovarian cancer
    at any age
    Close male relative with breast cancer
    Personal history of epithelial ovarian cancer
    Member of ethnicity with higher rate of mutations—Ashkenazi Jewish, Icelandic, Swedish,
    Hungarian, or other—no additional history required
  Personal history of epithelial ovarian cancer
    Member of ethnicity with higher rate of mutations—Ashkenazi Jewish, Icelandic, Swedish,
    Hungarian, or other—no additional history required
  Personal history of male breast cancer, particularly if one or more of the following is present:
    One or more close male relative with breast cancer
    One or more close female relative with breast or ovarian cancer
    Member of ethnicity with higher rate of mutations—Ashkenazi Jewish, Icelandic, Swedish,
    Hungarian, or other—no additional history required
  Family history only—close relative meeting any of the above criteria

professional with the appropriate training and time to ensure that the testing leads to informed decision making in an appropriately supportive environment. Genetic counseling is typically offered by professionals who have training at the Masters, MD, or PhD levels and have professional certification by organizations such as the American Board of Medical Genetics and American Board of Genetic Counseling (21). Referrals for genetic counseling professionals with expertise in cancer genetics can be obtained through professional organizations, as well as through the National Cancer Institute's Cancer Information Service. Resources for finding cancer genetics specialists are listed in Figure 4.

Masters prepared genetic counselors are generally trained in accredited genetic counseling training programs, and masters prepared nurses functioning in the genetic counseling role may also have such training as part of their master's or nurse practitioner preparation (1,22).

RISK ASSESSMENT

Multiple types of risk assessment models have been developed for breast, ovarian, and other cancers, and these models focus on two separate types of risk. The first type of risk information generally offered to patients describes their chance of developing a particular cancer. For example, breast cancer risk models currently being used include the Gail model (23), which incorporates epidemiologic risk factor information as well as family history information, and the Claus tables (24), which uses more detailed family history information but does not include other risk factors. Information derived from these models are often presented to patients as an estimated chance of developing

Table 2 Referral Criteria for Testing for Li–Fraumeni Syndrome (*p53*)

Patient meets one or more of the following criteria:

 Member of a family with a known *p53* mutation
 Meets classic Li–Fraumeni Syndrome criteria

 Personal history sarcoma diagnosed before age 45 and
  A first degree relative with cancer diagnosed before age 45 and
  An additional first- or second-degree relative in the same lineage with cancer diagnosed before age 45 or a sarcoma at any age
 Meets Li–Fraumeni–like criteria

 An affected individual with
  A childhood sarcoma OR
  Sarcoma, brain tumor, adrenocortical carcinoma diagnosed before age 45 AND a first- or second-degree relative with a typical LFS tumor at any age, AND another first- or second-degree relative with cancer diagnosed prior to age 60
 Cancers associated with LFS include but are not limited to
  Premenopausal breast cancer
  Bone and soft-tissue sarcomas
  Acute leukemia
  Brain tumor
  Adrenocortical carcinoma
  Unusually early onset of other adenocarcinomas or other childhood cancers

Abbreviation: LFS, Li-Fraumeni syndrome.

breast cancer in the next five years as well as the chance of developing breast cancer over their lifetime. It is not appropriate to apply these models to individuals when there is a known hereditary breast cancer syndrome in the family, since a woman's risk will largely depend on whether or not she has inherited the specific gene mutation underlying this syndrome.

The second type of risk information offered may be the chance that a patient carries a mutation in a particular cancer susceptibility gene. This risk, sometimes referred to as the "prior probability" or "pretest chance" of carrying a gene mutation, is particularly helpful in making genetic testing decisions. Further detailed information about using specific risk models are presented in the chapter 2 titled "Risk Prediction in Breast Cancer."

Patients may overestimate or underestimate their risks for developing cancer or their chance of having strong inherited genetic risk. Genetic counselors typically convey risk in more than one way, using quantitative estimates derived from risk models, and then setting those numbers in context, so patients can understand how their risks compare to the average risk individual. Using verbal descriptors of risk, such as low-, moderate-, or high-risk designations, in addition to numeric risks, can enhance the process of risk communication (25).

IDENTIFICATION OF GENETIC TESTING CANDIDATES

There are many publications, policy statements, and organizational recommendations that propose criteria for when an individual should be referred for genetic counseling

Table 3 Referral Criteria for Testing for Cowden Syndrome (*PTEN*)

Patient meets one or more of the following criteria:

 Member of a family with a known *PTEN* mutation

 Has one of the following pathognomonic features:

   Adult Lhermitte-Duclos disease (benign cerebellar tumor)

   Mucocutaneous lesions: trichilemmomas (facial), acral keratoses, papillomatous papules—
   mucocutaneous lesions alone are sufficient if

   There are six or more facial papules, of which three or more must be trichilemmoma or

   There are cutaneous facial papules and oral mucosal papillomatosis and acral
   keratosis, or

   There are palmoplantar keratoses, six or more

 Major criteria

   Breast cancer

   Thyroid cancer, especially follicular thyroid carcinoma, rarely papillary, never medullary

   Macrocephaly (equal or greater than the 97th percentile)

   Endometrial cancer

 Minor criteria

   Other thyroid lesions (e.g., adenoma multinodular goiter)

   Mental retardation (IQ < 75)

   GI hamartomas

   Fibrocystic disease of the breast

   Lipomas

   Fibromas

   GU tumors (especially renal-cell carcinoma)

   GU structural manifestations

   Uterine fibroids

 Two or more major criteria or

 One major and three or more minor criteria or

 Four or more minor criteria

Abbreviations: GI, gastrointestinal; GU, genitourinary.

regarding hereditary risk of breast and/or ovarian cancer, including the American Society of Clinical Oncology (26), the NCCN, the Preventive Services Task Force (27), the American College of Medical Genetics, and the National Institute for Clinical Excellence in the United Kingdom. Presented below as an example are the NCCN guidelines for who to refer for breast/ovarian cancer genetics services.

■ Early-onset breast cancer, usually defined as before age 50
■ Two breast primaries (bilateral disease or two or more clearly separate ipsilateral primary tumors)
■ Clustering of breast cancer with male breast cancer, thyroid cancer, sarcoma, adrenocortical carcinoma, endometrial cancer, pancreatic cancer, brain tumors, dermatologic manifestations, or leukemia/lymphoma on the same side of the family
■ Member of a family with a known mutation in a breast cancer susceptibility gene
■ Populations at risk—in these cases requirements for inclusion may be lessened, since the mutation frequency is higher. For example, all women of Ashkenazi Jewish descent with breast or ovarian cancer at any age

---

National Cancer Institute: Cancer Information Service

Phone: 1-800-4-CANCER

Website: http://www.cancer.gov/search/geneticsservices/

This American website contains a cancer genetics service provider search form. Services and contact information for specific cancer risk programs can be searched by geographic location. The listing is multidisciplinary, including physicians, genetic nurses and genetic counselors, and includes individual provider information about licensure and board certification.

National Society of Genetic Counselors

Phone: 312-321-6834

Website: http://www.nsgc.org/

This American website provides information about genetic counseling, and also lists genetic counselors, specialty areas of practice and contact information by geographic condition.

British Society for Human Genetics

Phone: +44(0) 121 627 2634

Website: http://www.bshg.org.uk/

This website contains a directory of the UK genetic centres, including laboratory referral information.

Canadian Society for Genetic Counselors

Phone: (905) 849-8299

Website: http://www.cagc-accg.ca/location/view/index.php?

This website allows one to search for genetic services throughout the provinces in both English and French

---

Figure 4   Referral sources for genetic counseling professionals.

For guidelines on who to refer specifically for genetic testing for *BRCA1/2*, Li–Fraumeni Syndrome, and Cowden Syndrome refer to Tables 1–3.

COUNSELING HIGH-RISK INDIVIDUALS FOR GENETIC TESTING

Cancer genetic testing programs are typically staffed by a multidisciplinary team of providers. These providers can include an oncology provider (physician or nurse practitioner), a genetics provider (a genetic counselor, geneticist, or genetics nurse), and support staff (clinical coordinator, phlebotomist). Typically such programs have a mental-heath provider such as a psychologist or social worker and other physician specialists such as a surgeon, gynecologic oncologist, or radiologist available in their own institution or by referral at other institutions. The most comprehensive cancer genetics programs can provide assessment, education, genetic counseling, facilitation of testing, medical recommendations for management based on individualized risk assessment, long term follow-up and support services, access to cancer prevention modalities, and research participation (10,21).

Components of the Genetic Counseling Session and Testing Process

Major components of a cancer genetic counseling session include collecting personal and family medical history, interpreting the pattern of cancer in the family, describing the features of the cancer syndrome, providing cancer risk assessment and pretest chances of finding a mutation in a cancer susceptibility gene, discussion of early detection and prevention strategies, and a discussion of genetic testing options (28). Logistical issues include the number of required genetic counseling visits, the test eligibility, the cost of testing, the informed consent process, the disclosure process, and the documentation of results.

Typical Clinical Flow

Many clinical cancer genetics programs require at least two visits to arrange for pretest counseling and discussion of the risk assessment and medical management in light of genetic testing results. A typical program may arrange visits according to the model outlined in Figure 5.

Pre-test Counseling Visit

The main purpose of the pre-test counseling visit is to assemble and assess the cancer pedigree and to provide individuals with sufficient information to allow them to provide appropriate and informed consent. The informed consent process includes the following: purpose of the test; information about their cancer risks and likelihood of harboring a detectable genetic risk; accuracy, limitations, cost, and logistics of the testing process; interpretation of all possible results; the implications of the results to the patient and other relatives; options for medical followup; risks and benefits of testing; emotional ramifications of learning the results; confidentiality issues; and alternatives to testing. In general, benefits of genetic testing include an enhanced understanding of one's personal cancer risks. Individuals who have already had a cancer diagnosis may be at risk for additional cancers and benefit from enhanced screening that might not otherwise be offered, and they may also benefit from prophylactic surgical interventions or chemoprevention. Some individuals consider genetic testing even at very advanced stages of disease. In this circumstance, such patients understand that identifying a cancer-associated mutation may have little or no impact on their own care but may benefit children, siblings, and other family members for generations to come. At-risk individuals can then receive more precise risk information, leading to enhanced decision making regarding their own care. Knowing about the presence of genetic risk allows informed decision making that can dramatically lower cancer risks and maximize screening opportunities. Limitations of testing include technology issues in not being able to identify all genetic risk for cancer and the possibility of having to deal with indeterminate or equivocal results.

Insurance preauthorization for genetic testing is also typically initiated at this first visit for those who desire testing and can take days to weeks for a determination to be made. If the genetic testing is likely to provide additional information, the patients then need to decide whether they want to proceed with testing. Many patients are also appreciative of information regarding their insurance coverage when considering whether or not to go forward with testing since the cost will vary from hundreds to thousands of dollars, depending on the test ordered. Countries with national health care will typically

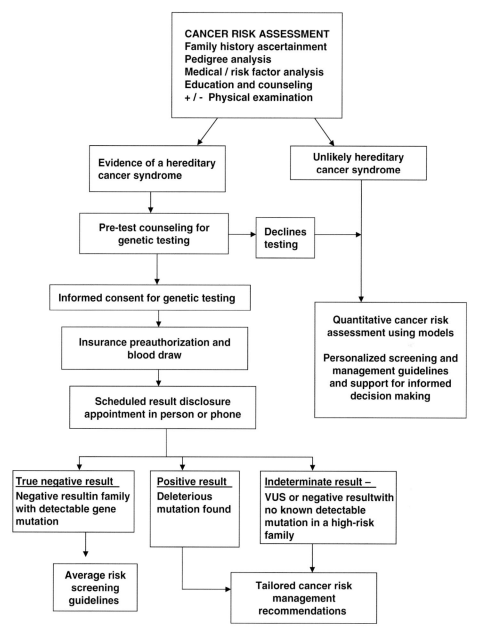

Figure 5 Clinical flow for genetic counseling and testing.

have clinical criteria for test eligibility, eliminating the cost of testing as a barrier for patients with significant likelihoods of testing positive. Written informed consent should be the culmination of this process (29), after which blood is drawn and typically sent to the testing laboratory. Typical turnaround times are two to four weeks but this time may be extended if insurance issues need to be clarified prior to releasing the specimen for analysis. Some laboratories offer an expedited option with results available in 7 to 10 business days for a substantial additional fee.

Test Eligibility

In general, individuals are offered testing if they are 18 years or older and have at least a 10% a priori likelihood of having a detectable mutation. Individuals with less than a 10% likelihood of having a mutation also have the option of being tested, although most third party payers will not cover the cost of testing if the likelihood is low. Testing for cancer predisposition that only manifests in adulthood leads most cancer genetics providers to restrict this testing to adults (at least age 18). Since testing would not affect medical management decisions in a child, there are concerns that the information provides a source of worry without the ability to act to lower cancer risk. In addition, many agree that individuals should decide for themselves whether and when to gain information about adult-onset cancer risks and these decisions are best made by an autonomous adult (30–32). Genetic testing for future cancer risk for children is appropriate when there are cancer risks that can manifest in childhood, such as the Li–Fraumeni Syndrome, which confers a high risk for childhood malignancy (33).

GENETIC TESTING COMPLEXITIES—WHERE TO START?

Careful assessment of the cancer pedigree allows the selection of the most appropriate candidate in whom to initiate testing. If possible, it is preferable to initially test a living affected family member (i.e., has had breast or ovarian cancer or a component tumor associated with the particular suspected syndrome) and select the individual who has the highest chance of having a detectable mutation. If a disease-conferring mutation is found in a family, then the source of cancer risk in the family is known. All other at-risk family members who desire testing for the known family mutation can then receive a highly informative result. Either the individual also inherited the known disease-conferring familial mutation and needs to consider high-risk management options or the individual did not inherit this mutation (true negative result) and can follow screening guidelines for average-risk individuals. If, on the other hand, one had first offered testing to an unaffected woman, a negative test result would not have carried the same meaning. In this instance, there are several possible interpretations of a negative test result including that (*i*) the proband did not inherit the mutation in her family, (*ii*) there is an as yet undefined high-penetrance cancer gene present in the family, (*iii*) current technology is unable to detect the *BRCA1* or *BRCA2* mutation present in the family, or (*iv*) the cluster of cancers occurring in the family were due to chance and not an inherited predisposition. Thus, one must be very careful not to assign average-risk status to an unaffected woman with negative genetic testing result, in the absence of a known detectable deleterious familial mutation. A negative genetic test result in this setting must be considered indeterminate.

Despite the preference to initiate testing in an affected relative, sometimes this is not possible, either due to the absence of any living affected relatives or due to the unwillingness of an affected relative to be tested. In these cases, testing may be considered for the unaffected relative with a significant prior probability of carrying a mutation. In this setting, finding a mutation will be extremely helpful, but the limitations of the negative result as described above must be conveyed in clear terms. Falsely reassuring a patient under this circumstance could lead to inappropriate dropping back in the intensity of surveillance and other cancer risk management strategies.

Complexities in arranging genetic testing can be illustrated by considering the pedigree in Figure 1 as an example. In this family, the proband is a 41-year-old unaffected woman who presents for risk assessment due to concern regarding her maternal family history of breast cancer. She tells you she is certain she will one day develop breast cancer since both her mother and maternal grandmother had breast cancer. After assessing the pedigree, it is clear that the paternal side is more concerning for strong genetic risk due to a mutation in *BRCA1* or *BRCA2*. A common misconception is that risk for "female cancers" can only be transmitted through the maternal side. Although the maternal side includes two generations of women with breast cancer, the ages of onset, well past menopause, are not highly suggestive of risk due to *BRCA1* or *BRCA2*. In addition, there are many at-risk women on the maternal side who have been cancer-free; there is no ovarian or other cancers suggesting an inherited cancer syndrome, there are no rare tumors or any individuals with multiple primary cancers. In contrast, the paternal side includes two women with breast cancer diagnosed at early ages and a first cousin with ovarian cancer. One paternal aunt, who lived to age 75 and was cancer-free, had a complete hysterectomy at age 38, which dramatically lowered her chances of developing both breast and ovarian cancer. Bilineal family histories of cancer are common, and in this situation, the astute cancer genetics provider would focus first on the paternal side when investigating the possibility of genetic risk, since this side has the higher chance of having detectable genetic risk.

After determining that genetic investigation of the paternal side is most appropriate, one can then focus on identifying the best candidate in whom to initiate testing. Certainly one could offer testing to the unaffected proband, but the limitations of this approach are significant as described above. There are two living affected women who would be good candidates for testing, either the proband's paternal first cousin with breast cancer at age 45 or her paternal first cousin with ovarian cancer at age 57. Since ovarian cancer is a less common malignancy, affecting only 1% to 2% of all women, compared with breast cancer, affecting 12% to 13% of all women in the United States, it is less likely that one would find a sporadic ovarian cancer in a family with a *BRCA1* or a *BRCA2* mutation. A final assessment of how to prioritize testing in this family is to first inquire about the cousin with ovarian cancer's interest in testing, followed by the cousin with breast cancer, and as a last resort, the unaffected proband. Cancer genetics providers can be quite helpful in conveying this complicated information to families, and then either arranging the relative's genetic counseling and testing or identifying a cancer genetics referral for the affected relative.

TYPES OF GENETIC TESTS

Genetic testing may examine the full length of the gene or look only for specific "founder" mutations based on the ethnic background of the patient. When there is a known mutation in the family, genetic testing of at-risk relatives focuses on that mutation only. One notable exception is in the Ashkenazi Jewish population where, due to the increased prevalence of all founder mutations, even when a particular founder mutation is detected, it is recommended that other at-risk family members undergo testing for all three founder mutations in *BRCA1/2* (34). This takes into account the possibility that a different founder mutation has descended from a different branch of the family. Other types of genetic tests are those that scan for mutations and may sacrifice a bit of sensitivity in exchange for a simpler, easier, and often less-expensive technique. Scanning for mutations may also be accomplished by using a technique such as Conformation Sensitive Gel Electrophoresis, Single-Strand Conformation Polymorphism, or Protein Truncation Testing, which are slightly less sensitive than sequencing. More recently, certain laboratories have added techniques in addition to full gene analysis such as southern blotting or Multiplex Ligation-dependent Probe Amplification to look for large genomic rearrangements or deletions that would be missed on sequencing. Information can be obtained from the laboratory performing the testing about sensitivity and specificity of the techniques used.

In order to determine the technique used, cancer genetics providers should obtain laboratory reports from affected individuals at high risk for having a mutation in whom testing in the past did not reveal a mutation. Sometimes, repeating the testing with a more sensitive technique is worthwhile and can finally identify the source of cancer risk missed in the past due to technology limitations.

Generally, the first person to be tested in the family must have full gene analysis spanning the entire gene. An exception to this situation is when the proband is a member of an ethnic group that has known founder mutations. These are specific alterations in the genetic code seen repeatedly in a particular ethnic population due to common ancestry. Examples of populations with founder mutations in *BRCA1* and *BRCA2* are the Ashkenazi Jews and individuals from Iceland, Sweden, and Hungary. A reasonable testing strategy for individuals derived from an ethnic group with founder mutations is to first start testing for those specific mutations. If this testing, which is typically a much easier laboratory procedure and, therefore, far less expensive, reveals a mutation, then much effort and expense can be spared. Referring back to Figure 1, if this were an Ashkenazi Jewish family, then testing could focus on the three founder mutations in *BRCA1/2*. However, in a high-risk family such as this one, if no mutation is found using this approach, then one would request that full gene analysis be performed to increase the sensitivity of the test.

POSSIBLE OUTCOMES OF GENETIC TESTING

As outlined in Figure 5, there are several types of genetic testing results: positive, negative, and indeterminate. A positive result reveals the presence of a deleterious mutation that is predicted to impair the function of the gene. This result is unambiguous and provides extraordinarily useful information for a family. All those at risk can now be informatively tested for the presence or absence of the known source of cancer risk in the family. If an unaffected family member then undergoes testing for the deleterious mutation and is found not have inherited it, this result is considered a true negative.

Other results are less clear, and correct interpretation of genetic testing results is an important function of the cancer genetics service. For example, it is possible that the proband's paternal cousin with ovarian cancer in Figure 1 could undergo full *BRCA1/2* testing, and even after sequencing, and screening for large rearrangements, still not have a detectable gene mutation. Such a finding would be considered indeterminate. The possible explanations for this finding include that there is a mutation in as yet undefined high-penetrance cancer gene, there is a *BRCA1* or *BRCA2* mutation in the family that cannot be detected with current technology, the cluster of cancers occurring in the family were due to chance and not an inherited predisposition, and finally the individual tested has sporadic cancer but is a member of a hereditary breast cancer family (i.e., a phenocopy). Since state-of-the-art genetic testing is unable to identify the source of breast and ovarian cancer risk in this suspicious family, the proband must be told she could still be at high risk for these cancers but that informative testing is not currently available to clarify her risk. Her cancer genetics providers should supply her with a risk assessment and options for management of cancer risk based on her family and personal medical history and encourage the family to periodically recontact the cancer genetics service since additional genetic testing opportunities could arise in the future. Clinicians must interpret results that consider the specific test ordered, whether or not the testing was performed on an affected individual, and whether or not there is a known mutation in the family.

Are All Negative Results Equal?

A true negative result is only possible when there is a known, detectable deleterious mutation in the family. For example, referring to the pedigree in Figure 1, if the proband's paternal cousin with ovarian cancer were tested and found to have a deleterious *BRCA1* mutation, one would surmise this mutation was inherited from her paternal grandmother since she had early onset breast cancer. Should the proband test negative for the same *BRCA1* mutation identified in her paternal cousin, then she did not inherit the known source of cancer risk on her father's side. This is a true negative result. Of note, one would have anticipated that the proband was at 25% risk of inheriting this mutation. *BRCA1* mutations are inherited in an autosomal-dominant manner; thus, the proband's father had a 50% chance of inheriting it from his mother, and the proband had a 50% chance of inheriting it from her father. By combining these probabilities $(0.50) \times (0.50) =$ 0.25, one arrives at the proband having a 25% risk of having inherited this mutation. One should always obtain a copy of the laboratory report documenting the specific familial mutation in order to know what test to order in the at-risk family member.

Additionally, since clinical scenarios are rarely straightforward, as in this example, one would not necessarily assign this 41-year-old unaffected proband the same risk for breast cancer as an average women, since she has a bilineal history of breast cancer. One of the breast cancer risk assessment models could be applied, taking into account her maternal family history, and then recommendations would be based on this assessment. Her assessment at this point would no longer need to consider the paternal history, since she did not inherit the known *BRCA1* mutation from her father's side. Although family history of postmenopausal breast cancer in one first- and one second-degree relative will influence her breast cancer risk, it will not raise her risk nearly as high as it would be had she inherited the known *BRCA1* mutation present in her paternal lineage. Therefore, the recommendations to manage her risk will also be different from the recommendations one would offer a *BRCA1* carrier. Although the chances of finding a *BRCA1* or *BRCA2* mutation on the maternal side are low, some clinicians might consider comprehensive testing for mutations in *BRCA1/2* due to the bilineal history. However, in the absence of insurance coverage for such testing, this strategy may be of sufficiently low yield to not justify a potentially significant financial burden.

The Dread Variant of Uncertain Significance

When screening the entire coding region of a gene, it is possible to detect sequence variations, typically but not limited to single base-pair alterations, or missense mutations. These alterations are of unknown clinical significance meaning it is unclear whether or not this sequence variant is a deleterious mutation conferring increased cancer risks or a harmless polymorphism representing normal interindividual variability. The chance of finding a variant of uncertain significance (VUS) depends to some degree on how many individuals from the patient's ethnic group have already been tested. For example, for women of African descent, who have been tested less frequently than those of Western

European ancestry, the rate of VUS was as high as 40% several years ago (35). However, as more African-American women are tested and their variants are categorized and tracked, the likelihood of finding a VUS has diminished.

To further investigate the clinical significance of a VUS, one can do variant tracking, evaluate if the variant has ever been reported in combination with a deleterious mutation, check for publications reporting the variant, and consider whether or not the sequence alteration has occurred in a highly conserved region of the gene (36). A clinical testing laboratory should be able to provide the referring clinician with assistance in interpreting the significance of the variant. Without proper genetic counseling, some women erroneously interpret these results as deleterious, associated with high cancer risks, and then choose inappropriate medical management that may not truly be reflective of their risk. Care and time must be taken to explain this significance of this indeterminate result.

For the family presented in Figure 1, variant tracking would be possible in the event that the proband were tested first and found to have a VUS. Since the most concerning history is present on the paternal side, one could test the paternal cousins with breast and ovarian cancer to see if one or both of these women also have it. If both women with cancer had the same VUS, the variant would be said to "track with cancer risk." On the other hand, if neither of these women carried the VUS, it would provide evidence against it being associated with elevated breast and ovarian cancer risks. Additional evidence against the variant being associated with cancer risk could be gained by testing the proband's maternal aunts who are cancer-free in their 70s and 80s. If the variant was present in these individuals, this would provide further evidence against it being associated with cancer risk. Certain variants will be classified as "suspected deleterious," and, typically, cancer genetics providers recommend that individuals with such a test result follow the management guidelines for those deleterious mutations as there is some laboratory or tracking evidence that the variant is harmful. Conversely, some VUS results are classified as "suspected polymorphism," and are therefore less likely to represent deleterious mutations. Although a VUS is a frustrating outcome of testing, it is recommended that individuals with such a result contact the provider who arranged the testing on an annual basis. This allows the status of the variant to be reassessed. Decisions about medical management of cancer risk may be altered based on a new interpretation of the significance of the VUS. It is critical that patients undergoing full screening of the coding sequence of a cancer susceptibility gene be informed during their pre-test counseling that this is a possible outcome and the limitation of testing.

Disclosure Process

During the initial counseling session, arrangements are typically made to share the result. Depending on the protocol of the cancer genetic center, the result may be given in person or by scheduled telephone appointment. Centers that provide the result by phone often schedule a followup visit in person to review medical management options, especially if the person is a carrier of a deleterious mutation. If the result session is scheduled in person, often, the patient is encouraged to bring a support person who is not also at risk (spouse or friend). It may take between 15 and 60 minutes to review the result of the genetic test, depending on the result and ease of interpretation, the response to the information, and the complexity of the cancer risk management alternatives being considered by the patient. The counseling session is focused on the specific issues relevant to the patient. For example, discussions regarding medical management with an unaffected young woman will differ considerably from discussions with a breast cancer patient who has already had bilateral mastectomies and previous oophorectomy. If the genetic testing result is positive, or if the result is the initial identification of the mutation in a family, the result session should also include a review of the pedigree to identify other genetic testing candidates and create a plan for communicating the result and local resources to them. In some centers, this may be spread into two or three follow-up sessions.

Documentation of Results

Typically, a personalized follow-up letter is provided to the patient after the result session. It includes a copy of the genetic test result as well as a review of the information discussed in the pre- and postcounseling sessions. When a clinician referred the individual for testing, either a copy of that letter or an additional cover letter should also be sent to the provider. Some centers have developed fact sheets summarizing key information and include them in the follow-up letter. In centers that provide consultation only, pertinent information regarding issues such as enhanced magnetic resonance imaging (MRI) screening or prophylactic surgical options are sent to the health-care providers who will be providing medical management to the patients.

UPTAKE OF GENETIC TESTING

Recent studies have shown variability in uptake of genetic testing, even in the setting of a known mutation. Keogh et al. (37) found in Australia that only 44% of at-risk individuals who had provided research blood samples for genetic testing for *BRCA1* or *BRCA2* mutations chose to receive results, despite the fact that testing and counseling were offered free of charge. Foster et al. (38) specifically studied decliners of genetic counseling and testing for *BRCA1/2* in Sutton, England, and found that decliners were more likely to be younger and have lower levels of cancer worry than seen in a national study of test acceptors. Brooks et al. (39) reported that uptake of testing in the setting of a known familial mutation varied depending on how actively at-risk family members were offered participation. They suggest that in general, one-third to one-half of at-risk family members will present for genetic counseling and testing once a family member has been informed about the presence of the mutation. Once an individual presents for genetic counseling, they are much more likely to proceed than decline, with 78% to 99% of those attending genetic counseling sessions proceeding with testing (40–42). People who agreed to be tested cite their interest in clarifying the risk of cancer for themselves and other relatives (especially sisters and daughters) and determining the need for additional surveillance or prophylactic surgery. People who decline *BRCA1* and *BRCA2* testing cite problems with access, finances, and logistics as well as concerns about possible insurance discrimination and increased emotional distress if they were to receive a positive result. Discrimination concerns are more a source of worry in the United States, since there is no guarantee of access to healthcare in the absence of insurance.

TIMING OF TESTING—SPECIAL CONSIDERATIONS

Genetic testing among recently diagnosed breast cancer patients is increasingly being considered, since finding a *BRCA1* or *BRCA2* mutation may influence definitive surgical decisions. Certain women may choose bilateral mastectomies rather than breast conservation in the setting of a deleterious mutation. In a study by Schwartz et al. (43), 48% of women tested at the time of diagnosis and found to have a *BRCA1* or *BRCA2* mutation chose bilateral mastectomies for their definitive surgery. These investigators point out that potential advantages to testing prior to completing local therapy are that carriers who choose immediate bilateral mastectomies can avoid a possible second surgery and unnecessary radiation therapy. Disadvantages to this approach include the additional stress of learning about genetic risk for additional cancers, as well as risk for other close family members, at a time when multiple difficult treatment decisions are being made. In addition, clinical testing including the possibility of insurance issues delays may not offer a fast enough turnaround time and could impose unacceptable surgical delay. Some also question the necessity of this aggressive approach for early-stage cancers in light of the low mortality rate and other alternatives for managing the risk for a second primary breast cancer. Others believe the benefit of bilateral mastectomy is greatest for those who have the longest life expectancy or early-stage disease. Quality of life is an important, highly individualized measure. A follow-up study by Tercyak et al. from 2007 indicated that women who underwent testing at the time of diagnosis and chose bilateral mastectomies did not report diminished quality of life or elevated distress in the first year after surgery when compared to those who chose breast conservation or unilateral mastectomy (44).

Although some individuals will be offered genetic testing in the timeframe immediately following their diagnosis, many will not be offered such testing until treatment has been completed or at some point down the road when an unaffected relative wonders about their own risk and is directed to this affected relative in order to arrange for the most informative testing in the family. Testing may also be offered to a patient who has completed treatment and is now concerned about developing a monitoring program that takes into account screening or prophylactic procedures to deal with possible additional cancer risks.

GENETIC DISCRIMINATION CONCERNS

For some patients concerned about genetic discrimination, medical record privacy remains an issue. Some elect to self-pay for the genetic consultation and testing and ask that the information be provided only to them. This strategy is generally ineffectual at maintaining privacy, since patients with a hereditary cancer syndrome typically want to discuss this highly relevant piece of information with their health-care providers. In addition, information about the presence of genetic risk for cancer often needs to be revealed to insurance companies in order to justify coverage for intensive screening, such as screening breast MRI, or to justify prophylactic procedures. Because the vast majority of cancer genetic centers are associated with tertiary care hospitals, the records are maintained in those hospital records, regardless of the reimbursement mechanism.

To date, there are no documented cases of health insurance or employment discrimination against carriers of *BRCA1* and *BRCA2* mutations in the United States (45), yet patients continue to be concerned. In one study from a high-risk clinic, investigators found that approximately 25% of patients declined testing due to concerns regarding insurance coverage in the event of a positive test result. These same investigators were unable to identify experiences of test result discrimination (46) and suggested that any adverse insurance underwriting was likelier due to a prior cancer diagnosis and not the identification of genetic risk. Concerns about possible genetic discrimination are voiced by clinicians, some of whom are misinformed about the existence of protective legislation or lack of published cases of genetic discrimination (47). Although patients seem most concerned about health insurance, they also express fear of genetic discrimination in other arenas, such as life or disability insurance, employment, arranged marriages, adoption, and child custody cases.

Even in countries with universal healthcare, patients remain concerned about access to life insurance. In the United Kingdom, a moratorium on the use of genetic test results by insurers until 2011 has been implemented. In other countries such as Australia, it is permissible for life insurance companies to ask their customers whether they have had any genetic testing, but the companies are only permitted to use this information in a "statistically relevant" way. Aldhous reported on a single case where an Australian woman with a *BRCA1* mutation was denied coverage for all forms of cancer in her life insurance policy (48). In 2003, Armstrong et al. reported that in the United States, concern about life insurance discrimination was inversely associated with the decision to undergo *BRCA1/2* genetic testing (49). However, in this survey of 636 women who participated in genetic counseling and testing, none reported having life insurance denied or cancelled based on their participation.

The U.S. Federal Health Insurance Portability and Accountability Act, passed in 1996, states that based on genetic information, a person who keeps continuous group health coverage can not be dropped, charged more, or denied access to a new group. This is a powerful national law that protects those Americans who have access to group health insurance but does leave some loopholes and thus individuals outside the scope of protection. It is hoped that the Genetic Information Nondiscrimination Act, which has been introduced at least six times over the last 12 years, may finally have the support needed to be enacted. It will provide more comprehensive protection to safeguard clinical and research genetic testing information from being used in both employment and insurance decisions.

COUNSELING ISSUES

This next section will highlight counseling issues that are typical of cancer genetic situations and include the patient's overall emotional status, reactions during the counseling session, timing issues, and ethical dilemmas.

Patient's Emotional Status

Living in a cancer family can be incredibly stressful, and many patients have described their lifelong fear of developing cancer after watching relatives go through diagnosis and treatment. The emotional distress engendered by the family's experiences with cancer or test results can sometimes be predicted based on the outcome of affected relatives. Those whose relatives have done poorly or have died may logically be more distressed about their cancer risk than those who have relatives who have been long-term survivors. Studies have shown that women whose mothers were diagnosed and died when they were children or adolescents may be at particular risk for ongoing distress (50,51).

Reactions During the Counseling Session

During any consultation, genetic counselors will assess the psychological ability of the individual and/or family to cope with the information, management, and testing choices being discussed. Within a counseling session, patients may exhibit a range of emotions, including anger, grief, guilt, and fear. Collecting information about the pattern of cancer in the family can evoke memories of relatives who have died and uncover family dysfunction. Discussing cancer risks and genetic testing options may be frightening prospects and can trigger a number of coping strategies from denial to over-intellectualization. Genetic counselors are well versed in counseling techniques that allow them to be empathetic and actively supportive throughout the session. Since emotional distress can detrimentally influence the capacity to learn, counselors will continually assess the patient's emotional state during the encounter and determine how best to proceed (52).

Timing Issues

Patients need to be emotionally ready to hear their genetic test results, which potentially can be a powerful piece of information. Genetic counselors are sensitive to the issue of timing in terms of how a test result might be interpreted. The timing issue may have to do with an anniversary date of when a close relative developed or died from cancer. Therefore, if a patient suddenly decides to have testing after years of declining it, it will be helpful to explore what brought about the change in mind. Perhaps the patient is approaching the age at which her mother or other relative developed cancer. Perhaps the patient's daughter is now the age she was when her mother first became sick. Or perhaps a new case of cancer in the family has galvanized her into action. The timing issues may have nothing to do with cancer—pregnancy, divorce, job stressors, relocation, or other big life events can all generate enormous amounts of stress and may influence the ability to process information about cancer risk or genetic test results.

Ethical Dilemmas

Balancing family rights when newly diagnosed is but one ethical dilemma that arises when offering genetic testing for cancer predisposition. Although most centers support the concept of voluntary testing, family situations can make the testing appear coercive. Males who are not at as great a risk of developing cancer may elect not to be tested, but in doing so, may compromise their daughter's access to care. Many centers are willing to test daughters if a father declines testing, with the understanding that a positive test result will reveal information about his mutation status if he is the link to the extended family that has the mutation.

In addition, parents often "encourage" their adult children to consider testing and some may not be ready or interested. Some young men and women who are not yet married and/or not candidates for medical management changes may not care, but appear willing to consider testing, especially if the parents are the source of the financial support for it.

Duty to warn other family members about cancer risks is a concern that seems to be minimized in most families. Several studies indicate that over 80% of families share mutation status with the family. The primary reason that information is not shared often is that individuals do not appreciate the importance of providing it, for example, to a young son who is not perceived to be at risk. Thus, as part of the post test counseling session, the clinician should identify the other at-risk relatives for whom testing would be appropriate. When family members are estranged, the counselor can explore other strategies to assure that the person who is not in regular communication can be provided the information, often by identifying a different family member who is in touch with the person (53,54).

POST TEST COUNSELING—REACTIONS TO THE RESULTS

Reactions to a Positive Result

For women who do not have cancer, a positive *BRCA1* or *BRCA2* test result typically engenders more emotional distress than a negative test result; however, the distress tends to be of short duration. Several studies have shown that mean anxiety and distress scores are not dramatically increased post disclosure (55). In fact, one study showed that the individuals with the highest anxiety levels were the ones who decided not to learn their results (56). These findings provide reassurance that learning one's *BRCA1* or *BRCA2* gene status does not cause overwhelming anxiety or depression. However, receiving a positive result can bring about feelings of sadness, exacerbate feelings of vulnerability, and retrigger grief responses. For these reasons, many programs have developed resources that target emotional as well as medical needs, such as the formation of support groups targeted to unaffected high-risk women (28).

Reactions of Women and Men with Breast Cancer, Who Have an Indeterminate Negative Result

Patients who are members of families in which no mutation has been identified can be frustrated by a negative result. If they were expecting that the genetic test would provide a reason for the development of cancer, especially if it occurred at an early age, anger at the continued uncertainty can manifest in a variety of ways. However, others may be pleased because they presume that a negative result means that the cancer in the family does not have an inherited component, which is often not the case.

Reactions to a True Negative Result

Patients who are in families with a known *BRCA1* or *BRCA2* mutation are almost always happy and relieved to learn that they do not carry the familial mutation and that their offspring are no longer at risk. However, many patients do express feelings of guilt regarding other relatives who have had cancer or have tested positive. These feelings of survivor guilt may temporarily strain family relationships. In addition, a subset of patients with true negative results may feel unsettled by the news, causing them to reevaluate all aspects of their lives.

Reactions to a VUS

This indeterminate result is a genetic change from the "normal" gene, but the significance of that change is not clear. Less is known about how people react to an indeterminate result. Indeterminate results can be very confusing to patients, especially if they have not been told about this possibility prior to the blood draw.

INFLUENCERS OF REACTIONS

Testing programs recognize that a small subset of patients will exhibit high levels of distress following the disclosure of their *BRCA1* and *BRCA2* result. For this reason, it is important for programs to have systems in place to assess levels of distress and to refer patients to the appropriate mental-health professional. A positive test result will engender more distress than a negative result, especially among individuals who have not yet had a cancer diagnosis.

Lack of Sufficient Social Support

People have varying social support needs, so it is helpful to ask if the patient has someone with whom they plan to share their result information. Patients who do not have anyone or who feel that their support is inadequate may benefit from having a referral or may need additional time to deal with their result.

Personal History of Untreated Depression or Anxiety, or Prior Suicidal Ideation or Attempt

When cancer genetic counseling was first offered, there were few other adult onset conditions for which predisposition testing was available. One was Huntington's disease (HD), and as part of the testing protocol for HD, most centers involve mental health-care providers. However, suicidal ideation is part of the biology of HD, and studies have demonstrated that learning cancer mutation status can cause anxiety but not to the degree that requires professional referrals (57,58).

However, because people who present for cancer genetic counseling are representative of the general population, about 10% to 25% may have a personal history of mental health problems, and some will be untreated (59). Many cancer genetic centers, as part of a larger facility, administer questionnaires that assess current mental health as part of the intake. However, it is also part of the psychosocial assessment during the initial counseling session, and when untreated mental health problems are identified, many counselors frame the conversation as one of "readiness" as they encourage patients to seek mental health-care services prior to learning their result. If the patient is already connected with a therapist, in some circumstances, with the permission of the patient, that therapist can be included in the provision of the result to assure that the patient response will be as healthy as possible.

CONCLUSION

The identification of the *BRCA1* and *BRCA2* genes has helped move genetics from rare disorders of childhood to common diseases of adulthood. Clinical testing programs are currently thriving but will need to identify more effective ways to bill for services and expand access without sacrificing quality. As genetic testing for breast cancer risk becomes more commonplace, it will be important to maintain high standards for providing pre- and post-test genetic counseling as well as proper informed consent. Without these core elements, the promise of genetic testing, and its potential to lessen morbidity and mortality from breast and other forms of cancer, will not be maximized. However, it is hoped that in families with hereditary risk, the cancer burden will continue to be reduced, as an increasing number of individuals take advantage of the cancer risk reduction and management strategies.

REFERENCES

1. Stopfer JE. Genetic counseling and clinical cancer genetics services. Semin Surg Oncol 2000; 18(4):347–357.

2. Peters JA, Stopfer JE. Role of the genetic counselor in familial cancer. Oncology (Williston Park) 1996; 10(2):159–166, 175; discussion 176–178.

3. Audrain J, et al. Psychological distress in women seeking genetic counseling for breast-ovarian cancer risk: the contributions of personality and appraisal. Ann Behav Med 1997; 19 (4):370–377.

4. Bennett IC, Gattas M, Teh BT. The management of familial breast cancer. Breast 2000; 9(5): 247–263.

5. Schneider KA, et al. Accuracy of cancer family histories: comparison of two breast cancer syndromes. Genet Test 2004; 8(3):222–228.

6. Kerber RA, Slattery ML. Comparison of self-reported and database-linked family history of cancer data in a case-control study. Am J Epidemiol 1997; 146(3):244–248.

7. Ziogas A, Anton-Culver H. Validation of family history data in cancer family registries. Am J Prev Med 2003; 24(2):190–198.

8. Severin MJ. Genetic susceptibility for specific cancers. Medical liability of the clinician. Cancer 1999; 86(11 suppl):2564–2569.

9. Bennett RL, et al. Recommendations for standardized human pedigree nomenclature. Pedigree Standardization Task Force of the National Society of Genetic Counselors. Am J Hum Genet 1995; 56(3):745–752.

10. Hoskins KF, et al. Assessment and counseling for women with a family history of breast cancer. A guide for clinicians. JAMA 1995; 273(7):577–585.

11. Domchek SM, et al. Application of breast cancer risk prediction models in clinical practice. J Clin Oncol 2003; 21(4):593–601.

12. Struewing JP, et al. The risk of cancer associated with specific mutations of *BRCA1* and *BRCA2* among Ashkenazi Jews. N Engl J Med 1997; 336(20):1401–1408.

13. Roa BB, et al. Ashkenazi Jewish population frequencies for common mutations in *BRCA1* and *BRCA2*. Nat Genet 1996; 14(2):185–187.

14. Antoniou AC, et al. Risk models for familial ovarian and breast cancer. Genet Epidemiol 2000; 18(2):173–190.

15. Verhoog LC, et al. Large regional differences in the frequency of distinct *BRCA1/BRCA2* mutations in 517 Dutch breast and/or ovarian cancer families. Eur J Cancer 2001; 37(16): 2082–2090.

16. Tonin PN, et al. Founder *BRCA1* and *BRCA2* mutations in French Canadian breast and ovarian cancer families. Am J Hum Genet 1998; 63(5):1341–1351.

17. Thorlacius S, et al. A single *BRCA2* mutation in male and female breast cancer families from Iceland with varied cancer phenotypes. Nat Genet 1996; 13(1):117–119.

18. Johannsson O, et al. Founding *BRCA1* mutations in hereditary breast and ovarian cancer in southern Sweden. Am J Hum Genet 1996; 58(3):441–450.

19. Claus EB, et al. The genetic attributable risk of breast and ovarian cancer. Cancer 1996; 77(11): 2318–2324.

20. Resta R, et al. A new definition of Genetic Counseling: National Society of Genetic Counselors' Task Force report. J Genet Couns 2006; 15(2):77–83.

21. Calzone KA, et al. Establishing a cancer risk evaluation program. Cancer Pract 1997; 5(4): 228–233.

22. Calzone KA, Jenkins J, Masny A. Core competencies in cancer genetics for advanced practice oncology nurses. Oncol Nurs Forum 2002; 29(9):1327–1333.

23. Gail MH, et al. Projecting individualized probabilities of developing breast cancer for white females who are being examined annually. J Natl Cancer Inst 1989; 81(24):1879–1886.

24. Claus EB, Risch N, Thompson WD. Autosomal dominant inheritance of early-onset breast cancer. Implications for risk prediction. Cancer 1994; 73(3):643–651.

25. Trepanier A, et al. Genetic cancer risk assessment and counseling: recommendations of the national society of genetic counselors. J Genet Couns 2004; 13(2):83–114.

26. American Society of Clinical Oncology policy statement update: genetic testing for cancer susceptibility. J Clin Oncol 2003; 21(12):2397–2406.

27. Nelson HD, et al. Genetic risk assessment and *BRCA* mutation testing for breast and ovarian cancer susceptibility: systematic evidence review for the U.S. Preventive Services Task Force. Ann Intern Med 2005; 143(5):362–379.
28. Schneider K. Counseling About Cancer. 2nd ed. New York: Wiley-Liss, Inc, 2002.
29. Durfy SJ, Buchanan TE, Burke W. Testing for inherited susceptibility to breast cancer: a survey of informed consent forms for *BRCA1* and *BRCA2* mutation testing. Am J Med Genet 1998; 75(1):82–87.
30. Grosfeld FJ, et al. Psychological risks of genetically testing children for a hereditary cancer syndrome. Patient Educ Couns 1997; 32(1–2):63–67.
31. Laxova R. Testing for cancer susceptibility genes in children. Adv Pediatr 1999; 46:1–40.
32. Patenaude AF. The genetic testing of children for cancer susceptibility: ethical, legal, and social issues. Behav Sci Law 1996; 14(4):393–410.
33. Eng C, et al. Third international workshop on collaborative interdisciplinary studies of *p53* and other predisposing genes in Li-Fraumeni syndrome. Cancer Epidemiol Biomark Prev 1997; 6(5): 379–383.
34. Liede A, et al. A family with three germline mutations in *BRCA1* and *BRCA2*. Clin Genet 1998; 54(3):215–218.
35. Nanda R, et al. Genetic testing in an ethnically diverse cohort of high-risk women: a comparative analysis of *BRCA1* and *BRCA2* mutations in American families of European and African ancestry. JAMA 2005; 294(15):1925–1933.
36. Petrucelli N, et al. Clinical interpretation and recommendations for patients with a variant of uncertain significance in *BRCA1* or *BRCA2*: a survey of genetic counseling practice. Genet Test 2002; 6(2):107–113.
37. Keogh LA, et al. Uptake of offer to receive genetic information about *BRCA1* and *BRCA2* mutations in an Australian population-based study. Cancer Epidemiol Biomark Prev 2004; 13(12): 2258–2263.
38. Foster C, et al. Non-uptake of predictive genetic testing for *BRCA1/2* among relatives of known carriers: attributes, cancer worry, and barriers to testing in a multicenter clinical cohort. Genet Test 2004; 8(1):23–29.
39. Brooks L, et al. *BRCA1/2* predictive testing: a study of uptake in two centres. Eur J Hum Genet 2004; 12(8):654–662.
40. Watson M, et al. Genetic testing in breast/ovarian cancer (*BRCA1*) families. Lancet 1995; 346 (8974):583.
41. Lerman C, et al. *BRCA1* testing in families with hereditary breast-ovarian cancer. A prospective study of patient decision making and outcomes. JAMA 1996; 275(24):1885–1892.
42. Julian-Reynier C, et al. Uptake of hereditary breast/ovarian cancer genetic testing in a French national sample of *BRCA1* families. The French Cancer Genetic Network. Psychooncology 2000; 9(6):504–510.
43. Schwartz MD, et al. Impact of *BRCA1/BRCA2* counseling and testing on newly diagnosed breast cancer patients. J Clin Oncol 2004; 22(10):1823–1829.
44. Tercyak KP, et al. Quality of life after contralateral prophylactic mastectomy in newly diagnosed high-risk breast cancer patients who underwent *BRCA1/2* gene testing. J Clin Oncol 2007; 25(3):285–291.
45. Hall MA, Rich SS. Laws restricting health insurers' use of genetic information: impact on genetic discrimination. Am J Hum Genet 2000; 66(1):293–307.
46. Peterson EA, et al. Health insurance and discrimination concerns and *BRCA1/2* testing in a clinic population. Cancer Epidemiol Biomark Prev 2002; 11(1):79–87.
47. Nedelcu R, et al. Genetic discrimination: the clinician perspective. Clin Genet 2004; 66(4): 311–317.
48. Aldhous P. Victims of genetic discrimination speak up. New Sci 2005; 188(2524):7.
49. Armstrong K, et al. Life insurance and breast cancer risk assessment: adverse selection, genetic testing decisions, and discrimination. Am J Med Genet A 2003; 120(3):359–364.
50. Wellisch DK, et al. Psychological functioning of daughters of breast cancer patients. Part I: daughters and comparison subjects. Psychosomatics 1991; 32(3):324–336.

51. Wellisch DK, et al. Psychological functioning of daughters of breast cancer patients. Part II: characterizing the distressed daughter of the breast cancer patient. Psychosomatics 1992; 33(2): 171–179.

52. Hopwood P, et al. Psychological support needs for women at high genetic risk of breast cancer: some preliminary indicators. Psychooncology 1998; 7(5):402–412.

53. Harris M, Winship I, Spriggs M. Controversies and ethical issues in cancer-genetics clinics. Lancet Oncol 2005; 6(5):301–310.

54. Hallowell N, et al. Communication about genetic testing in families of male *BRCA1/2* carriers and non-carriers: patterns, priorities and problems. Clin Genet 2005; 67(6):492–502.

55. Lerman C, Croyle R. Psychological issues in genetic testing for breast cancer susceptibility. Arch Intern Med 1994; 154(6):609–616.

56. Lerman C, et al. What you don't know can hurt you: adverse psychologic effects in members of *BRCA1*-linked and *BRCA2*-linked families who decline genetic testing. J Clin Oncol 1998; 16(5):1650–1654.

57. Paulsen JS, et al. Critical periods of suicide risk in Huntington's disease. Am J Psychiatry 2005; 162(4):725–731.

58. Schwartz MD, et al. Impact of *BRCA1/BRCA2* mutation testing on psychologic distress in a clinic-based sample. J Clin Oncol 2002; 20(2):514–520.

59. Coyne JC, et al. Distress and psychiatric morbidity among women from high-risk breast and ovarian cancer families. J Consult Clin Psychol 2000; 68(5):864–874.

60. http://www.nccn.org/professionals/physician_gls/default.asp

61. http://www.health.state.ny.us/nysdoh/cancer/obcancer/contents.htm

62. http://www.nice.org.uk/guidance/CG41

11

Molecular Diagnostics: Methods and Limitations

Sean V. Tavtigian and Florence LeCalvez-Kelm
International Agency for Research on Cancer, Lyon, France

INTRODUCTION

The discovery and complete sequencing of *BRCA1* and *BRCA2* (1–3) and the subsequent clinical application of genetic testing for these genes have generated a series of questions of research and clinical importance. For example, what is the mutation spectrum of these genes? Are the cancer susceptibility mutations found in these genes gain of function mutations? Are they loss of function mutations? Are their effects dominant negative? How many different mutations are there in the population? How many different kinds of mutations are there in breast cancer families? These questions were important for basic biological understanding and because of their implications for therapeutic and diagnostic uses of the genetic data.

BRCA1 and *BRCA2* both encode relatively large proteins, and the majority of predisposing mutations in these genes are protein-truncating mutations that cause substantial loss of function (4,5); that is to say, they are tumor-suppressor genes. Prediscovery aspirations that there would be an easy route from the function of *BRCA1* and *BRCA2* to anti-tumor drugs that would be effective in a large fraction of breast cancer patients were shattered by the observation that these genes are tumor suppressors. Most drugs either inhibit an enzyme or else mimic/antagonize a small molecule that is involved in signal transduction. Had it turned out that the predisposing mutations in these genes were gain-of-function ones, then it might have been straightforward to develop inhibitors that would have therapeutic potential. However, the most direct therapeutic approach to a loss-of-function syndrome requires either repairing the gene defect or replacing the protein function, either of which is an extremely difficult task.

On the other hand, tumor-suppressor genes that contribute to cancer susceptibility syndromes are suitable for application in predisposition diagnostic testing. The basic rules that govern gene structure, splicing of hnRNA to make mRNA and translation of mRNA to make protein, are well known. Consequently, many of the possible classes of loss-of-function mutation are understood and many (but certainly not all) loss-of-function mutations are readily identifiable from simple DNA sequence analysis. However, there is a gulf between finding that a gene is suitable for predisposition diagnostic testing and building a test that can be applied to a clinical setting. The majority of laboratory approaches available for predisposition diagnostic testing fall into one of five categories: (*i*) conformational analyses; (*ii*) mismatch/heteroduplex analyses; (*iii*) protein truncation assays; (*iv*) tests for rearrangements; and (*v*) sequencing. In addition to detecting the presence of a genetic variant in a patient sample, there are two additional requirements on the testing process: (*vi*) sample tracking, which is necessary to ensure that sequence variants are correctly ascribed to the sample in which they occur and (*vii*) genetic variant classification, which is necessary to distinguish between deleterious and neutral genetic variants.

CONFORMATIONAL ANALYSES

Single-Strand Conformation Polymorphism

Intrastrand base pairing drives single-stranded DNA (ssDNA) into a sequence-specific secondary structure of stems, loops, and more complex structures, resulting in a unique three-dimensional (3D) conformation (6). Single-strand conformation polymorphism (SSCP) takes advantage of the fact that two ssDNA molecules differing in sequence at a single nucleotide may form slightly different patterns of intrastrand base pairs and consequently assume slightly different 3D conformations. As molecules of the same size but different conformation often have different electrophoretic mobility, these differences can be detected by gel electrophoresis.

As first described by Orita et al. in 1989 (7), SSCP was a somewhat complex protocol based on the Southern blot. Whole genomic DNA was digested with a restriction enzyme, denatured, fractionated on an acrylamide gel, and blot transferred to a membrane. The membrane was then probed with a radiolabeled DNA fragment from the gene of interest. Fragments carrying sequence variants were recognized by shifts in gel mobility as compared to wild-type samples. However, after SSCP was adapted to polymerase chain reaction (PCR) (8,9), the protocol became much more efficient. Segments of target genes were PCR-amplified using a ^{32}P labelled nucleotide mix. After PCR, the fragments were denatured and then snap cooled to favor formation of intrastrand structures over double-stranded DNA (dsDNA) duplexes. After electrophoresis, fragments carrying sequence variants were again recognized by shifts in gel mobility as compared to wild-type samples. Because the protocol is fast, inexpensive, and does not require specialized equipment, it has been used in a variety of research settings (10–13).

Multiple improvements have been described to increase the sensitivity, reproducibility, and throughput of SSCP. Radioactive labeling or silver staining have been replaced by fluorescent primers or fluorescently labeled nucleotide mixes. Fluorescent labeling has in turn enabled transfer of the protocols to capillary electrophoresis (14). In addition, combination of multicolor multiplexing to improve throughput and improved electrophoretic sieving matrices combine to make fluorescent capillary electrophoresis single-strand conformation polymorphism (CE-SSCP) an attractive alternative to conventional slab gel–based SSCP methods for simple, low-cost, high throughput scanning of genetic variants (14,15).

Despite its strengths, SSCP faces some non-negligible limitations. Most importantly, not all of the nucleotides in an ssDNA molecule are involved in intrastrand base pairing. Consequently, some nucleotide substitutions have little or no effect on intrastrand base pairing and hence little or no effect on DNA folding or structure. In addition, sequence variation can lead to structures with either higher or lower gel mobility than canonical sequences, complicating analysis and interpretation of SSCP data. Moreover, ssDNA secondary structures depend strongly upon the physical environment and are altered by variables including temperature, gel polymer composition, buffer composition, and additives such as glycerol. Thus, optimal conditions (e.g., in terms of temperature and polyacrylamide gel composition) differ from fragment to fragment and may have to be optimized by experiment.

Given these weaknesses, it is not surprising that a number of investigators have reported that the sensitivity and reproducibility of SSCP are not completely satisfying. Using *BRCA1* as the target gene, several groups have carried out mutation-screening techniques' comparisons in which SSCP was among the techniques tested (16–18). In each case, SSCP was found to be one of the least sensitive of the techniques compared. For example, the Breast Cancer Information Core (BIC) coordinated a mutation-screening techniques comparison in which the screening centers were blinded to the true mutation status of the samples examined. SSCP had a sensitivity for detecting substitutions and small insertion–deletion variants of 72% (17). Accordingly, some investigators who included SSCP analysis as a mutation-screening technique in large mutation surveys of *BRCA1*, *BRCA2*, and/or *ATM* actually adjusted their observed results for an assumed systematic false-negative detection rate of 30%. This is a clear acknowledgment of the limited sensitivity of this protocol (13,19).

MISMATCH/HETERODUPLEX ANALYSES

When dsDNA is PCR amplified from an individual who is heterozygous at a single polymorphic position located within the amplicon, the PCR product will ideally consist of a 1:1 mixture of two populations of perfectly complementary dsDNA molecules, one containing the first allele of the genetic variant and the other containing the second allele. If this mixture is heat denatured and then allowed to slowly cool back below its melting temperature (T_m), it will ideally form a 1:1:1:1 mixture of four populations of double-stranded molecules: two of these will be the original perfectly complementary double-stranded molecules (i.e., "homoduplexes") and two will be double-stranded molecules that contain a single mismatched base pair (i.e., "heteroduplexes"). Heteroduplexes differ from homoduplexes in a number of physical characteristics, and these differences have been exploited to develop a variety of methods for identifying genetic variants.

Methods Relying on Gel Electrophoresis to Resolve Heteroduplexes from Homoduplexes

Two somewhat distinct families of mutation-screening techniques rely on gel electro-phoresis to resolve heteroduplexes from homoduplexes. The first family is based on electrophoresis of samples in a denaturing gradient, and its basic implementation is referred to as denaturing gradient gel electrophoresis (DGGE). The second relies on the gel matrix itself to achieve separation between homoduplexes and heteroduplexes. Its basic implementation is referred to as conformation-sensitive gel electrophoresis (CSGE).

Denaturing Gradient Gel Electrophoresis

The DGGE protocol arose from studies of the biophysical and electrophoretic properties of dsDNA molecules and was not originally intended for mutation screening per se. In 1979, Fischer and Lerman found that the gel mobility of dsDNA molecules drops dramatically when these molecules become partially denatured and that this gel mobility transition varies according to the denaturant concentration (20). It was also observed that two dsDNA molecules differing by only a single nucleotide substitution could be resolved by electrophoresis into a denaturing gradient of urea and formamide because the lower T_m member of the pair would reach its mobility transition earlier in the denaturing gradient than the higher T_m member of the pair (21). However, if the DNA fragment of interest contains two or more domains with distinct T_m, this approach was somewhat insensitive to nucleotide substitutions in the domain that had the highest T_m. That limitation was overcome by fusing the target sequence to a very high GC-content sequence referred to as a "GC-clamp," yielding a DGGE procedure that should have had over 90% sensitivity for single nucleotide substitutions and higher sensitivity for small insertion–deletion variants (22,23). The initial GC-clamp experiments were performed with cloned DNAs and gel purified fragments digested by restriction endonucleases, which would not have been amenable to high-throughput mutation screening. However, PCR provided a natural strategy for adding the GC clamp to target DNA segments, yielding a relatively sensitive mutation-screening strategy (24). Although the combined complications of developing GC-clamped amplicons and pouring denaturing gradient gels have historically limited the application of pure DGGE to mutation screening of breast cancer susceptibility genes, a Dutch research group has recently developed a comprehensive DGGE-based screen for *BRCA1* and *BRCA2*. Preliminary indications are that the screen has excellent sensitivity and may well be adopted by other labs (25).

The original DGGE studies were an example of two-dimensional (2D) gel electrophoresis. A large number of DNA fragments (e.g., a complete restriction digest of *Escherichia coli* genomic DNA) was loaded into a single lane of a standard agarose gel and fractionated by size. The lane was then cut out of the gel, loaded at the top of an acrylamide denaturing gradient gel, and fractionated perpendicular to the original direction of electrophoresis. Electrophoresis in the second direction fractionated on the basis of fragment stability, and the 2D electrophoresis could resolve several hundred distinct DNA fragments. In 1996, Van Orsouw et al. took advantage of the fragment resolving power of the 2D DGGE to achieve complete mutation screening of the tumor-suppressor *RB1* on a single gel (26). The same group went on to develop 2D DGGE assays, which they refer to as 2D gene scanning (TDGS), for many other susceptibility genes including *PTEN*, *TP53*, *BRCA1*, and *BRCA2* (27–30). By combining software for selecting GC-clamped amplicons that can be amplified in multiplex, multiplex PCR, three colors of fluorescent PCR primers, and a semiautomated 2D gel apparatus, the same team built an efficient and powerful mutation-screening system (28,30,31). In a blinded methods comparison, TDGS was found to have better than 90% sensitivity for a wide variety of mutations in *BRCA1* (17). Even so, perhaps due to the inherent difficulty in casting 2D gels and the technical skill required to read those gels, TDGS has not been widely used for screening breast cancer susceptibility genes outside of the lab where it was developed.

Two closely related techniques, temporal temperature gradient electrophoresis (TTGE) and temperature gradient capillary electrophoresis (TGCE), harness an increasing temperature gradient during electrophoresis to resolve homoduplex from heteroduplex DNAs (32,33). In principle, both should share the relatively high sensitivity of DGGE without the complication of having to pour gradient gels, and TGCE run with multiple colors of fluorescent primers on a capillary electrophoresis system with 96 or more capillaries should achieve very high throughput. To date, neither of these techniques has seen widespread use in the analysis of breast cancer susceptibility genes.

Heteroduplex Analysis and CSGE

Resolving homoduplexes from heteroduplexes by gel electrophoresis does not necessarily require electrophoresis in a denaturing gradient. In 1989, Bhattacharyya and Lilley conducted a series of electrophoretic mobility and chemical reactivity experiments intended to probe the physical structure of dsDNA molecules containing mismatches. As a by-product of their studies, they found that artificial heteroduplexes containing insertion–deletion mismatches are easily resolved from homoduplexes on native tris borate EDTA (TBE) acrylamide gels. Artificial heteroduplexes containing multiple single-base mismatches are also resolved, but not so robustly (34). Shortly thereafter, Nagamine et al. noticed that heteroduplexes in PCR products cause alterations in gel mobility and suggested that this phenomenon could be used as a mutation-screening method. Rommens et al. showed that heterozygous carriers of the 3 bp cystic fibrosis mutation *deltaF508* are easily detected by electrophoresis of heteroduplexes on native acrylamide gels (35,36). Further protocol development experiments yielded the observations that hydrolink gels "mutation detection enhancement (MDE) Gel matrix" have better sensitivity for mismatches than do standard acrylamide gels. Alternatively, acrylamide gels polymerized with bis-acrolylpiperazine (BAP) instead of the more usual N'-N'-methylene-bisacrylamide (BIS) and containing ethylene glycol = formamide also outperform standard acrylamide gels (37–40).

Thus were born two closely related mutation-screening protocols: heteroduplex analysis (HA) based on hydrolink MDE gels, and Conformation Sensitive Gel Electrophoresis (CSGE) based on acrylamide/BAP gels with a modified runnning buffer. Both require little more than PCR of the target sequence, denaturation, and renaturation to form heteroduplexes and electrophoresis on an easily prepared gel. Accordingly, both have been used to screen *BRCA1*, *BRCA2*, and many other genes in labs around the world.

As fluorescent sequencing instruments such as the ABI 377 became widespread, it was inevitable that these two protocols would be transformed into higher throughput multicolor fluorescent assays. Indeed, Ganguly et al. developed four-color fluorescent conformation sensitive gel electrophoresis (F-CSGE) by 1998 and Edwards et al. reported fluorescent HA [fluorescent mutation detection (F-MD)] in 2001 (41,42). Development of F-CSGE did not require any special modifications of the fluorescent sequencer. Consequently, mutation screening of *BRCA1* and *BRCA2* by this protocol has spread beyond the lab where it was developed (43,44) and has also been further adapted for capillary electrophoresis [conformation-sensitive capillary electrophoresis (CSCE)] (45,46). On the other hand, development of F-MD required cooling the gel to below room temperature during electrophoresis, dehumidifying the electrophoresis room to prevent condensation on the gel, and modifying the sequencer's run software. Thus, one would predict that F-MD will spread more slowly than F-CSGE and will be more difficult to adapt to capillary electrophoresis.

Just after heteroduplex detection on native TBE gels was first reported, Bhattacharyya and Lilley also conducted a systematic test of gel mobility effects due to single-base mismatches and reported that many of these mobility effects were very subtle (47). Since then, many investigators have found that this family of techniques is quite sensitive to insertion–deletion mutations but has an appreciable false-negative rate for single nucleotide substitutions. For example, the sensitivity of CSGE reported in the blinded BIC methods comparison was 76% (17). The teams that developed F-CSGE techniques report sensitivities in the range of 90% to 95%. Fluorescent sequencers require that samples migrate the full length of the gel or capillary before detection, and this can improve sensitivity compared to regular gels. Software-aided detection of abnormal peak shapes may also improve heteroduplex detection. Still, the improved sensitivity of these protocols remains to be confirmed in a blinded or independent test format.

Denaturing High Performance Liquid Chromatography

Gel electrophoresis is not the only technique able to resolve heteroduplex from homoduplex DNAs. Britten and Smith demonstrated in 1970 that dsDNA binds much more tightly to hydroxyapatite than does ssDNA. Davidson et al. then used hydroxyapatite column chromatography as a method to separate ssDNA from dsDNA in sheared genomic DNA that had been denatured and allowed to partially renature as a method to estimate the fraction of the genome that is present in single copy versus repetitive sequence (48,49). During the late 1970s and 1980s, reversed phase chromatography was sometimes used as an alternative to gel electrophoresis to separate and purify different length DNA restriction fragments (50,51). It was also known that dsDNA fragments with blunt ends elute from such columns at lower salt concentrations than do dsDNA fragments of similar size that have the short single-stranded "sticky ends" left by some restriction enzymes such as Eco RI or Hind III (50).

Given this background, it is not surprising that column chromatography would eventually be tested as a method for heteroduplex detection. Thus, in 1993, Huber et al. developed denaturing high performance liquid chromatography (DHPLC) as a high-resolution reversed phase chromatography method for separation of dsDNA fragments. In 1995, Oefner and Underhill demonstrated mutation detection using DHPLC (52,53). It quickly became clear that DHPLC has better sensitivity for detecting single nucleotide substitutions in heteroduplexes than methods such as SSCP, HA, and CSGE (53–55).

As with other heteroduplex detection methods, DHPLC analysis begins with denaturation and renaturation of PCR products to form the usual mixture of homoduplexes and heteroduplexes (assuming that the sample contains a heterozygous sequence variant). The sample is then fractionated by ion-pair–reversed phase liquid chromatography in a hydrophobic column containing alkylated particles. Partial heteroduplex denaturation associated with a linear gradient of acetonitrile causes early elution of the heteroduplexes as compared to their homoduplex counterparts (53). Advantages of DHPLC include an automated chromatography system with relative rapid analysis time, no need for radioactive labeling or ethidium bromide staining, and very good sensitivity and specificity (54,56). Mutation analysis of inherited breast cancer susceptibility genes by DHPLC was demonstrated within a few years of the method's introduction and has earned a reputation as being relatively sensitive, fast, reliable, and cost-effective (16,55,57). DHPLC has better than 95% sensitivity for single nucleotide substitutions and, in the blinded BIC methods comparison, found 100% of the mutations present in the sample series (17). However, DHPLC remains a complex assay and requires thorough knowledge of the instrument to correctly perform the analyses. Furthermore, interpretation of DHPLC data is not computerized but is based on a subjective visual inspection of abnormal chromatograms. Indeed, operator experience is by far the most reliable tool for DHPLC data analysis. For these reasons, maintenance of high accuracy and precision in DHPLC analysis requires strict adherence to quality control measures. Accordingly, an initiative has begun within the genetic testing community to develop standardized DHPLC operating procedures (58).

Mismatch Cleavage Methods

Mismatches in DNA duplexes can also be detected by enzymatic or chemical methods that cleave ssDNA or mismatched DNA strands. In order for such protocols to be useful, they have to combine high sensitivity and specificity for nucleotide mismatches with low differential sensitivity due to sequence context. The requirement for low sequence specificity may seem paradoxical. What is meant is that if a reagent is specific for mismatched dC residues (as one example of four), then it must have similar activity toward all mismatched dC and this must be much higher than its activity toward proper CG base pairs. If, due to sequence context, the reagent has differential sensitivity among mismatched dC, then no single treatment condition will find all dC-containing mismatches efficiently and the method will not compare favorably with other mutation detection methods.

During the 1980s and 1990s, a variety of nuclease-based or chemical reagent–based methods were tested for their ability to cleave either mismatch-containing DNA duplexes or RNA–DNA heteroduplexes. Many of these relied on single-strand endonucleases such as nuclease S1 or ribonuclease A (59–61). Largely because of enzymatic sequence specificity, none of these achieved high enough sensitivity to be useful as general mutation-screening strategies. However, in 1988, Cotton et al. made a systematic comparison of chemical cleavage reagents in a search for conditions that combined high sensitivity for mismatches with low sequence context specificity (62). In their screen of chemical reagents that were known to react with RNA or DNA nucleotides such that subsequent treatment with piperidine leads to strand cleavage, they found that hydroxylamine has good specificity for mismatched dC residues and osmium tetroxide has good specificity for mismatched T residues. Although neither has perfect sequence context independence, their sequence context dependencies are somewhat complementary (63). Thus, used in parallel, these two reagents are able to cleave at least one strand of all naturally occurring single nucleotide substitutions or small insertion–deletion mutations, giving rise to the chemical cleavage of mismatch (CCM) protocol. Six years after development of the original ^{32}P labelled CCM protocol, Verpy et al. converted it to its fluorescent incarnation, fluorescence-assisted mismatch analysis (FAMA) (63,64).

Compared to most other mutation-scanning techniques, CCM and FAMA have the advantages that they work with relatively long amplicons, up to approximately 1.4 kb, can detect more than one genetic variant in the same PCR product, and provide an indication of the location of each genetic variant located within each individual PCR product. The sensitivity of the method is also reported at above 95% (64,65). Given the large size of exon 11 of *BRCA1* and exon 11 of *BRCA2*, and that both these genes have several consecutive small exons that are close enough together to analyze in single amplicons, FAMA provides an attractive approach to mutation scanning these genes. Accordingly, Ricevuto et al. first reported complete FAMA-based mutation scanning of *BRCA1* and Pages et al. reported combined FAMA and DGGE mutation scanning of *BRCA2* (65,66). Others have also used FAMA to mutation scan *TP53* (67,68).

The main disadvantage of FAMA is that the procedure involves multiple sample manipulations including the use of somewhat toxic chemicals. Thus, the procedure is somewhat labor intensive and relatively more expensive than other mutation-scanning techniques and will remain so unless it becomes adapted to laboratory automation.

High-Resolution Melt Curve Analysis

High-resolution melt curve analysis (HRM or MCA) has been recently introduced as a promising technique for high throughput genotyping (69) and mutation scanning (70). The method rests on three biophysical principles and is elegant in its simplicity. First, certain dyes bind to double-strand DNA, fluoresce under ultraviolet light when bound, and are compatible with PCR at saturating concentrations. This makes possible high-resolution fluorescence versus temperature, or melting curve, analysis of PCR products by optical methods. Second, if a particular amplicon is polymorphic, PCR of that amplicon from a heterozygote sample followed by denaturation and reannealing results in four DNA duplexes: two homoduplexes of opposite genotype and two mismatched heteroduplexes. Each of these duplexes has a characteristic melting curve, and the sum of all of the melting curves of the PCR products present in a single sample can be observed by a HRM analysis. Third, because mismatched heteroduplexes have a lower T_m than either homoduplex, a heterozygote in the sample (and resulting mismatch duplex) shifts the melting curve profile. This shift can be detected reliably by a suitably sensitive HRM instrument.

MCA/HRM offers several obvious advantages as compared to traditional mutation-scanning methods. First, it is a rapid and secure method because its closed-tube nature avoids the time-consuming separation step on a gel or other matrix while minimizing any potential risk of contamination or sample handling error. Second, MCA/HRM is easy to implement, as it does not require any post-PCR sample manipulation other than the closed-tube melting analysis. Third, the protocol is extremely easy to automate because it involves so few steps. Fourth, the melt curve analysis is nondestructive; individual samples can be reanalyzed several times and the same sample that was subject to melt curve analysis can also be sequenced. Fifth, the protocol is relatively inexpensive because it requires only PCR reagents plus a small amount of fluorescent dye. Finally, MCA/HRM seems to be suitable for high-throughput mutation screening as the latest instruments enable the simultaneous acquisition of up to 384 fluorescent melting signals in less than five minutes.

Specificity and sensitivity of MCA/HRM for mutation scanning of single-base substitutions were evaluated using an assay specifically developed to assess the effect of PCR product size, GC content, and the nature and the position of the base change within the PCR product (70). The authors reported 100% sensitivity for single nucleotide substitutions in fragments of less than 300 bp and over 95% sensitivity in fragments with length between 400 and 1000 bp. The false-negative error rate tended to increase with fragment length and for the identification of A:A or T:T mismatches. Although complete mutation screening of breast cancer susceptibility genes by MCA/HRM has not yet been reported, a recent technical assessment of the protocol by the UK National Genetics Reference Laboratory also reported over 98% sensitivity for a mix of small insertion–deletion mutations and single nucleotide substitutions in a variety of sequence contexts (71). Although investigators interested in using MCA/HRM to screen breast cancer susceptibility genes will clearly have to pay attention to amplicon size, there is a strong probability that this will become a popular mutation-screening method.

PROTEIN TRUNCATION TEST

There are a number of disease susceptibility genes whose mutation spectra are dominated by protein truncating mutations such as nonsense substitutions and small insertion–deletion mutations that cause frame shifts to the open reading frame. In 1993, Roest et al., working with the Duchenne muscular dystrophy gene, and Powell et al., working with the colon cancer susceptibility gene *APC*, both recognized that in vitro translation of RNA that is heterozygous for a truncating mutation will lead to a mix of normal and truncated protein products and that this could form the basis of a mutation-screening method (72,73). In the protein truncation test (PTT), PCR is performed from either patient cDNA or patient genomic DNA using a primer pair in which the gene-specific component of the sense-strand primer has a 5' extension that contains a T7 RNA polymerase promoter sequence and eukaryotic translation initiator site. Protein products are synthesized from this DNA construct by programming a commercially available coupled in vitro transcription/translation assay with the PCR product and a radioactive amino acid mix. The translation products are then analyzed by polyacrylamide gel electrophoresis. Truncating mutations are recognized by shorter than expected translation products. As with the CCM assay, the size of the truncated translation product gives an indication of where in the gene the mutation is located.

The PTT assay has three main advantages: it is relatively easy to implement, it has very high sensitivity and specificity for truncating mutations, and it can be used to screen larger amplicons than almost any other method. As the mutation spectra of BRCA1 and BRCA2 are both dominated by truncating mutations (74,75), it was natural that a number of research groups built PTT assays for these genes. For BRCA1 and BRCA2, the main question was whether to screen the whole gene by PTT or just to screen the large exons (exon 11 of BRCA1 and exons 10 and 11 of BRCA2).

Hogervorst et al. reported complete PTT mutation screening of the BRCA1 open reading frame in 1995 (76). This test was sensitive to both nonsense/frameshift mutations and splice junction mutations. Exons 2 to 10 and 12 to 23 were screened from cDNA while exon 11 was screened from genomic DNA. By 1997, a PTT test had also been designed for BRCA2. Later, a single PTT test for both BRCA1 and BRCA2 was developed using just nine amplicons (77,78). However, it was already clear by this time that the actual achieved sensitivity of PTT was less than its theoretical sensitivity.

Although the PTT assays for BRCA1 and BRCA2 are quite efficient, they have three main limitations. One of the limitations is caused by nonsense-mediated mRNA decay (NMD). The NMD pathway in mammalian cells recognizes and destroys mRNA transcripts that contain a stop codon before the last splice junction. Presumably, the NMD pathway functions to prevent the synthesis of truncated proteins, which may have dominant negative effects in vivo (79). Because of NMD, transcripts from alleles containing a protein truncating mutation are usually less abundant than transcripts from normal alleles. For PTT assays that start with RNA, this means that the truncated protein product will be less abundant than the full-length product, which can reduce the sensitivity of the PTT assay. PTT assays that start with genomic DNA are not affected by this limitation. A second limitation arises if the truncating mutation is very close to the forward PCR primer. In this case, the truncated translation product will be small and may either be poorly resolved from the unincorporated amino acids or disproportionately elute from the gel during washing. The combination of poor gel resolution for low molecular weight peptides and NMD makes detection from cDNA of truncating mutations that are located near the forward PCR primer particularly difficult (80). Finally, missense substitutions are by definition invisible to PTT. As a consequence, most contemporary BRCA1 and BRCA2 mutation screening efforts that include PTT use the procedure to detect mutations in the large exons 11 but use other methods to screen the smaller coding exons of these genes.

SEQUENCING METHODS

All of the previously described mutation-scanning methods detect the presence of genetic variants without revealing the exact underlying sequence variant. Defining the precise genetic change requires sequencing. The first truly effective DNA sequencing methods were described by Maxam and Gilbert and Sanger and Coulson, both in 1977 (81,82). The Maxam and Gilbert sequencing method depends on base-specific chemical cleavage of DNA, whereas the Sanger sequencing method relies on incorporation of chain-terminating dideoxy nucleotides (or, alternatively, arabinotides) to reveal DNA sequences. The Sanger method has become much more popular than the Maxam and Gilbert method, probably because the Maxam and Gilbert method relied on rather toxic chemicals such as dimethyl sulfate and hydrazine, whereas Sanger sequencing evolved into a single-tube enzymatic/fluorescent reaction. More recently, chip-based sequencing by hybridization has also become a viable alternative to sequencing methods that require electrophoresis.

Gel Electrophoresis–Based Sequencing Methods

During the period of the *BRCA1* and *BRCA2* positional cloning projects, the most efficient sequencing based mutation-screening strategy was in fact dideoxy cycle sequencing of PCR products using ^{32}P labeled nucleotides to label the sequencing products. Mutation screening by radioactive cycle sequencing required four lanes of a slab sequencing gel, corresponding to the A, C, G, and T sequence reactions, for each sample. However, instead of running the four lanes representing each sample adjacently to each other, the A lanes for all of the samples were run in a group, the C lanes for all of the samples were run in a group, etc. This strategy took advantage of the human eye's ability to spot individual lanes that differed from neighboring lanes on the X-ray film image of the mutation-screening gel, providing a sensitive and reasonably efficient mutation-screening method.

By the time *BRCA1* was discovered, fluorescent Sanger dideoxy sequencing was well on its way to replacing its radiolabeled progenitor for most de novo sequencing applications but was not yet widely used for mutation screening. There are two basic protocols for fluorescent dideoxy sequencing, dye terminator (83,84) and dye primer (85); each has its advantages and disadvantages. Dye-terminator sequencing has the advantage of simplicity. In this protocol, each of the four dideoxy-nucleotide terminators is labeled with a different fluorescent dye. Thus, all four can be premixed in a single sequencing reagent, resulting in a single reaction per sample sequenced (or two reactions if sequencing is to be carried out in both directions). Dye terminator has the added advantage of relatively low background because the only sequencing extension products that are labeled are those that have incorporated a fluorescent dideoxy terminator. The disadvantage of dye-terminator sequencing is that DNA polymerases seem to have considerable sequence-specific differential affinity for deoxy nucleotides versus dye-labelled dideoxy nucleotides. The result is that one regularly observes individual base positions in dye-terminator sequences where the peak is disproportionately weak compared to surrounding peaks (86). In mutation screening, if the minor allele base corresponding to a mutation happens to be disproportionately weak because of its sequence context, then the mutation is very easy to miss in the resulting chromatogram (86–88).

Since the mid-1990s, sequencing reagent manufacturers have both engineered the polymerases to reduce sequence-specific differential selectivity between deoxy and dideoxy nucleotides (89,90) and modified the fluorescent dideoxynucleotides themselves to reduce this problem (91,92).

As the name implies, the fluorescent labels in dye-primer sequencing are placed on the primers. Reactions are terminated with normal dideoxy nucleotides, resulting in the advantage of superior peak height uniformity and better sensitivity for heterozygous positions than that achieved by dye-terminator sequencing. However, this advantage is offset by the added complexity of having to set up and then consolidate four reactions (e.g., A, C, G, T) for each sample. Consequently, dye primer is for the most part only used in highly automated laboratory settings such as Myriad Genetic Laboratory's BRACAnalysis platform. Still, because of the volume of testing that Myriad performs, dye-primer sequencing may be the dominant technique in terms of the number of samples processed.

One common approach to define mutations is to first use one of the mutation-scanning techniques [see sections entitled Conformational Analyses, Mismatch/Heteroduplex

Analyses, and Protein Truncation Test (PTT)] to identify individual samples that contain sequence variants, and then sequence just those samples that appear to contain such a variant. This approach relies on the sequencing instrument's base calling software and visual inspection of chromatograms to identify heterozygous nucleotide changes in the sequence (87,93); as long as both forward and reverse chromatograms are examined from samples that are thought to contain heterozygous positions, this approach is generally sufficient. However, when full sequencing is used as the primary mutation-screening technique, the number of chromatograms that must be analyzed becomes enormous and requires more efficient chromatogram management software.

For example, Myriad Genetic Laboratory's BRACAnalysis platform uses a laboratory information management system (LIMS), into which their mutation-screening software has been integrated, to track the entire mutation-screening process. Patient samples are tracked by barcode through each step from sample accession through PCR and sequencing until chromatograms have been created and analyzed. Similarly, laboratory reagents are tracked from receipt through preparation of PCR or sequencing reagent plates to completion of electrophoresis (94). The mutation-screening software is a particularly important component of this workflow. Instead of analyzing single chromatograms, Myriad's mutation-screening application operates by making a comparison between the forward–reverse chromatogram pair generated from each patient amplicon and a synthetic "averaged" forward–reverse chromatogram pair from that amplicon. In doing so, the software makes use of data not available to standard base callers such as (*i*) the presence of a new, approximately half-height peak that does not correspond to the canonical sequence of the amplicon, (*ii*) a decrease to approximately half-height of the corresponding wild-type sequence peak, and (*iii*) the joint data from each forward and reverse chromatogram pair. Although the Myriad mutation-screening application is proprietary, many of these features are also present in the genome assembly program 4 (GAP4) heterozygote detection module of the Staden chromatogram analysis package as well as in the heterozygote detection software single nucleotide polymorphism (SNP) detector (95–97). The combination of LIMS and integrated mutation-screening software provides an advantage at the level of process troubleshooting because chromatograms are linked in the database to all the lots of reagents and specific laboratory instruments that were used in their production, providing the opportunity to rapidly associate quality control problems to specific reagent lots or instruments. Additionally, all of the chromatograms derived from each individual patient sample are linked to each other, which means that the output of the mutation-screening process can be viewed as a nucleotide-by-nucleotide genotype across the open reading frame and proximal splice junctions of both *BRCA1* and *BRCA2*.

Array-Based Sequencing Strategies

High-density microarray fabrication techniques have now made it possible to manufacture slides or chips on which the reference sequence of a target gene, and every possible single nucleotide substitution from that reference sequence, are present as features on the chip. Two basic approaches can be used for mutation screening with these chips: sequencing by hybridization (SBH) and arrayed primer extension (APEX).

SBH requires a chip prepared with oligonucleotide features that completely tile the sequence to be interrogated in steps of one nucleotide. If we think of the center nucleotide of each feature as the nucleotide that is being interrogated by that feature, then the chip will actually have four versions of each feature: one that matches the reference sequence and three others representing each of the possible single nucleotide substitution variants of the target nucleotide. In addition, the chip may have features representing deletions of

1, 2, ..., N nucleotides at the target and features representing insertions at the target. Several different protocols have been tested with such chips. The most sensitive appears to be a two-color assay that is closely similar to array-competitive genome hybridization (98). In this assay, a test probe is prepared from an experimental DNA sample in one fluorescent color, and a reference probe is prepared from a control DNA sample in a second fluorescent color. The two probes are mixed and hybridized to the chip. After washing and reading, the relevant signal is the ratio of test:reference fluorescence at each feature on the chip. A decreased test:reference fluorescence ratio at a wild-type feature coupled with an increased test:reference fluorescence ratio at a corresponding variant sequence feature is indicative of a sequence variant in the experimental sample. Hacia and coworkers (99–101) have investigated performance characteristics for mutation screening *BRCA1* and *ATM* with these chips in a very controlled environment and report that the sensitivity of the approach may exceed 95%. However, the ability of SBH chips to detect sequence alterations that are not specifically included as features on the array is limited, and few groups have as yet used SBH in production mutation-screening projects.

The APEX technique can be thought of as a cross between Sanger sequencing and sequencing by hybridization. In this application, a series of oligonucleotide primers that tile across the target gene in steps of one nucleotide are arrayed on a slide or chip with the 5′ ends linked to the solid support and their 3′ ends free to serve as a substrate for primer extension. Target gene sequences are PCR amplified; then the PCR products are fragmented and allowed to hybridize to the oligonucleotide primers on the arrays. Hybridization is followed by a one-nucleotide sequencing reaction using dideoxy nucleotides only. As with dye-terminator sequencing, each of the four dideoxy nucleotides is fluorescently labeled a different color so that the identity of the extended nucleotides at each feature on the array, corresponding to each nucleotide of the target sequence, can be assigned by their fluorescent signal (102,103). Compared to SBH, APEX has the advantage that the complexity of the array is decreased by at least an order of magnitude because the oligonucleotide features need encode only the reference sequence of the target gene in order to detect single nucleotide substitutions. APEX arrays should also signal the presence of insertion–deletion mutations by virtue of interrogating their endpoints; however, APEX cannot reveal the sequence within an insertion mutation and would consequently need to be supplemented by some standard sequencing (98). An APEX prototype has been developed and tested for the identification of *BRCA1* mutations at 42 common sites across six exons (104) but so far, no comprehensive arrays capable of screening the entire gene have been developed. The only breast cancer susceptibility gene for which a comprehensive APEX resequencing array has been developed is *TP53*. The performance of the *TP53* APEX resequencing array (sensitivity and detection limits) in detecting somatic mutations in tumor DNAs has been extensively assessed and compared with both TTGE and DHPLC (105–107). The authors reported that APEX offered a flexible, sensitive, and low-cost resequencing approach suitable for large-scale studies; however, potential insertion–deletion mutations identified by APEX sometimes need to be sequenced by more traditional means in order to determine their exact sequence.

SCREENING FOR PRIMER POLYMORPHISMS AND GROSS GENE REARRANGEMENTS

All of the above described mutation detection techniques, whether based on conformational analysis, mismatch detection, or direct sequencing, share two limitations: inability to detect primer polymorphisms and inability to detect gross gene rearrangements.

Primer Polymorphisms

Primer polymorphisms are genetic variants that lie within the sequence that is recognized by an oligonucleotide that is required for PCR amplification. If such a polymorphism is heterozygous, it can result in differential amplification of the two alleles, with the perfectly matched allele amplified more efficiently than the mismatched allele. If the amplicon also contains a heterozygous genetic variant that should be detected as part of the mutation-screening process, and that genetic variant is on the poorly amplified allele, then the genetic variant will be underrepresented in the amplified product. As underrepresentation of a genetic variant in the amplified product can lead to failure to detect the variant during the mutation-screening step, primer polymorphisms can lead to false-negative mutation-screening results. There are only two real defenses against primer polymorphisms. The first is for investigators to keep track of all known genetic variants in target genes of interest and redesign the oligonucleotides being used for PCR amplification when genetic variants contained in those oligos are reported. The other is to watch for an excess of homozygous signals at polymorphic positions or unequal heterozygous signals at those positions, both of which can provide evidence that the two alleles of some samples are being differentially amplified.

Gross Gene Rearrangements

From the perspective of mutation screening, gross gene rearrangements are deletions or duplications that, at minimum, span a primer-binding site but often include deletion or duplication of an entire exon or even an entire gene. Large-scale deletions are not easily detected by the techniques described in the previous sections because only one allele may be amplified, and this monoallelic amplification product will appear to not be mutated. Similarly, large-scale duplications are not easily detected because three copies of the target will be amplified instead of two, and these will also usually appear to not be mutated. As described below, a number of techniques are sensitive to the presence of gross gene rearrangements, and several of these have been applied to breast cancer susceptibility genes.

Southern Blot

Southern blot (108) usually begins with fragmentation of whole genomic DNA by restriction digest followed by fractionation on an agarose gel. After electrophoresis, the DNA is blot transferred to a solid support such as a nitrocellulose or nylon membrane. The membrane is then probed with a radioactive DNA fragment(s) containing the sequence(s) of interest, washed thoroughly, and exposed to X-ray film. The size(s) of restriction fragment(s) carrying the sequence(s) of interest are then revealed on the resulting autoradiogram. Within three years of its development, the Southern blot had been adapted for detection of length polymorphisms in human disease susceptibility genes (109).

Within two years of the discovery of *BRCA1*, it was clear that some families with very high log odds (LOD) scores at the *BRCA1* locus did not harbor deleterious nucleotide substitutions or small insertion–deletion mutations in or around the protein coding exons of the gene. Accordingly, several research groups began using the Southern blot technique to identify larger insertion or deletion mutations in or around the gene. In 1997, Puget et al. reported the first deletion of an entire *BRCA1* exon, an inter-Alu recombination mediated deletion of exon 17 (110). Shortly thereafter, Swensen et al. reported the first deletion that destroyed the *BRCA1* promoter without altering the coding sequence (111). Thereafter, many other large-scale *BRCA1* rearrangements, and a few *BRCA2* rearrangements, have been found by Southern blot.

Although Southern blots provide an effective technique for finding gross gene rearrangements in genes such as *BRCA1* and *BRCA2*, the technique is rather laborious, requires a relatively large quantity of good quality DNA, is not particularly amenable to automation, and is therefore difficult to use in a high-throughput laboratory environment. In response to these shortcomings, several research groups have developed higher throughput DNA amplification–dependent techniques for detection of large-scale rearrangements or copy number variation.

Semiquantitative Fluorescent Multiplex PCR

The detection of large rearrangements has been substantially facilitated by the introduction of a simple approach called semiquantitative multiplex fluorescent PCR. The method consists of a simultaneous amplification of multiple exonic DNA fragments with fluorescently labeled primers located within target exons and allows comparisons between electropherograms generated from test samples and nonrearranged reference samples. An analysis of experimental DNA samples is then made by calculating the ratio of normalized peak data from the test sample against the same normalized peak data from the reference sample; a 1.5-fold increase and a twofold decrease indicate a heterozygous duplication or deletion, respectively. This method has been successfully applied and validated for the identification of large deletions and duplications in *BRCA1* (112,113). An improvement has been achieved with the introduction of the quantitative multiplex PCR of short fluorescent fragments (QMPSF). Because the complete quantitative copy number analysis of large genes such as *BRCA1* and *BRCA2* requires many amplification products, Charbonnier et al. modified the method by shortening PCR product lengths in order to provide favorable conditions for quantitative multiplex PCR (114). The modified method has been applied to both *BRCA1* and *BRCA2* (115,116). The authors argue that QMPSF is a suitable low-cost approach for the search of large rearrangements in breast cancer families owing to its simplicity, rapidity, and sensitivity. However, they also discuss limitations associated with QMPSF such as the possibility of missing rearrangements that involve only portions of exons because the design of the method is based on the amplification of short-target sequences (116). As with other PCR-based techniques, specificity may be decreased by primer polymorphisms interfering with amplification of affected fragments and thereby generating false positives (115). Finally, DNA quality is critically important to all methods that rely on quantitative DNA amplification, and poor quality DNA can definitely lead to false-positive deletion or duplication signals (114). Although it may not always be practical to exactly map and sequence the breakpoints of a duplication or deletion, prudent practice is to confirm candidate duplications or deletions with a second, independent, primer set if not a second, independent, assay method.

Multiplex Ligation–Dependent Probe Amplification

Multiplex ligation–dependent probe amplification (MLPA) is a high-resolution method specifically designed to measure copy number for up to 45 nucleic acid sequences in a single reaction (117). The MLPA protocol is based on the interrogation of target sequences by hybridization of pairs of MLPA probes that are then joined by ligation and amplified by PCR. Many exon-specific MLPA probes can be ligated in a single reaction and then PCR amplified simultaneously using a single pair of universal primers. As each probe is designed to have a different length, the resulting mix of amplification products can be fractionated by gel electrophoresis. In the resulting chromatogram, the peak area of each amplification product reflects the relative copy number of the corresponding target exon, enabling detection of copy number changes. For copy number measurements, peak areas for test probes from the gene of interest are normalized against peak areas of probes from a control gene. These peak area ratios are then compared to the ratios obtained from control samples with known gene copy numbers. Decreased peak area ratios are indicative of deletions, and increased peak area ratios are indicative of duplications. MLPA has rapidly gained acceptance both in genetic diagnostic laboratories and in the research community due to its simplicity, relatively low cost, capacity for high throughput screening, and perceived robustness. Available evidence suggests that MLPA offers several advantages over existing techniques (118). Implementation of the method in laboratories is facilitated by the existence of commercial MLPA kits that include all the required reagents with detailed protocols, minimal hands-on time, and the possibility to analyze MLPA data with free spreadsheets available for a number of genes. Furthermore, inclusion in each MLPA kit of probes for sequences outside of the target gene plus internal quality controls reduce the risk of false-positive reporting.

MLPA kits are available for both *BRCA1* and *BRCA2*, and use of MLPA to detect genetic variants is spreading rapidly through the breast cancer genetics community (119–122). Caveats associated with MLPA are essentially identical to those associated with QMPSF. In particular, prudent practice is to confirm candidate duplications or deletions with a second, independent, primer set if not a second, independent, assay method.

Prevalence of Gross Rearrangements

As assays for gross rearrangements in *BRCA1* and *BRCA2* became more efficient, it became possible to estimate the fraction of high-risk mutations that this class of sequence variants accounts for. Estimates based on analyses of high-risk families in which no other mutation had been found put this fraction in the range of 10% to 15% (123–125), underlining the importance of including a test for gross rearrangements as an integral part of systematic mutation screening of these genes. In order to estimate the fraction of mutations represented by gross rearrangements in a clinically representative outbred population, Myriad Genetic Laboratories developed allele-specific PCR tests for one *BRCA1* duplication and five *BRCA1* deletions that had been reported in two or more independent families in the literature. After screening more than 21,000 BRACAnalysis subjects, the Myriad authors concluded that these five rearrangements account for about 2.5% of high-risk *BRCA1* mutations in their test population (126). This allele-specific PCR test became a standard component of BRACAnalysis. In addition, in 2006, Myriad added a BRACAnalysis rearrangement Test (BART) to their menu of testing options. BART is from the semiquantitative multiplex fluorescent PCR/QMPSF assay family, but its exact specifications have not been described to date.

CLASSIFICATION OF SEQUENCE VARIANTS

In the course of mutation screening, investigators will find truncating mutations that clearly alter protein function. They may also find intronic or splice junction variants that may or may not interfere with splicing and missense substitutions that may or may not interfere with protein function. Classification of these sequence variants into clinically useful categories such as "clinically important" or "neutral or of little clinical importance (neutral/ LCI)" is part of the mutation-screening process. We discuss three classes of mutations: truncating mutations, splice junction mutations, and missense substitutions.

Truncating Mutations

The overwhelming majority of protein truncating mutations in *BRCA1* and *BRCA2* are clinically important high-risk mutations. However, it has long been known that some truncating mutations located near the carboxy termini of these proteins are neutral/LCI. For example, Mazoyer et al. found that the *BRCA2* nonsense variant *K3326X*, which has an allele frequency of approximately 1% in NW European populations, does not confer high risk of breast or ovarian cancer even though it results in deletion of the last 93 amino acids of *BRCA2* (127). In practice, the positions of the furthest downstream high-risk truncating mutation, and the first non–high-risk truncating mutation, have been mapped rather precisely. At this time, these positions are amino acid positions 1853 and 1854 for *BRCA1*, and approximately amino acid positions 3310 and 3325 for *BRCA2* (Amie Deffenbaugh, Myriad Genetic Laboratories, Personal Communication). Thus, mutation-screening services will sometimes observe truncating mutations that are not high-risk mutations, providing a strong research rationale to collect pedigrees that segregate truncating mutations in or around these gray zones.

Splice Junction Mutations

Mutations within splice donor or splice acceptor consensus sequences can interfere with splicing, leading to exon skipping (i.e., loss of the expression of an exon), failure to splice excise an intron (i.e., retention of an intron after completion of mRNA processing), or activation of cryptic splice junctions. In addition, mutations within exons or even deep within introns can activate cryptic splice junctions, leading to aberrant splicing. The vast majority of introns, including all of the introns of *BRCA1*, *BRCA2*, *TP53*, and *PTEN* are of the GT–AG type, meaning that the first two base pairs of the intron are GT and the last two base pairs are AG. These four nucleotides form the core of the GT–AG splice junction consensus. The first intron of *PTEN* is one of the very rare AT–AC type introns that actually use GT–AG at the splice junctions (SV Tavtigian unpublished observation). Mutations at any one of these four canonical splice junction nucleotides are sufficiently suspicious that they are often presumed to interfere with splicing. However, splice donors and acceptors have extended consensus sequences that include roughly 8 and 20 bp, respectively. Many sequence variants within the consensus sequences interfere with splicing but many others do not and spice junction prediction algorithms are not sufficiently accurate to use their results in a clinical setting.

Fortunately, there is a relatively straightforward experimental strategy to identify splice junction mutations that interfere with splicing. Briefly, a reverse transcription polymerase chain reaction (RT-PCR) amplicon is designed with a forward primer located one or more exons upstream of the suspicious splice junction variant and a reverse primer located one or more exons downstream. The amplicon is also designed to contain at least one common exonic polymorphism, which will be used to discriminate between the two alleles in the patient sample. Peripheral blood is obtained from one or more carriers of the suspicious splice junction variant, and these are used to prepare both DNA and RNA. The exonic polymorphism is genotyped from the genomic DNA in order to find an individual who carries the suspicious splice junction variant and is heterozygous for the exonic polymorphism. RNA from this individual(s) is then subjected to RT-PCR. The RT-PCR products are fractionated by gel electrophoresis and both the expected canonical length product and any notable alternative length product(s) are gel purified. These RT-PCR products are then sequenced to determine three things: (*i*) whether both alleles of the polymorphism are equally represented in the canonical PCR product, (*ii*) the exon structure of any aberrant product(s), and if present, (*iii*) whether both alleles of the polymorphism are equally represented in the aberrant PCR product(s). If the splice junction mutation does not interfere with splicing, then the two alleles of the exonic polymorphism will be approximately equally represented in the canonical PCR product. In contrast, if the splice junction mutation does interfere with splicing, then there will be skewed representation of the two alleles of the exonic polymorphism in the canonical PCR product. If disequilibrium (or phase) between the splice junction mutation and the exonic polymorphism are known, then the allele of the exonic polymorphism that is on the same chromosome as the splice junction mutation will be underrepresented or absent in the canonical PCR product. Depending on the nature of the splice defect, the RT-PCR may detect an aberrant splice product; representation of the two alleles of the exonic polymorphism in the aberrant product should be skewed in the opposite sense to what was observed in the canonical product. The combined data of one allele preferentially represented in the canonical splice product and the other allele preferentially represented in the aberrant splice product is diagnostic of a splice junction mutation that interferes with splicing.

A significant fraction of the high-risk mutations in breast cancer susceptibility genes are indeed splice junction mutations. However, because there is a relatively straightforward assay to determine whether or not newly observed splice junction variants interfere with gene expression, they do not constitute a large fraction of overall pool of unclassified variants.

Missense Substitutions

More than 1500 distinct missense substitutions have been observed in *BRCA1* and *BRCA2*. But, only a small fraction, less than 10%, have been classified as either clinically important or neutral/LCI (128–130). There are two basic reasons that only a small number have been classified. First, most of the missense substitutions are exceedingly rare in the population and, therefore, difficult to classify by standard human genetics approaches. Second, although functional assays have been developed for several of the recognized structural domains of *BRCA1* and *BRCA2*, these assays have not yet been demonstrated to distinguish between clinically important and neutral/*LCS* variants with sufficient sensitivity and specificity to justify their use for clinical classification of missense substitutions. In order to overcome the limited information content of the individual types of data that are available to classify rare missense substitutions, Goldgar et al. developed a multifactorial method of analysis of unclassified sequence variants that integrates several disparate data types (128).

As initially presented, Goldgar's method integrated five data types: (*i*) co-occurrence between unclassified variants and known deleterious mutations in trans in the same gene; (*ii*) co-segregation between unclassified variants and breast cancer in pedigrees; (*iii*) summary of family history across multiple pedigrees in which a specific unclassified variant was observed; (*iv*) a sequence analysis–based assessment of the probability that the position in the protein at which a variant is observed is functionally constrained or not; and (*v*) the Grantham score, which is a measure of the severity of a missense substitution. The key to this multifactorial method was that the analysis of each data type was quantified as a likelihood ratio related to the risk for a carrier of a missense substitution of interest to develop cancer. Because the five data types are independent or very nearly so, the likelihood ratios derived from each data type can be multiplied to produce a summary likelihood ratio for that substitution. A second strength of this multifactorial method is that it can be extended to include other data types so long as analysis of those data types can be formulated into a likelihood ratio and the data are independent of the data types already integrated. Indeed, Chenevix-Trench et al. integrated tumor histopathology into this multifactorial method (131), and the method can be expected to continue to evolve as additional data become available and are integrated into the model.

Clinically important high-risk truncating mutations and splice junction mutations are distributed fairly evenly across the exons and splice junctions of *BRCA1* and *BRCA2*. There are no obvious hotspots for these types of mutations (75,132). In contrast, the few *BRCA1* missense substitutions that have been classified as clinically relevant high-risk mutations are located in either the really-interesting-new-gene (RING) or the *BRC*A1 *C-t*erminal (BRCT) domains of the BRCA1 protein. Some have argued that missense substitutions located in other domains of the protein are likely to confer increased risk of disease (133–135), but this point remains to be tested rigorously. On the other hand, as only one *BRCA2* missense substitution, *D2723H*, has so far been classified as a clinically important high-risk variant (128), the distribution of deleterious missense substitutions across the open reading frame of this gene remains unclear. What is clear is that *BRCA1* does harbor a substantial number of deleterious missense substitutions, but most of these are currently unclassified (129,130,135). Whether or not *BRCA2* harbors a substantial number of deleterious missense substitutions remains to be determined. But, the tools required to classify these missense substitutions have been developed and are being improved.

Expert Opinion on Unclassified Variants in *BRCA1* and *BRCA2*

The Breast Cancer Information Core (BIC) maintains a website (136) that contains a central repository of information on sequence variation in *BRCA1* and *BRCA2*. In late 2005, the BIC steering committee took the decision to begin conducting expert opinion evaluations of some of the *BRCA1* and *BRCA2* sequence variants recorded in the BIC. The method of evaluation adopted by the BIC steering committee is essentially a qualitative implementation of the multifactorial method described by Goldgar et al. (128). From January 2007, these expert opinion classifications, along with summaries of the discussions that informed those classifications, will be available at the BIC website.

SUMMARY

A wide variety of mutation-screening techniques has been developed (Table 1), and many of these have been applied to the major known breast cancer susceptibility genes. Each method has its strengths and weaknesses, and no one method is perfect. Still, several trends are apparent.

First, SSCP and derivative methods that detect conformational polymorphism were popular in the 1990s because they are inexpensive and technically straightforward. However, the sensitivity of this family of methods is fundamentally limited because an appreciable fraction of single nucleotide substitutions does not result in conformational changes. Some heteroduplex detection methods match the cost and ease-of-use of conformational polymorphism methods while delivering superior sensitivity. For this reason, pure conformational polymorphism detection methods are likely to disappear from use.

Second, some groups continue to use PTT to screen exon 11 of *BRCA1* and *BRCA2* because the method is very efficient and, when based on DNA rather than RNA, has very

Table 1 Diagnostic Methods

Conformational polymorphism detection methods	
SSCP	Single Strand Conformational Polymorphism
CE-SSCP	Capillary Electrophoresis SSCP
Heteroduplex methods	
DGGE	Denaturing Gradient Gel Electrophoresis
TDGS	Two-Dimensional Gene Scanning
TTGE	Temporal Temperature Gradient Electrophoresis
TGCE	Temperature Gradient Capillary Electrophoresis
CSGE	Conformation Sensitive Gel Electrophoresis
F-CSGE	Fluorescent-CSGE
CSCE	Conformation Sensitive Capillary Electrophoresis
HA	Heteroduplex Analysis
F-MD	Fluorescent Mutation Detection
DHPLC	Denaturing High Performance Liquid Chromatography
CCM	Chemical Cleavage of Mismatch
FAMA	Fluorescence Assisted Mismatch Analysis
HRM or MCA	High Resolution Melt Curve Analysis
Mutation detection by translation of RNA to protein	
PTT	Protein Truncation Test
Sequencing methods	
–	Maxam and Gilbert sequencing
–	Sanger sequencing
–	Radioactive cycle sequencing
–	Dye-terminator sequencing
–	Dye-primer sequencing
SBH	Sequencing by hybridization
APEX	Arrayed Primer Extension
Detection of large scale gene rearrangements	
–	Southern blot
QMPSF	Quantitative Multiplex PCR of Short Fluorescent Fragments
MLPA	Multiplex Ligation-Dependent Probe Amplification

good sensitivity for truncating mutations. But, PTT is flawed because it cannot detect missense substitutions. As interest in identifying deleterious missense substitutions in these genes increases, that interest will weigh against the use of PTT. Moreover, two of the keys to classifying missense substitutions have been to identify families in which the substitutions of interest segregate and also to find individuals who carry both a missense substitution of interest and another clearly high-risk mutation in the same gene. As PTT does not contribute to this research activity, one could argue that use of the protocol results in a slight net reduction in the data available to the research community for classification of missense substitutions.

Third, heteroduplex detection methods can have very good sensitivity, and methods of development over the last few years have resulted in inexpensive high-throughput techniques, such as FMD, TGCE, and MCA/HRM, which maintain very good sensitivity. One challenge posed by this generation of techniques is that it is very difficult to make comparisons of sensitivity, specificity, and cost-effectiveness that can actually make statistically significant distinctions between protocols that have real-world sensitivities of 95% and above.

Fourth, mutation-scanning techniques have to be followed by sequencing in order to identify and eventually classify the sequence variants that were found. Although it is often said that sequencing is the gold standard against which other techniques are measured, a more precise statement would be that double-stranded dye-primer sequencing is the gold standard. Double-stranded dye-terminator sequencing also has extremely high sensitivity, but single-stranded dye-terminator sequencing will result in some false negatives due to sequence-specific peak height variation in the chromatograms. In large-scale mutation-screening projects, and especially clinical mutation-screening work, chromatogram management and analysis becomes a critical challenge. With very robust software, complete open reading frame mutation screening can be achieved by resequencing alone. This strategy results in a workflow that has fewer steps than mutation scanning followed by sequencing, but the tradeoff is a more expensive test.

Finally, even if 100% sensitivity for nucleotide substitutions and small insertion–deletion mutations is achieved, mutation-screening protocols that are based on amplification of individual exons will miss insertion–deletion mutations that involve whole exons or larger regions. Although effective, Southern blots were a very tedious approach to finding these mutations. Fortunately, refinements in quantitative multiplex PCR and the development of MLPA have provided efficient and sensitive protocols for the discovery of these mutations.

Over the last decade, the combined sensitivity and throughput of mutation-scanning techniques have improved substantially. The advent of capillary sequencing has improved the throughput of resequencing and also reduced sample tracking problems that could arise from electrophoresis irregularities on slab gels. Whether a modern, high-sensitivity testing workflow incorporates mutation scanning before double-stranded sequencing probably has a smaller impact on the overall sensitivity of the test than does whether or not the test workflow incorporates a systematic screen for duplications and deletions. Still, challenges remain. The problem of primer polymorphism will contribute to false-negative test results from any method that requires oligonucleotide-dependent target amplification and could contribute to false-positive results for measurements of copy number. It is possible for nucleotide substitutions or small insertion–deletion mutations located deep in introns to activate cryptic splice junctions, thus interfering with proper splicing and mRNA maturation. Moreover, the mechanisms of gene regulation are not yet well understood. Sequence variation in proximal promoters or more distant transcriptional enhancers can lead to differential allelic expression, and underexpressed alleles that encode otherwise normal RNA and protein could in turn confer increased risk of breast cancer. Finally, the problem of unclassified sequence variants remains. Encouragingly, the challenge of classifying missense substitutions has led to international collaborations that transcend academic/industry barriers and benefit breast cancer patients and their relatives everywhere.

REFERENCES

1. Miki Y, Swensen J, Shattuck-Eidens D, et al. A strong candidate for the breast and ovarian cancer susceptibility gene BRCA1. Science 1994; 266(5182):66–71.
2. Wooster R, Bignell G, Lancaster J, et al. Identification of the breast cancer susceptibility gene BRCA2. Nature 1995; 378(6559):789–792.
3. Tavtigian SV, Simard J, Rommens J, et al. The complete BRCA2 gene and mutations in chromosome 13q-linked kindreds. Nat Genet 1996; 12(3):333–337.
4. Ford D, Easton DF, Stratton M, et al. Genetic heterogeneity and penetrance analysis of the BRCA1 and BRCA2 genes in breast cancer families. The Breast Cancer Linkage Consortium. Am J Hum Genet 1998; 62(3):676–689.

5. Venkitaraman AR. Cancer susceptibility and the functions of BRCA1 and BRCA2. Cell 2002; 108(2):171–182.

6. Nielsen DA, Novoradovsky A, Goldman D. SSCP primer design based on single-strand DNA structure predicted by a DNA folding program. Nucleic Acids Res 1995; 23(12): 2287–2291.

7. Orita M, Iwahana H, Kanazawa H, et al. Detection of polymorphisms of human DNA by gel electrophoresis as single-strand conformation polymorphisms. Proc Natl Acad Sci U S A 1989; 86(8):2766–2770.

8. Suzuki Y, Orita M, Shiraishi M, et al. Detection of ras gene mutations in human lung cancers by single-strand conformation polymorphism analysis of polymerase chain reaction products. Oncogene 1990; 5(7):1037–1043.

9. Berta P, Hawkins JR, Sinclair AH, et al. Genetic evidence equating SRY and the testis-determining factor. Nature 1990; 348(6300):448–450.

10. Friedman LS, Ostermeyer EA, Szabo CI, et al. Confirmation of BRCA1 by analysis of germline mutations linked to breast and ovarian cancer in ten families. Nat Genet 1994; 8(4): 399–404.

11. Langston AA, Malone KE, Thompson JD, et al. BRCA1 mutations in a population-based sample of young women with breast cancer. N Engl J Med 1996; 334(3):137–142.

12. Phelan CM, Lancaster JM, Tonin P, et al. Mutation analysis of the BRCA2 gene in 49 site-specific breast cancer families. Nat Genet 1996; 13(1):120–122.

13. Renwick A, Thompson D, Seal S, et al. ATM mutations that cause ataxia-telangiectasia are breast cancer susceptibility alleles. Nat Genet 2006; 38(8):873–875.

14. Andersen PS, Jespersgaard C, Vuust J, et al. High-throughput single strand conformation polymorphism mutation detection by automated capillary array electrophoresis: validation of the method. Hum Mutat 2003; 21(2):116–122.

15. Doi K, Doi H, Noiri E, et al. High-throughput single nucleotide polymorphism typing by fluorescent single-strand conformation polymorphism analysis with capillary electrophoresis. Electrophoresis 2004; 25(6):833–838.

16. Gross E, Arnold N, Goette J, et al. A comparison of BRCA1 mutation analysis by direct sequencing, SSCP, and DHPLC. Hum Genet 1999; 105(1-2):72–78.

17. Eng C, Brody LC, Wagner TM, et al. Interpreting epidemiological research: blinded comparison of methods used to estimate the prevalence of inherited mutations in BRCA1. J Med Genet 2001; 38(12):824–833.

18. Andrulis IL, Anton-Culver H, Beck J, et al. Comparison of DNA- and RNA-based methods for detection of truncating BRCA1 mutations. Hum Mutat 2002; 20(1):65–73.

19. Basham VM, Lipscombe JM, Ward JM, et al. BRCA1 and BRCA2 mutations in a population-based study of male breast cancer. Breast Cancer Res 2002; 4(1):R2.

20. Fischer SG, Lerman LS. Length-independent separation of DNA restriction fragments in two-dimensional gel electrophoresis. Cell 1979; 16(1):191–200.

21. Fischer SG, Lerman LS. DNA fragments differing by single base-pair substitutions are separated in denaturing gradient gels: correspondence with melting theory. Proc Natl Acad Sci U S A 1983; 80(6):1579–1583.

22. Myers RM, Fischer SG, Lerman LS, et al. Nearly all single base substitutions in DNA fragments joined to a GC-clamp can be detected by denaturing gradient gel electrophoresis. Nucleic Acids Res 1985; 13(9):3131–3145.

23. Myers RM, Fischer SG, Maniatis T, et al. Modification of the melting properties of duplex DNA by attachment of a GC-rich DNA sequence as determined by denaturing gradient gel electrophoresis. Nucleic Acids Res 1985; 13(9):3111–3129.

24. Sheffield VC, Cox DR, Lerman LS, et al. Attachment of a 40-base-pair G + C-rich sequence (GC-clamp) to genomic DNA fragments by the polymerase chain reaction results in improved detection of single-base changes. Proc Natl Acad Sci U S A 1989; 86(1):232–236.

25. van der Hout AH, van den Ouweland AM, van der Luijt RB, et al. A DGGE system for comprehensive mutation screening of BRCA1 and BRCA2: application in a Dutch cancer clinic setting. Hum Mutat 2006; 27(7):654–666.

26. Van Orsouw NJ, Li D, van der Vlies P, et al. Mutational scanning of large genes by extensive PCR multiplexing and two-dimensional electrophoresis: application to the RB1 gene. Hum Mol Genet 1996; 5(6):755–761.

27. Marsh DJ, Roth S, Lunetta KL, et al. Exclusion of PTEN and 10q22-24 as the susceptibility locus for juvenile polyposis syndrome. Cancer Res 1997; 57(22):5017–5021.

28. Rines RD, van Orsouw NJ, Sigalas I, et al. Comprehensive mutational scanning of the p53 coding region by two-dimensional gene scanning. Carcinogenesis 1998; 19(6):979–984.

29. van Orsouw NJ, Dhanda RK, Elhaji Y, et al. A highly accurate, low cost test for BRCA1 mutations. J Med Genet 1999; 36(10):747–753.

30. Bounpheng M, McGrath S, Macias D, et al. Rapid, inexpensive scanning for all possible BRCA1 and BRCA2 gene sequence variants in a single assay: implications for genetic testing. J Med Genet 2003; 40(4):e33.

31. McGrath SB, Bounpheng M, Torres L, et al. High-speed, multicolor fluorescent two-dimensional gene scanning. Genomics 2001; 78(1–2):83–90.

32. Marsh DJ, Dahia PL, Caron S, et al. Germline PTEN mutations in Cowden syndrome-like families. J Med Genet 1998; 35(11):881–885.

33. Li Q, Liu Z, Monroe H, et al. Integrated platform for detection of DNA sequence variants using capillary array electrophoresis. Electrophoresis 2002; 23(10):1499–1511.

34. Bhattacharyya A, Lilley DM. The contrasting structures of mismatched DNA sequences containing looped-out bases (bulges) and multiple mismatches (bubbles). Nucleic Acids Res 1989; 17(17):6821–6840.

35. Nagamine CM, Chan K, Lau YF. A PCR artifact: generation of heteroduplexes. Am J Hum Genet 1989; 45(2):337–339.

36. Rommens J, Kerem BS, Greer W, et al. Rapid nonradioactive detection of the major cystic fibrosis mutation. Am J Hum Genet 1990; 46(2):395–396.

37. Keen J, Lester D, Inglehearn C, et al. Rapid detection of single base mismatches as heteroduplexes on Hydrolink gels. Trends Genet 1991; 7(1):5.

38. Perry DJ, Carrell RW. Hydrolink gels: a rapid and simple approach to the detection of DNA mutations in thromboembolic disease. J Clin Pathol 1992; 45(2):158–160.

39. Soto D, Sukumar S. Improved detection of mutations in the p53 gene in human tumors as single-stranded conformation polymorphs and double-stranded heteroduplex DNA. PCR Methods Appl 1992; 2(1):96–98.

40. Ganguly A, Rock MJ, Prockop DJ. Conformation-sensitive gel electrophoresis for rapid detection of single-base differences in double-stranded PCR products and DNA fragments: evidence for solvent-induced bends in DNA heteroduplexes. Proc Natl Acad Sci U S A 1993; 90(21):10325–10329.

41. Ganguly T, Dhulipala R, Godmilow L, et al. High throughput fluorescence-based conformation-sensitive gel electrophoresis (F-CSGE) identifies six unique BRCA2 mutations and an overall low incidence of BRCA2 mutations in high-risk BRCA1-negative breast cancer families. Hum Genet 1998; 102(5):549–556.

42. Edwards SM, Kote-Jarai Z, Hamoudi R, et al. An improved high throughput heteroduplex mutation detection system for screening BRCA2 mutations-fluorescent mutation detection (F-MD). Hum Mutat 2001; 17(3):220–232.

43. Spitzer E, Abbaszadegan MR, Schmidt F, et al. Detection of BRCA1 and BRCA2 mutations in breast cancer families by a comprehensive two-stage screening procedure. Int J Cancer 2000; 85(4):474–481.

44. Seo JH, Cho DY, Ahn SH, et al. BRCA1 and BRCA2 germline mutations in Korean patients with sporadic breast cancer. Hum Mutat 2004; 24(4):350.

45. Rozycka M, Collins N, Stratton MR, et al. Rapid detection of DNA sequence variants by conformation-sensitive capillary electrophoresis. Genomics 2000; 70(1):34–40.

46. Davies H, Dicks E, Stephens P, et al. High throughput DNA sequence variant detection by conformation sensitive capillary electrophoresis and automated peak comparison. Genomics 2006; 87(3):427–432.

47. Bhattacharyya A, Lilley DM. Single base mismatches in DNA. Long- and short-range structure probed by analysis of axis trajectory and local chemical reactivity. J Mol Biol 1989; 209(4):583–597.

48. Britten RJ, Smith J. A bovine genome. Carnegie Inst Wash Yearbook 1970; 68:378–386.

49. Davidson EH, Hough BR, Amenson CS, et al. General interspersion of repetitive with non-repetitive sequence elements in the DNA of Xenopus. J Mol Biol 1973; 77(1):1–23.

50. Hardies SC, Wells RD. Preparative fractionation of DNA restriction fragments by reversed phase column chromatography. Proc Natl Acad Sci U S A 1976; 73(9): 3117–3121.

51. Usher DA. Reverse-phase HPLC of DNA restriction fragments and ribooligonucleotides on uncoated Kel-F powder. Nucleic Acids Res 1979; 6(6):2289–2306.

52. Huber CG, Oefner PJ, Preuss E, et al. High-resolution liquid chromatography of DNA fragments on non-porous poly(styrene-divinylbenzene) particles. Nucleic Acids Res 1993; 21(5):1061–1066.

53. Oefner PJ, Underhill PA. Comparative DNA sequencing by denaturing high-performance liquid chromatography (DHPLC). Am J Hum Genet 1995; 57s:A266.

54. O'Donovan MC, Oefner PJ, Roberts SC, et al. Blind analysis of denaturing high-performance liquid chromatography as a tool for mutation detection. Genomics 1998; 52(1): 44–49.

55. Wagner T, Stoppa-Lyonnet D, Fleischmann E, et al. Denaturing high-performance liquid chromatography detects reliably BRCA1 and BRCA2 mutations. Genomics 1999; 62(3): 369–376.

56. Underhill PA, Jin L, Lin AA, et al. Detection of numerous Y chromosome biallelic polymorphisms by denaturing high-performance liquid chromatography. Genome Res 1997; 7(10):996–1005.

57. Sevilla C, Moatti JP, Julian-Reynier C, et al. Testing for BRCA1 mutations: a cost-effectiveness analysis. Eur J Hum Genet 2002; 10(10):599–606.

58. Schollen E, Dequeker E, McQuaid S, et al. Diagnostic DHPLC Quality Assurance (DDQA): a collaborative approach to the generation of validated and standardized methods for DHPLC-based mutation screening in clinical genetics laboratories. Hum Mutat 2005; 25(6): 583–592.

59. Shenk TE, Rhodes C, Rigby PW, et al. Biochemical method for mapping mutational alterations in DNA with S1 nuclease: the location of deletions and temperature-sensitive mutations in simian virus 40. Proc Natl Acad Sci U S A 1975; 72(3):989–993.

60. Myers RM, Larin Z, Maniatis T. Detection of single base substitutions by ribonuclease cleavage at mismatches in RNA:DNA duplexes. Science 1985; 230(4731):1242–1246.

61. Winter E, Yamamoto F, Almoguera C, et al. A method to detect and characterize point mutations in transcribed genes: amplification and overexpression of the mutant c-Ki-ras allele in human tumor cells. Proc Natl Acad Sci U S A 1985; 82(22):7575–7579.

62. Cotton RG, Rodrigues NR, Campbell RD. Reactivity of cytosine and thymine in single-base-pair mismatches with hydroxylamine and osmium tetroxide and its application to the study of mutations. Proc Natl Acad Sci U S A 1988; 85(12):4397–4401.

63. Verpy E, Biasotto M, Meo T, et al. Efficient detection of point mutations on color-coded strands of target DNA. Proc Natl Acad Sci U S A 1994; 91(5):1873–1877.

64. Verpy E, Biasotto M, Brai M, et al. Exhaustive mutation scanning by fluorescence-assisted mismatch analysis discloses new genotype-phenotype correlations in angioedema. Am J Hum Genet 1996; 59(2):308–319.

65. Ricevuto E, Sobol H, Stoppa-Lyonnet D, et al. Diagnostic strategy for analytical scanning of BRCA1 gene by fluorescence-assisted mismatch analysis using large, bifluorescently labeled amplicons. Clin Cancer Res 2001; 7(6):1638–1646.

66. Pages S, Caux V, Stoppa-Lyonnet D, et al. Screening of male breast cancer and of breast-ovarian cancer families for BRCA2 mutations using large bifluorescent amplicons. Br J Cancer 2001; 84(4):482–488.

67. Tessitore A, Di Rocco ZC, Cannita K, et al. High sensitivity of detection of TP53 somatic mutations by fluorescence-assisted mismatch analysis. Genes Chromosomes Cancer 2002; 35(1):86–91.

68. De Galitiis F, Cannita K, Tessitore A, et al. Novel P53 mutations detected by FAMA in colorectal cancers. Ann Oncol 2006; 17(Suppl 7):vii78–vii83.

69. Liew M, Pryor R, Palais R, et al. Genotyping of single-nucleotide polymorphisms by high-resolution melting of small amplicons. Clin Chem 2004; 50(7):1156–1164.

70. Reed GH, Wittwer CT. Sensitivity and specificity of single-nucleotide polymorphism scanning by high-resolution melting analysis. Clin Chem 2004; 50(10):1748–1754.

71. http://www.ngrl.org.uk/Wessex/downloads.htm

72. Roest PA, Roberts RG, van der Tuijn AC, et al. Protein truncation test (PTT) to rapidly screen the DMD gene for translation terminating mutations. Neuromuscul Disord 1993; 3(5–6):391–394.

73. Powell SM, Petersen GM, Krush AJ, et al. Molecular diagnosis of familial adenomatous polyposis. N Engl J Med 1993; 329(27):1982–1987.

74. Neuhausen SL, Ostrander EA. Mutation testing of early-onset breast cancer genes BRCA1 and BRCA2. Genet Test 1997; 1(2):75–83.

75. Blackwood MA, Weber BL. BRCA1 and BRCA2: from molecular genetics to clinical medicine. J Clin Oncol 1998; 16(5):1969–1977.

76. Hogervorst FB, Cornelis RS, Bout M, et al. Rapid detection of BRCA1 mutations by the protein truncation test. Nat Genet 1995; 10(2):208–212.

77. Garvin AM, Attenhofer-Haner M, Scott RJ. BRCA1 and BRCA2 mutation analysis in 86 early onset breast/ovarian cancer patients. J Med Genet 1997; 34(12):990–995.

78. Garvin AM. A complete protein truncation test for BRCA1 and BRCA2. Eur J Hum Genet 1998; 6(3):226–234.

79. Baker KE, Parker R. Nonsense-mediated mRNA decay: terminating erroneous gene expression. Curr Opin Cell Biol 2004; 16(3):293–299.

80. Ozcelik H, Antebi YJ, Cole DE, et al. Heteroduplex and protein truncation analysis of the BRCA1 185delAG mutation. Hum Genet 1996; 98(3):310–312.

81. Maxam AM, Gilbert W. A new method for sequencing DNA. Proc Natl Acad Sci U S A 1977; 74(2):560–564.

82. Sanger F, Nicklen S, Coulson AR. DNA sequencing with chain-terminating inhibitors. Proc Natl Acad Sci U S A 1977; 74(12):5463–5467.

83. Smith LM, Fung S, Hunkapiller MW, et al. The synthesis of oligonucleotides containing an aliphatic amino group at the 5′ terminus: synthesis of fluorescent DNA primers for use in DNA sequence analysis. Nucleic Acids Res 1985; 13(7):2399–2412.

84. Smith LM, Sanders JZ, Kaiser RJ, et al. Fluorescence detection in automated DNA sequence analysis. Nature 1986; 321(6071):674–679.

85. Prober JM, Trainor GL, Dam RJ, et al. A system for rapid DNA sequencing with fluorescent chain-terminating dideoxynucleotides. Science 1987; 238(4825):336–341.

86. Parker LT, Zakeri H, Deng Q, et al. AmpliTaq DNA polymerase, FS dye-terminator sequencing: analysis of peak height patterns. Biotechniques 1996; 21(4):694–699.

87. Chadwick RB, Conrad MP, McGinnis MD, et al. Heterozygote and mutation detection by direct automated fluorescent DNA sequencing using a mutant Taq DNA polymerase. Biotechniques 1996; 20(4):676–683.

88. Yan H, Kinzler KW, Vogelstein B. Techsight. Genetic testing–present and future. Science 2000; 289(5486):1890–1892.

89. Tabor S, Richardson CC. A single residue in DNA polymerases of the Escherichia coli DNA polymerase I family is critical for distinguishing between deoxy- and dideoxyribonucleotides. Proc Natl Acad Sci U S A 1995; 92(14):6339–6343.

90. Reeve MA, Fuller CW. A novel thermostable polymerase for DNA sequencing. Nature 1995; 376(6543):796–797.

91. Rosenblum BB, Lee LG, Spurgeon SL, et al. New dye-labeled terminators for improved DNA sequencing patterns. Nucleic Acids Res 1997; 25(22):4500–4504.

92. Duthie RS, Kalve IM, Samols SB, et al. Novel cyanine dye-labeled dideoxynucleoside triphosphates for DNA sequencing. Bioconjug Chem 2002; 13(4):699–706.

93. Phelps RS, Chadwick RB, Conrad MP, et al. Efficient, automatic detection of heterozygous bases during large-scale DNA sequence screening. Biotechniques 1995; 19(6):984–989.

94. Tavtigian SV, Oliphant A, Shattuck-Eidens D, et al. Genomic organization, functional analysis, and mutation screening of BRCA1 and BRCA2. In: Fortner JG, Sharp PA, eds. Accomplishments in Cancer Research 1996. Philadelphia, New York: Lippincott-Raven, 1997: 189–204.

95. Bonfield JK, Rada C, Staden R. Automated detection of point mutations using fluorescent sequence trace subtraction. Nucleic Acids Res 1998; 26(14):3404–3409.

96. Staden R, Beal KF, Bonfield JK. The Staden package, 1998. Methods Mol Biol 2000;; 132: 115–130.

97. Zhang J, Wheeler DA, Yakub I, et al. SNPdetector: a software tool for sensitive and accurate SNP detection. PLoS Comput Biol 2005; 1(5):e53.

98. Hacia JG. Resequencing and mutational analysis using oligonucleotide microarrays. Nat Genet 1999; 21(1 suppl):42–47.

99. Hacia JG, Brody LC, Chee MS, et al. Detection of heterozygous mutations in BRCA1 using high density oligonucleotide arrays and two-colour fluorescence analysis. Nat Genet 1996; 14(4):441–447.

100. Hacia JG, Sun B, Hunt N, et al. Strategies for mutational analysis of the large multiexon ATM gene using high-density oligonucleotide arrays. Genome Res 1998; 8(12): 1245–1258.

101. Karaman MW, Groshen S, Lee CC, et al. Comparisons of substitution, insertion and deletion probes for resequencing and mutational analysis using oligonucleotide microarrays. Nucleic Acids Res 2005; 33(3):e33.

102. Shumaker JM, Metspalu A, Caskey CT. Mutation detection by solid phase primer extension. Hum Mutat 1996; 7(4):346–354.

103. Kurg A, Tonisson N, Georgiou I, et al. Arrayed primer extension: solid-phase four-color DNA resequencing and mutation detection technology. Genet Test 2000; 4(1):1–7.

104. Tonisson N, Kurg A, Kaasik K, et al. Unravelling genetic data by arrayed primer extension. Clin Chem Lab Med 2000; 38(2):165–170.

105. Tonisson N, Zernant J, Kurg A, et al. Evaluating the arrayed primer extension resequencing assay of TP53 tumor suppressor gene. Proc Natl Acad Sci U S A 2002; 99(8):5503–5508.

106. Kringen P, Bergamaschi A, Due EU, et al. Evaluation of arrayed primer extension for TP53 mutation detection in breast and ovarian carcinomas. Biotechniques 2005; 39(5): 755–761.

107. Le Calvez F, Ahman A, Tonisson N, et al. Arrayed primer extension resequencing of mutations in the TP53 tumor suppressor gene: comparison with denaturing HPLC and direct sequencing. Clin Chem 2005; 51(7):1284–1287.

108. Southern EM. Detection of specific sequences among DNA fragments separated by gel electrophoresis. J Mol Biol 1975; 98(3):503–517.

109. Kan YW, Dozy AM. Polymorphism of DNA sequence adjacent to human beta-globin structural gene: relationship to sickle mutation. Proc Natl Acad Sci U S A 1978; 75(11): 5631–5635.

110. Puget N, Torchard D, Serova-Sinilnikova OM, et al. A 1-kb Alu-mediated germ-line deletion removing BRCA1 exon 17. Cancer Res 1997; 57(5):828–831.

111. Swensen J, Hoffman M, Skolnick MH, et al. Identification of a 14 kb deletion involving the promoter region of BRCA1 in a breast cancer family. Hum Mol Genet 1997; 6(9): 1513–1517.

112. Robinson MD, Chu CE, Turner G, et al. Exon deletions and duplications in BRCA1 detected by semiquantitative PCR. Genet Test 2000; 4(1):49–54.

113. Hofmann W, Gorgens H, John A, et al. Screening for large rearrangements of the BRCA1 gene in German breast or ovarian cancer families using semi-quantitative multiplex PCR method. Hum Mutat 2003; 22(1):103–104.

114. Charbonnier F, Raux G, Wang Q, et al. Detection of exon deletions and duplications of the mismatch repair genes in hereditary nonpolyposis colorectal cancer families using multiplex polymerase chain reaction of short fluorescent fragments. Cancer Res 2000; 60(11): 2760–2763.

115. Casilli F, Di Rocco ZC, Gad S, et al. Rapid detection of novel BRCA1 rearrangements in high-risk breast-ovarian cancer families using multiplex PCR of short fluorescent fragments. Hum Mutat 2002; 20(3):218–226.

116. Tournier I, Paillerets BB, Sobol H, et al. Significant contribution of germline BRCA2 rearrangements in male breast cancer families. Cancer Res 2004; 64(22):8143–8147.

117. Schouten JP, McElgunn CJ, Waaijer R, et al. Relative quantification of 40 nucleic acid sequences by multiplex ligation-dependent probe amplification. Nucleic Acids Res 2002; 30(12):e57.

118. Taylor CF, Charlton RS, Burn J, et al. Genomic deletions in MSH2 or MLH1 are a frequent cause of hereditary non-polyposis colorectal cancer: identification of novel and recurrent deletions by MLPA. Hum Mutat 2003; 22(6):428–433.

119. Montagna M, Dalla Palma M, Menin C, et al. Genomic rearrangements account for more than one-third of the BRCA1 mutations in northern Italian breast/ovarian cancer families. Hum Mol Genet 2003; 12(9):1055–1061.

120. Hogervorst FB, Nederlof PM, Gille JJ, et al. Large genomic deletions and duplications in the BRCA1 gene identified by a novel quantitative method. Cancer Res 2003; 63(7):1449–1453.

121. Bunyan DJ, Eccles DM, Sillibourne J, et al. Dosage analysis of cancer predisposition genes by multiplex ligation-dependent probe amplification. Br J Cancer 2004; 91(6):1155–1159.

122. Agata S, Dalla Palma M, Callegaro M, et al. Large genomic deletions inactivate the BRCA2 gene in breast cancer families. J Med Genet 2005; 42(10):e64.

123. Puget N, Stoppa-Lyonnet D, Sinilnikova OM, et al. Screening for germ-line rearrangements and regulatory mutations in BRCA1 led to the identification of four new deletions. Cancer Res 1999; 59(2):455–461.

124. Gad S, Caux-Moncoutier V, Pages-Berhouet S, et al. Significant contribution of large BRCA1 gene rearrangements in 120 French breast and ovarian cancer families. Oncogene 2002; 21(44):6841–6847.

125. Walsh T, Casadei S, Coats KH, et al. Spectrum of mutations in BRCA1, BRCA2, CHEK2, and TP53 in families at high risk of breast cancer. JAMA 2006; 295(12):1379–1388.

126. Hendrickson BC, Judkins T, Ward BD, et al. Prevalence of five previously reported and recurrent BRCA1 genetic rearrangement mutations in 20,000 patients from hereditary breast/ovarian cancer families. Genes Chromosomes Cancer 2005; 43(3):309–313.

127. Mazoyer S, Dunning AM, Serova O, et al. A polymorphic stop codon in BRCA2. Nat Genet 1996; 14(3):253–254.

128. Goldgar DE, Easton DF, Deffenbaugh AM, et al. Integrated evaluation of DNA sequence variants of unknown clinical significance: application to BCA1 and BRCA2. Am J Hum Genet 2004; 75(4):535–544.

129. Tavtigian SV, Deffenbaugh AM, Yin L, et al. Comprehensive statistical study of 452 BRCA1 missense substitutions with classification of eight recurrent substitutions as neutral. J Med Genet 2006; 43(4):295–305.

130. Tavtigian SV, Samollow PB, de Silva D, et al. An analysis of unclassified missense substitutions in human BRCA1. Fam Cancer 2006; 5(1):77–88.

131. Chenevix-Trench G, Healey S, Lakhani S, et al. Genetic and histopathologic evaluation of BRCA1 and BRCA2 DNA sequence variants of unknown clinical significance. Cancer Res 2006; 66(4):2019–2027.

132. Thompson D, Easton D. The genetic epidemiology of breast cancer genes. J Mammary Gland Biol Neoplasia 2004; 9(3):221–236.

133. Fleming MA, Potter JD, Ramirez CJ, et al. Understanding missense mutations in the BRCA1 gene: an evolutionary approach. Proc Natl Acad Sci U S A 2003; 100(3):1151–1156.

134. Ramirez CJ, Fleming MA, Potter JD, et al. Marsupial BRCA1: conserved regions in mammals and the potential effect of missense changes. Oncogene 2004; 23(9):1780–1788.
135. Abkevich V, Zharkikh A, Deffenbaugh A, et al. Analysis of missense variation in human BRCA1 in the context of interspecific sequence variation. J Med Gen 2004; 41:492–507.
136. http://research.nhgri.nih.gov/bic/

12
Breast Cancer Risk Modifiers

Roger Milne and Georgia Chenevix-Trench
Queensland Institute of Medical Research, Brisbane, Queensland, Australia

INTRODUCTION

The incomplete penetrance associated with mutations in *BRCA1* and *BRCA2* suggests that environmental or genetic risk-modifying factors may exist that affect the phenotype of *BRCA1* and *BRCA2* mutation carriers. Initial estimates from clinic-based data indicated that around 80% of carriers of mutations in *BRCA1* and *BRCA2* from multiple-case families would develop breast cancer (1,2), whereas a later pooled analysis from population-based studies has suggested that for the great majority of mutation carriers, their average lifetime risk is closer to 45% to 66% (3). This pooled-analysis of *BRCA1* and *BRCA2* carriers also showed that in *BRCA1* mutation carriers, the breast cancer penetrance for relatives ascertained through a breast cancer case was significantly higher than for those ascertained through an ovarian cancer case, and even higher if the index case was diagnosed before the age of 35 (3). Conversely, the ovarian cancer risk was higher in families ascertained through an ovarian cancer index case. Similar differences in risk, depending on the cancer site in the index case, were also reported by Simchoni et al. in an Ashkenazi Jewish population (4). These variations in risk between different studies, and according to the phenotype of the proband, are consistent with the presence of modifying factors. There is also a recent report that the phenocopy rate in *BRCA1* and *BRCA2* families is increased over the population rate, further suggesting the existence of environmental or genetic modifiers (5).

ENVIRONMENTAL MODIFIERS

Environmental or lifestyle factors may be important in explaining the variation in breast cancer risk among *BRCA1* and *BRCA2* mutation carriers. Estimates of risk in carriers may vary between countries for cultural reasons. For example, parity (number of full-term pregnancies), oral contraceptive use, and oophorectomy all influence the risks of breast cancer, and these factors vary between countries (6). That the risk of breast cancer for *BRCA1* and *BRCA2* mutation carriers appears to have increased over calendar time (7–9) strengthens the argument for the existence of environmental determinants of risk in the carrier population (10).

    Options to reduce of breast cancer risk which are available to unaffected carriers of mutations in *BRCA1* and *BRCA2* are discussed elsewhere in this volume. Briefly, they include chemoprevention, and surveillance [by regular self-examination of the breasts, clinical breast examination, mammography, ultrasound and/or magnetic resonance imaging (MRI)] as well as prophylactic bilateral mastectomy and prophylactic bilateral oophorectomy (105). Apart from prophylactic mastectomy and oophorectomy, there is little consistent information about what *BRCA1* and *BRCA2* carriers can do to reduce their risk. If modifiable environmental or lifestyle factors were identified that affected breast cancer risk in carriers, a perhaps more acceptable alternative would be to inform these women of how they can change their habits or lifestyle to reduce their risk. It cannot necessarily be assumed that the widely recognized risk factors for breast cancer in the general population, such as reproductive and hormonal factors, operate in the same way in women who carry mutations in *BRCA1* and *BRCA2*. While there have been number of relatively recent publications addressing this issue by studying mutation carriers, a variety of methodological challenges complicate our ability to draw strong inferences from these studies. Thus, few firm conclusions have been drawn about the role of modifiers to date.

Methodological Issues

In most studies of mutation carriers, recruitment of subjects is largely carried out by testing an affected family member from a multiple-case family. Considering the first identified carrier in a family as the "proband," only probands are selected directly on the basis of disease outcome (consistent with standard case–control designs), whereas nonprobands may fall into two other categories with regard to selection. First, those who are selected independently of disease outcome (consistent with standard retrospective cohort designs). Second, those who have decided whether or not to be tested for the identified familial mutation based on whether or not they have cancer (which is not consistent with either design). Many of the affected carriers are prevalent cases, while virtually all unaffected carriers are relatives of cases. Members of the same family are likely to have correlated exposures (both environmental and genetic), and are likely to have correlated disease risks that may be independent of the mutation carried in *BRCA1* or *BRCA2*. In addition, environmental exposures are typically assessed retrospectively, the recall of which may vary by affected status as well. These conditions mean that standard analytical methods cannot necessarily be applied, and it is not immediately obvious how these potential biases may influence estimates of relative risk (RR) obtained from these methods.

However, until data are available from large, prospective cohort studies of unaffected carriers (keeping in mind that such studies may be limited by subjects avoiding much of the disease risk by choosing to undergo prophylactic surgical intervention), we must endeavor to analyze the available data and make appropriate inferences in order to inform mutation carriers, clinicians, and genetic counselors about the possible effect of environmental factors on cancer risk. It is therefore important that multiple, independent studies are conducted, using different analytical approaches that address different potential biases. Indeed, there are several collaborations of researchers currently studying potential environmental modifiers of breast cancer risk in mutation carriers. These include at least four international consortia, each applying different analytical models: the studies led by Narod involving approximately 55 centers from around the world (11,12); the International *BRCA1/2* Carrier Cohort Study (IBCCS) (13); the PROSE and MAGIC consortia involving approximately 24 centers in Europe and North America (14); and another, led by the Breast Cancer Family Registry (BCFR) (15), which has combined its carrier data with those of the Kathleen Cuningham Foundation Consortium for Research into Familial Breast Cancer (KConFab) (16) and the Ontario Cancer Genetics Network (OCGN) (17).

The analytical approach adopted by the Narod et al. group has matched affected carriers to unaffected carriers on potential confounders such as age, year of birth, and gene in which the mutation occurs (ignoring familial relationships), and applied conditional logistic regression to matched sets. Apart from being subject to the potential biases mentioned above, this matching approach has resulted in up to 40% of carriers being excluded from the analyses because of the lack of an appropriate match (12), and this may introduce an additional bias. Nevertheless, theirs is currently the largest sample set and represents the largest geographic spectrum. The BCFR-led consortium has not used this matching approach, but has instead applied unconditional logistic regression, adjusting for family history and other potential confounders. The degree to which this approach adequately deals with ascertainment bias depends on how well the family history variable used acts as a surrogate for the familial phenotypes that led to inclusion in the study. In an effort to minimize recall and other biases due to the inclusion of prevalent cases, the BCFR group has also restricted inclusion to cases diagnosed within five years of interview, which has resulted in a reduced dataset in their analyses. The IBCCS and PROSE/MAGIC studies have taken a cohort approach, including all carriers for whom exposure information was available and applying Cox regression models to time to breast cancer diagnosis from birth. The IBCCS study has used a weighted regression approach, with weights determined to account for ascertainment biases due to age-specific preferential sampling of cases relative to controls. This weighting results in reduced power to detect associations (18). All groups have used robust estimates of variance to account for correlations within families. It is clear that each analytic approach adopted has its advantages and disadvantages, and so the most informative and clinically applicable results will be those that are consistent across studies.

A review of the studies assessing environmental modifiers of breast cancer risk among *BRCA1* and *BRCA2* mutation carriers published to date is presented, by exposure, in the following subsections and summarized in Table 1.

Parity

It is well established that parity reduces the risk of female breast cancer in the general population in the longer term, with the degree of protection increasing with the number of births (19). The largest dataset analyzed estimated the risk reduction to be around 7% per additional birth (20). Each full-term pregnancy is associated with a transient increase in risk, so that the protective effect of parity is most apparent in women over the age of 40 years (21). Women who have their first birth at a younger age are also at reduced risk (19).

It has been suggested that the protective effect of parity is reduced, or not evident, in women who are carriers of mutations in *BRCA1* and *BRCA2* (22–25), but few of the studies on which this was based compared affected and unaffected mutation carriers separately by gene. Jernstrom et al. (24) found that being parous increased the risk of breast cancer before the age of 41 years [odds ratio (OR) = 1.71; 95% confidence interval (CI) = 1.13–2.62] among pooled samples of 472 *BRCA1* and *BRCA2* mutation carriers, and that risk increased with each additional birth ($p = 0.007$). These results were not confirmed in a subsequent analysis of an expanded dataset (including 2520 carriers from 55 collaborating centers) by the group led by Narod (26), which found that the associations differed by mutation. Risk was found to increase with parity among *BRCA2* carriers under the age of 50 years, who represented only 20% of the sample in the earlier study (OR = 1.17 per birth; 95% CI = 1.01–1.36), but not among older carriers. On the other hand, among *BRCA1* carriers, having four or more children was associated with a

Table 1 Summary of Large Studies of Environmental Modifiers of Breast Cancer Risk Comparing Exposures of Affected Carriers to Unaffected Carriers

Authors, year (Consortium)	Methodology	N^a	Exposure(s) assessed	RR (95% CI)
Jernstrom et al., 1999 (24) (Narod Consortium)	Conditional logistic regression analysis of matched case–control data from pooled female *BRCA1* and *BRCA2* mutation carriers aged ≤40 years	189/189 (*BRCA1*); 47/47 (*BRCA2*)	*Pooled carriers* Parity (ever) Per birth	1.71 (1.13–2.62) 1.24 (1.04–1.47)
Cullinane et al., 2005 (26) (Narod Consortium)	Conditional logistic regression analysis of matched case–control data from female *BRCA1* and *BRCA2* mutation carriers of all ages, by gene and by age (divided at age 50 years)	934/934 (*BRCA1*); 326/326 (*BRCA2*)	*BRCA1* carriers Parity (ever) ≥4 births vs. never Per birth *BRCA2* carriers Parity (ever) ≥2 births vs. never Per birth Per birth, women aged <50 years Per birth, women aged ≥50 years	0.94 (0.75–1.19) 0.62 (0.41–0.94) 0.94 (0.86–1.02) 1.37 (0.93–2.03) 1.53 (1.01–2.32) 1.15 (1.00–1.33) 1.17 (1.01–1.36) 0.97 (0.58–1.53)
Gronwald et al., 2006 (27) (data may be included in the Narod Consortium studies)	Conditional logistic regression analysis of matched case–control data from female *BRCA1* mutation carriers of all ages with mutations in *BRCA1*	348/348 (*BRCA1*)	*BRCA1* carriers Parity (per birth) Breastfeeding (≥12 months vs. never) Age at menarche (per year) Oral contraceptive use (ever)	1.2 (P^{bc} = 0.02) 0.5 (P^c = 0.02) 0.9 (P^c = 0.004) 0.8 (P^c = 0.3)

Reference	Method	Cases/Controls	Factor	Estimate (95% CI)
Andrieu et al., 2006 (28) (IBCCS Consortium)	Weighted Cox regression analysis of affected and unaffected female BRCA1 and BRCA2 mutation carriers of all ages, by gene and by age (divided at age 40 years)	602/585 (BRCA1) 251/163 (BRCA2)	*BRCA1* carriers	
			Parity (ever)	0.86 (0.64–1.15)
			Age at first birth (<20 years vs. ≥30 years)	1.72 (1.06–2.78)
			Induced abortion (ever)	0.92 (0.56–1.51)
			Miscarriage (ever)	0.84 (0.51–1.39)
			Breastfeeding (≥12 months vs.never)	1.07 (0.81–1.40)
			BRCA2 carriers	
			Parity (ever)	0.79 (0.46–1.37)
			Age at first birth (<20 years vs. ≥20 years)	0.5 (not given)
			Induced abortion (ever)	0.34 (0.11–1.08)
			Miscarriage (ever)	0.56 (0.21–1.48)
			Breastfeeding (≥12 months vs. never)	0.79 (0.44–1.39)
			Pooled carriers	
			Parity (per birth)	0.86 (0.78–0.94)
			(Per birth, women aged ≤40 years)	1.10 (0.90–1.34)
			(Per birth, women aged >40 years)	0.85 (0.77–0.95)
Rebbeck et al., 2001 (29) (PROSE/ MAGIC Consortium)	Unconditional logistic regression analysis of affected and unaffected female BRCA1 and BRCA2 mutation carriers of all ages pooled	278/170 (BRCA1 and BRCA2 pooled)	Pooled carriers	
			Age at first birth (<30 years vs. ≥30 years or nulliparous)	0.33 (0.16–0.66)
			Age at menarche (≥13 years vs. <13 years)	0.82 (0.55–1.23)

(Continued)

Table 1 Summary of Large Studies of Environmental Modifiers of Breast Cancer Risk Comparing Exposures of Affected Carriers to Unaffected Carriers (*Continued*)

Authors, year (Consortium)	Methodology	N^a	Exposure(s) assessed	RR (95% CI)
Friedman et al., 2006 (31) (Narod Consortium)	Conditional logistic regression analysis of matched case–control data from female *BRCA1* and *BRCA2* mutation carriers of all ages, by gene	1,313/1,313 (*BRCA1*) 380/380 (*BRCA2*)	*BRCA1* carriers Induced abortion (ever) Miscarriage (ever) *BRCA2* carriers Induced abortion (ever) Miscarriage (ever)	0.98 (0.78–1.22) 1.09 (0.89–1.32) 0.64 (0.41–1.00) 0.75 (0.55–1.04)
Jernstrom et al., 2004 (32) (Narod Consortium)	Conditional logistic regression analysis of matched case–control data from female *BRCA1* and *BRCA2* mutation carriers of all ages, by gene	685/685 (*BRCA1*) 280/280 (*BRCA2*)	*BRCA1* carriers Breastfeeding (≥12 months vs. never) (Per month) *BRCA2* carriers Breastfeeding (≥12 months vs. never) (Per month)	0.55 (0.38–0.80) 0.98 (0.97–0.99) 0.95 (0.56–1.59) 0.99 (0.98–1.01)
Narod et al., 2002 (12) (Narod Consortium)	Conditional logistic regression analysis of matched case–control data from female *BRCA1* and *BRCA2* mutation carriers of all ages, by gene	981/981 (*BRCA1*) 330/330 (*BRCA2*)	*BRCA1* carriers Oral contraceptive use (ever) (Ever, women aged <40 years) (≥5 years use vs. never) (Use before the age of 30 years vs. never) (Use before 1975 vs. never) (Per year) *BRCA2* carriers Oral contraceptive use (ever)	1.20 (1.02–1.40) 1.38 (1.11–1.72) 1.33 (1.11–1.60) 1.29 (1.09–1.52) 1.42 (1.17–1.75) 1.02 (1.00–1.03) 0.94 (0.72–1.24)

Reference	Description of analysis	Sample sizes	Exposure / carriers	Result
Haile et al., 2006 (17) (BCFR Consortium)	Unconditional logistic regression analysis of affected and unaffected female *BRCA1* and *BRCA2* mutation carriers aged <50 years, by gene	195/302 (*BRCA1*); 128/179 (*BRCA2*)	*BRCA1* carriers: Oral contraceptive use (ever); *BRCA2* carriers: Oral contraceptive use (ever) (≥5 years use vs. never) (Per year)	0.77 (0.53–1.12); 1.62 (0.90–2.92); 2.06 (1.08–3.94); 1.08 ($P^c = 0.008$)
McGuire et al., 2006 (44) (BCFR Consortium)	Unconditional logistic regression analysis of affected and unaffected female *BRCA1* and *BRCA2* mutation carriers aged <50 years, by gene	195/302 (*BRCA1*); 128/179 (*BRCA2*)	*BRCA1* carriers: Alcohol use (ever); *BRCA2* carriers: Alcohol use (ever)	1.06 (0.73–1.52); 0.66 (0.45–0.97)
Brunet et al., 1998 (45) (Narod Consortium)	Conditional logistic regression analysis of matched case–control data from pooled female *BRCA1* and *BRCA2* mutation carriers of all ages	186/186 (*BRCA1* and *BRCA2* pooled)	Pooled carriers: Cigarette smoking (ever)	0.54 (0.34–0.84)
Ghadirian et al., 2004 (46) (Narod Consortium)	Conditional logistic regression analysis of matched case–control data from female *BRCA1* and *BRCA2* mutation carriers of all ages, by gene	806/806 (*BRCA1*); 291/291 (*BRCA2*)	*BRCA1* carriers: Cigarette smoking (ever); *BRCA2* carriers: Cigarette smoking (ever)	1.09 (0.87–1.33); 0.97 (0.68–1.38)
Colilla et al., 2006 (48) (PROSE/MAGIC Consortium)	Cox regression analysis of affected and unaffected female *BRCA1* mutation carriers of all ages	176/140 (*BRCA1*)	*BRCA1* carriers: Cigarette smoking (ever)	0.63 (0.47–0.87)
King et al., 2003 (7)	Cox regression analysis of affected female carriers (of all ages) of one of three ancient mutations in *BRCA1* and *BRCA2*	104/0 (*BRCA1* and *BRCA2* pooled)	Pooled carriers: Weight at menarche (normal); Physical activity as teenager; Body mass index at the age of 21 years (per unit)	0.46 ($P^c = 0.02$); 0.63 ($P^c = 0.03$); 1.02 ($P^c = 0.01$)

(Continued)

Table 1 Summary of Large Studies of Environmental Modifiers of Breast Cancer Risk Comparing Exposures of Affected Carriers to Unaffected Carriers (*Continued*)

Authors, year (Consortium)	Methodology	N^a	Exposure(s) assessed	RR (95% CI)
Kotsopoulos et al., 2005 (50) (Narod Consortium)	Conditional logistic regression analysis of matched case–control data from pooled female *BRCA1* and *BRCA2* mutation carriers aged >30 years, by gene and by age (divided at age 40 years)	797/797 (*BRCA1*) 276/276 (*BRCA2*)	Weight change at ages 18–30 (loss of ≥10 lb vs. loss/gain within 10 lb) Pooled carriers Pooled carriers aged ≤40 years Pooled carriers aged >40 years *BRCA1* carriers aged ≤40 years *BRCA2* carriers aged ≤40 years	0.66 (0.46–0.93) 0.47 (0.28–0.79) 0.97 (0.52–1.65) 0.35 (0.18–0.67) 0.88 (0.35–2.23)
Narod et al., 2006 (11) (Narod Consortium)	Conditional logistic regression analysis of matched case–control data from pooled female *BRCA1* and *BRCA2* mutation carriers of all ages, by gene and by age (divided at age 40 years)	1260/1260 (*BRCA1*) 340/340 (*BRCA2*)	Mammography (ever) Pooled carriers Pooled carriers aged ≤40 years Pooled carriers aged >40 years *BRCA1* carriers *BRCA2* carriers	1.03 (0.85–1.25) 1.18 (0.89–1.55) 0.87 (0.66–1.15) 1.04 (0.84–1.29) 1.06 (0.67–1.66)
Andrieu et al., 2006 (53) (IBCCS Consortium)	Weighted Cox regression analysis of affected and unaffected female *BRCA1* and *BRCA2* mutation carriers of all ages, by gene, by age (divided at age 40 years), and by year of birth (divided at 1950)	602/585 (*BRCA1*) 251/163 (*BRCA2*)	Chest X rays (ever) Pooled carriers Pooled carriers aged ≤40 years Pooled carriers born ≥1950 Exposed before the age of 20 years *BRCA1* carriers *BRCA2* carriers	1.54 (1.1–2.1) 1.97 (1.3–2.9) 2.56 (1.8–3.7) 4.64 (2.2–10.9) 1.42 (1.0–2.0) 2.33 (1.1–5.0)

| Kotsopoulos et al., 2005 (56) (Narod Consortium) | Weighted Cox regression analysis of affected and unaffected female *BRCA1* and *BRCA2* mutation carriers of all ages, by gene | 945/945 (*BRCA1*) 366/366 (*BRCA2*) | *BRCA1* carriers Age at menarche (≥15 vs. ≤11) (Trend[b]—per year) *BRCA2* carriers Age at menarche (≥15 vs. ≤11) (Trend [b]—per year) | 0.46 (0.30–0.69) $P^c = 0.0002$ 0.72 (0.37–1.38) $P^c = 0.5$ |
| Mitchell et al., 2006 (58) | Unconditional logistic regression analysis of affected and unaffected female *BRCA1* and *BRCA2* mutation carriers, by gene | 52/72 (*BRCA1*) 44/38 (*BRCA2*) | Breast density (Dense area ≥50% vs. <50%) *BRCA1* carriers *BRCA2* carriers | 2.77 (1.15–6.67) 2.24 (0.84–6.00) |

[a]Number of affected carriers/number of unaffected carriers (gene in which a mutation is carried in parenthesis).
[b]*P*-value for trend only, as elative risk estimate was not provided.
[c]*P*, *p*-value (95% CI not provided).
Abbreviations: BCFR, Breast Cancer Family Registry; CI, confidence interval; IBCCS, International *BRCA1/2* Carrier Cohort Study; PROSE/MAGIC; RR, estimate of relative risk associated with the exposure.

modest reduction in risk relative to being nulliparous (OR = 0.62; 95% CI = 0.41–0.94), and this effect did not appear to differ by age. The investigators also analyzed time since last birth and found some evidence that while for *BRCA2* mutation carriers, there was a nonsignificant transient increase in breast cancer risk following each birth, for *BRCA1* mutation carriers, there was a modest nonsignificant decrease in risk in the two years immediately following a full-term pregnancy. Gronwald et al. (27) recently published results based on an analysis of 696 Polish *BRCA1* (mostly founder) mutation carriers in which they reported that the risk of breast cancer increased with each live birth (OR = 1.2 per birth; $p = 0.02$). It is possible, though not certain, that this Polish dataset is a subset of the larger collaboration led by Narod.

Using a different analytical approach, the IBCCS consortium has also recently published its analysis of 1187 *BRCA1* and 414 *BRCA2* mutation carriers in which it found that while breast cancer risk did not appear to differ between parous and nulliparous women, among parous women, an increasing number of full-term pregnancies was associated with protection from breast cancer [hazard ratio (HR) = 0.86; 95% CI = 0.78–0.94] (28). This effect appeared to be restricted to women over the age of 40 years, with some evidence that risk increased with number of pregnancies in younger parous women. These results were seen consistently in both *BRCA1* and *BRCA2* mutation carriers analyzed separately, although the effects appeared to be slightly stronger among *BRCA2* mutation carriers. The IBCCS consortium also evaluated the risk associated with age at first birth, and found that among *BRCA2* mutation carriers, women who first gave birth before the age of 20 years were found to be at approximately 50% reduced risk of breast cancer, but that the opposite was the case for *BRCA1* mutation carriers, with risk appearing to be higher for those with an earlier age at first birth.

Rebbeck et al. (29) also assessed the effect of age at first live birth among a pooled sample of 448 female *BRCA1* and *BRCA2* mutation carriers of all ages, most of whom had *BRCA1* mutations, and found that women who had their first live birth before the age of 30 years were at a reduced risk compared to nulliparous and other parous women (OR = 0.33; 95% CI = 0.16–0.66).

Although these various findings appear to be contradictory and certainly require further investigation to clarify exactly how full-term pregnancies influence breast cancer risk in carriers of mutations in *BRCA1* and *BRCA2*, some preliminary conclusions can be drawn that may have relevance for genetic counseling of mutation carriers. The effects of parity on breast cancer risk may not be the same for *BRCA1* and *BRCA2* mutation carriers, and so studies that pool them may be less informative. Having many children is possibly associated with an increased risk of breast cancer among younger (aged less than 40 years) female carriers of mutations in either gene, but particularly *BRCA2* mutation carriers. This is perhaps consistent with the observation that the transient increase in risk associated with a full-term pregnancy seen in the general population may occur in *BRCA2* mutation carriers but not *BRCA1* mutation carriers. While the protection associated with having a first birth at a young age (before the age of 20 years) among women in the general population may also be present among *BRCA2* mutation carriers, it is not clear whether this is the case for *BRCA1* mutation carriers.

Spontaneous and Induced Abortions

A recent, very large collaborative reanalysis of data from 53 epidemiological studies found that, in the general population, having a spontaneous abortion is not associated with breast cancer risk and induced abortions are associated with a slightly reduced risk (RR = 0.93; 95% CI = 0.89–0.96) (30). Both the IBCCS and the Narod-led consortium have recently published findings from analyses of abortion and breast cancer risk in *BRCA1* and *BRCA2* mutation carriers (28,31). Results were consistent in the two studies, the former including 1601 carriers and the latter 2828. Among *BRCA1* mutation carriers, neither spontaneous nor induced abortions were found to be associated with breast cancer risk. For *BRCA2* carriers, as observed in the general population, spontaneous abortions were not associated with risk, and induced abortions seemed to, if anything, be associated with reduced risk. It seems relatively clear that neither spontaneous nor induced abortions increase breast cancer risk among carriers of mutations in either gene.

Breastfeeding

A collaborative reanalysis of data from 47 epidemiological studies has established that, in the general population, women who breastfeed are at a slightly lower risk of breast cancer, and that each cumulative year of breastfeeding reduces risk by 4.3% (20). This association is independent of parity. Three published studies have investigated this association among *BRCA1* and *BRCA2* mutation carriers. Based on analyses of 1930 carriers of both mutations from a subset of collaborators in the consortium led by Narod (32), it was found that increasing the duration of breastfeeding was associated with increasing protection from breast cancer among carriers of mutations in *BRCA1* (approximately 22% per year of breastfeeding). However, this effect was not seen for *BRCA2* mutation carriers, although the latter group consisted of fewer (560) carriers. The Polish study of 696 *BRCA1* mutation carriers previously mentioned, which may have included some of the data in the paper by Jernstrom et al. (32), also found a protective effect of breastfeeding for at least 12 months (OR $= 0.5; p = 0.02$) (27). An Icelandic study found evidence that *BRCA2* mutation carriers were afforded greater protection from breastfeeding than noncarriers, but they did not compare the breastfeeding behavior of affected carriers to that of unaffected carriers directly (25). The IBCCS study found no evidence of an association between breastfeeding and breast cancer risk among 1601 carriers of mutations in either gene (HR $= 1.04$; 95% CI $= 0.81$–1.34 for the pooled data) (28), although they acknowledged that they had limited power to detect the modest effect found in the general population [4.3% risk reduction per year of breastfeeding according to the Collaborative Group on Hormonal Factors in Breast Cancer (20)]. Based on these studies, it seems that the protective effect of breastfeeding seen in the general population may also apply to carriers of *BRCA1* and *BRCA2* mutations, but this is yet to be confirmed.

Oral Contraceptive Use

It is generally accepted, based on a large collaborative study published in 1996, that women taking oral contraceptives (OCs) have about a 20% increased risk of breast cancer and that the increased risk persists for up to 10 years after ceasing OC use (33). However, it should be noted that a large case–control study has subsequently found no evidence of increased risk, at least in women over the age of 35 years (34). The consortium led by Narod published analyses based on a subset of 2622 carriers of mutations in *BRCA1* and *BRCA2*. They found that while OC use was not associated with risk of breast cancer for *BRCA2* mutation carriers, use of OCs by *BRCA1* mutation carriers was associated with a 20% increase in risk, and that this increase was greater for those who had used OCs for at least five years, used OCs before the age of 30 years, were diagnosed with breast cancer before the age of 40 years, or first used OCs before 1975 (12). The Polish study of 696 *BRCA1* mutation carriers found no evidence of an association between OC use and breast cancer risk (27). Most recently, the

BCFR-led consortium studied 804 affected and unaffected carriers of mutations in both genes, all under the age of 50 years, and found no significant association between risk of breast cancer and use of OCs for *BRCA1* mutation carriers (OR = 0.77; 95% CI = 0.53–1.12) (17). However, for *BRCA2* mutation carriers, OC use for at least five years was associated with an increased risk (OR = 2.06; 95% CI = 1.08–3.94) as was duration of use (OR = 1.08 per year of use; $p = 0.008$).

It is particularly important to resolve the issue of whether OC use might increase breast cancer risk among *BRCA1* and *BRCA2* mutation carriers, because OC use is relatively common and there is reasonable evidence that OC use is associated with reduced *ovarian* cancer risk among mutation carriers (27,35–37). Consideration of the studies of mutation carriers published to date suggests that for *BRCA1* mutation carriers, the use of current OC formulations (i.e., those produced after 1975) is most likely not associated with an increased risk of breast cancer. The evidence is less clear for *BRCA2* mutation carriers.

Hormone Replacement Therapy

It is well established that women who use hormone replacement therapy (HRT) are at a slightly increased risk of breast cancer and that risk increases with duration of use (by 2–3% per year of use), but decreases when use is ceased (38). Rebbeck et al. have reported that use of HRT in mutation carriers who had undergone a bilateral prophylactic oophorectomy (BPO) did not significantly alter the reduction in breast cancer risk associated with BPO. These data suggest that short-term HRT does not negate the protective effect of BPO on subsequent breast cancer risk in *BRCA1* or *BRCA2* mutation carriers. In addition, the Narod-led collaboration have reported that HRT use by carriers does not appear to adversely influence their risk of *ovarian* cancer (OR = 0.93; 95% CI = 0.56–1.56) (39). Despite these encouraging results, additional research on the use of HRT and its role in breast cancer risk among women with *BRCA1* or *BRCA2* mutations is warranted.

Nutrition

Although a number of dietary factors have been investigated to varying degrees with respect to their effects on breast cancer risk, it is generally understood that the only established risk factor in the general population is alcohol consumption (40–42). The Collaborative Group on Hormonal Factors in Breast Cancer has clearly established that daily consumption of more than one standard alcoholic drink is associated with a slight increase in breast cancer risk, with an average 7% increase in risk per standard drink, per day (43). The BCFR-led consortium studied 804 carriers of mutations in *BRCA1* and *BRCA2* aged less than 50 years, and found no evidence that alcohol intake was associated with increased breast cancer risk among carriers of mutations in either gene (OR = 1.06; 95% CI = 0.73–1.52 for *BRCA1* mutation carriers), and weak evidence that it may even reduce the risk among *BRCA2* mutation carriers (OR = 0.66; 95% CI 0.45–0.97) (44). However, this study was probably underpowered to detect an association of the magnitude observed among predominantly noncarriers. No other studies of carriers investigating alcohol consumption have been published to date.

Smoking

Cigarette smoking has been found not to be associated with breast cancer risk in the general population after adjusting for the confounding effects of alcohol consumption (43).

Nevertheless, smoking has been investigated among *BRCA1* and *BRCA2* mutation carries by members of the consortium of Narod et al. Brunet et al. (45) published results based on just 372 carriers of mutations in either gene (pooled) showing evidence of a protective effect of cigarette smoking. However, a subsequent publication by the same group reported that this was no longer observed for carriers of mutations in either gene after recruitment of additional carriers (to a combined total of 2194) into their study (OR = 1.05; 95% CI = 0.88–1.25) (46,47). An additional study has recently reported a protective effect of cigarette smoking on breast cancer risk for *BRCA1* mutation carriers (HR = 0.63; 95% CI = 0.47–0.87) (48), but this was based on relatively few carriers (just 316) and therefore requires confirmation. The weight of evidence to date indicates that smoking is not associated with *increased* risk of breast cancer among carriers of mutations in either gene.

Physical Exercise and Body Weight

Physical exercise is known to be associated with reduced breast cancer risk in the general population, although the degree of protection afforded in relation to the amount and intensity of exercise is not entirely clear (41). The relationship between body weight and breast cancer risk is more complex, with an interaction repeatedly observed with menopausal status. A pooled analysis of data from seven prospective cohort studies has confirmed that while being overweight increases breast cancer risk among postmeno-pausal women by around 25%, obesity is associated with *protection* from breast cancer in premenopausal women (49). Only two studies have investigated weight-related factors among *BRCA1* and *BRCA2* mutation carriers. In a study including just 104 Ashkenazi Jewish carriers of one of three ancient mutations, King et al. (7) found evidence that physical exercise during teenage years was associated with reduced breast cancer risk among *BRCA1* and *BRCA2* mutation carriers (RR = 0.63; $p = 0.03$), as was being normal weight at menarche (RR = 0.46; $p = 0.02$) and a lighter weight at the age of 21 years. The group led by Narod reported findings from a study of 2146 carriers suggesting that weight loss of at least 10 pounds between the ages of 18 and 30 years was associated with a reduction in breast cancer risk in mutation carriers under the age of 40 years (OR = 0.47; 95% CI = 0.28–0.79), though not in later life (50). The variables assessed in the former study were not clearly defined, and the results of both studies clearly require confirmation by other independent groups. However, these findings suggest that engaging in physical exercise and maintaining a healthy weight, both from a young age, should be encouraged in mutation carriers, as in the general population.

Screening Mammography and Chest X Rays

It is well established that moderate-to-high-dose medical radiation to the chest increases breast cancer risk (51). Screening mammography involves the administration of a small dose of radiation to the breast that is not thought to be sufficient to increase the risk of breast cancer in the general population. However, it has been suggested that women with mutations in *BRCA1* and *BRCA2* may be more sensitive to the potentially DNA-damaging effects of this exposure and therefore be at higher risk from mammography (52). Some members of the consortium led by Narod analyzed data from 3200 *BRCA1* and *BRCA2* mutation carriers and found no evidence of an association between having at least one screening mammography and breast cancer risk for carriers of mutations in either gene (OR = 1.03; 95% CI = 0.85–1.25) (11). However, the ability to assess the impact of cumulative exposure was very limited, and so further studies are required before clear conclusions can be drawn.

There is limited published information on whether occasional exposure to low-dose radiation in chest X rays influences breast cancer risk in the general population (53) carried out a pooled analysis of eight cohort studies and found that the risk was modest for protracted low-dose exposures, but higher for exposures at younger ages. They estimated that breast cancer risk was twofold for exposures of at least 1 Gy before the age of 25 years. The IBCCS study of 1601 *BRCA1* and *BRCA2* mutation carriers found that any reported exposure to X rays was associated with increased breast cancer risk (HR = 1.54; $p = 0.007$). The increase in risk was even higher for women born after 1949 (HR = 2.56; $p < 0.001$) and higher again for those exposed before the age of 20 years (HR = 4.64; $p < 0.001$) (54). Although recall bias may explain at least part of the observed association, the pattern of risk by age at exposure is consistent with that observed in the general population, but at much lower doses (estimated to be between 0.0005 and 0.02 Gy). If confirmed, these findings will have important implications for the use of otherwise routine X-ray imaging in young carriers of mutations in *BRCA1* and *BRCA2*.

Nonmodifiable Factors

Additional established risk factors for breast cancer in the general population that have been studied in carriers of mutations in *BRCA1* and *BRCA2*, but which are not modifiable, are later age, early age at menarche, and increasing mammographic density (19,55,56). The magnitude of age-specific RRs of breast cancer for mutation carriers versus noncarriers appears to differ by gene. An analysis of pooled data from 22 population-based studies of families of unselected mutation carriers found that while *BRCA2* mutation carriers appear to be at a fairly stable 10- to 15-fold increased risk of breast cancer relative to noncarriers over all ages, the RR for *BRCA1* carriers drops with age, from more than 30 before the age of 50 years down to around 11 after the age of 60 years (3). The effect of age at menarche may also differ by gene. Two possibly overlapping studies from the Narod and Polish groups have found that later age at menarche was associated with reduced breast cancer risk among 1890 and 696 *BRCA1* mutation carriers, respectively (OR = 0.90 per delayed year of menarche, $p = 0.004$) (27,58). However, no association was seen in smaller studies of 732 *BRCA2* mutation carriers (57) or in 448 *BRCA1* or *BRCA2* mutation carriers (29).

Mammographic density is a particularly strong risk factor in the general population, with women with dense tissue in more than 75% of the breast being at between four- and fivefold risk of breast cancer compared to women with little or no density in the breast (56). Investigators from the Epidemiological Study of *BRCA1* and *BRCA2* mutation carriers (EMBRACE), which is part of the larger IBCCS consortium, studied the mammograms of 206 carriers and found that high density was associated with increased breast cancer risk (OR = 2.29 for a density of ≥50%; 95% CI = 1.23–4.26). The RR did not appear to differ by the gene in which the mutation was carried and was considered to be of similar magnitude to that observed in the general population (58). The authors argued that mammographic density could therefore be used to improve breast cancer risk prediction in carriers.

GENETIC MODIFIERS

As discussed at the start of this chapter, the variation in the risk of breast and ovarian cancer for *BRCA1* and *BRCA2* mutation carriers between different studies, and according to the phenotype of the proband, is consistent with the presence of either environmental or genetic modifiers. Genetic modifiers are probably more likely than shared environment to account for familial clustering of cancer sites in Ashkenazi Jewish mutation carriers, for example, since intrafamilial differences in environment are large in such families with recent immigration histories (4). Although there has also been considerable interest in finding genetic modifiers of cancer risk in *BRCA1* and *BRCA2* mutation carriers, the number of published studies is still fairly modest. The underlying reason for this may be that there is still a paucity of validated "low-risk common alleles" for breast or ovarian cancer in the general population, and until such alleles are identified, testing candidate single nucleotide polymorphisms (SNPs) as modifiers of *BRCA1* and *BRCA2* remains a fairly high-risk endeavor. Candidate modifier genes include those involved in detoxification of environmental carcinogens, in DNA repair, and in steroidogenesis.

Most studies of genetic modifiers of cancer risk in *BRCA1* and *BRCA2* mutation carriers have focused on SNPs for which there has been some evidence for modification of breast cancer risk in the general population. Given the apparent relationship between the cancer site in the proband and risk in relatives, it is likely that at least some genetic modifiers influence the risk of breast or ovarian cancer, but not both (4). Thus, a viable strategy would also be to examine polymorphisms that affect ovarian cancer risk in the general population, once they have been convincingly identified. However, given the lower penetrance for ovarian cancer in *BRCA1* and *BRCA2* carriers, extremely large studies will be necessary to identify genes that modify ovarian cancer risk in these carriers.

Methodological Issues

Studies of genetic modifiers use samples of carriers that are collected from multiple-case families, in the same way as for environmental modifiers, and are therefore subject to the same, mostly unpredictable biases as described above. One obvious exception is that recall bias is not an issue, unless environmental factors are also considered. An additional consideration is that genetic factors are always (rather than possibly) correlated within families, and the use of robust estimates of variance are therefore essential in order to avoid inflated type I errors. The application of Cox proportional hazards regression models without correction for preferential selection of cases versus controls by age has been shown to give biased estimates of RR, and so results from such analyses should be interpreted with caution (18). Furthermore, the use of prevalent cases will be particularly problematic if the variant being studied is associated with survival, which may more often be the case than for environmental exposures. In addition, the approach of picking candidate SNPs or genes to evaluate as modifiers of *BRCA1* and *BRCA2* suffers from the same general problems that face all candidate-based genetic association studies, such as the choice of candidate genes and variants, the small a priori likelihood that any of them are true modifiers, and the ability to identify relevant interactions that may involve complex biochemical pathways (59). These issues may be overcome in the future by linkage analyses (60) and genome-wide association studies (61).

As mentioned above for studies of modifying exposures, a number of consortia have been developed to study the role of genetic modifiers of risk in *BRCA1* and *BRCA2* mutation carriers, including some of those mentioned previously. An important development in the evolution of these studies is the creation of the Consortium of Investigators of Modifiers of *BRCA1* and *BRCA1* (CIMBA). This consortium was established in 2005 to generate sample sets of sufficient statistical power to identify modifier genes. There are currently 24 groups from Australia, North America, and Europe who plan to contribute to some or all of the planned, collaborative CIMBA projects, and collectively, they have DNA and data from more than 10,000 *BRCA1* and *BRCA2* carriers. This consortium may also provide a mechanism for conducting genome-wide association studies to identify novel modifier genes (61).

Androgen Receptor

The CAG repeat length polymorphism in the androgen receptor (*AR*) gene, the length of which has been shown to be inversely correlated with the strength of AR signaling, has been found to be associated with prostate, breast, and ovarian cancer risks. However, the data from different studies are contradictory, and no firm conclusions can be drawn as to the magnitude of such an effect, if any (62–67). Several groups have evaluated this polymorphism as a modifier of breast cancer risk in mutation carriers. The first published study was of 304 female *BRCA1* mutation carriers from North America, and it reported that women who had at least one *AR* allele with 29 CAG repeats were diagnosed with breast cancer an average of 4.7 years earlier than women with no such allele (68). Women with at least one allele containing 30 or more CAG repeats were diagnosed with breast cancer an average of 10.3 years earlier than women who did not carry any such allele ($p = 0.0002$). They used Cox regression and robust estimates of variance to correct for nonindependence of observations from related carriers. This association between long *AR* allele and increased breast cancer risk has not been replicated in a smaller study of 188 female Ashkenazi Jewish carriers from Israel and the United Kingdom, most of whom had mutations in *BRCA1*. *BRCA1* and *BRCA2* carriers were pooled for the analysis, which was conducted using a variant of the log rank test as well as Cox regression (69). Dagan et al. also evaluated AR CAG repeat length in 227 Israeli Jewish *BRCA1* ($n = 169$) and *BRCA2* ($n = 58$) mutation carriers and found an association between the *shorter* allele and increased risk of early onset breast cancer, but no overall effect (70). The largest study to date, of 376 *BRCA1* and 219 *BRCA2* carriers from 376 Australian and British families, also found no evidence that the presence of one allele of 28 or more CAG repeats affects breast cancer risk in *BRCA1* carriers (RR = 0.74; 95% CI 0.42–1.29) or in *BRCA2* carriers (RR = 1.12; 95% CI 0.55–2.25) (65). This study used a weighted Cox regression method to account for the fact that the disease status of the carriers may have affected the likelihood of ascertainment, and applied robust estimates of variance to allow for the nonindependence of genotypes from related carriers.

The amino terminal domain of AR, which contains the glutamine repeat encoded by the CAG triplet, binds directly to the amino acid 758–1064 region of *BRCA1*. Spurdle et al. therefore considered the possibility that AR-dependent modification of cancer risk in carriers may differ according to the mutation position relative to the AR binding site but found no compelling evidence for an effect of mutation position on risk in their relatively small sample. Analysis of the AR repeat polymorphism is complicated by the fact that this locus is on the X-chromosome and undergoes X-inactivation, and so only one allele is active in any one cell, but which particular allele is active in the relevant cell types of any one individual is not known. Given the conflicting results from these relatively large studies from different ethnic groups, as well as two smaller ones (71,72), a large collaborative study which takes into account mutation position may be needed to resolve the issue of whether the CAG repeat in *AR* modifies risk in *BRCA1*, or *BRCA2*, carriers.

Amplified in Breast Cancer 1

BRCA1 is a coactivator of AR, and this activation is mediated in part through an estrogen-receptor coactivator, amplified in breast cancer 1 (*AIB1*) (73). Rebbeck et al. studied the effect of a glutamine repeat polymorphism at the *AIB1* locus, whose functional effect is unknown, using a matched case–control sample of 448 women with germline *BRCA1* (*n* = 370) or *BRCA2* (*n* = 78) mutations (29). These women were at a significantly higher breast cancer risk if they carried alleles with at least 28 or 29 polyglutamine repeats in *AIB1*, compared with women who carried alleles with fewer repeats (OR = 1.59; 95% CI 1.03–2.47 or OR = 2.85; 95% CI 1.64–4.96, respectively). This effect was also seen when analysis was restricted to only *BRCA1* mutation carriers. Women were at an even higher risk if they had *AIB1* alleles with at least 28 polyglutamine repeats and were either nulliparous or had had a late age at first live birth (OR = 4.62; 95% CI 2.02–10.56) compared to women with none of these risk factors. The unconditional logistic regression analysis used in this study did not take into account the relatedness of carriers, nor did the study have sufficient power to examine the effect on *BRCA2* carriers alone. Colilla et al. (48) appeared to confirm this result and found an interaction with smoking, using a different method to categorize repeat lengths. Three further studies have since attempted to replicate this result, with little success. Kadouri et al. (74) genotyped 311 carriers, 257 of which were of Jewish origin, and, using a maximum likelihood approach to account for ascertainment, found that there was a nonsignificant elevation of breast cancer risk (OR = 1.29; 95% CI 0.85–1.96) in *BRCA1* mutation carriers with at least 29 AIB1 repeats. However, when the repeat was analyzed as a continuous variable, the effect was significant, particularly among *BRCA1* carriers (RR = 1.25; 95% CI 1.09–1.42). Hughes et al. (75) genotyped 851 *BRCA1* and 324 *BRCA2* female carriers from 678 families from France, Greece, and the United States, and used a standard Cox proportional hazards model for the analysis. No effect of the *AIB1* repeat polymorphisms was found regardless of whether the *BRCA1* and *BRCA2* carriers were analyzed together (HR = 1.10; 95% CI 0.92–1.11 when analyzed as a continuous variable) or separately. The largest study of the role of the *AIB1* repeat polymorphism as a modifier of *BRCA1* or *BRCA2* evaluated 1090 *BRCA1* and 661 *BRCA2* carriers from Australia, Europe, and North America (76). The association between genotype and disease risk was assessed using weighted Cox regression analysis, which adjusts for the fact that disease status of the carriers may have affected the likelihood of ascertainment. Robust variance estimates were used to calculate confidence limits, taking into account relatedness between carriers from the same family. There was no evidence for an increased risk of breast cancer associated with the AIB1 glutamine repeat length, whether the repeat was evaluated as a continuous variable, or with cut points of ≥28 or ≥29 repeats, for *BRCA1* or *BRCA2* carriers. This study was sufficiently large to detect risk ratios of 1.56 and 2.85 with 91% and 100% power respectively for *BRCA1* carriers, and 58% and 100% power for *BRCA2* carriers, and so we can confidently exclude any substantial risk of this polymorphism in *BRCA1* or *BRCA2* carriers.

TP53

Somatic mutations in *TP53* are the most frequent events in human cancer, and germline mutations of *p53* cause Li Fraumeni syndrome, of which early onset breast cancer is a feature. Polymorphisms of *TP53* are therefore good candidates as modifiers of *BRCA1* and *BRCA2*, in particular Pro72Arg, which appears to be a functional SNP (77). There are also multiple intronic polymorphisms in *TP53*, two of which were examined by Wang-Gohrke et al. (78) in 400 German *BRCA1* and *BRCA2* carriers but were not found to be associated with risk of ovarian cancer, despite some evidence to the contrary in unselected ovarian cancer cases. The largest study to evaluate *TP53* as a modifier of *BRCA1* and *BRCA2* was of 447 Spanish carriers (including 88 males) from 170 families (79). Osorio et al. genotyped the Pro72Arg SNP, as well as a 16 bp insertion in intron 3, and used unconditional logistic regression to compare haplotype frequencies between early onset breast or ovarian cancer cases and other carriers. They also used robust estimators of variance to take into account the relatedness of the carriers. They found that the "No Ins-72 Pro" haplotype was associated with early age of onset (before age 35) of breast or ovarian cancer in *BRCA2* mutation carriers ($n = 119$) (OR = 2.69; 95% CI 1.15–6.29), but not in *BRCA1* carriers ($n = 146$). This apparent differential effect on *BRCA1* versus *BRCA2* carriers may be because the penetrance of *BRCA2* mutations is lower. They repeated the analyses, including just the 170 index cases from each family (who were therefore unrelated) and found that the results were consistent when the *BRCA1* and *BRCA2* carriers were combined. Osorio et al. also reported that No Ins-72Arg homozygous cells are more efficient at inducing apoptosis than genotypes with at least one mutant *72Pro* allele. A larger study of both *BRCA1* and *BRCA2* carriers is now warranted to try and validate this association between *TP53* haplotypes and risk of cancer in *BRCA2* mutation carriers, and to determine whether they also modify risk in *BRCA1* mutation carriers.

RAD51

RAD51 currently provides the most convincing evidence for the existence of a modifier gene for cancer risk in *BRCA2* mutation carriers. *RAD51* is the homolog of bacterial RecA, which is required for recombinational repair of double-strand DNA breaks, in particular for *BRCA2*-mediated repair (80). Both *BRCA1* and *BRCA2* interact with *RAD51* (81,82), and the *RAD51* mouse knockout phenotype resembles the *BRCA1* and *BRCA2* knockout phenotypes (82). The $-135G > C$ SNP in the 5' untranslated regions (UTR) of *RAD51* was first published in a study of 257 female Ashkenazi Jewish carriers from 141 *BRCA1* and 64 *BRCA2* families (83). Using logistic regression and Cox proportional hazard analysis, no effect was seen on *BRCA1* carriers, but the HR for cancer (breast or ovarian) associated with heterozygosity for the C allele in *BRCA2* carriers was 4.0 (85% CI 1.3–9.2), largely because of its effect on breast cancer risk. The results were similar when the analysis was restricted to unrelated cases. Three additional studies of this *RAD51* SNP as a modifier of *BRCA1/2* have been published. Wang et al. (85) genotyped two sets of carriers; in the first set of 186 carriers, the C allele was more common in affected women with a mutation in either *BRCA1* or *BRCA2*. However, when this dataset was combined with a larger set of 466 carriers ascertained by three centers in Australia and the United States, an increased risk of breast cancer was only found among *BRCA2* carriers ($n = 216$; OR = 3.2; 95% CI 1.4–40), while their risk of ovarian cancer appeared to be decreased. Logistic regression was used to determine the effect of the *RAD51* SNP on risk, and a bootstrapping resampling technique was employed to calculate CIs and *P*-values that accounted for the nonindependence of genotypes from related carriers. Kadouri et al. (86) genotyped 297 *BRCA1* and *BRCA2* carriers from Israel and the United Kingdom for the same SNP in the *RAD51* promoter and, using Cox regression, also found an increased risk of breast cancer (HR = 2.09; 95% CI 1.04–4.18) for *BRCA2* carriers, and that the median age of breast cancer in *BRCA2* carriers with the *RAD51* C allele was seven years less than that in *RAD51* wild-type carriers. In contrast, Jakubowska et al. (87) evaluated this *RAD51* SNP in just 83 pairs of (affected and unaffected) female carriers of the Polish *BRCA1* founder mutation, *5382insC*. They reported a *reduced* risk of breast cancer among *RAD51* C allele carriers (OR = 0.23; 95% CI 0.07–0.62). If confirmed, *RAD51* $-135G > C$ would be the first SNP found to have opposite effects in *BRCA1* and *BRCA2* carriers. The function of the $-135G > C$ SNP in *RAD51* is not clear, but being located in the 5' UTR, it could affect mRNA stability or translational efficiency.

Other Genes

There are several other genes for which there has been a single report evaluating their role as genetic modifiers of *BRCA1* and *BRCA2*, but without any subsequent validation. Phelan et al. (88) examined a variable number of tandem repeats (VNTR) polymorphism downstream of the *HRAS1* gene in a panel of 307 *BRCA1* carriers from 79 different families, of whom 173 were affected with breast cancer, 42 with ovarian cancer, and 20 with both cancers. Carrier status for 41 of these carriers was inferred on the basis of linkage analysis, but not proven by mutation analysis. Using a Cox proportional hazards model, this study reported that the risk of ovarian cancer in these carriers was 2.11 times greater in those who harbored one or two rare alleles of this VNTR ($P = 0.015$), but that the risk of breast cancer was not changed. However, this study did not take into account the relatedness of the carriers, which could have biased the estimates of risk. Its significance is further reduced by the fact that the mechanism of action of the *HRAS1* VNTR alleles is not clear, and there is only weak evidence from one small study that this polymorphism is associated with ovarian cancer in the general population (89).

Runnebaum et al. (90) examined the PROGINS haplotype in the progesterone receptor gene (*PGR*) in 591 *BRCA1* carriers and 183 *BRCA2* carriers from 405 breast–ovarian cancer families. Overall, there was no association between disease status and presence of the *PROGINS* allele. However, among the 214 carriers (of either *BRCA1* or *BRCA2* mutations) who reported no past history of OC use, the presence of one or more *PROGINS* alleles was associated with a 2.4-fold increased risk of ovarian cancer ($P = 0.004$). Given the multiple comparisons performed in this analysis, independent replication is particularly necessary. The *PROGINS* allele has been associated with the risk of ovarian cancer in the general population, but the most comprehensive study to date found that although variation in *PGR* was associated with ovarian cancer risk, the strongest result was not with the *PROGINS* allele itself (91). The C677T (Ala225Val) SNP in the methylenetetrahydrofolate reductase (*MTHFR*) gene is associated with reduced enzyme activity and has been evaluated in 205 *BRCA1* and *BRCA2* carriers as a modifier of breast and ovarian cancer risk (92). No effect was found, but power was very limited.

Ginolhac et al. (93) hypothesized that wild-type alleles of *BRCA1* might modify the cancer risk in *BRCA1* carriers because of its effect on DNA repair rates in $BRCA1^{+/-}$ cells. A set of 591 *BRCA1* carriers from 282 families were genotyped for multiple *BRCA1* SNPs, but in order to account for the fact that some of the carriers were from the same family, only one carrier per sister-set was included in the analysis, resulting in the selection of 388 carriers for analysis using Cox regression. Among these 388 mutation carriers, carriers of the more common allele (glycine) at the Gly1038Glu SNP had a higher risk of ovarian cancer (HR = 1.50; 95% CI 1.03–2.19), but not of breast cancer. This effect appeared to be independent of the haplotype on which the *Gly1038* allele was carried, suggesting a direct effect of this SNP itself, although it does not appear to affect breast or ovarian cancer risk in the general population.

The same group, based at the International Agency for Research on Cancer (IARC), also hypothesized that common variants in *BRCA2* might modify cancer risk in *BRCA1* carriers (94). Using a set of 788 carriers from 403 families, they evaluated the Arg372His SNP of *BRCA2*. This SNP had previously been associated with both breast and ovarian cancer risk in the general population (95–97), although a large international consortium has recently failed to validate the effect on breast cancer risk in approximately 15,000 cases and 15,000 controls (98). The IARC group did not find any effect of this SNP in the *BRCA1* carriers on either breast or ovarian cancer risk (94).

The BARD1 protein exists with *BRCA1* in a heterodimeric complex that is involved in homologous-recombination-directed and transcription-coupled DNA repair. *BARD1* is therefore a good candidate *BRCA1* risk modifier. A large population-based Icelandic study recently evaluated the Cys557Ser missense SNP in *BARD1* in 992 unselected cases, which included 53 999del5 *BRCA2* carriers and 703 controls (99). The rare variant was associated with an overall increased risk of breast cancer in cases (OR = 1.82; $P = 0.014$) and also in *BRCA2* carriers (OR = 3.11; $P = 0.046$). However, Vahteristo et al. (100) previously found no increased risk associated with this *BARD1* variant in 1181 familial and 1565 unselected breast cancer cases compared to 1083 controls from Finland.

Even though some of these studies have been conducted in quite large carrier sets, until their findings have been validated independently, the results should be interpreted with caution.

Cytogenetic Abnormalities in *BRCA1* and *BRCA2* Carriers

Most studies aimed at identifying genetic modifiers of *BRCA1* and *BRCA2* have evaluated polymorphisms in candidate genes, but Nathanson et al. have taken a different approach, applying linkage analysis to *BRCA1* positive families, and targeting chromosomes 4 and 5 which have been shown by comparative genomic hybridization to be frequently altered in tumors from *BRCA1* mutation carriers (60). No significant linkage was observed for chromosome 4, but significant linkage was found to a maker on the long arm of chromosome 5 ($P = 0.009$), suggesting that one or more modifier genes may be located at 5q33-34. There is also some evidence from cytogenetic studies that germline abnormalities of 9p23-24 might occur in some *BRCA2* families with male breast cancer and harbor modifying genes (101,102).

SUMMARY

In summary, evidence to date suggests that the effects of environmental exposures on breast cancer risk may not be the same for mutation carriers as for the general population, and, furthermore, may differ between *BRCA1* versus *BRCA2* mutation carriers (Table 1). Having many children may be associated with increased risk for carriers under the age of 40 years, particularly in carriers of mutations in *BRCA2*. Exposure to chest X rays may also increase risk. Breastfeeding appears to offer protection from breast cancer among carriers, as in the general population. Exposures that do not appear to increase risk of breast cancer among mutation carriers include spontaneous and induced abortions, smoking, and OC use, the latter among *BRCA1* mutation carriers only. The effect of OC use remains unclear for *BRCA2* mutation carriers.

Some progress has been made in identifying genetic modifiers of breast cancer risk in *BRCA1* and *BRCA2* mutation carriers, but large, collaborative analyses will be needed though consortia such as CIMBA to provide convincing evidence for their existence. Identification of bona fide modifier genes will help to understand the biology of hereditary breast tumors and, in the case of *BRCA1* modifiers, will also provide candidate low-penetrance genes for "sporadic" basal cell breast cancers because of their similarity to *BRCA1*-related breast tumors (103,104). In the long term, it might be possible to include information on genetic modifiers in risk prediction models, and to give individualized advice on personal cancer risks to mutation carriers.

References

1. Easton DF et al. "Breast and ovarian cancer incidence in BRCA1-mutation carriers. Breast Cancer Linkage Consortium." Am J Hum Genet 1995; 56(1):265–271.

2. Ford D et al. "Genetic heterogeneity and penetrance analysis of the BRCA1 and BRCA2 genes in breast cancer families. The Breast Cancer Linkage Consortium." Am J Hum Genet 1998; 62(3):676–689.

3. Antoniou A et al. "Average risks of breast and ovarian cancer associated with BRCA1 or BRCA2 mutations detected in case Series unselected for family history: a combined analysis of 22 studies." Am J Hum Genet 2003; 72(5):1117–1130.

4. Simchoni S et al. "Familial clustering of site-specific cancer risks associated with BRCA1 and BRCA2 mutations in the Ashkenazi Jewish population." Proc Natl Acad Sci U S A 2006; 103(10):3770–3774.

5. Evans D et al. "The trouble with phenocopies: are those testing negative for a family BRCA1/2 really at population risk?" Am J Hum Genet 2005, Abstract 71.

6. Narod SA, Foulkes WD. "BRCA1 and BRCA2: 1994 and beyond." Nat Rev Cancer 2004; 4(9):665–676.

7. King MC et al. "Breast and ovarian cancer risks due to inherited mutations in BRCA1 and BRCA2." Science 2003; 302(5645):643–646.

8. Narod S et al. "Increasing incidence of breast cancer in family with BRCA1 mutation." Lancet 1993; 341(8852):1101–1102.

9. Tryggvadottir L et al. "Population-based study of changing breast cancer risk in Icelandic BRCA2 mutation carriers, 1920–2000." J Natl Cancer Inst 2006; 98(2):116–122.

10. Narod SA. "Modifiers of risk of hereditary breast and ovarian cancer." Nat Rev Cancer 2002; 2(2):113–123.

11. Narod SA et al. "Screening mammography and risk of breast cancer in BRCA1 and BRCA2 mutation carriers: a case-control study." Lancet Oncol 2006; 7(5):402–406.

12. Narod SA et al. "Oral contraceptives and the risk of breast cancer in BRCA1 and BRCA2 mutation carriers." J Natl Cancer Inst 2002; 94(23):1773–1779.

13. Goldgar D et al. "The International BRCA1/2 Carrier Cohort Study Collaborators Group: The International BRCA1/2 Carrier Cohort Study: purpose, rationale, and study design." Breast Cancer Res 2000; 2:E010.

14. www.cceb.med.upenn.edu/PROSE.

15. http://epi.grants.cancer.gov/CFR/about_breast.html.

16. kConFab, www.kconfab.org.

17. Haile RW et al. "BRCA1 and BRCA2 mutation carriers, oral contraceptive use and breast cancer before age 50." Cancer Epidemiol Biomarkers Prev 2006; 15(10):1863–1870.

18. Antoniou AC et al. "A weighted cohort approach for analysing factors modifying disease risks in carriers of high-risk susceptibility genes." Genet Epidemiol 2005; 29(1):1–11.

19. Kelsey JL et al. "Reproductive factors and breast cancer." Epidemiol Rev 1993; 15(1): 36–47.

20. Collaborative Group on Hormonal Factors in Breast Cancer. "Breast cancer and breastfeeding: collaborative reanalysis of individual data from 47 epidemiological studies in 30 countries, including 50,302 women with breast cancer and 96,973 women without the disease." Lancet 2002; 360(9328):187–195.

21. Lambe M et al. "Transient increase in the risk of breast cancer after giving birth." N Engl J Med 1994; 331(1):5–9.

22. Becher H et al. "Reproductive factors and familial predisposition for breast cancer by age 50 years. A case-control-family study for assessing main effects and possible gene-environment interaction." Int J Epidemiol 2003; 32(1):38–48.

23. Hartge P et al. "Breast cancer risk in Ashkenazi BRCA1/2 mutation carriers: effects of reproductive history." Epidemiology 2002; 13(3):255–261.

24. Jernstrom HC et al. "Pregnancy and risk of early breast cancer in carriers of BRCA1 and BRCA2." Lancet 1999; 354(9193):1846–1850.

25. Tryggvadottir L et al. "BRCA2 mutation carriers, reproductive factors and breast cancer risk." Breast Cancer Res 2003; 5(5):R121–R128.

26. Cullinane CA et al. "Effect of pregnancy as a risk factor for breast cancer in BRCA1/BRCA2 mutation carriers." Int J Cancer 2005; 117(6):988–991.

27. Gronwald J et al. "Influence of selected lifestyle factors on breast and ovarian cancer risk in BRCA1 mutation carriers from Poland." Breast Cancer Res Treat 2006; 95(2):105–109.

28. Andrieu N et al. "Pregnancies, breast-feeding, and breast cancer risk in the International BRCA1/2 Carrier Cohort Study (IBCCS)." J Natl Cancer Inst 2006; 98(8):535–544.

29. Rebbeck TR et al. "Modification of BRCA1- and BRCA2–associated breast cancer risk by AIB1 genotype and reproductive history." Cancer Res 2001; 61(14):5420–5424.

30. Beral V et al. "Breast cancer and abortion: collaborative reanalysis of data from 53 epidemiological studies, including 83,000 women with breast cancer from 16 countries." Lancet 2004; 363(9414):1007–1016.

31. Friedman E et al. "Spontaneous and therapeutic abortions and the risk of breast cancer among BRCA mutation carriers." Breast Cancer Res 2006; 8(2):R15.

32. Jernstrom H et al. "Breast-feeding and the risk of breast cancer in BRCA1 and BRCA2 mutation carriers." J Natl Cancer Inst 2004; 96(14):1094–1098.

33. Collaborative Group on Hormonal Factors in Breast Cancer. "Breast cancer and hormonal contraceptives: collaborative reanalysis of individual data on 53,297 women with breast cancer and 100,239 women without breast cancer from 54 epidemiological studies. Collaborative Group on Hormonal Factors in Breast Cancer." Lancet 1996; 347(9017): 1713–1727.

34. Marchbanks PA et al. "Oral contraceptives and the risk of breast cancer." N Engl J Med 2002; 346(26):2025–2032.

35. McGuire V et al. "Relation of contraceptive and reproductive history to ovarian cancer risk in carriers and noncarriers of BRCA1 gene mutations." Am J Epidemiol 2004; 160(7): 613–618.

36. Narod SA et al. "Oral contraceptives and the risk of hereditary ovarian cancer. Hereditary Ovarian Cancer Clinical Study Group." N Engl J Med 1998; 339(7):424–428.

37. Whittemore AS et al. "Oral contraceptive use and ovarian cancer risk among carriers of BRCA1 or BRCA2 mutations." Br J Cancer 2004; 91(11):1911–1915.

38. Collaborative Group on Hormonal Factors in Breast Cancer. "Breast cancer and hormone replacement therapy: collaborative reanalysis of data from 51 epidemiological studies of 52,705 women with breast cancer and 108,411 women without breast cancer. Collaborative Group on Hormonal Factors in Breast Cancer." Lancet 1997; 350(9084):1047–1059.

39. Kotsopoulos J et al. "Hormone replacement therapy and the risk of ovarian cancer in BRCA1 and BRCA2 mutation carriers." Gynecol Oncol 2006; 100(1):83–88.

40. Hanf V, Gonder U. "Nutrition and primary prevention of breast cancer: foods, nutrients and breast cancer risk." Eur J Obstet Gynecol Reprod Biol 2005; 123(2):139–149.

41. McTiernan A. "Behavioral risk factors in breast cancer: can risk be modified?" Oncologist 2003; 8(4):326–334.

42. Nkondjock A, Ghadirian P. "Epidemiology of breast cancer among BRCA mutation carriers: an overview." Cancer Lett 2004; 205(1):1–8.

43. Hamajima N et al. "Alcohol, tobacco and breast cancer—collaborative reanalysis of individual data from 53 epidemiological studies, including 58,515 women with breast cancer and 95,067 women without the disease." Br J Cancer 2002; 87(11):1234–1245.

44. McGuire V et al. "No increased risk of breast cancer associated with alcohol consumption among carriers of BRCA1 and BRCA2 mutations under age 50 years." Cancer Epidemiol Biomarkers Prev 2006; 15:1565–1567.

45. Brunet JS et al. "Effect of smoking on breast cancer in carriers of mutant BRCA1 or BRCA2 genes." J Natl Cancer Inst 1998; 90(10):761–766.

46. Ghadirian P et al. "Smoking and the risk of breast cancer among carriers of BRCA mutations." Int J Cancer 2004; 110(3):413–416.

47. Hopper JL, Baron JA. "Re: oral contraceptives and the risk of breast cancer in BRCA1 and BRCA2 mutation carriers." J Natl Cancer Inst 2003; 95(13):1010–1011; author reply 1012–1013.

48. Colilla S et al. "The joint effect of smoking and AIB1 on breast cancer risk in BRCA1 mutation carriers." Carcinogenesis 2006; 27(3):599–605.

49. van den Brandt PA et al. "Pooled analysis of prospective cohort studies on height, weight, and breast cancer risk." Am J Epidemiol 2000; 152(6):514–527.

50. Kotsopoulos J et al. "Changes in body weight and the risk of breast cancer in BRCA1 and BRCA2 mutation carriers." Breast Cancer Res 2005; 7(5):R833–R843.

51. Ron E. "Cancer risks from medical radiation." Health Phys 2003; 85(1):47–59.

52. Friedenson B. "Is mammography indicated for women with defective BRCA genes? Implications of recent scientific advances for the diagnosis, treatment, and prevention of hereditary breast cancer." MedGenMed 2000; 2(1):E9.

53. Breast cancer association consortium. Commonly studied single-nucleotide polymorphisms and breast cancer: results from the breast cancer association consortium. J Natl Cancer Inst 2006 Oct 4; 98(19):1382–96.

54. Andrieu N et al. "Effect of chest X-Rays on the risk of breast cancer among BRCA1/2 mutation carriers in the international BRCA1/2 carrier cohort study." J Clin Oncol 2006; 24: 3361–3366.

55. Bernstein L et al. "Ethnicity-related variation in breast cancer risk factors." Cancer 2003; 97 (1 suppl):222–229.

56. Boyd NF et al. "Mammographic breast density as an intermediate phenotype for breast cancer." Lancet Oncol 2005; 6(10):798–808.

57. Kotsopoulos J et al. "Age at menarche and the risk of breast cancer in BRCA1 and BRCA2 mutation carriers." Cancer Causes Control 2005; 16(6):667–674.

58. Mitchell G et al. "Mammographic density and breast cancer risk in BRCA1 and BRCA2 mutation carriers." Cancer Res 2006; 66(3):1866–1872.

59. Pharoah PD et al. "Association studies for finding cancer-susceptibility genetic variants." Nat Rev Cancer 2004; 4(11):850–860.

60. Nathanson KL et al. "CGH-targeted linkage analysis reveals a possible BRCA1 modifier locus on chromosome 5q." Hum Mol Genet 2002; 11(11):1327–1332.

61. Hirschhorn JN, Daly MJ. "Genome-wide association studies for common diseases and complex traits." Nat Rev Genet 2005; 6(2):95–108.

62. Giguere Y et al. "Short polyglutamine tracts in the androgen receptor are protective against breast cancer in the general population." Cancer Res 2001; 61(15):5869–5874.

63. Haiman CA et al. "The androgen receptor CAG repeat polymorphism and risk of breast cancer in the Nurses' Health Study." Cancer Res 2002; 62(4):1045–1049.

64. Modugno F. "Ovarian cancer and polymorphisms in the androgen and progesterone receptor genes: a HuGE review." Am J Epidemiol 2004; 159(4):319–335.

65. Spurdle AB et al. "The androgen receptor CAG repeat polymorphism and modification of breast cancer risk in BRCA1 and BRCA2 mutation carriers." Breast Cancer Res 2005; 7(2): R176–R183.

66. Suter NM et al. "Androgen receptor (CAG)n and (GGC)n polymorphisms and breast cancer risk in a population-based case-control study of young women." Cancer Epidemiol Biomarkers Prev 2003; 12(2):127–135.

67. Zeegers MP et al. "How strong is the association between CAG and GGN repeat length polymorphisms in the androgen receptor gene and prostate cancer risk?" Cancer Epidemiol Biomarkers Prev 2004; 13(11 Pt 1):1765–1771.

68. Rebbeck TR et al. "Modification of BRCA1-associated breast cancer risk by the polymorphic androgen-receptor CAG repeat." Am J Hum Genet 1999; 64(5):1371–1377.

69. Kadouri L et al. "CAG and GGC repeat polymorphisms in the androgen receptor gene and breast cancer susceptibility in BRCA1/2 carriers and non-carriers." Br J Cancer 2001; 85(1): 36–40.

70. Dagan E et al. "Androgen receptor CAG repeat length in Jewish Israeli women who are BRCA1/2 mutation carriers: association with breast/ovarian cancer phenotype." Eur J Hum Genet 2002; 10(11):724–728.

71. Kim SC et al. "CAG repeat length in exon 1 of the androgen receptor gene is related to age of diagnosis but not germ line BRCA1 mutation status in ovarian cancer." Int J Gynecol Cancer 2006; 16(suppl 1):190–194.

72. Menin C et al. "Lack of association between androgen receptor CAG polymorphism and familial breast/ovarian cancer." Cancer Lett 2001; 168(1):31–36.

73. Irvine RA et al. "Inhibition of p160-mediated coactivation with increasing androgen receptor polyglutamine length." Hum Mol Genet 2000; 9(2):267–274.

74. Kadouri L et al. "Polyglutamine repeat length in the AIB1 gene modifies breast cancer susceptibility in BRCA1 carriers." Int J Cancer 2004; 108(3):399–403.

75. Hughes DJ et al. "Breast cancer risk in BRCA1 and BRCA2 mutation carriers and polyglutamine repeat length in the AIB1 gene." Int J Cancer 2005; 117(2):230–233.

76. Spurdle AB et al. "The AIB1 polyglutamine repeat does not modify breast cancer risk in BRCA1 and BRCA2 mutation carriers." Cancer Epidemiol Biomarkers Prev 2006; 15(1): 76–79.

77. Thomas M et al. "Two polymorphic variants of wild-type p53 differ biochemically and biologically." Mol Cell Biol 1999; 19(2):1092–1100.

78. Wang-Gohrke S et al. "Intron variants of the p53 gene are associated with increased risk for ovarian cancer but not in carriers of BRCA1 or BRCA2 germline mutations." Br J Cancer 1999; 81(1):179–183.

79. Osorio A et al. "A haplotype containing the p53 polymorphisms Ins16bp and Arg72Pro modifies cancer risk in BRCA2 mutation carriers." Hum Mutat 2006; 27(3):242–248.

80. Karran P. "DNA double strand break repair in mammalian cells." Curr Opin Genet Dev 2000; 10(2):144–150.

81. Scully R et al. "Association of BRCA1 with Rad51 in mitotic and meiotic cells." Cell 1997; 88(2):265–275.

82. Wong AK et al. "RAD51 interacts with the evolutionarily conserved BRC motifs in the human breast cancer susceptibility gene BRCA2." J Biol Chem 1997; 272(51):31941–31944.

83. Shu Z et al. "Disruption of muREC2/RAD51L1 in mice results in early embryonic lethality which can Be partially rescued in a p53(-/-) background." Mol Cell Biol 1999; 19(12): 8686–8693.

84. Levy-Lahad E et al. "A single nucleotide polymorphism in the RAD51 gene modifies cancer risk in BRCA2 but not BRCA1 carriers." Proc Natl Acad Sci USA 2001; 98(6):3232–3236.

85. Wang WW et al. "A single nucleotide polymorphism in the 5' untranslated region of RAD51 and risk of cancer among BRCA1/2 mutation carriers." Cancer Epidemiol Biomarkers Prev 2001; 10(9):955–960.

86. Kadouri L et al. "A single-nucleotide polymorphism in the RAD51 gene modifies breast cancer risk in BRCA2 carriers, but not in BRCA1 carriers or noncarriers." Br J Cancer 2004; 90(10):2002–2005.

87. Jakubowska A et al. "Breast cancer risk reduction associated with the RAD51 polymorphism among carriers of the BRCA1 5382insC mutation in Poland." Cancer Epidemiol Biomarkers Prev 2003; 12(5):457–459.

88. Phelan CM et al. "Ovarian cancer risk in BRCA1 carriers is modified by the HRAS1 variable number of tandem repeat (VNTR) locus." Nat Genet 1996; 12(3):309–311.

89. Weitzel JN et al. "The HRAS1 minisatellite locus and risk of ovarian cancer." Cancer Res 2000; 60(2):259–261.

90. Runnebaum IB et al. "Progesterone receptor variant increases ovarian cancer risk in BRCA1 and BRCA2 mutation carriers who were never exposed to oral contraceptives." Pharmacogenetics 2001; 11(7):635–638.

91. Pearce CL et al. "Clarifying the PROGINS allele association in ovarian and breast cancer risk: a haplotype-based analysis." J Natl Cancer Inst 2005; 97(1):51–59.

92. Gershoni-Baruch R et al. "Association of the C677T polymorphism in the MTHFR gene with breast and/or ovarian cancer risk in Jewish women." Eur J Cancer 2000; 36(18): 2313–2316.

93. Ginolhac SM et al. "BRCA1 wild-type allele modifies risk of ovarian cancer in carriers of BRCA1 germ-line mutations." Cancer Epidemiol Biomarkers Prev 2003; 12(2):90–95.

94. Hughes DJ et al. "Common BRCA2 variants and modification of breast and ovarian cancer risk in BRCA1 mutation carriers." Cancer Epidemiol Biomarkers Prev 2005; 14(1):265–267.

95. Auranen A et al. "BRCA2 Arg372Hispolymorphism and epithelial ovarian cancer risk." Int J Cancer 2003; 103(3):427–430.

96. Healey CS et al. "A common variant in BRCA2 is associated with both breast cancer risk and prenatal viability." Nat Genet 2000; 26(3):362–364.

97. Spurdle AB et al. "The BRCA2 372 HH genotype is associated with risk of breast cancer in Australian women under age 60 years." Cancer Epidemiol Biomarkers Prev 2002; 11(4): 413–416.

98. Consortium T. B. C. A. "Commonly studies SNPs and breast cancer: negative results from 12,000–32,000 cases and controls from the Breast Cancer Association Consortium." J Natl Cancer Inst 2006. In press.

99. Stacey SN et al. "The BARD1 Cys557Ser Variant and Breast Cancer Risk in Iceland." PLoS Med 2006; 3(7):e217.

100. Vahteristo P et al. "BARD1 variants Cys557Ser and Val507Met in breast cancer predisposition." Eur J Hum Genet 2006; 14(2):167–172.

101. Savelyeva L et al. "An interstitial tandem duplication of 9p23-24 coexists with a mutation in the BRCA2 gene in the germ line of three brothers with breast cancer." Cancer Res 1998; 58 (5):863–866.

102. Savelyeva L et al. "Constitutional genomic instability with inversions, duplications, and amplifications in 9p23-24 in BRCA2 mutation carriers." Cancer Res 2001; 61(13): 5179–5185.

103. Lakhani SR et al. "Multifactorial analysis of differences between sporadic breast cancers and cancers involving BRCA1 and BRCA2 mutations." J Natl Cancer Inst 1998; 90(15): 1138–1145.

104. Lakhani SR et al. "Prediction of BRCA1 status in patients with breast cancer using estrogen receptor and basal phenotype." Clin Cancer Res 2005; 11(14):5175–5180.

105. Antill Y et al. "Risk-reducing surgery in women with familial susceptibility for breast and/or ovarian cancer." Eur J Cancer 2006; 42(5):621–628.

106. Calderon-Margalit R, Paltiel O. "Prevention of breast cancer in women who carry BRCA1 or BRCA2 mutations: a critical review of the literature." Int J Cancer 2004; 112(3):357–364.

107. U.S. Preventive Services Task Force. "Genetic risk assessment and BRCA mutation testing for breast and ovarian cancer susceptibility: recommendation statement." Ann Intern Med 2005; 143(5):355–361.

13

BRCA1 and *BRCA2* in Underserved and Special Populations

Bifeng Zhang and Olufunmilayo I. Olopade

Section of Hematology/Oncology, Department of Medicine, University of Chicago, Chicago, Illinois, U.S.A.

INTRODUCTION

Breast cancer incidence rate is low among African American, Asian American, Hispanic, and American Indian women compared with White women (Table 1) (1). However, the death rate from breast cancer is higher among African/African American women than among White women. Breast cancer is often diagnosed at an advanced stage among African/African American women and Hispanic women (2). The advanced stage at diagnosis is a major factor leading to high mortality rates among underserved populations. Whether genetic factors in part explain these observations is unclear.

It is estimated that 5% to 10% of breast cancer cases are attributed to pathogenic germline mutations or alterations in breast cancer susceptibility genes (3) including *BRCA1* and *BRCA2* (Table 2) (6,7), as well as *CHK2, TP53, PTEN, ATM,* and *STK11* (8–15). *BRCA1* and *BRCA2* are by far the most clinically relevant of these genes. Information about the distribution and clinical relevance of these genes in non-European populations is only beginning to be understood. Yet such information could improve our cancer control efforts.

BRCA1 AND *BRCA2* IN UNDERSERVED AND SPECIAL POPULATIONS

African Americans

African Americans comprise 12.9% of American population (16). Although the incidence rate of breast cancer is lower in African and African American women compared with White females, breast cancer in black women is often early onset and has a high mortality. According to Myriad Genetic Laboratories, Inc., only 3% of individuals undergoing *BRCA1/2* testing are self-reported to be African American (17).

There are striking similarities between *BRCA1* associated breast cancer and breast cancer in young African and African American women. Both cancers are often poorly differentiated, hormone receptor negative and have increased S-phase fraction (17–23).

To date, 1536 distinct *BRCA1* mutations, polymorphisms, and unclassified variants and 878 alterations have been reported in the Open Access Online Breast Cancer Mutation Database (24–27). Also, 1885 distinct *BRCA2* mutations, polymorphisms, and

233

Table 1 Female Breast Cancer Incidence and Death Rates by Race and Ethnicity, United States, 1998–2002

	Breast cancer incidence (per 100,000)	Breast cancer death rates (per 100,000)
White	141.1	25.9
African American	119.4	34.7
Asian American/Pacific Islander	96.6	12.7
Hispanic/Latina	89.9	16.7
American Indian/Alaska Native	54.8	13.8

Note: Rates are age-adjusted to the 2000 U.S. standard population.
Source: From Ref. 1.

variants and 1140 alterations have been reported (27). Of this, 36.5% of the *BRCA1* and 38.7% of *BRCA2* variants are deleterious (27). Of these pathogenic mutations, only 51 *BRCA1* and 40 *BRCA2* deleterious mutations have been reported in individuals of African and African American descent. The findings are summarized in Table 3 (24,27–30,32–37,42,43). In the Open Access Online Breast Cancer Mutation Database, 30 of 51 (60%) *BRCA1* mutations and 21 of 40 (53%) *BRCA2* mutations are confined to African and African American descendents (27). Nanda et al. compared African Americans with non-Hispanic, non-Jewish whites and reported that African Americans had a low rate of *BRCA1* and *BRCA2* deleterious mutations but a high rate of sequence variations (8).

There are 53 *BRCA1* unclassified variants and polymorphisms reported in African and African American females and among them, 24 (45%) are confined to African and African American descendents (27). There are 100 *BRCA2* unclassified variants reported in African and African American females and among them, 52 (52%) unclassified variants are confined to African and African American descendents (27). *BRCA1* and *BRCA2* variants in Africans and African Americans demonstrate a distinctive overall spectrum.

Some recurrent *BRCA1* and *BRCA2* mutations are of founder effects in a specific ethnic group: recurrent mutations arose from a common ancestral mutation and constituted a frequent allele in the current population (31,38–40). The high frequency of recurrent and founder mutations can expedite genetic testing in a specific ethnicity group and their identification is of special clinical significance in underserved populations. However, few founder mutations have been identified in women of African ancestry. The *BRCA1* 943ins10 mutations shared a single haplotype in five families from the Ivory Coast, South Carolina, Washington, D.C., Florida, and the Bahamas (41). Thus, *BRCA1* 943ins10 mutation represents a founder mutation of West African origin.

Table 2 Risks of Breast Cancer

Lifetime risk	Breast cancer
General female	13%
Females carrying germline mutations in *BRCA1*	56–87%
Females carrying germline mutations in *BRCA2*	37–85%

Source: From Refs. 4,5.

Table 3 *BRCA1* and *BRCA2* Deleterious Mutations in African and African Americans

BRCA1 mutations	Mutation effect	No. of observations in Af or Af Am	No. of non-Af	Refs.	BRCA2 mutations	Mutation effect	No. of observations in Af or Af Am	No. of non-Af	Refs.
1505delG	F	1 Af	0	27	*1536del4*	F	1 Af Am	0	25
1755del19	F	2 Af	0	27	*1646del4*	F	Af Am	0	27
2333delT	F	1 Af	0	27	*1882 del T*	F	1 Af Am	2	27, 26
2508delGA	F	1 Af	0	27	*1991delATAA*	F	1 Af Am	0	26, 33
2883del4	F	1 Af Am	0	27	*1993delAA*	F	1 Af Am	0	26
3405delC	F	1 Af	0	27	*2001delTTTAT*	F	1 Af Am	0	26
4035delTT	F	1 Af	5	27	*2320delC*	F	1 Af	0	27
4184del4	F	1 Af	41	27	*2816insA*	F	2 Af Am	5	25, 26, 27, 33
4241delTG	F	1 Af	0	27	*3034del4*	F	2 Af	35	25, 27
4730insG	F	2 Af	0	27	*3185insG*	F	1 Af	1	27
155del4	F	1 Af Am	0	42	*3910del4*	F	1 Af	0	27
1625del5	F	1 Af Am	0	28	*4075delGT*	F	1 Af Am	25	25, 26, 27
1742insG	F	1 Af	0	27	*4088delA*	F	1 Af Am	2	26, 27
1832del5	F	2 Af Am	0	42	*491delT*	F	1 Af	0	27
2418delA	F	3 Af, 2 Af Am	0	27	*5579insA*	F	1 Af	5	27
3331insG	F	1 Af Am	0	129	*5844del5*	F	3 Af, 2 Af Am	0	27
3450del4	F	1 Af Am	9	27, 34, 35	*5849del4*	F	2 Af	7	27
3875delGTCT	F	2 Af, 1 Af Am	35	27, 28	*6633del5*	F	1 Af Am	7	27
3883insA	F	1 Af Am	0	25	*6696delTC*	F	1 Af Am	10	25, 27
3888delGA	F	1 Af Am	1	27, 43	*6828delTT*	F	2 Af	0	27
4160delAG	F	1 Af Am	0	43	*7436del4*	F	1 Af Am	0	43
4730insG	F	1 Af Am	0	27	*7795delCT*	F	2 Af Am	0	25, 27
4794insA	F	1 Af Am	0	43	*7907delTT*	F	1 Af Am	0	43
5296del4	F	2 Af Am	9	27, 25	*802delAT*	F	1 Af Am	19	27
943ins10	F	7 Af Am, 6 Af	2	27, 41	*8075delC*	F	1 Af	0	27
C61G	M	2 Af Am	65	27	*8643 delAT*	F	1 Af Am	0	26

(Continued)

Table 3 *BRCA1* and *BRCA2* Deleterious Mutations in African and African Americans (*Continued*)

BRCA1 mutations	Mutation effect	No. of observations in Af or Af Am	No. of non-Af	Refs.	BRCA2 mutations	Mutation effect	No. of observations in Af or Af Am	No. of non-Af	Refs.
C64G	M	1 Af Am	2	27, 29	9326insA	F	1 Af Am	9	27
M1775R	M	6 Af, 5 Af Am	7	6, 27, 47	9481insA	F	2 Af, 2 Af Am	6	27
W1718C	M	1 Af Am	1	27, 35	K3326X	N	1 Af Am	111	27
C274X	N	1 Af	0	27	K944X	N	1 Af Am	0	27
E1535X	N	1Af, 2 Af Am	0	27	L164X	N	1 Af	0	27
E673X	N	1 Af Am	0	27	Q1886X	N	Af Am	0	27
K1290X	N	1 Af Am	1	27	Q2042X	N	3 Af	0	27
Q1090X	N	1 Af	0	25	Q2342X	N	1 Af Am	0	27
Q1447X	N	1 Af	0	27	R3128X	N	1 Af Am	26	27
Q491X	N	1 Af	1	27	S2372X	N	1 Af	0	27
R1443X	N	1 Af,	89	27	W2990X	N	1 Af	1	27
R1751X	N	1 Af, 1 Af Am	15	27	IVS13 − 2A/G	S	1 Af Am	0	43
S1796X	N	1 Af,	0	27	IVS16 + 1G>A	S	1 Af	1	27
Y1463X	N	1 Af Am	2	27	P3039P	S	1 Af	5	27
Y101X	N	4 Af	0	36					
D1692N	S	1 Af Am	3	27					
IVS13 + IG/A	S	6 Af, 1 Af Am	0	27					
IVS16 + 6T>C	S	3 Af, 1 Af Am	3	27					
IVS19 + 3del13	S	1 Af	0	27					
IVS22 + 5G/T	S	1 Af, 1 Af Am	0	35					
IVS23 + 1G>A	S	1 Af, 1 Af Am	1	27					
IVS4 − IG/T	S	1 Af Am	9	27, 43					
IVS5 − 11T > G	S	1 Af	39	27					
IVS6 + 2insT	S	1 Af Am	0	27					
IVS8 + 1G > A	S	1 Af	0	27					

Abbreviations: Af, African; Af Am, African American; F, frameshift mutation; M, missense mutation; N, nonsense mutation; S, splicing variant.

Hispanics

Hispanics account for 12.5% of the U.S. population (44). Hispanics mean persons of Latin American descent, especially of Mexican, Cuban, and Puerto Rican origin and may be of any ethnicity group (White, Black, Asian, etc.) (16).

Breast cancer is the most common cancer and the leading cause of cancer death in Hispanic women (45). Breast cancer in Hispanics is often at an advanced stage. About 60 *BRCA1* and 46 *BRCA2* deleterious mutations have been reported in individuals of Hispanic descent (Table 4) (27,47). In this, 25 of 60 (42%) *BRCA1* mutations and 16 of 46 (35%) *BRCA2* mutations are confined to Hispanic descendants (27). In this ethnic group, 51 *BRCA1* unclassified variants, two *BRCA1* polymorphisms, and 96 *BRCA2* unclassified variants have been reported (27). In this, 22 *BRCA1* unclassified variants and 38 *BRCA2* unclassified variants are confined to Hispanic descendants (27). *BRCA1* and *BRCA2* variants in Hispanics demonstrate a distinctive overall spectrum. The *BRCA1* and *BRCA2* mutations in Hispanics are summarized in Table 4.

Weitzel et al. studied 110 probands of Hispanic origin with a personal or family history of breast and/or ovarian cancer and reported that 34 out of the 110 (30.9%) probands had deleterious mutations including 25 *BRCA1* mutations and nine *BRCA2* mutations and that 25 (22.7%) probands had one or more unclassified variants (47). In this cohort, six recurrent mutations were also identified: *BRCA1 185delAG* ($n = 4$), *IVS5 + 1G* > A ($n = 2$), *S955X* ($n = 3$), *R1443X* ($n = 3$), *2552delC* ($n = 2$), and *BRCA2 3492insT* ($n = 2$). Further, the genotype analysis of recurrent mutations *BRCA1 185delAG*, *IVS5 + 1G* > A, *S955X*, *R1443X*, and *2552delC* suggested they have founder effects. The *BRCA1 185delAG* mutation in Hispanics has the same mutation haplotype as the corresponding Ashkenazi Jewish mutation (47). In this study, the six recurrent mutations accounted for 47% of the deleterious mutations (47). Such a high ratio of recurrent mutations suggests that genetic testing is feasible in Hispanic females at risk of developing breast cancer.

BRCA1 1205del56 and *BRCA2 3492insT* have also been observed over three times in Hispanic populations (Table 4) (27). Mexicans consist of 60% Amerindian-Spanish and 9% white; Cubans have 37% white and 11% black; Puerto Ricans consist of 80.5% white (mostly Spanish origin) and 8% black (16). Therefore, some *BRCA1* and *BRCA2* mutations in Hispanic women have exogenous origins. *BRCA1 185delAG*, *R1443X*, *5382insC*, and *BRCA2 6174delT* have been observed many times in Hispanics and possibly derived from European ancestry.

Asians

Asian Americans account for 4.2% of the population in the United States and 57% of the world population (16). The prevalence and mortality rate of breast cancer in Asian populations vary significantly across various countries (48,49). Breast cancer in East Asia generally features a low incidence rate and an early age onset. However, Asians living in North America have much higher incidence and mortality rates of breast cancer. The change of lifestyle is probably the culprit of the increased rates. Genetic epidemiological studies of *BRCA1* and *BRCA2* are rare in American Asians. However, there have been several reports in Asian countries. The *BRCA1* and *BRCA2* mutations in Asian populations are summarized in Table 5 (46,49–70,74–76).

Japanese

Breast cancer incidence rate is low in Japanese population. Katagiri et al. examined *BRCA1* in 103 patients either having an early age onset (< 35 years) or having multiple

(Text continues on p. 244.)

Table 4 *BRCA1* and *BRCA2* Mutations in Hispanics

BRCA1 mutations	Mutation effect	No. of observations in Hispanic	No. of non-Hispanic	Refs.	*BRCA2* mutations	Mutation effect	No. of observations in Hispanic	No. of non-Hispanic	Refs.
1135insA	F	2	26	27, 47	*1538del4*	F	1	6	27
1205del56	F	3	0	27, 47	*2059delT*	F	1	0	27
2415delAG	F	1	0	27, 47	*3036del4*	F	1	46	27
2525del4	F	1	0	27, 47	*3070insG*	F	1	0	27
2925del4	F	2	0	27, 47	*3185insG*	F	1	1	27
5382insC	F	5	>500	27, 47	*3417del4*	F	1	0	27, 47
943ins10	F	2	8	27	*3492insT*	F	13	0	27, 47
2552delC	F	8	0	27	*3908delTTG*	F	1	2	27
185delAG	F	30	>500	27, 47	*5164del4*	F	1	6	27, 47
1207delA	F	1	0	27	*5578delAA*	F	1	20	27
1508delAAinsG	F	1	0	27	*5579insA*	F	1	4	27
1793delA	F	2	0	27	*5770delA*	F	1	0	27
183delT	F	1	0	27	*5950delCT*	F	1	16	27
188insAG	F	2	0	27	*6027del4*	F	1	1	27
2080insA	F	1	4	27	*6174delT*	F	3	>500	27
2594delC	F	1	18	27	*6252insG*	F	2	0	27
2800delAA	F	1	31	27	*6503delTT*	F	1	45	27
3034delG	F	1	0	27	*7640del10*	F	1	0	27
3124delA	F	1	3	27	*7753insA*	F	1	0	27
3127delTT	F	1	1	27	*7784insC*	F	1	1	27

Mutation			References	Mutation			References
3148delCT	2	F	0	27	8550insT	1	F	0	27, 47
3450del4	2	F	16	27	8803delC	1	F	8	27
3746insA	1	F	4	27	8821ins T	1	F	1	27
3790ins4	1	F	5	27	886delGT	6	F	10	27
3875del4	1	F	45	27	8976ins4	1	F	1	27
3878delTTA	2	F	0	27	9254del5	4	F	3	27, 47
3949insC	1	F	0	27	9326insA	1	F	9	27
4160delAG	1	F	3	27	9481insA	1	F	10	27
4184del4	3	F	48	27	957del4	1	F	0	27, 47
4204delA	1	F	0	27	984delCA	1	F	0	27
5055delG	1	F	0	27	9927del4	1	F	0	27
589delCT	1	F	1	27	999del5	2	F	4	27
917delTT	3	F	8	27	M1R	1	M	1	27
exon-13-ins-6 kb	1	F	54	27	E1308X	7	N	2	27
A1708E	12	M	23	27, 47	E218X	2	N	0	27
C44Y	1	M	1	27	E49X	3	N	9	27
C61Y	1	M	2	27	Q742X	2	N	0	27, 47
M1775R	1	M	8	27	Q92X	2	N	0	27
M1I-(122G>T)	1	M	0	27	R2520X	1	N	19	27
R71G	5	M	6	27	R3128X	5	N	17	27
K654X	2	N	2	27, 47	S1442X	3	N	2	27
Q1200X	1	N	12	27, 47	S2022X	1	N	1	27
R1443X	5	N	80	27, 47	W2586X	1	N	3	27, 47
S955X	4	N	4	27	Y1313X	1	N	2	27
C944X	1	N	0	27	Y3308X	1	N	4	27
E1339X	1	N	0	27	E2918E	1	S	0	27
E1754X	1	N	3	27					

(Continued)

Table 4 *BRCA1* and *BRCA2* Mutations in Hispanics (*Continued*)

BRCA1 mutations	Mutation effect	No. of observations in Hispanic	No. of non-Hispanic	Refs.	*BRCA2* mutations	Mutation effect	No. of observations in Hispanic	No. of non-Hispanic	Refs.
E765X	N	1	0	27					
Q1518X	N	1	0	27					
Q169X	N	1	3	27					
S451X	N	1	0	27					
IVS5 + 1G>A	S	2	3	27, 47					
D1692N	S	1	3	27					
IVS13 + 1G>A	S	1	12	27					
IVS16 + 6T>C	S	3	6	27					
IVS20 + 1delG	S	1	0	27					
IVS20 + 1G>A	S	1	21	27					
IVS4 – 1G>T	S	1	3	27					
IVS6 – 1G>A	S	1	0	27					
R1495M	S	2	9	27					

Abbreviations: F, frameshift mutation; M, missense mutation; N, nonsense mutation; S, splicing variant.

Table 5 *BRCA1* and *BRCA2* Mutations in Asians

Asian populations	*BRCA1* mutations	Mutation effect	No. of observations within the population	No. outside the population	*BRCA2* mutations	Mutation effect	No. of observations within the population	No. outside the population
Japanese	2509delAA	F	4	0	S2834X	F	6	0
	2508delAG	F	5	0	5802del4	F	7	0
	4237delAG	F	2	0	6633del5	F	2	8
	Q934X	N	13	1	S1882X	N	1	12
	E1214X	N	6	5	E2877X	N	1	0
	L63X	N	18	0				
Korean	IVS7+1G>A	S	1	0	3972del4	F	2	2
	1041delAGCinsT	F	2	1	4994delC	F	1	0
	1835insA	F	1	>500	5057del2	F	1	0
	2080delA	F	1	9	9481insA	F	1	11
	1942delA	F	1	0	R2494X	N	2	0
	2167delA	F	1	0	S2984X	N	1	0
	2552delC	F	2	8	Y2997X	N	1	0
	3746insA	F	3	3	K467X	N	3	0
	4184del4	F	2	50				
	3413delC	F	1	0				
	5589del8	F	3	0				
	5615del11insA	F	3	0				
	5672insC	F	1	0				
	3452delA	F	2	0				
	Q538X	N	1	0				
	G972X	N	1	0				
	L1198X	N	1	0				
	E1661X	N	2	0				
Mongolian	589delCT	F	3	2	Q1037X	N	1	3
Chinese	IVS7-2del10	F	1	0	2041delA	F	1	8
	1081delG	F	2	0	6382delT	F	1	0
	2371delTG	F	1	0				

(*Continued*)

Table 5 *BRCA1* and *BRCA2* Mutations in Asians (*Continued*)

Asian populations	*BRCA1* mutations	Mutation effect	No. of observations within the population	No. outside the population	*BRCA2* mutations	Mutation effect	No. of observations within the population	No. outside the population
Filipino	*3690ins4*	F	1	0				
	3975del4	F	1	0				
	E879X	N	1	0				
	5454delC	F	5	0	*3827delGT*	F	2	3
	R1835X	N	1	18	*4265delCT*	F	3	1
	Q1538X	N	1	0	*4859delA*	F	7	1
					2042insA	F	1	3
					6083insAGTT	F	1	0
					3798delG	F	1	0
					Q940X	N	1	0
					S1121X	N	2	0
Thai	*3300delA*	F	2	0	*2041delA*	F	1	9
	744ins20	F	1	0	*6382delT*	F	1	0
Malay	*2846insA*	F	2	0				
	5447insC	F	1	1				
Iranian	*185delAG*	F	2	>500	*6261insGT*	F	1	0
	1359del7	F	1	0	*3979insA*	F	1	0
	5154delC	F	1	0				
	Y978X	N	1	3				

Indian and Pakistani

Mutation	Type		
1014delGT	F	1	2
1616delAAAT	F	1	0
1701del7	F	2	0
185delAG	F	1	>500
1956delA	F	2	0
2080insA	F	1	3
2388delG	F	1	2
2524delTG	F	1	3
2828delT	F	1	0
2885delA	F	1	0
3227delT	F	1	0
4184del4	F	3	51
4284delAG	F	1	3
804delT	F	2	0
894delG	F	1	0
2674delG	F	1	0
3913delG	F	1	0
4773insA	F	1	0
5057delTG	F	1	2
5302insA	F	1	2
9140delA	F	1	0
Q1037X	N	2	2

Abbreviations: F, frameshift mutation; M, missense mutation; N, nonsense mutation; S, splicing variant.
Source: Japanese data is from Refs. 27, 46, 49–54, 74–76; Korean data is from Refs. 27; Mongolian data is from Refs. 27; Chinese data is from Refs. 27, 49, 56; Chinese data is from Refs. 27, 49, 57–59; Malay data is from Refs. 27, 49, 60, 61; Thai data is from Refs. 27, 49, 62; Filipino data is from Refs. 27, 49, 63; Iranian data is from Refs. 27, 49, 64–66; Indian data is from Refs. 27, 49, 67; Pakistani data is from Refs. 27, 49, 70.

affected family members or with bilateral breast cancers and found *BRCA1* mutations in four patients (3.9%) (74). Ikeda et al. reported a much higher frequency of *BRCA1/2* mutations among at-risk Japanese women. They identified 15 *BRCA1* deleterious mutations (13.3%) and 21 *BRCA2* deleterious mutations (18.6%) in 113 breast cancer patients with at least one breast cancer or ovarian cancer case in their first-degree relatives (75).

BRCA1 *Q934X, L63X, 2509delAA, E1214X* and *BRCA2 S2834X, 5802del4* are responsible for multiple breast and ovarian cancer cases in Japanese population (46,49–52,76). *L63X* is believed to be the most common *BRCA1* mutation in Japanese population and reported in 18 unrelated Japanese families (49). The Haplotype analysis of *BRCA1 Q934X* and *L63X* suggested that these two mutations were likely to derive from the same ancestors (49,52).

Korean

Breast cancer incidence rate in Korean females is low but breast cancer has become the most common cancer in Korean women (48,49). Ahn et al. analyzed 354 Korean breast cancer patients with at least two first- or second-degree relatives with breast and/or ovarian cancer and found that 40 patients (11.3%) carried 25 *BRCA1/2* mutations including 12 novel mutations (55).

Chinese

Breast cancer incidence rate in Chinese women from China is among the lowest recorded (48,49). The Chinese Diaspora is widespread in East and South East Asia including Malaysia, Thailand, the Philippines, Singapore, etc. Tang et al. studied *BRCA1* in 130 breast cancer cases and identified five *BRCA1* mutations among which *589delCT* was observed twice (57). Khoo et al. reported *BRCA1 1081delG* in two unrelated Chinese ovarian cancer patients and both share the same mutation-linked haplotype (59). However, mutation analysis of *BRCA2* has not been conducted often among Chinese populations.

Malay and Thai

By protein truncation test, Lee et al. examined *BRCA1* in 49 unrelated Malay breast cancer patients unselected for age of early onset and found *BRCA1 2845insA* in three patients who had the same mutation haplotype for the flanking markers (49,60). Patmasiriwat et al. examined *BRCA1* and *BRCA2* in 12 Thai breast and/or ovarian cancer families and six early-onset breast or breast/ovarian cancer cases without a family history of cancer (62). Four mutations including *BRCA1 744ins20* and *3300delA* and *BRCA2 2041delA* and *6382delT* were identified (49,62).

Filipino

Breast cancer incidence rate in Philippine women is high among Asian populations. De Leon Matsuda et al. estimated a prevalence of 5.1% (15 out of 294) for *BRCA1/2* mutations in unselected breast cancer cases (49,63). The *BRCA2* mutations accounted for over 80% (12 out of 15) of the *BRCA1 and 2* mutations. In the study, three founder mutations, *BRCA1 5454delC* ($n = 2$) and *BRCA2 4859delA* ($n = 4$) and *4265delCT* ($n = 2$), were responsible for over half of the mutations (63). The penetrance of *BRCA1 and 2* mutations in this study was comparable to those in European populations (63).

Iranian

Yassaee et al. analyzed *BRCA1* exons 11 and *BRCA2* exons 10 and 11 by protein truncation test, and *BRCA1* exons 2, 3, 5, 13, and 20 and *BRCA2* exons 9, 17, 18, and 23 with single-strand conformation polymorphism assay among 83 early-onset breast cancer patients in Tehran (49,64). They found five frameshift mutations (6%) including *BRCA1 185delAG, 181insT, 2335delAA* and *BRCA2 6261insGT, 3979insA* (49,64). The Ashkenazi Jewish founder mutation *BRCA1 185delAG* was reported several times in Iranian Jewish descendents (49,65,66).

Indian and Pakistani

Saxena et al. studied a series of 20 breast cancer patients from North India either with a family history of breast and/or ovarian cancer or having an early age of onset and identified two splice variants $331 + 1G > T$ and $4476 + 2T > C$ in *BRCA1* (67).

Pakistan has the highest incidence rate of breast cancer among Asian populations (excluding Jewish) and breast cancer in Pakistan often features early age of onset (49,68,69).

The frequently reported European *BRCA1 4184del4* mutation and Ashkenazi Jewish *BRCA1 185delAG* mutation were also identified in Indian and Pakistani women but the mutation-linked haplotypes are different from those in European and Jewish women (38,49). This suggests that the *BRCA1 185delAG* mutations identified in Indian and Pakistani women have an independent origin.

Liede et al. studied 341 subjects with breast cancer and 120 subjects with ovarian cancer (both unselected for age of onset or family history) and reported 6.7% *BRCA1/2* mutations in breast cancer patients and 15.8% *BRCA1/2* mutations in ovarian cases (49,70). In the study, six recurrent mutations were identified including five *BRCA1* mutations (*2080insA, 3889delAG, 4184del4, 4284delAG*, and *IVS14* 1ArG) and one *BRCA2* mutation, *Q1037X* (70). The penetrance of *BRCA1/2* mutations in Pakistanis is close to that in Western populations (49,70).

American Indians/Alaska Natives

Amerindian and Alaska Natives are about 1% of American population (16). American Indian breast cancer incidence and mortality rates are of the lowest recorded in American populations (1). There are few studies of *BRCA1* and *BRCA2* in Native American women with breast and ovarian cancer. Liede et al. reported a *BRCA1* mutation *1510insG* (1506A > G) in two families of aboriginal tribes Cree and Ojibwe in Canada. This mutation has not been found in other populations (71).

About 21 *BRCA1* and 32 *BRCA2* deleterious mutations have been reported in individuals of Native American ancestry (Table 6) (27,47). It was found that 2 out of 22 (9%) *BRCA1* mutations and 5 of 32 (16%) *BRCA2* mutations are confined to Native American descendents (27). There are 11 *BRCA1* unclassified variants reported in American Indian/ Alaska Native females and, among them, only *BRCA1 IVS11 − 10G > A* is confined to this ethnicity (27). There are 66 *BRCA2* unclassified variants and two polymorphisms reported in American Indians/Alaska Natives and, among them, ten unclassified variants and one polymorphism are confined to Native American descendents (27).

Genomic Alterations in *BRCA*

BRCA1 rearrangements such as IVS12-1643del3835, exon-13-ins-6 kb, exon-22-del-510 bp, exon 8 to 9 del7.1 kb, and exon-14-20-del-26 kb are used in genetic testing based on the

Table 6 *BRCA1* and *BRCA2* Mutations in American Indians/Alaska Natives

BRCA1 mutations	Mutation effect	No. of observations in Native American	No. of non-Native	*BRCA2* mutations	Mutation effect	No. of observations in Native American	No. of non-Native
1137delG	F	1	2	*1493delA*	F	1	5
1406insA	F	1	3	*1983del5*	F	1	9
1506A > G	F	1	2	*2041insA*	F	2	26
185delAG	F	4	>500	*2117delC*	F	1	3
2072del4	F	2	8	*3036del4*	F	1	48
2798del4	F	1	17	*379delG*	F	1	1
3124delA	F	1	3	*4075delGT*	F	2	22
3227delT	F	1	0	*5531delTT*	F	1	1
3604delA	F	1	19	*5804del4*	F	2	13
3884insA	F	1	0	*5849del4*	F	2	8
4184del4	F	1	40	*6056delC*	F	2	1
4744delCT	F	1	2	*6085delG*	F	1	0
4873delCA	F	1	2	*6503delTT*	F	3	46
5256delG	F	1	7	*6714del4*	F	1	>500
5382insC	F	1	>500	*6985delCT*	F	1	0

Mutation	Type	No. 1	No. 2
C61G	M	102	1
C64Y	M	6	1
E1250X	N	50	1
E1373X	N	4	1
R1443X	N	89	1
S1298X	N	4	1
IVS4 – 1G > T	S	15	1
802delAT	F	5	15
8765delAG	F	1	31
9132delC	F	1	12
983delCAGT	F	1	0
9927del4	F	1	2
999del5	F	2	>500
XG1377ins(4359ins6)	F	1	8
E1308X	N	1	8
K1530X	N	2	1
Q3066X	N	1	1
R245X	N	1	0
S611X	N	1	3
Y3098X	N	1	6
IVS15 – 1G > A	S	1	10
IVS7 + 2T > G	S	1	8

Abbreviations: F, frameshift mutation; M, missense mutation; N, nonsense mutation; S, splicing variant.
Source: From Refs. 27, 71.

commercial standard in Myriad Genetic Laboratories. In Table 7, the observations of these alterations in different populations are summarized (27,47).

GENETIC COUNSELING AND TESTING

Genetic testing for *BRCA1/2* mutations became available in 1996 (72). Women carrying *BRCA1* have a 56% to 87% probability of developing breast cancer and women carrying *BRCA2* mutations have a 37% to 85% cumulative lifetime risk (Table 2) (4,5,73). The genetic testing for deleterious *BRCA1/2* variants provides not only the cancer-risk information to the individuals who are tested but also the link to other at-risk family members (77,78). The detection of risk-conferring *BRCA1/2* mutations will help physicians to develop strategies to reduce breast cancer mortality rate and risk in mutation carriers and their family members.

Minority women at moderate or high risk for *BRCA1/2* mutations have favorable attitudes about genetic testing (77). However, several studies reported the existence of racial disparity in the use of genetic testing for *BRCA1/2* mutations (8). For example, African American women have limited interest in genetic testing and are much less likely to undergo genetic testing for *BRCA1/2* than White women (77,78). According to Myriad Genetic Laboratories, Inc., only 3% of individuals undergoing *BRCA1* and *2* testing are self-reported as African American (22). The reasons for these disparities still remain unclear and many factors might be involved. One reason for this might be the poor access to specialized cancer prevention among minority groups (79,80). In one study, Weissman et al suggested that absence of health insurance coverage could keep minority women from receiving comprehensive cancer care (81). Another explanation for the racial disparities in the use of genetic testing is perceived risk and knowledge about genetic testing (79,82). In the 2000 National Health Interview Survey, 49.9% of White women had heard of genetic testing for cancer risk while only 32.69% of African American women and 20.6% of Hispanic women knew about genetic testing (79,83). Furthermore, in the study by Matthews et al., none of the African American participants with strong family history of cancer had knowledge of genetic counseling (79,84). The average African American woman underestimates her risk of breast cancer and the role of genetic testing as a means of assessing cancer risk and reducing cancer mortality rate (79).

However, the disparities of using the genetic counseling and testing do not arise only from the side of patients. The role of physicians in identifying and referring high-risk patients to genetic counseling is significant (79). The average oncologist is more effective at recruiting African Americans to participate in genetic counseling and testing than the average general medical practitioner (85,86). On the other hand, underserved

Table 7   Number of Observations of *BRCA1* Alterations Used by Myriad Inc. in the Open Access Online Breast Cancer Mutation Database

BRCA1 alterations	White	Hispanic	African and African American	Asian	Native American
Exon-13-ins-6 kb	58	1	1	0	2
IVS12-1643del3835	19	0	0	0	0
Exon-22-del-510bp	8	0	0	0	0
Exon-14-20-del-26 kb	15	0	0	0	0

Source: From Ref. 28.

populations are likely to have less trust in healthcare providers than are White women and less likely to report their perceptions of personal risk after their relative is diagnosed with breast cancer. This might aggravate the existing disparities in the use of genetic testing for cancer risk (87). Furthermore, ethnic differences in spiritual faith, cancer-specific distress, and demographic factors may also be related to the disparities (77,88,89).

Greater efforts are needed to intensify and integrate genetic counseling and testing into the clinical care of African American women and other minority women (77). Nationwide education among minority populations is needed to increase the awareness of inherited breast cancer risk and the benefits of genetic counseling and testing. On the other side, education about hereditary breast cancer needs to be enhanced among healthcare practitioners who provide referral of minority women to genetic testing for *BRCA1/2* (85). Physicians also should pay greater attention to minority women's psychological issues, including concerns about breast cancer, distress during genetic testing, and trust on physicians (82).

CONCLUSION

In general, there are limited genetic epidemiological reports of *BRCA1* and *BRCA2* in underserved populations, especially in American Indian/Alaska Native, Hispanic, and African American women. Based on the available data, underserved populations have distinctive spectrums of *BRCA1* and *BRCA2* variants and alterations. Some frequent *BRCA1/2* mutations in these ethnic groups are good candidates for targets of genetic testing.

The racial disparities in the use of *BRCA1/2* genetic testing widely exist, and compared with non-Hispanic White women, the underserved populations benefit less from the advance in translational research of *BRCA1* and *BRCA2*. Thus, greater efforts are needed to intensify genetic testing in the clinic care of high breast cancer risk women of underserved ethnicity background (77).

More efforts in genetic epidemiological study of *BRCA1/2* among underserved populations and research of racial disparities regarding genetic counseling and testing are needed in order to reduce breast cancer mortality rate in these ethnic groups.

REFERENCES

1. American_Cancer_Society, Breast Cancer Facts and Figures: 2005–2006. 2006, The American Cancer Society.
2. Hunter CP. Epidemiology, stage at diagnosis, and tumor biology of breast carcinoma in multiracial and multiethnic populations. Cancer 2000; 88(5 suppl):1193–1202.
3. Claus EB et al. The genetic attributable risk of breast and ovarian cancer. Cancer 1996; 77 (11):2318–2324.
4. Fackenthal J, Olopade O. Inherited susceptibility to breast and ovarian cancer. Adv Oncol 2000; 16:10–18.
5. Ford D et al. Genetic heterogeneity and penetrance analysis of the BRCA1 and BRCA2 genes in breast cancer families. The Breast Cancer Linkage Consortium. Am J Hum Genet 1998; 62 (3):676–689.
6. Miki Y et al. A strong candidate for the breast and ovarian cancer susceptibility gene BRCA1. Science 1994; 266(5182):66–71.

7. Wooster R et al. Localization of a breast cancer susceptibility gene, BRCA2, to chromosome 13q12-13. Science 1994; 265(5181):2088–2090.

8. Nanda R et al. Genetic testing in an ethnically diverse cohort of high-risk women: a comparative analysis of BRCA1 and BRCA2 mutations in American families of European and African ancestry. JAMA 2005; 294(15):1925–1933.

9. Giardiello FM et al. Very high risk of cancer in familial Peutz-Jeghers syndrome. Gastroenterology 2000; 119(6):1447–1453.

10. Vahteristo P et al. A CHEK2 genetic variant contributing to a substantial fraction of familial breast cancer. Am J Hum Genet 2002; 71(2):432–438.

11. Liaw D et al. Germline mutations of the PTEN gene in Cowden disease, an inherited breast and thyroid cancer syndrome. Nat Genet 1997; 16(1):64–67.

12. Lim W et al. Further observations on LKB1/STK11 status and cancer risk in Peutz-Jeghers syndrome. Br J Cancer 2003; 89(2):308–313.

13. Li FP et al. A cancer family syndrome in twenty-four kindreds. Cancer Res 1988; 48(18): 5358–5362.

14. Brownstein MH, Wolf M, Bikowski JB. Cowden's disease: a cutaneous marker of breast cancer. Cancer 1978; 41(6):2393–2398.

15. Boardman LA et al. Increased risk for cancer in patients with the Peutz-Jeghers syndrome. Ann Intern Med 1998; 128(11):896–899.

16. The World Factbook 2005. 2006, Central Intelligence Agency.

17. Pal T et al. BRCA1 and BRCA2 mutations in a study of African American breast cancer patients. Cancer Epidemiol Biomarkers Prev 2004; 13(11 Pt 1):1794–1799.

18. Marcus JN et al. Hereditary breast cancer: pathobiology, prognosis, and BRCA1 and BRCA2 gene linkage. Cancer 1996; 77(4):697–709.

19. Verhoog LC et al. Survival and tumour characteristics of breast-cancer patients with germline mutations of BRCA1. Lancet 1998; 351(9099):316–321.

20. Marcus JN et al. BRCA2 hereditary breast cancer pathophenotype. Breast Cancer Res Treat 1997; 44(3):275–277.

21. Chen VW et al. Histological characteristics of breast carcinoma in blacks and whites. Cancer Epidemiol Biomarkers Prev 1994; 3(2):127–135.

22. Joslyn SA, West MM. Racial differences in breast carcinoma survival. Cancer 2000; 88(1): 114–123.

23. Ikpatt OF et al. Breast cancer in Nigeria and Finland: epidemiological, clinical and histological comparison. Anticancer Res 2002; 22(5):3005–3012.

24. Panguluri RC et al. BRCA1 mutations in African Americans. Hum Genet 1999; 105(1–2): 28–31.

25. Gao Q et al. Prevalence of BRCA1 and BRCA2 mutations among clinic-based African American families with breast cancer. Hum Genet 2000; 107(2):186–191.

26. Kanaan Y et al. Inherited BRCA2 mutations in African Americans with breast and/ or ovarian cancer: a study of familial and early onset cases. Hum Genet 2003; 113(5): 452–460.

27. (BIC), B.C.I.C. An Open Access On-Line Breast Cancer Mutation Data Base. 2006 [cited; Available from: http://www.nhgri.nih.gov/Intramural_research/Lab_transfer/Bic/].

28. Arena JF et al. BRCA1 mutations in African American women. Am J Hum Genet (Suppl) 1996; 59:A34.

29. Shen D et al. Mutation analysis of BRCA1 gene in African-American patients with breast cancer. J Natl Med Assoc 2000; 92(1):29–35.

30. Arena J et al. BRCA1 mutation analysis in 20 at-risk African-American families supports a low frequency of germ-line mutation. Am J Hum Genet 1998; 63(suppl 4):A62.

31. Barkardottir RB et al. Haplotype analysis in Icelandic and Finnish BRCA2 999del5 breast cancer families. Eur J Hum Genet 2001; 9(10):773–779.

32. Castilla LH et al. Mutations in the BRCA1 gene in families with early-onset breast and ovarian cancer. Nat Genet 1994; 8(4):387–391.

33. Whitfield-Broome C, Dunston GM, Brody LC. BRCA2 mutations in African Americans. Proc Am Assoc Cancer Res 1999; 40:269, abstract #1788.

34. Blesa JR, Garcia JA, Ochoa E. Frequency of germ-line BRCA1 mutations among Spanish families from a Mediterranean area. Hum Mutat 2000; 15(4):381–382.

35. Kedar-Barnes I et al. Intronic BRCA1 mutations in two highly affected kindreds. Am J Hum Genet (Suppl 2) 2000; 67(99):A484.

36. Zhang B, Fackenthal J, Niu Q, et al. BRCA1 Y101X, a recurrent mutation with potential founder effect in Nigerian breast cancer patients. Proc Am Assoc Cancer Res 2006; 2006:264.

37. Olopade OI et al. Breast cancer genetics in African Americans. Cancer 2003; 97(1 suppl): 236–245.

38. Neuhausen SL et al. Haplotype and phenotype analysis of six recurrent BRCA1 mutations in 61 families: results of an international study. Am J Hum Genet 1996; 58(2):271–280.

39. Friedman LS et al. Novel inherited mutations and variable expressivity of BRCA1 alleles, including the founder mutation 185delAG in Ashkenazi Jewish families. Am J Hum Genet 1995; 57(6):1284–1297.

40. Roa BB et al. Ashkenazi Jewish population frequencies for common mutations in BRCA1 and BRCA2. Nat Genet 1996; 14(2):185–187.

41. Mefford HC et al. Evidence for a BRCA1 founder mutation in families of West African ancestry [letter]. Am J Hum Genet 1999; 65(2):575–578.

42. Dangel J et al. Novel germline BRCA1 mutation (155del4) in an African American with early-onset breast cancer. Hum Mutat 1999; 14(6):545.

43. Gao Q et al. Contribution of recurrent BRCA1 (B1) and BRCA2 (B2) mutations to breast cancer in African American (AA) women. Proc Am Assoc Cancer Res 1998; 39:475, abstract #3229.

44. Census 2000 Summary File 1 (SF 1) 100-Percent Data. 2000, U.S. Census Bureau.

45. American_Cancer_Society, Cancer Facts and Figures 2006. 2006, Atlanta.

46. Inoue R et al. Germline mutation of BRCA1 in Japanese breast cancer families. Cancer Res 1995; 55(16):3521–3524.

47. Weitzel JN, et al. Prevalence of BRCA mutations and founder effect in high-risk Hispanic families. Cancer Epidemiol Biomarkers Prev 2005; 14(7):1666–1671.

48. Parkin DM, Whelan SL, Ferlay J, Raymond L, Young J. Cancer Incidence in Five Continents. Vol. 7. Lyon: Scientific Publication, 1997.

49. Liede A, Narod SA. Hereditary breast and ovarian cancer in Asia: genetic epidemiology of BRCA1 and BRCA2. Hum Mutat 2002; 20(6):413–424.

50. Noguchi S et al. Clinicopathologic analysis of BRCA1- or BRCA2-associated hereditary breast carcinoma in Japanese women. Cancer 1999; 85(10):2200–2205.

51. Schehl CM, Ostrander GK. Identification of BRCA1 germline mutation, 797delAA, in a Japanese breast-ovarian cancer patient. J Natl Cancer Inst 1997; 89(20):1547–1548.

52. Sekine M et al. Mutational analysis of BRCA1 and BRCA2 and clinicopathologic analysis of ovarian cancer in 82 ovarian cancer families: two common founder mutations of BRCA1 in Japanese population. Clin Cancer Res 2001; 7(10):3144–3150.

53. Takano M et al. Mutational analysis of BRCA1 gene in ovarian and breast-ovarian cancer families in Japan. Jpn J Cancer Res 1997; 88(4):407–413.

54. Emi M et al. Multiplex mutation screening of the BRCA1 gene in 1000 Japanese breast cancers. Jpn J Cancer Res 1998; 89(1):12–16.

55. Ahn SH et al. BRCA1 and BRCA2 germline mutations in Korean breast cancer patients at high risk of carrying mutations. Cancer Lett 2006; 245(1–2):90–5.

56. Elit L et al. A unique BRCA1 mutation identified in Mongolia. Int J Gynecol Cancer 2001; 11 (3):241–243.

57. Tang NL et al. Prevalence of mutations in the BRCA1 gene among Chinese patients with breast cancer. J Natl Cancer Inst 1999; 91(10):882–885.

58. Zhi X et al. BRCA1 and BRCA2 sequence variants in Chinese breast cancer families. Hum Mutat 2002; 20(6):474.

59. Khoo US et al. Recurrent BRCA1 and BRCA2 germline mutations in ovarian cancer: a founder mutation of BRCA1 identified in the Chinese population. Hum Mutat 2002; 19(3): 307–308.

60. Lee AS et al. Founder mutation in the BRCA1 gene in Malay breast cancer patients from Singapore. Hum Mutat 2003; 22(2):178.

61. Ho GH et al. Novel germline BRCA1 mutations detected in women in Singapore who developed breast carcinoma before the age of 36 years. Cancer 2000; 89(4):811–816.

62. Patmasiriwat P et al. Analysis of breast cancer susceptibility genes BRCA1 and BRCA2 in Thai familial and isolated early-onset breast and ovarian cancer. Hum Mutat 2002; 20(3):230.

63. De Leon Matsuda ML et al. BRCA1 and BRCA2 mutations among breast cancer patients from the Philippines. Int J Cancer 2002; 98(4):596–603.

64. Yassaee VR et al. Novel mutations in the BRCA1 and BRCA2 genes in Iranian women with early-onset breast cancer. Breast Cancer Res 2002; 4(4):R6.

65. Bar-Sade RB et al. The 185delAG BRCA1 mutation originated before the dispersion of Jews in the diaspora and is not limited to Ashkenazim. Hum Mol Genet 1998; 7(5):801–805.

66. Levy-Lahad E et al. Founder BRCA1 and BRCA2 mutations in Ashkenazi Jews in Israel: frequency and differential penetrance in ovarian cancer and in breast-ovarian cancer families. Am J Hum Genet 1997; 60(5):1059–1067.

67. Saxena S et al. BRCA1 and BRCA2 in Indian breast cancer patients. Hum Mutat 2002; 20(6)): 473–474.

68. Bhurgri Y et al. Cancer incidence in Karachi, Pakistan: first results from Karachi Cancer Registry. Int J Cancer 2000; 85(3):325–329.

69. Usmani K et al. Breast carcinoma in Pakistani women. J Environ Pathol Toxicol Oncol 1996; 15(2–4):251–253.

70. Liede A et al. Contribution of BRCA1 and BRCA2 mutations to breast and ovarian cancer in Pakistan. Am J Hum Genet 2002; 71(3):595–606.

71. Liede A et al. A BRCA1 mutation in Native North American families. Hum Mutat 2002; 19 (4):460.

72. Armstrong K et al. Racial differences in the use of BRCA1/2 testing among women with a family history of breast or ovarian cancer. JAMA 2005; 293(14):1729–1736.

73. Schubert EL et al. BRCA2 in American families with four or more cases of breast or ovarian cancer: recurrent and novel mutations, variable expression, penetrance, and the possibility of families whose cancer is not attributable to BRCA1 or BRCA2 (see comment). Am J Hum Genet 1997; 60(5):1031–1040.

74. Katagiri T et al. Mutations in the BRCA1 gene in Japanese breast cancer patients. Hum Mutat 1996; 7(4):334–339.

75. Ikeda N et al. Frequency of BRCA1 and BRCA2 germline mutations in Japanese breast cancer families. Int J cancer 2001; 91(1):83–88.

76. Kijima G et al. Nonsense mutation at codon 63 of the BRCA1 gene in Japanese breast cancer patients. Jpn J Cancer Res 1998; 89(8):837–841.

77. Ikpatt OF, Olopade OI. Genetics of breast cancer in women of African descent: an overview. In: Olopade OI, Williams CKO, Falkson CI, eds. Breast Cancer in Women of African Descent. The Netherlands: Springer, Dordrecht, 2006:23–37.

78. Kessler L et al. Attitudes about genetic testing and genetic testing intentions in African American women at increased risk for hereditary breast cancer. Genet Med 2005; 7(4): 230–238.

79. Hall M, Olopade OI. Confronting genetic testing disparities: knowledge is power (see comment). JAMA 2005; 293(14):1783–1785.

80. Kelley E et al. The national healthcare quality and disparities reports: an overview. Med Care 2005; 43(3 suppl):13–18.

81. Weissman JS, Schneider EC. Social disparities in cancer: lessons from a multidisciplinary workshop. Cancer Causes Control 2005; 16(1):71–74.

82. Armstrong K et al. Interest in BRCA1/2 testing in a primary care population. Prev Med 2002; 34(6):590–595.

83. Wideroff L et al. Awareness of genetic testing for increased cancer risk in the year 2000 National Health Interview Survey. Community Genet 2003; 6(3):147–156.

84. Matthews AK, Cummings S, Thompson S, et al. Genetic testing of African Americans for susceptibility to inherited cancers. J Psychosoc Oncol 2000; 18:1–13.

85. Halbert CH et al. Recruiting African American women to participate in hereditary breast cancer research. J Clin Oncol 2005; 23(31):7967–7973.

86. Freedman AN et al. US physicians' attitudes toward genetic testing for cancer susceptibility. Am J Med Genet Part A 2003; 120(1):63–71.

87. Halbert C, Armstrong K, Gandy O, Shaker L. Racial differences in trust in health care providers. Arch Intern Med 2006; 166:896–901.

88. Halbert C et al. Psychological functioning in African American women at an increased risk of hereditary breast and ovarian cancer. Clin Genet 2005; 68(3):222–227.

89. Schlich-Bakker KJ, ten Kroode HF, Ausems MG. A literature review of the psychological impact of genetic testing on breast cancer patients. Patient Educ Couns 2006; 62(1):13–20.

14

Psychological and Behavioral Impact of *BRCA1/2* Genetic Testing

Kristi Graves and Marc D. Schwartz
Cancer Control Program, Lombardi Comprehensive Cancer Center,
Georgetown University, Washington, D.C., U.S.A.

INTRODUCTION

Prior to the widespread availability of *BRCA1* and *BRCA2* (*BRCA1/2*) testing, researchers and clinicians identified a number of potential benefits and risks in receiving test results (1–3). Key benefits included reassurance for individuals testing negative and opportunities for risk reduction among those testing positive. Risks included the potential for adverse psychosocial outcomes among carriers, false reassurance for noncarriers, family conflict, and insurance discrimination (2–5).

In the 10 years since the advent of *BRCA1/2* testing, Myriad Genetics has tested well over 100,000 individuals. Research has begun to address the questions first raised by investigators in anticipation of genetic testing for cancer susceptibility. Much of this research has focused on the psychosocial and behavioral outcomes of *BRCA1/2* testing. In this chapter, we review the empirical research that has examined whether the putative benefits and risks of genetic testing have been realized and identify areas that need further research.

PSYCHOSOCIAL IMPACT OF *BRCA1/2* GENETIC TESTING

When *BRCA1/2* gene testing became available, many of the initial concerns were related to the potential for adverse psychological reactions to receiving a positive *BRCA1/2* test result. These concerns centered on the possibility of depression and anxiety among women who learn they carry a *BRCA1/2* mutation (1,6,7). Other concerns involved the possibility of guilt following a negative test result or the potential for testing to adversely impact the family (8). For example, familial conflict could stem from disagreements between family members regarding communication of test results or willingness to undergo testing (9,10). Below, we highlight key quantitative findings examining the short-, intermediate-, and long-term impact of *BRCA1/2* testing on psychosocial and family functioning outcomes.

Short-Term Psychosocial Impact

Key studies examining distress following *BRCA1/2* testing are displayed in Table 1. Research evaluating the short-term psychological impact of genetic testing (i.e., outcomes

Table 1   Research Studies of the Psychosocial Impact of *BRCA1/2* Genetic Testing

Author	Sample	Design	Outcomes	Follow-up	Results
Lerman et al., 1996 (11)	279 affected and unaffected	P	Depression, functional health	1 mo	Positives: no change in depression or functional impairment Negatives: reduced depression and functional impairment
Croyle et al., 1997 (4)	60 affected and unaffected	P	Anxiety, testing distress	1–2 wk	Positives: higher test-related distress and anxiety compared to negatives. Unaffected positives reported highest levels of distress. Anxiety declined for all participants at follow-up
Lerman et al., 1998 (12)	327 affected and unaffected	P	Cancer distress, depression	1 and 6 mo	Positives: no change in depression Negatives: decrease in depression Females, unmarried individuals, and those with high baseline distress were at greatest risk for distress
Smith et al., 1999 (13)	212 affected and unaffected	P	Testing distress, anxiety	1–2 wk	Positives: female positives more distressed than female negatives. Greatest distress in female positives whose siblings were negatives. Male positives did not differ from male negatives. Male positives more distressed if first sibling tested in family
Dorval et al., 2000 (14)	41 affected and unaffected	P	General distress	6 mo	Positives who accurately anticipated their psychological response to their test results reported less sadness, anger, and worry than positives who underestimated their response to the test result
Wagner et al., 2000 (15)	138 affected and unaffected	P	Depression	6–8 wk	Positives: no change in depression; depression higher in affected positives than unaffected positives Negatives: increase in depression

Author	Design	Sample	Measures	Time	Findings
Wood et al., 2000 (16)	P	35 affected women	Anxiety, depression, cancer distress	1 mo	All: decrease in anxiety. Negatives: decrease in cancer distress. Distress highest among women most recently diagnosed with cancer
Lodder et al., 2001 (17)	P	78 unaffected women	General and cancer distress	1–3 wk	Positives: slight increase in anxiety, depression, and cancer distress. Negatives: decrease in anxiety, depression, and cancer distress. After adjusting for baseline anxiety and depression, mutation status unrelated to anxiety and depression
Tercyak et al., 2001 (18)	P	107 affected and unaffected women	Anxiety	Post disclosure	Positives: more distressed than uninformatives/negatives at postdisclosure. Postdisclosure anxiety predicted by education, predisclosure anxiety, and mutation status
Cella et al., 2002 (19)	P	158 affected and unaffected women	General, cancer, and testing distress	1 mo	Positives: test distress and intrusions higher than in other groups. Negatives and uninformatives did not differ on distress
Meiser et al., 2002 (20)	P	90 unaffected women carriers and noncarriers and 53 low-risk women	Cancer distress, anxiety, depression	7–10 days, 4 and 12 mo	Positives: higher cancer distress in the short- and long-term; decreased anxiety at 12 mo compared to untested women. Negatives: decrease in anxiety at 7–10 days and decrease in depression at 4 mo compared to untested women
Schwartz et al., 2002 (21)	P	279 affected and unaffected women	Cancer and general distress	6 mo	Positives: no change over time. Negatives: decrease in distress. Uninformatives: no change over time
Hagoel et al., 2003 (22)	CS	165 affected and unaffected women	General distress	4–6 wk	Positives did not differ from uninformatives/negatives on any measured variables. Probands did not differ from relatives

(Continued)

Table 1 Research Studies of the Psychosocial Impact of *BRCA1/2* Genetic Testing (*Continued*)

Author	Sample	Design	Outcomes	Follow-up	Results
van Oostrom et al., 2003 (23)	65 unaffected women	P	Anxiety, depression, cancer distress, body image, sexual functioning	4–6 yr	Positives: no difference from negatives on distress outcomes; poorer body image and sexual relationships compared to negatives Cancer distress predicted by baseline distress, having younger children, more relatives who died from breast/ovarian cancer, poor family communication, doubt over validity of result
Arver et al., 2004 (24)	66 unaffected women	P	Anxiety, depression, QOL	1 wk; 2, 6, and 12 mo	Positives: no change in QOL; decrease in anxiety and depression Negatives: decrease in anxiety and increase in depression over time
Claes et al., 2004 (25)	62 affected and unaffected women	CS	General distress, cancer distress	3 mo to 5+ yr	Positives: did not differ from negatives on general and cancer distress at least 6 mo postresult
Manne et al., 2004 (26)	153 affected and unaffected women	P	General and cancer distress	6 mo	No differences in distress by mutation status. General distress predicted by pretest distress, age, more partner support, and less partner protective buffering. Cancer distress predicted by pretest, distress, age, and protective buffering
Reichelt et al., 2004 (27)	395 affected and unaffected women	P	Anxiety, depression, general and cancer distress	6 wk	Positives: did not differ from negatives on distress postresult Regardless of test result, participants with clinical anxiety at baseline reported decrease in anxiety postresult
Smith et al., 2004 (28)	101 members of linked kindred	P	Testing and cancer distress	4 mo, 1 and 2 yr	Positives: higher cancer distress at 4 mo than negatives
van Dijk et al., 2004 (29)	241 affected and unaffected women	P	Cancer distress	1 mo	Positives: no changes in distress VUCS/uninformatives: decrease in cancer distress Negatives: no change in distress (lower at all time points than positives or VUCS/uninformatives)

Study	Sample	Design	Variables	Timepoint	Results
van Roosmalen et al., 2004 (30)	368 affected and unaffected women	P	Anxiety, depression, cancer distress, general health	2 wk	Positives: increased anxiety, depression, cancer-related distress, and decreased general health compared to uninformatives/negatives. Affected positives had highest levels of anxiety and cancer distress
Watson et al., 2004 (31)	261 unaffected men and women	P	General health, cancer distress	1, 4, and 12 mo	Positives: greater cancer distress than negatives; positive females: more health symptoms than negatives at 1 and 4 mo. Younger positives: higher cancer worry than older positives at 1 mo
Claes et al., 2005 (32)	68 unaffected women	P	Cancer distress, general distress	1 yr	Positives: no change in distress with the exception of decreased ovarian cancer distress. Negatives: decrease in cancer distress and anxiety. Mean levels of distress were within population norm ranges for entire sample
Lynch et al., 2006 (33)	395 affected and unaffected men and women	CS	Test distress	Mean = 5 yr	Positives: affected positives had higher distress than unaffected negatives. Affected and unaffected positives had more worries and concerns compared to all negatives
van Dijk et al., 2006 (34)	238 affected and unaffected women	P	Cancer distress	1 and 7 mo	Positives: no change in distress. Negatives: decrease in distress over time. Uninformatives: decrease in distress 1 and 7 mo postresult

Note: All studies also assessed demographic and clinical variables.

Abbreviations: CS, cross-sectional study design; P, prospective study design; QOL, quality of life; VUCS, variant of uncertain clinical significance.

assessed within one to two months of receiving test results) provide little evidence for adverse outcomes among mutation carriers (11,15,16,22,24,27,29). The majority of these studies indicate that distress among carriers neither increases nor decreases from pretesting levels (11,12,15). However, there are exceptions in which distress or anxiety either increased slightly (18–20) or decreased (16,24,27) in the immediate aftermath of receiving a positive test result.

In contrast to individuals who learn that they carry a deleterious *BRCA1/2* mutation, those who receive a definitive negative result typically exhibit decreased distress (4,11,29,34). The combination of decreased distress among those receiving negative test results and stable distress in those receiving positive test results has, in some cases, led to distress differences between these groups (4,34). Such differences reflect the reassurance that comes with a definitive negative result.

Studies evaluating the impact of receiving uninformative test results have found either no change or slight decreases in short-term distress. For example, while Bish et al. (35) reported no change in distress following uninformative test results, van Dijk et al. (29,34) found distress decreased among women who carried a variant of uncertain clinical significance or who received uninformative results. Interestingly, in this study, distress decreased only among those women with uninformative results and a less suggestive family history of breast cancer (34). These results make clinical sense, as women who receive an uninformative test result despite a strong family history of breast/ovarian cancer remain at substantially elevated risk.

Despite little evidence of significant adverse psychological reactions, specific individual characteristics, such as younger age, affected status, and high pretest anxiety and distress may place one at risk for elevated distress following *BRCA1/2* testing (30,31). For example, among *BRCA1/2* carriers younger than 50 years of age, cancer-related distress increased in the month following receipt of a positive test result (31). Although this heightened worry decreased over time, it remained significantly higher than among noncarriers. Participants in another study (30), particularly women affected with breast cancer, reported increased anxiety, depression, and cancer-specific distress two weeks after receipt of a positive test result. Although some individuals may be at a greater risk for short-term increases in psychological distress after receipt of a positive *BRCA1/2* test result, in most cases, the overall level of distress does not appear to be clinically significant (24,33,36,37).

Intermediate and Long-Term Psychosocial Outcomes

Consistent with research on the short-term impact of testing, studies that have evaluated the intermediate (3–12 months) and long-term (one year or more) impact of testing have found little evidence of significant adverse psychosocial outcomes. These studies have typically reported no change or a decrease in distress within the first six months to two years following genetic testing (21,22,25,34,38). For example, in a study that included women with and without breast cancer, we found that six months after receiving test results, distress decreased in women who received negative test results, but remained stable for women with positive or uninformative test results (21). Studies with longer follow-up periods (one to five years) also found stable distress in positives and decreased distress in negatives (23,24,32).

As with short-term distress, there are subgroups of patients who are at higher risk for long-term distress. For example, women with a prior psychiatric history or those who have been more recently diagnosed with breast cancer appear to be at increased risk for adverse psychological reactions to a positive *BRCA1/2* test result (15,16,30,39,40).

However, such findings are not uniform, as other studies indicate no differences between affected and unaffected women, regardless of test result (27).

Thus, despite the absence of serious adverse outcomes, there is some evidence of ongoing, albeit mild, distress among mutation carriers. While negative results typically lead to long-term reduction in distress, positive test results may not. It is not clear whether such mild but stable distress will have an impact on physical or mental health over the long term. Future research will need to address the psychosocial, physical, and behavioral impact of such distress over the long term. Moreover, relatively few studies have prospectively evaluated factors that predict adverse psychosocial outcomes. Individuals at highest risk for adverse outcomes could be identified and targeted for increased posttest monitoring or enhanced/adjunct counseling interventions designed to minimize distress and facilitate decision-making related to the test results (41–43).

Family Communication and Functioning

Clinical guidelines recommend that predictive testing be made available to family members if a risk-conferring mutation is identified in a proband (44). Thus, the impact of *BRCA1/2* genetic counseling and testing extends beyond the individual to family communication and psychosocial reactions in family members. A number of studies have examined the communication of test results within families. Evidence from these studies suggests that the majority of probands share their test results with at least some of their relatives (45–47). For example, in a study investigating communication of test results between sisters, 85% of probands communicated test results to their sisters (46). Carriers were significantly more likely to communicate results than those who received uninformative test results. Evidence from this and other studies suggests that results are most commonly shared with sisters and spouses (46,48). Male first-degree relatives and all second-degree relatives are less likely to be informed than female first-degree relatives (47–49).

Beyond the communication of test results, family factors may also play a role in how individuals respond to *BRCA1/2* test results. Smith et al. (13) found that the order of testing within a sibship was strongly associated with individual outcomes. For men, carrier status, by itself, had little impact on distress. However, male carriers were more likely to report more distress if they were the first sibling tested and when all other siblings tested negative. For women, carrier status did impact distress; women with positive results reported more distress than women with negative results. However, like men, the impact of testing was moderated by siblings' test results. Specifically, the highest levels of distress were reported in female carriers whose siblings all tested negative. Not surprisingly, outcomes of genetic testing are also influenced by the reactions of partners (26). Among women who received positive *BRCA1/2* test results, partner support was unrelated to distress outcomes six months following testing; however, women who reported that they did not openly share their concerns about testing with their partners (called protective buffering) reported more distress. For women with uninformative results, more protective buffering was also related to more distress, whereas more partner support was associated with less participant distress in this group.

Summary/Future Directions/Clinical Implications

Evidence to date suggests that serious adverse psychosocial outcomes among *BRCA1/2* carriers are rare. Although there may be some distress among carriers in the short term, it typically dissipates quickly. Individuals who learn that they do not carry a deleterious mutation frequently benefit from this information in the form of significantly reduced distress. To place our current understanding of the nature and course of distress following *BRCA1/2* testing within a broader context, future work could use case–control designs to compare long-term outcomes of high-risk women who pursue testing to high-risk women who do not pursue testing. Moreover, because much of the work to date has been conducted with fairly homogeneous and self-selected populations, future efforts should include individuals of diverse ethnic, racial, and socioeconomic backgrounds to expand the generalizability of the results.

Despite generally positive adjustment following genetic testing, a number of factors have been demonstrated to predict distress among mutation carriers, including family-level factors such as order of testing in a sibship and partner's level of support. Although these variables have been found to predict distress, the level of distress in these carriers has typically been low. Thus, while it may be possible to identify individuals who are at risk for psychological distress following testing, more research is needed to determine the long-term course and implications of this low-level distress. If such research demonstrates a significant physical, behavioral, or quality of life impact over the long term, then it may be possible to target at-risk individuals for enhanced psychosocial support during and perhaps following genetic counseling. Recent efforts toward this end include tailored genetic counseling sessions and additional recognition of and investigation into the impact of *BRCA1/2* counseling and testing on the family (41,43).

BEHAVIORAL OUTCOMES OF *BRCA1/2* TESTING

The promise of *BRCA1/2* testing lies in the potential for this information to lead to breast and ovarian cancer risk reduction on an individual level. However, in order for *BRCA1/2* testing to realize this promise, the receipt of a positive *BRCA1/2* test result must be followed by the adoption of appropriate and effective risk-management strategies. Strong evidence documents the risk-reducing benefit of prophylactic mastectomy and oophorectomy among mutation carriers and individuals at risk for carrying a mutation. Prophylactic mastectomy has been shown to reduce breast cancer risk by about 90% (50–53). Prophylactic oophorectomy (PO) reduces ovarian cancer risk by over 90% and can reduce breast cancer risk by over 50% (54,55). Evidence for risk reduction is less clear-cut for chemopreventive options such as tamoxifen and raloxifene (56). Similarly, the efficacy of enhanced breast [i.e., mammography and magnetic resonance imaging (MRI)] and ovarian cancer screening [CA-125 and transvaginal ultrasound (TVUS)] has not yet been established. In this section, we review the evidence on the adoption of specific breast and ovarian cancer risk–management strategies following *BRCA1/2* testing.

Bilateral Prophylactic Mastectomy Among Women Unaffected with Breast Cancer

Studies that have evaluated the use of bilateral prophylactic mastectomy (BLM) among *BRCA1/2* mutation carriers who have not been affected with breast cancer are summarized in Table 2. Despite the clear efficacy of BLM, U.S. studies suggest that healthy mutation carriers are reluctant to undergo this procedure (57,59,60,62). Rates of BLM among mutation carriers in these studies have ranged from 0% to 3% in samples drawn from hereditary cancer registries (57,62) and only slightly higher (5–15%) in clinical samples (59,60). Outside the United States, rates of BLM among unaffected

Table 2 Studies of Prophylactic Mastectomy Following *BRCA1/2* Testing

Author	Sample	Design	Outcome	Follow-up	Results
Lerman et al., 2000 (57)	29 unaffected carriers	P	BLM	12 mo	3% rate of BLM
Meijers-Heijboer et al., 2000 (58)	411 unaffected women from HBOC families	P	BLM	16–62 mo ($M = 26$ mo)	51% rate of BLM among carriers
Peshkin et al., 2002 (59)	107 unaffected carriers and noncarriers	P	BLM	12 mo	5% rate of BLM among carriers; 0% among noncarriers
Scheuer et al., 2002 (60)	251 affected and unaffected carriers	CS	BLM	<1–35 mo ($M = 5$ mo)	15% rate of BLM among carriers. BLM predicted by: young age and strong family history
Lodder et al., 2002 (61)	63 unaffected carriers and noncarriers	P	BLM	12 mo	54% rate of BLM among carriers
Botkin et al., 2003 (62)	129 unaffected carriers and noncarriers	P	BLM	24 mo	0% rate of BLM among carriers and noncarriers
Meijers-Heijboer et al., 2003 (63)	101 affected carriers	P	CPM	2–8 yr	35% rate of CPM. CPM predicted by younger age and being aware of carrier status at the time of diagnosis
Weitzel et al., 2003 (64)	35 newly diagnosed breast cancer patients	CS	CPM		100% rate of CPM among carriers; 9% among uninformatives
Schwartz et al., 2004 (65)	194 newly diagnosed breast cancer patients	P	CPM	To definitive breast cancer treatment	48% rate of CPM for carriers; 24% for uninformatives; 4% for decliners. CPM predicted by physician recommendation and test result
Watson et al., 2004 (31)	261 carriers and noncarriers	P	BLM	12 mo	28% rate of BLM for carriers; 0% among noncarriers
Claes et al., 2005 (32)	34 unaffected carriers and 34 unaffected noncarriers	P	BLM	12 mo	6% rate of BLM among carriers; 0% among noncarriers
Metcalfe et al., 2005 (66)	81 unaffected carriers	CS	BLM	2–110 mo	27% rate of BLM
Evans et al., 2005 (67)	20 affected carriers	CS	CPM		65% rate of CPM
van Sprundel et al., 2005 (53)	148 affected carriers	CS	CPM	$M = 7.4$ yr postdiagnosis	53% rate of CPM

(*Continued*)

Table 2 Studies of Prophylactic Mastectomy Following *BRCA1/2* Testing (*Continued*)

Author	Sample	Design	Outcome	Follow-up	Results
Stolier et al., 2005 (68)	46 affected women who had genetic testing following breast-conserving surgery	CS	CPM		88% rate of CPM among carriers who knew their mutation status at diagnosis
Phillips et al., 2006 (69)	134 unaffected carriers with intact breasts	P	BLM	33–59 mo (M = 39 mo)	11% rate of BLM among carriers aware of mutation status; 0% among carriers unaware of status
Graves et al., 2006 (70)	452 affected carriers and uninformatives	P	CPM	12 mo	18% rate of CPM among carriers; 3% among uninformatives. CPM predicted by positive test result, younger age, higher distress

Abbreviations: BLM, bilateral prophylactic mastectomy; CPM, contralateral prophylactic mastectomy; CS, cross-sectional study design; HBOC, hereditary breast ovarian cancer; P, prospective study design.

BRCA1/2 mutation carriers are variable, ranging from 9% to 54% (32,61,66,69). In particular, studies conducted in the United Kingdom and the Netherlands have reported substantially higher rates of BLM (28–54%) (31,58,61). The reasons for the discrepancies between U.S. women and women from other countries are not clear, but likely are related to cultural differences, differing physician attitudes toward prophylactic surgery, and differences across healthcare systems (69,71).

Contralateral Prophylactic Mastectomy Among Women Affected with Breast Cancer

Although the use of BLM is relatively rare among unaffected mutation carriers in the United States, the rate of contralateral prophylactic mastectomy (CPM) among previously affected mutation carriers is substantially higher. For example, among a group of breast cancer survivors (i.e., women previously diagnosed and treated for breast cancer) who sought genetic testing at varying times following their diagnosis, we found that 18% of *BRCA1/2* mutation carriers opted for CPM in the year following testing. This is in addition to the 16% of participants who had already had prophylactic mastectomy *prior* to undergoing testing (70). In European studies, the rates of CPM among previously diagnosed breast cancer survivors have ranged from 35% to 65% (58,61,67). Studies that have directly compared rates of mastectomy among affected and unaffected carriers have yielded mixed results. A small study reported a higher rate of prophylactic mastectomy among previously affected women (72), while a larger study did not detect a difference between these two groups (60).

Recent research suggests that those most likely to choose CPM are newly diagnosed breast cancer patients who learn their carrier status at the time of diagnosis or shortly thereafter (i.e., prior to definitive local breast cancer treatment). Although data are limited, rates of CPM within this population have ranged from 48% to 100% (63–65,68). In the largest study to date, we found that 48% of newly diagnosed breast cancer patients who received positive *BRCA1/2* test results at the time of diagnosis chose immediate mastectomy of the affected breast along with CPM of the unaffected breast (65). Although newly diagnosed women in our sample self-referred to genetic counseling and thus may be a select group, at least two smaller studies have reported higher rates of bilateral mastectomy (88–100%) among women who learn that they carry a *BRCA1/2* mutation at the time of their breast cancer diagnosis (64,68). These findings are consistent with results from another study that indicated that breast cancer patients who are aware that they carry a *BRCA1/2* mutation at the time of diagnosis are more likely to choose CPM compared to women who learn of their carrier status later (63).

Predictors and Outcomes of Prophylactic Mastectomy

Studies examining the factors associated with the use of prophylactic mastectomy and the psychosocial outcomes of such surgery are limited. Among unaffected women, being younger than 50 years and having children are associated with opting for BLM (58,61). Among women affected with breast cancer, receipt of a positive *BRCA1/2* test result at diagnosis or *prior to* diagnosis is associated with CPM (63–65,73). Other factors that have been associated with CPM include younger age, physician recommendation to consider CPM, greater distress, and more extensive family history (60,63,65,70).

Studies examining psychosocial and quality of life outcomes following BLM or CPM have reported generally high levels of satisfaction, little distress, and overall quality of life comparable to women who chose not to undergo prophylactic surgery (74–77).

For example, at one year postdiagnosis, we found no differences in distress or quality of life among affected women who did and did not opt for prophylactic mastectomy at the time of their initial diagnosis (78). Despite these generally positive outcomes, some women do report an adverse impact of BLM or CPM. Among breast cancer patients who opted for CPM, one-third reported a negative impact on body appearance, 26% reported a diminished sense of femininity, 23% reported negative effects on sexual relationships, and 17% reported diminished self-esteem. Patients who reported such outcomes also reported greater dissatisfaction with their decision to have prophylactic mastectomy (74,76). These data are consistent with an earlier study of BLM outcomes among high-risk women (74). Compared to carriers who chose surveillance, carriers who chose BLM reported increased distress at one and six months following testing. However, most of these differences had disappeared by 12 months postdisclosure (61). Taken together, these data suggest that while a minority of women choosing CPM or BLM report adverse effects on body image and sexual functioning, there is little long-term evidence for an adverse effect on overall quality of life.

Prophylactic Oophorectomy

In addition to reducing the risk of ovarian cancer, PO also reduces the risk of breast cancer when performed premenopausally (54,55). Recent studies have suggested that PO may also reduce overall and cancer-specific mortality among *BRCA1/2* mutation carriers (79). Given these benefits, plus the lack of evidence for the efficacy of ovarian cancer screening, it is not surprising that PO is chosen by mutation carriers far more frequently than prophylactic mastectomy.

Studies that have examined the use of PO among mutation carriers are summarized in Table 3. Although initial reports from registry-based samples suggested relatively low rates of PO following the receipt of a positive test result (57), more recent clinical reports indicate substantially higher rates of PO. In U.S. studies, rates have ranged from 21% to 57% (54,57,60,62,80). U.S. studies that reported lower rates of PO generally had the shortest follow-up periods. For example, in our own study, we found that 27% of mutation carriers opted for PO in the first year after receiving their test result (80). In contrast to studies of BLM and CPM, results from studies that examined PO over periods of two years or more indicate that a significant number of carriers obtain PO beyond the first year after genetic testing. These studies have reported cumulative rates of PO ranging from 46% to 57% (54,60,62). European studies have reported slightly higher rates of PO, ranging from 31% (31) to over 70% (32,53). Again, studies that follow women for a longer period of time report higher cumulative rates of PO. Of course, this is consistent with clinical recommendations for PO in which carriers are advised to obtain PO between the ages of 35 and 40 or after the completion of child bearing.

Predictors and Outcomes of PO

A few studies have examined factors that are associated with the decision to obtain PO. Unsurprisingly, women who carry a *BRCA1/2* mutation are more likely to obtain a PO than women who do not (21). Further, *BRCA1* carriers are more likely to opt for PO than *BRCA2* carriers (21). Older age, family history of ovarian cancer, personal history of breast cancer (particularly early-stage breast cancer), elevated perceived risk for ovarian cancer, and having children, have all been found in one or more studies to predict receipt of PO (31,60,63,80,81).

Table 3 Studies of Prophylactic Oophorectomy Following *BRCA1/2* Testing

Author	Sample	Design	Outcomes	Follow-up	Results
Lerman et al., 2000 (57)	84 carriers	P	BPO	12 mo	13% rate of BPO
Kauff et al., 2002 (54)	170 carriers	P	BPO	<1–76 mo ($M = 24$ mo)	57% rate of BPO
Meijers-Heijboer et al., 2000 (58)	411 women from HBOC families	P	BPO	16–62 mo ($M = 26$ mo)	64% rate of BPO among carriers
Scheuer et al., 2002 (60)	251 carriers	CS	BPO	2–66 mo ($M = 25$ mo)	50% rate of BPO; BPO predicted by: older age and previous breast cancer diagnosis
Schwartz et al., 2003 (80)	79 carriers, 44 negatives, and 166 uninformatives	P	BPO	12 mo	27% rate of BPO among carriers; 9% rate of BPO among uninformatives; BPO predicted by: positive test result, higher perceived risk for ovarian cancer, and stronger family history
Botkin et al., 2003 (62)	26 carriers, 69 noncarriers	P	BPO	24 mo	46% rate of BPO among carriers; 4% rate of BPO among noncarriers; BPO predicted by older age
Meijers-Heijboer et al., 2003 (63)	101 carriers	P	BPO	2–8 yr	49% rate of BPO; BPO predicted by having an earlier stage breast cancer
Watson et al., 2004 (31)	91 carriers and 170 noncarriers	P	BPO	12 mo	31% rate of BPO among carriers; 0% rate of BPO among noncarriers; BPO predicted by: older age
Claes et al., 2005 (32)	16 carriers age 35+ with intact ovaries at the time of testing	P	BPO	12 mo	75% rate of BPO among carriers; BPO predicted by: older age and higher ovarian cancer risk perceptions

(Continued)

Table 3 Studies of Prophylactic Oophorectomy Following *BRCA1/2* Testing (*Continued*)

Author	Sample	Design	Outcomes	Follow-up	Results
Madalinska et al., 2005 (81)	846 members of HBOC families	CS	BPO		44% rate of BPO overall; 72% rate of BPO among women who were aware that they were *BRCA1/2* carriers; BPO predicted by carrier status, older age, having had breast cancer, having had BLM, having children, less education
van Sprundel et al., 2005 (53)	148 carriers	CS	BPO		73% rate of BPO
Metcalfe et al., 2005 (66)	81 unaffected carriers	CS	BPO	2–110 mo	67% rate of BPO
Phillips et al., 2006 (69)	123 carriers with at least one ovary (56 aware of mutation status)	P	BPO	33–59 mo ($M = 39$ mo)	29% rate of BPO among carriers who were aware of their mutation status; 6% rate of BPO among carriers unaware of their status

Abbreviations: BLM, bilateral prophylactic mastectomy; BPO, bilateral prophylactic oophorectomy; CS, cross-sectional study design; HBOC, hereditary breast ovarian cancer; P, prospective study design.

Fewer studies have evaluated psychosocial outcomes and quality of life following PO. Madalinska et al. (81) compared psychosocial and quality of life outcomes among over 800 high-risk women who did and did not opt for PO. There were no differences in overall quality of life between the two groups. Patients who opted for PO reported less worry about cancer compared to those who decided against PO. However, there were adverse sexual and endocrine side effects that were associated with PO. Specifically, patients who received PO reported more discomfort, less sexual pleasure, and a greater number of endocrine symptoms compared to those who did not obtain PO.

Chemoprevention

The little data available on the clinical use of chemopreventive agents (i.e., tamoxifen and raloxifene) among *BRCA1/2* carriers suggest extremely low use. Metcalfe et al. (66) reported that 12% of mutation carriers used tamoxifen. Phillips et al. (69) reported that only 1% of Australian mutation carriers reported using tamoxifen as a chemopreventive agent. This is consistent with previous research documenting low rates of participation in chemoprevention trials (82–84). Additional research is needed to better characterize the use of chemopreventive agents among mutation carriers and to understand the apparent barriers to the use of these agents.

Breast Cancer Surveillance

Carriers who do not opt for prophylactic surgery are advised to participate in breast cancer screening beginning at the age of 25 to 35 years (85,86). Initial studies among *BRCA1/2* carriers suggested suboptimal adherence to these guidelines. Lerman et al. (57) reported that at six months following testing, only 60% of carriers who were due for a mammogram reported receiving one. In a separate, clinic-based study, we found that only 59% of mutation carriers obtained a mammogram in the year following testing (59). In this study, use of mammography was highly related to age. Seventy-four percent of carriers aged 40 years and above obtained a mammogram compared to only 39% of carriers aged 25 to 39 years. These results are consistent with findings from a recent study in which carriers over the age of 40 years obtained mammograms at high rates, but only 59% of younger carriers obtained the recommended two mammograms during the two-year follow-up period (62). Other recent studies have reported substantially higher rates of mammography for carriers, ranging from 82% to 95% (32,60). Studies directly comparing mammography adherence among carriers and noncarriers have found increased adherence among carriers (32,57,59,60,62).

Evidence to date does not support initial concerns about the possibility of false reassurance among women who receive negative test results. For example, Plon et al. (87) found that 88% of Ashkenazi women who tested negative for one of the Ashkenazi Jewish founder mutations were adherent to mammography recommendations one year after testing, and 92% were adherent two years after testing. Other studies have found no decreases in screening among noncarriers over the age of 40 years (62) and appropriate decreases in screening among noncarriers under the age of 40 years (59).

Recent evidence has suggested that MRI may be more sensitive than mammography and that the combination of MRI and mammography may be particularly sensitive in this population (88,89). Despite the increased sensitivity of MRI, questions still remain about its impact on mortality and its cost-effectiveness (89,90). As more centers begin to recommend annual MRI to mutation carriers, the use of MRI within this population will need to be evaluated.

Ovarian Cancer Surveillance

Given the low sensitivity and specificity of current ovarian cancer screening approaches, most centers recommend PO to *BRCA1/2* carriers. However, for those women who are under 35 years and have not completed child bearing, or for women who decide not to pursue PO, many providers recommend TVUS and CA-125 testing. The low rates of ovarian cancer screening reported among carriers reflect the lack of acceptance of ovarian cancer screening among most health professionals. In our own research, 43% of carriers reported an annual CA-125 and 40% an annual TVUS (80). Lower rates have been reported in previous studies (57). Among noncarriers, rates of CA-125 and TVUS, low prior to testing, remain low following the receipt of negative test results (80). Across these studies, variables associated with the use of ovarian cancer screening include a positive *BRCA1/2* test result, higher perceived risk for ovarian cancer, and higher anxiety prior to testing (80).

Medical Decision-Making Summary and Conclusions

Although some discrepancies exist among the data published to date, most carriers appear to obtain either prophylactic surgery or recommended surveillance. Rates of prophylactic surgery are generally lower in the United States compared to Europe, Canada, and Australia. Although most *BRCA1/2* carriers do take action to reduce their cancer risk, a substantial minority do not choose prophylactic surgery and do not obtain regular screening. Predictors of nonadherence are not well understood. Future research must identify factors that are associated with nonadherence in order to develop strategies that maximize the medical benefit of receiving a positive *BRCA1/2* test result. In terms of noncarriers, there is little evidence suggesting a false reassurance effect. The screening practices of noncarriers and women who receive uninformative test results appear to be consistent with medical recommendations.

OVERALL SUMMARY AND CONCLUSIONS

Significant progress has been made in increasing our understanding of the psychosocial and behavioral impact of *BRCA1/2* genetic counseling and testing since the discovery of the *BRCA1/2* genes. Evidence indicates that *BRCA1/2* counseling and testing does not result in adverse psychological responses for most individuals, and there does not appear to be any long-term negative impact for the majority of carriers. Short-term distress, if present, typically dissipates quickly, and noncarriers frequently seem to psychologically benefit through reduced distress. Certain subgroups, such as individuals with high levels of pretest anxiety or distress, may be more at risk for negative sequelae following testing. Despite the substantial gains in knowledge surrounding the psychological outcomes of *BRCA1/2* testing, questions remain. Future efforts to clearly identify specific risk factors for distress after testing are warranted, as are studies designed to evaluate how slight increases in distress may impact long-term psychological and behavioral outcomes in mutation carriers. Such information could be critical to developing more individually tailored genetic counseling practices. It is important to note that much of the research to date has been based upon individuals who actively sought out genetic testing. Such testing was typically provided by highly trained genetic counselors in a research setting. As genetic testing becomes more integrated into clinical medicine, it will be essential to determine whether the positive outcomes seen in these initial studies generalize to patients who do not actively seek out genetic testing, and to patients who receive genetic counseling in alternative settings and from alternative providers.

In terms of behavioral outcomes following genetic testing, evidence clearly indicates that women are much more willing to obtain PO compared to prophylactic mastectomy. However, recent studies demonstrate that women who learn their carrier status at the time of their breast cancer diagnosis may be more willing to take preventive action than unaffected women or those who do not learn their carrier status until after they have completed breast cancer treatment. The implications of such findings need to be explored further. However, these data certainly suggest that the integration of genetic counseling and testing into routine oncologic care for high-risk individuals could impact subsequent cancer risks. Finally, given the sufficient evidence documenting generally positive psychosocial and behavioral outcomes following *BRCA1/2* testing, it is certainly reasonable to begin to evaluate the impact that such testing may have on subsequent cancer and mortality risks.

REFERENCES

1. Biesecker BB, Boehnke M, Calzone K, et al. Genetic counseling for families with inherited susceptibility to breast and ovarian cancer. JAMA 1993; 269(15):1970–1974.
2. Collins FS. *BRCA1*—lots of mutations, lots of dilemmas. N Engl J Med 1996; 334(3): 186–188.
3. Lerman C, Croyle R. Psychological issues in genetic testing for breast cancer susceptibility. Arch Intern Med 1994; 154(6):609–616.
4. Croyle RT, Smith KR, Botkin JR, Baty B, Nash J. Psychological responses to *BRCA1* mutation testing: preliminary findings. Health Psychol 1997; 16(1):63–72.
5. Hubbard R, Lewontin RC. Pitfalls of genetic testing. N Engl J Med 1996; 334(18):1192–1194.
6. Lerman C, Rimer BK, Engstrom PF. Cancer risk notification: psychosocial and ethical implications. J Clin Oncol 1991; 9(7):1275–1282.
7. Botkin JR, Croyle RT, Smith KR, et al. A model protocol for evaluating the behavioral and psychosocial effects of BRCA1 testing. J Natl Cancer Inst 1996; 88(13):872–882.
8. Josten DM, Evans AM, Love RR. The Cancer Prevention Clinic: a service program for cancer-prone families. J Psychosocial Oncol 1985; 3:5–20.
9. Vries-Kragt K. The dilemmas of a carrier of *BRCA1* gene mutations. Patient Educ Couns 1998; 35(1):75–80.
10. Foster C, Eeles R, Ardern-Jones A, Moynihan C, Watson M. Juggling roles and expectations: dilemmas faced by women talking to relatives about cancer and genetic testing. Psychology Health 2004; 19(4):439–455.
11. Lerman C, Narod S, Schulman K, et al. BRCA1 testing in families with hereditary breast-ovarian cancer. A prospective study of patient decision making and outcomes. JAMA 1996; 275(24):1885–1892.
12. Lerman C, Hughes C, Lemon SJ, et al. What you don't know can hurt you: adverse psychologic effects in members of BRCA1-linked and *BRCA2*-linked families who decline genetic testing. J Clin Oncol 1998; 16(5):1650–1654.
13. Smith KR, West JA, Croyle RT, Botkin JR. Familial context of genetic testing for cancer susceptibility: moderating effect of siblings' test results on psychological distress one to two weeks after *BRCA1* mutation testing. Cancer Epidemiol Biomarkers Prev 1999; 8(4 Pt 2): 385–392.
14. Dorval M, Patenaude AF, Schneider KA, et al. Anticipated versus actual emotional reactions to disclosure of results of genetic tests for cancer susceptibility: findings from p53 and BRCA1 testing programs. J Clin Oncol 2000; 18(10):2135–2142.
15. Wagner TM, Moslinger R, Langbauer G, et al. Attitude towards prophylactic surgery and effects of genetic counselling in families with *BRCA* mutations. Austrian Hereditary Breast and Ovarian Cancer Group. Br J Cancer 2000; 82(7):1249–1253.
16. Wood ME, Mullineaux L, Rahm AK, Fairclough D, Wenzel L. Impact of *BRCA1* testing on women with cancer: a pilot study. Genet Test 2000; 4(3):265–272.

17. Lodder L, Frets PG, Trijsburg RW, et al. Psychological impact of receiving a BRCA1/BRCA2 test result. Am J Med Genet 2001; 98(1):15–24.

18. Tercyak KP, Lerman C, Peshkin BN, et al. Effects of coping style and BRCA1 and BRCA2 test results on anxiety among women participating in genetic counseling and testing for breast and ovarian cancer risk. Health Psychol 2001; 20(3):217–222.

19. Cella D, Hughes C, Peterman A, et al. A brief assessment of concerns associated with genetic testing for cancer: the Multidimensional Impact of Cancer Risk Assessment (MICRA) questionnaire. Health Psychol 2002; 21(6):564–572.

20. Meiser B, Butow P, Friedlander M, et al. Psychological impact of genetic testing in women from high-risk breast cancer families. Eur J Cancer 2002; 38(15):2025–2031.

21. Schwartz MD, Peshkin BN, Hughes C, Main D, Isaacs C, Lerman C. Impact of BRCA1/BRCA2 mutation testing on psychologic distress in a clinic-based sample. J Clin Oncol 2002; 20(2):514–520.

22. Hagoel L, Neter E, Dishon S, Barnett O, Rennert G. BRCA1/2 mutation carriers: living with susceptibility. Community Genet 2003; 6(4):242–248.

23. van Oostrom I, Meijers-Heijboer H, Lodder LN, et al. Long-term psychological impact of carrying a BRCA1/2 mutation and prophylactic surgery: a 5-year follow-up study. J Clin Oncol 2003; 21(20):3867–3874.

24. Arver B, Haegermark A, Platten U, Lindblom A, Brandberg Y. Evaluation of psychosocial effects of pre-symptomatic testing for breast/ovarian and colon cancer pre-disposing genes: a 12–month follow-up. Fam Cancer 2004; 3(2):109–116.

25. Claes E, Evers-Kiebooms G, Boogaerts A, Decruyenaere M, Denayer L, Legius E. Diagnostic genetic testing for hereditary breast and ovarian cancer in cancer patients: women's looking back on the pre–test period and a psychological evaluation. Genet Test 2004; 8(1):13–21.

26. Manne S, Audrain J, Schwartz M, Main D, Finch C, Lerman C. Associations between relationship support and psychological reactions of participants and partners to BRCA1 and BRCA2 testing in a clinic-based sample. Ann Behav Med 2004; 28(3):211–225.

27. Reichelt JG, Heimdal K, Moller P, Dahl AA. BRCA1 testing with definitive results: a prospective study of psychological distress in a large clinic-based sample. Fam Cancer 2004; 3(1):21–28.

28. Smith KR, Ellington L, Chan AY, Croyle RT, Botkin JR. Fertility intentions following testing for a BRCA1 gene mutation. Cancer Epidemiol Biomarkers Prev 2004; 13(5):733–740.

29. van Dijk S, van Asperen CJ, Jacobi CE, et al. Variants of uncertain clinical significance as a result of BRCA1/2 testing: impact of an ambiguous breast cancer risk message. Genet Test 2004; 8(3):235–239.

30. van Roosmalen MS, Stalmeier PF, Verhoef LC, et al. Impact of BRCA1/2 testing and disclosure of a positive test result on women affected and unaffected with breast or ovarian cancer. Am J Med Genet A 2004; 124(4):346–355.

31. Watson M, Foster C, Eeles R, et al. Psychosocial impact of breast/ovarian (BRCA1/2) cancer-predictive genetic testing in a UK multi-centre clinical cohort. Br J Cancer 2004; 91(10): 1787–1794.

32. Claes E, Evers-Kiebooms G, Decruyenaere M, et al. Surveillance behavior and prophylactic surgery after predictive testing for hereditary breast/ovarian cancer. Behav Med 2005; 31(3): 93–105.

33. Lynch HT, Snyder C, Lynch JF, et al. Patient responses to the disclosure of BRCA mutation tests in hereditary breast-ovarian cancer families. Cancer Genet Cytogenet 2006; 165(2): 91–97.

34. van Dijk S, Timmermans DR, Meijers-Heijboer H, Tibben A, van Asperen CJ, Otten W. Clinical characteristics affect the impact of an uninformative DNA test result: the course of worry and distress experienced by women who apply for genetic testing for breast cancer. J Clin Oncol 2006; 24(22):3672–3677.

35. Bish A, Sutton S, Jacobs C, Levene S, Ramirez A, Hodgson S. No news is (not necessarily) good news: impact of preliminary results for BRCA1 mutation searches. Genet Med 2002; 4(5):353–358.

36. Coyne JC, Benazon NR, Gaba CG, Calzone K, Weber BL. Distress and psychiatric morbidity among women from high-risk breast and ovarian cancer families. J Consult Clin Psychol 2000; 68(5):864–874.

37. Palmer SC, Kagee A, Kruus L, Coyne JC. Overemphasis of psychological risks of genetic testing may have "dire" consequences. Psychosomatics 2002; 43(1):86–87.

38. Loader S, Shields CG, Rowley PT. Impact of genetic testing for breast-ovarian cancer susceptibility. Genet Test 2004; 8(1):1–12.

39. Hamann HA, Somers TJ, Smith AW, Inslicht SS, Baum A. Posttraumatic stress associated with cancer history and BRCA1/2 genetic testing. Psychosom Med 2005; 67(5): 766–772.

40. Pasacreta JV. Psychosocial issues associated with increased breast and ovarian cancer risk: findings from focus groups. Arch Psychiatr Nurs 1999; 13(3):127–136.

41. Miller SM, Roussi P, Daly MB, et al. Enhanced counseling for women undergoing BRCA1/2 testing: impact on subsequent decision making about risk reduction behaviors. Health Educ Behav 2005; 32(5):654–667.

42. Shoda Y, Mischel W, Miller SM, Diefenbach M, Daly MB, Engstrom PF. Psychological interventions and genetic testing: facilitating informed decisions about BRCA1/2 cancer susceptibility. J Clin Psychol Med Settings 1998; 5(1):3–17.

43. McInerney-Leo A, Biesecker BB, Hadley DW, et al. BRCA1/2 testing in hereditary breast and ovarian cancer families: effectiveness of problem-solving training as a counseling intervention. Am J Med Genet A 2004; 130(3):221–227.

44. Nelson HD, Huffman LH, Fu R, Harris EL. Genetic risk assessment and BRCA mutation testing for breast and ovarian cancer susceptibility: systematic evidence review for the U.S. Preventive Services Task Force. Ann Intern Med 2005; 143(5):362–379.

45. d'Agincourt-Canning L. Experiences of genetic risk: disclosure and the gendering of responsibility. Bioethics 2001; 15(3):231–247.

46. Hughes C, Lerman C, Schwartz M, et al. All in the family: evaluation of the process and content of sisters' communication about BRCA1 and BRCA2 genetic test results. Am J Med Genet 2002; 107(2):143–150.

47. Costalas JW, Itzen M, Malick J, et al. Communication of BRCA1 and BRCA2 results to at-risk relatives: a cancer risk assessment program's experience. Am J Med Genet 2003; 119:11–18.

48. Smith KR, Zick CD, Mayer RN, Botkin JR. Voluntary disclosure of BRCA1 mutation test results. Genet Test 2002; 6(2):89–92.

49. Claes E, Evers-Kiebooms G, Boogaerts A, Decruyenaere M, Denayer L, Legius E. Communication with close and distant relatives in the context of genetic testing for hereditary breast and ovarian cancer in cancer patients. Am J Med Genet A 2003; 116(1): 11–19.

50. Herrinton LJ, Barlow WE, Yu O, et al. Efficacy of prophylactic mastectomy in women with unilateral breast cancer: a cancer research network project. J Clin Oncol 2005; 23(19): 4275–4286.

51. McDonnell SK, Schaid DJ, Myers JL, et al. Efficacy of contralateral prophylactic mastectomy in women with a personal and family history of breast cancer. J Clin Oncol 2001; 19(19): 3938–3943.

52. Peralta EA, Ellenhorn JD, Wagman LD, Dagis A, Andersen JS, Chu DZ. Contralateral prophylactic mastectomy improves the outcome of selected patients undergoing mastectomy for breast cancer. Am J Surg 2000; 180(6):439–445.

53. van Sprundel TC, Schmidt MK, Rookus MA, et al. Risk reduction of contralateral breast cancer and survival after contralateral prophylactic mastectomy in BRCA1 or BRCA2 mutation carriers. Br J Cancer 2005; 93(3):287–292.

54. Kauff ND, Satagopan JM, Robson ME, et al. Risk-reducing salpingo-oophorectomy in women with a BRCA1 or BRCA2 mutation. N Engl J Med 2002; 346(21):1609–1615.

55. Rebbeck TR, Lynch HT, Neuhausen SL, et al. Prophylactic oophorectomy in carriers of BRCA1 or BRCA2 mutations. N Engl J Med 2002; 346(21):1616–1622.

56. King MC, Wieand S, Hale K, et al. Tamoxifen and breast cancer incidence among women with inherited mutations in BRCA1 and BRCA2: National Surgical Adjuvant Breast and Bowel Project (NSABP-P1) Breast Cancer Prevention Trial. JAMA 2001; 286(18): 2251–2256.

57. Lerman C, Hughes C, Croyle RT, et al. Prophylactic surgery decisions and surveillance practices one year following BRCA1/2 testing. Prev Med 2000; 31(1):75–80.

58. Meijers-Heijboer EJ, Verhoog LC, Brekelmans CT, et al. Presymptomatic DNA testing and prophylactic surgery in families with a BRCA1 or BRCA2 mutation. Lancet 2000; 355(9220): 2015–2020.

59. Peshkin BN, Schwartz MD, Isaacs C, Hughes C, Main D, Lerman C. Utilization of breast cancer screening in a clinically based sample of women after BRCA1/2 testing. Cancer Epidemiol Biomarkers Prev 2002; 11(10 Pt 1):1115–1118.

60. Scheuer L, Kauff N, Robson M, et al. Outcome of preventive surgery and screening for breast and ovarian cancer in BRCA mutation carriers. J Clin Oncol 2002; 20(5):1260–1268.

61. Lodder LN, Frets PG, Trijsburg RW, et al. One year follow-up of women opting for presymptomatic testing for BRCA1 and BRCA2: emotional impact of the test outcome and decisions on risk management (surveillance or prophylactic surgery). Breast Cancer Res Treat 2002; 73(2):97–112.

62. Botkin JR, Smith KR, Croyle RT, et al. Genetic testing for a BRCA1 mutation: prophylactic surgery and screening behavior in women 2 years post testing. Am J Med Genet A 2003; 118 (3):201–209.

63. Meijers-Heijboer H, Brekelmans CT, Menke-Pluymers M, et al. Use of genetic testing and prophylactic mastectomy and oophorectomy in women with breast or ovarian cancer from families with a BRCA1 or BRCA2 mutation. J Clin Oncol 2003; 21(9):1675–1681.

64. Weitzel JN, McCaffrey SM, Nedelcu R, MacDonald DJ, Blazer KR, Cullinane CA. Effect of genetic cancer risk assessment on surgical decisions at breast cancer diagnosis. Arch Surg 2003; 138(12):1323–1328.

65. Schwartz MD, Lerman C, Brogan B, et al. Impact of BRCA1/BRCA2 counseling and testing on newly diagnosed breast cancer patients. J Clin Oncol 2004; 22(10):1823–1829.

66. Metcalfe KA, Snyder C, Seidel J, Hanna D, Lynch HT, Narod S. The use of preventive measures among healthy women who carry a BRCA1 or BRCA2 mutation. Fam Cancer 2005; 4(2):97–103.

67. Evans DG, Lalloo F, Hopwood P, et al. Surgical decisions made by 158 women with hereditary breast cancer aged <50 years. Eur J Surg Oncol 2005; 31(10):1112–1118.

68. Stolier AJ, Corsetti RL. Newly diagnosed breast cancer patients choose bilateral mastectomy over breast-conserving surgery when testing positive for a BRCA1/2 mutation. Am Surg 2005; 71(12):1031–1033.

69. Phillips KA, Jenkins MA, Lindeman GJ, et al. Risk-reducing surgery, screening and chemoprevention practices of BRCA1 and BRCA2 mutation carriers: a prospective cohort study. Clin Genet 2006; 70(3):198–206.

70. Graves KD, Peshkin BN, Halbert CH, Demarco TA, Isaacs C, Schwartz MD. Predictors and outcomes of contralateral prophylactic mastecomy. Breast Cancer Res Treat 2006 Oct 26 [Epub ahead of print].

71. Julian-Reynier CM, Bouchard LJ, Evans DG, et al. Women's attitudes toward preventive strategies for hereditary breast or ovarian carcinoma differ from one country to another: differences among English, French, and Canadian women. Cancer 2001; 92(4):959–968.

72. Ray JA, Loescher LJ, Brewer M. Risk-reduction surgery decisions in high-risk women seen for genetic counseling. J Genet Couns 2005; 14(6):473–484.

73. Stolier AJ, Fuhrman GM, Mauterer L, Bolton JS, Superneau DW. Initial experience with surgical treatment planning in the newly diagnosed breast cancer patient at high risk for BRCA-1 or BRCA-2 mutation. Breast J 2004; 10(6):475–480.

74. Frost MH, Schaid DJ, Sellers TA, et al. Long-term satisfaction and psychological and social function following bilateral prophylactic mastectomy. JAMA 2000; 284(3):319–324.

75. Schwartz MD. Contralateral prophylactic mastectomy: efficacy, satisfaction, and regret. J Clin Oncol 2005; 23(31):7777–7779.

76. Frost MH, Slezak JM, Tran NV, et al. Satisfaction after contralateral prophylactic mastectomy: the significance of mastectomy type, reconstructive complications, and body appearance. J Clin Oncol 2005; 23(31):7849–7856.

77. Geiger AM, West CN, Nekhlyudov L, et al. Contentment with quality of life among breast cancer survivors with and without contralateral prophylactic mastectomy. J Clin Oncol 2006; 24(9):1350–1356.

78. Tercyak KP, Peshkin BN, Isaacs C, et al. Impact of contralateral prophylactic mastectomy on quality of life. J Clin Oncol 2007; 25(3):285–291.

79. Domchek SM, Stopfer JE, Rebbeck TR. Bilateral risk-reducing oophorectomy in BRCA1 and BRCA2 mutation carriers. J Natl Compr Canc Netw 2006; 4(2):177–182.

80. Schwartz MD, Kaufman E, Peshkin BN, et al. Bilateral prophylactic oophorectomy and ovarian cancer screening following BRCA1/BRCA2 mutation testing. J Clin Oncol 2003; 21(21):4034–4041.

81. Madalinska JB, Hollenstein J, Bleiker E, et al. Quality-of-life effects of prophylactic salpingo-oophorectomy versus gynecologic screening among women at increased risk of hereditary ovarian cancer. J Clin Oncol 2005; 23(28):6890–6898.

82. Isaacs C, Peshkin BN, Schwartz M, Demarco TA, Main D, Lerman C. Breast and ovarian cancer screening practices in healthy women with a strong family history of breast or ovarian cancer. Breast Cancer Res Treat 2002; 71(2):103–112.

83. Evans D, Lalloo F, Shenton A, Boggis C, Howell A. Uptake of screening and prevention in women at very high risk of breast cancer. Lancet 2001; 358(9285):889–890.

84. Miller HH, Bauman LJ, Friedman DR, DeCosse JJ. Psychosocial adjustment of familial polyposis patients and participation in a chemoprevention trial. Int J Psychiatry Med 1986; 16 (3):211–230.

85. Burke W, Daly M, Garber J, et al. Recommendations for follow-up care of individuals with an inherited predisposition to cancer. II. BRCA1 and BRCA2. Cancer Genetics Studies Consortium. JAMA 1997; 277(12):997–1003.

86. National Comprehensive Cancer Network. NCCN Clinical Practice Guidelines in Oncology – version 1.2006. Genetic/Familial High-Risk Assessment: Breast and Ovarian. Available at http://www.nccn.org/professionals/physician_gls/PDF/genetics_screening.pdf. Retrieved Sept. 18, 2006.

87. Plon SE, Peterson LE, Friedman LC, Richards CS. Mammography behavior after receiving a negative BRCA1 mutation test result in the Ashkenazim: a community-based study. Genet Med 2000; 2(6):307–311.

88. Leach MO, Boggis CR, Dixon AK, et al. Screening with magnetic resonance imaging and mammography of a UK population at high familial risk of breast cancer: a prospective multicentre cohort study (MARIBS). Lancet 2005; 365(9473):1769–1778.

89. Warner E, Plewes DB, Hill KA, et al. Surveillance of BRCA1 and BRCA2 mutation carriers with magnetic resonance imaging, ultrasound, mammography, and clinical breast examination. JAMA 2004; 292(11):1317–1325.

90. Plevritis SK, Kurian AW, Sigal BM, et al. Cost-effectiveness of screening BRCA1/2 mutation carriers with breast magnetic resonance imaging. JAMA 2006; 295(20):2374–2384.

15

Breast Cancer Screening and Prevention Options in *BRCA1* and *BRCA2* Mutation Carriers

Karen Lisa Smith
Washington Cancer Institute, Washington Hospital Center, Washington, D.C., U.S.A.

Claudine Isaacs
Fisher Center for Familial Cancer Research, Lombardi Comprehensive Cancer Research, Georgetown University, Washington, D.C., U.S.A.

INTRODUCTION

Although less than 5% to 10% of breast cancer cases are attributable to *BRCA1* and *BRCA2* mutations, the risk of breast cancer in known *BRCA1* and *BRCA2* heterozygotes is substantial. Estimates vary, but the recently reported lifetime breast cancer risk for *BRCA1* mutation carriers in a combined analysis of data from 22 studies of case series unselected for family history is 65% (1–3). The burden of this risk in *BRCA1* mutation carriers begins at a young age with premenopausal *BRCA1* mutation carriers facing between 17- and 32-fold higher breast cancer risk than age-matched controls in the general population. The risk plateaus as age increases but continues through the post-menopausal years, with *BRCA1* mutation carriers aged 60 to 69 facing 14-fold higher risk than age-matched controls in the general population. The estimated lifetime breast cancer risk in *BRCA2* mutation carriers from the combined analysis is lower, at approximately 45%, although still significantly greater than that of the general population. For *BRCA2* mutation carriers, the breast cancer risk increases with age and is greatest during the postmenopausal years (3). This significant extent of breast cancer penetrance in *BRCA1/2* mutation carriers has led to the development of prevention and early detection interventions for this high-risk population. These interventions are reviewed in this chapter.

In addition to the risk of developing de novo breast cancer described above, *BRCA1/2* mutation carriers already affected with breast cancer face the continued risk of developing new primary breast cancers. Reported risks for metachronous primary contralateral breast cancer (CBC) in *BRCA1/2* mutation carriers range from approximately 25% to 40%, which is significantly higher than that noted in women with sporadic breast cancer (4–8). In addition, late ipsilateral recurrences, often in different quadrants from the original tumors, have been observed in affected women with *BRCA1/2* mutations who undergo breast conserving therapy, leading many to suspect that these represent new primary breast cancers in this high-risk population (7,9). Some of the therapeutic interventions that aim to reduce the risk of breast cancer recurrence also reduce the risk of the development of new primary breast cancers (6,7,10–12). These therapeutic interventions, as relevant to the management of affected *BRCA1/2* mutation carriers, are reviewed elsewhere in this book; however, their impact on prevention of new primary breast cancers is discussed in this chapter. In addition, screening interventions for unaffected women with *BRCA1/2* mutations are generally applied to affected women who retain breast tissue after the completion of their breast cancer treatment such that new primary breast cancers may be detected. Thus screening interventions discussed in this chapter pertain not only to unaffected women with *BRCA1/2* mutations but also to affected women who have completed treatment for their breast cancer and are under surveillance both for the detection of recurrence of their breast cancer and for new primary breast cancers.

Although not the focus of this chapter, it must be noted that *BRCA1/2* mutation carriers face risks for other cancers besides breast cancer. In particular, the risk for ovarian cancer is substantial with recently reported lifetime risk of 39% among *BRCA1* mutation carriers and 11% among *BRCA2* mutation carriers (3). There is some overlap between the prevention options for breast cancer and those of ovarian cancer in this high-risk population and the ovarian cancer risk reduction associated with the breast cancer prevention interventions reviewed in this chapter is discussed as appropriate.

BREAST CANCER SCREENING IN UNAFFECTED *BRCA1/2* MUTATION CARRIERS

The standard of care for breast cancer screening in *BRCA1/2* mutation carriers is currently evolving. Until recently, clinical breast examination (CBE), self-breast examination and yearly mammography beginning at approximately age 25 to 35 were recommended for women at risk for hereditary breast cancer (13). However, there are multiple limitations to the use of yearly mammography as a sole imaging modality in this high-risk population and new research has demonstrated improved results with the incorporation of breast magnetic resonance imaging (MRI) in screening programs for women at risk for hereditary breast cancer.

Limitations of yearly mammography as a sole screening modality in *BRCA1/2* mutation carriers include inadequate sensitivity, the frequency of interval cancers, and the theoretical potential for radiation-induced carcinogenesis. With regard to sensitivity, a higher false-negative rate for mammography in *BRCA1/2* mutation carriers compared with women without mutations has been demonstrated in a case-control study (62% vs. 29%, $p = 0.01$) (14). In addition, a prospective trial identified a nonsignificant trend toward reduced sensitivity of mammography in *BRCA1/2* mutation carriers compared with noncarriers (46.2% vs. 31.6%, $p = 0.32$) (15).

Part of the explanation for the reduced sensitivity of mammography screening in women with *BRCA1/2* mutations may be breast density. It is well known that the sensitivity of mammography varies inversely with breast density (16). In addition, increased breast density has been associated with increased breast cancer risk in both the general population and the *BRCA1/2* mutation carriers (17,18). Younger women tend to have more dense breasts than older women, a finding that is thought to contribute to reduced sensitivity of mammography in young women (19,20). Since *BRCA1/2* mutation carriers start breast cancer screening at a young age, it is likely that increased breast density contributes to the suboptimal sensitivity of screening mammography in this population.

BRCA1/2 mutation–associated breast cancers are known to have faster doubling times than sporadic breast cancers, a finding that may explain the relatively high frequency of interval malignancies identified in *BRCA1/2* mutation carriers. Interval malignancies are those that are diagnosed between regularly scheduled imaging studies and usually present with symptoms or palpable lesions. Although rates vary, the frequency of interval cancers identified in mammography-based screening programs in women with *BRCA1/2* mutations has been reported to be as high as approximately 50% (21–23).

In addition to the above concerns regarding the potential inadequacy of screening mammography to identify breast cancers in *BRCA1/2* mutation carriers, the suggestion that screening mammography may actually be harmful to *BRCA1/2* mutation carriers has recently been raised. This concern is based on the hypothesis that *BRCA1/2* mutation carriers may be particularly sensitive to the carcinogenic effects of ionizing radiation (24–26). Since screening begins at a young age in *BRCA1/2* mutation carriers, some have suggested that, in an attempt to identify malignancies at an early stage, yearly mammography may result in a significant amount of radiation exposure that may, itself, promote carcinogenesis (27). Andrieu et al. performed a retrospective cohort study evaluating the effect of radiation exposure on cancer risk in approximately 1600 *BRCA1/2* mutation carriers. In this cohort, radiation exposure, in the form of chest X-rays, was associated with a 1.5-fold higher risk of breast cancer. Subgroup analysis revealed that this risk is particularly high among those exposed to chest X-rays at a young age (26). Although this finding is subject to recall bias and is based on chest X-ray exposure instead of mammogram exposure, it suggests the potential consequences of early and consistent radiation exposure through routine screening mammography in this high-risk population. Despite these findings, two recent retrospective studies have not identified exposure to mammograms as a risk factor for breast cancer in *BRCA1/2* mutation carriers. In the first, a history of screening mammography and the age at which it was first performed was compared among 1600 *BRCA1/2* mutation carriers with breast cancer and 1600 *BRCA1/2* mutation carriers without breast cancer. No association between ever having had screening mammography and risk of breast cancer was identified (28). More recently, a retrospective cohort study of a smaller group of *BRCA1/2* mutation carriers did not identify an association between the number of screening mammograms a woman had undergone and her breast cancer risk (29).

Despite the potential concern that radiation exposure may increase the risk of breast cancer in *BRCA1/2* mutation carriers, mammography has not definitively been demonstrated to do so. In addition, mammography is the only breast cancer screening modality to date demonstrated to impact breast cancer mortality in the general population (30). Thus, it is not currently recommended that screening mammography be avoided in *BRCA1/2* mutation carriers. Rather, recent developments focus on the addition of other screening modalities to yearly mammography.

MRI has recently been shown to be a powerful tool for the identification of breast cancer. To date, seven prospective trials evaluating MRI for breast cancer screening have been performed in high-risk women (Table 1).

Although only one of the trials has been limited to women with known *BRCA1/2* mutations, the findings from these trials have led to the incorporation of MRI as a developing new standard for breast cancer screening in this population.

In the first study, Tilanus–Linthorst et al. performed MRI and CBE in 109 women with above 25% lifetime risk of breast cancer in whom mammography six months earlier had revealed dense breast tissue but no suspicious lesion. In the cohort, 12 women had known *BRCA1/2* mutations. MRI led to the identification of three breast cancers (2.8%) in this cohort, whereas only two were expected. There were, however, six false-positive MRI results, all of which necessitated further diagnostic evaluation (31).

Table 1   Results of Prospective Trials Evaluating Screening Breast Magnetic Resonance Imaging in Conjunction with Mammography in Women with Increased Breast Cancer Risk

Study (N)	Key inclusion criteria (% with known BRCA1/2 mutations)	Screening program	Mammography		MRI	
			Sensitivity[a]	Specificity	Sensitivity[a]	Specificity
Tilanus–Linthorst et al. (31) (109)	>25% breast cancer risk; >50% breast density on mammography (11%)	CBE q 6 mo / Annual mammo[b] / Annual MRI[b]	Not reported	Not reported	100%	94%
Kriege et al. (32) (1909)	≥15% breast cancer risk (18.5%)	CBE q 6 mo / Annual mammo / Annual MRI	40%	95%	71%	90%
Warner et al. (33) (236)	BRCA1/2 mutation (100%)	CBE q 6 mo / Annual mammo / Annual MRI / Annual US	36%	99.8%	77%	95%
Lehman et al. (34) (367)	>25% breast cancer risk (unknown)	MRI once / CBE once / Mammo once	Not reported	Not reported	100%	95%
Leach et al. (35) (649)	Carriers of BRCA1/2 or p53 mutations or their first-degree relatives or patients with family history consistent with hereditary breast ovarian cancer syndrome or family history consistent with Li-Fraumeni syndrome (18.5%)	Annual mammo / Annual MRI	40%	93%	77%	81%

			CBE	US	Mammo	MRI
Kuhl et al. (36) (529)	≥20% breast cancer risk (8.1%)	CBE q 6 mo US q 6 mo Annual mammo Annual MRI	33%	97%	91%	97%
Sardanelli et al. (37) (278)	*BRCA1/2* mutation carriers or their first-degree relatives or patients with strong family history of breast or ovarian cancer	Annual CBE Annual US Annual mammo Annual MRI	59%	Not reported	94%	Not reported

[a] Sensitivity for the detection of all breast cancers (both invasive and in situ).

[b] MRI and mammo performed 6 mo apart from one another.

Abbreviations: CBE, clinical breast examination; mammo, mammography; MRI, magnetic resonance imaging; US, ultrasound.

The second study evaluated a screening program consisting of yearly MRI and mammography in addition to CBE every six months in a population of women whose cumulative lifetime breast cancer risk exceeded 15%. Among the screening cohort of 1909 women, 354 had known *BRCA1/2* mutations. During a median 2.9 years of followup, the screening program identified 41 cancers. The highest rate of detection (26.5 per 1000) was observed in women with germline mutations predisposing to breast cancer, most of whom had *BRCA1/2* mutations. Four interval malignancies were observed. The sensitivity of MRI for the detection of invasive breast cancer was 79.5% in comparison to 33.3% for mammography. However, the specificity of MRI was lower than that of mammography (89.8% vs. 95%), with a positive predictive value of only 7.1% for MRI. The malignancies identified with this screening program were compared to those of two historical control groups and were more likely to be smaller and node negative. Notably, several cases of ductal carcinoma in situ (DCIS) were missed by MRI in this trial (32).

The third study, which was limited to women with known *BRCA1/2* mutations, evaluated a Canadian screening program consisting of yearly MRI, mammography, and ultrasound performed the same day and CBE performed every six months. All women underwent one to three rounds of screening. The screening program identified a total of 22 breast cancers, 16 of which were invasive. The sensitivity of MRI was noted to be 77%, whereas the sensitivity of the MRI, mammography, ultrasound, and CBE performed together in accordance with the protocol was 95%. False-positive MRI rates were noted to be higher on the first round of screening in this study and to decline thereafter. The overall specificity of MRI was 95.4% with a positive predictive value of 46%. Only one interval malignancy was noted during this study. Of all the malignancies that occurred in the participants of this study, only two were associated with axillary lymph node metastases (33).

In the fourth study, Lehman et al. evaluated an MRI-based screening program in a heterogeneous international group of 367 women with above 25% lifetime breast cancer risk based on family history or genetic testing. The proportion of participants with *BRCA1/2* mutations is not reported. The screening program consisted of MRI, mammography, and CBE performed once within 90 days of each other. A total of four malignancies were identified, all of which were small and node negative. Notably, MRI detected all four of these malignancies whereas mammography detected only one. The sensitivity and specificity of MRI were 100% and 94.5%, respectively, but the positive predictive value was only 16.7%, with MRI resulting in multiple false-positive reports, which led to further imaging and/or biopsies (34).

The fifth prospective MRI screening study performed to date was a multicenter British study evaluating a program consisting of annual MRI, mammography, and CBE all performed on the same day [Magnetic Resonance Imaging for Breast Screening (MARIBS) trial]. The participants were known carriers of *BRCA1/2* mutations, *p53* mutations, their first-degree relatives or women with family histories consistent with hereditary breast–ovarian cancer syndrome or Li–Fraumeni syndrome. Of the 649 participants, 120 had known *BRCA1/2* mutations. The study population underwent two to seven screening cycles. The sensitivity and specificity of MRI in this study were 77% and 81%, respectively, in comparison to 40% and 93% for mammography. The sensitivity and specificity of the combined screening program using MRI, mammography, and CBE were 94% and 77%, respectively. Thus, the addition of MRI to mammography in this study increased sensitivity but reduced specificity. Notably, subgroup analysis revealed that the increase in sensitivity from the addition of MRI was significant in women with *BRCA1* mutations or with relatives with *BRCA1* mutations but not significant in women with *BRCA2* mutations or with relatives with *BRCA2* mutations. False-positive MRI assessments in this study required further evaluation at a rate of 10.7% per woman-year, with a reported positive predictive value of MRI of only 7.3%. A total of 35 malignancies were identified in women participating in this study, only two of which presented as interval malignancies. The overwhelming proportion of invasive malignancies identified in this study was small and node negative. There were three cases of DCIS that were identified by mammography but not by MRI in this trial (35).

The sixth prospective screening study of MRI to date evaluated 529 women with at least 20% lifetime risk of breast cancer with annual CBE, MRI, ultrasound, and mammography, all performed within eight weeks of one another. In addition, half-yearly CBE and ultrasound were performed between annual surveillance rounds. In the cohort, 43 women had known *BRCA1/2* mutations. Each woman underwent two to seven screening cycles. A total of 43 malignancies were identified, only one of which was diagnosed between scheduled screening intervals. The sensitivity, specificity, and positive predictive value of MRI in this study were 90.7%, 97.2%, and 50%, respectively. Notably, the addition of MRI to mammography alone resulted in an increase in sensitivity from 32.6% for mammography alone to 93% for the two modalities combined. However, among the subgroup with known *BRCA1/2* mutations, the sensitivity of the two modalities combined was 100%. The decrement in specificity with the addition of MRI to mammography was minimal, dropping from 96.8% for mammography alone to 96.1% for the two modalities combined in the cohort as a whole. However, in *BRCA1/2* mutation carriers, the specificity of the two modalities combined was 94.4%. Notably, there was one case of DCIS, which was missed by MRI and diagnosed by mammography alone in this trial. As with the other MRI screening studies described above, most of the cancers diagnosed were of an early stage (36).

The final prospective MRI screening study to date was a nonrandomized prospective trial performed at multiple centers throughout Italy (High Breast Cancer Risk Italian Trial). Two hundred and seventy eight women and men with known *BRCA1/ 2* mutations or first-degree relatives with known *BRCA1/2* mutations or strong family histories of breast and/or ovarian cancer were enrolled. Among the study population, 63% had either known *BRCA1/2* mutations or were the first-degree relatives of *BRCA1/2* mutation carriers. The screening protocol consisted of CBE, mammography, ultrasound, and MRI performed annually. The interim results reported to date describe the results of the first one or two screening rounds for each subject. A total of 18 malignancies have been identified to date (11 in the first round and 7 in the second round), 6 of which were detected by MRI only. Among these, 4 are in situ and 14 are invasive. Among those for which axillary lymph nodes have been assessed, only 23% are positive. No interval cancers have been reported to date. The sensitivity and positive predictive value of MRI are reported to be 94% and 63%, respectively (37).

In sum, these trials demonstrate that MRI offers greater sensitivity but lower specificity than mammography for the diagnosis of breast cancer in high-risk women. As noted above, sensitivities of MRI for the detection of invasive breast cancer range from 71% to 100% whereas specificities range from 81% to 97.2%. False-positive MRI results, however, are not infrequent, as demonstrated by the positive predictive values reported in the above studies, which range from 7% to 63%. In general, the breast cancers identified through screening programs involving MRI have been small and have not metastasized to the axillary lymph nodes (31–37). It should be noted, however, that despite improved sensitivity for the detection of invasive breast cancer, several of the studies to date have demonstrated that MRI is not as sensitive for the detection of DCIS as mammography (32,35,36). In addition, it is important to note that the sensitivity and specificity of MRI differs depending on the criteria used to define a positive imaging study and slightly different criteria have been reported in the MRI screening trials performed to date (32).

Based on these results, the addition of MRI to a screening program already involving mammography and CBE is the growing standard of care for *BRCA1/2* mutation carriers. However, many unanswered questions regarding the optimal screening regimen for *BRCA1/2* mutation carriers remain.

There have been no randomized studies assessing the role of MRI in breast cancer screening in this population, although it is unlikely that such studies could accrue participants now as MRI is widely available and recommended by a number of organizations (38–41). In addition, unlike mammography, the trials to date have not demonstrated a mortality benefit for screening breast MRI (39,42).

Furthermore, the screening regimens in each of the recent prospective screening trials for high-risk women have differed with regard to imaging modalities and schedule. Some have incorporated ultrasound, although the role of ultrasound in screening programs for high-risk women currently remains undefined. With regard to schedule, breast cancer screening has traditionally been performed annually. However, since *BRCA1/2* mutation–associated breast cancers have shorter doubling times than sporadic breast cancers and the diagnosis of breast cancer between regularly scheduled screening intervals is not uncommon in *BRCA1/2* mutation carriers, some have considered shortening the screening interval in this population (22,43). Although the MRI-based screening trials above all involved annual mammography and MRI, some also involved more frequent ultrasound and CBE (32,33,36). In addition, in the first trial, Tilanus–Linthorst et al. staggered the MRI and mammography such that the interval between imaging studies was six months (31). At this time, the optimal schedule and combination of imaging modalities for screening women with *BRCA1/2* mutations for breast cancer is still unknown (39).

In addition, technical issues still limit the widespread use of MRI for breast cancer screening. Optimizing breast MRI requires a dedicated breast coil, a well-established technique, radiologist expertise, and the ability to perform MRI-guided breast biopsies, which are not yet available at all centers (39,41). Furthermore, variations in enhancement throughout the menstrual cycle make timing important to the interpretation of MRI. Mid-cycle is thought to be the optimal time to perform breast MRI (42).

A further concern that may limit uptake of breast MRI for screening is its cost. Cost-effectiveness assessments are currently under way. One recent report suggested that the cost-effectiveness of MRI varies with age and *BRCA* mutation. Using a threshold of US$100,000 per quality adjusted life year added, MRI was found to be cost-effective for *BRCA1* mutation carriers aged 35 to 54 and for *BRCA2* mutation carriers with dense breasts in whom mammography is not very sensitive. The cost-effectiveness of MRI is thought to differ for *BRCA1* and *BRCA2* mutation carriers because the incidence of breast cancer differs by gene mutation. In addition, the cost-effectiveness is thought to vary by age based on the frequency of breast cancer at different ages in mutation carriers and based on the frequency of comorbid medical conditions at different ages (44). Despite these cost-effectiveness findings, MRI is currently recommended for breast cancer screening for all women with *BRCA1/2* mutations after approximately age 25 (41).

In addition to differential cost-effectiveness by *BRCA* mutation, the MARIBS trial suggested that the sensitivity of MRI may also vary by *BRCA* mutation. In this trial, subgroup analysis revealed that the addition of MRI to mammography resulted in a statistically significant improvement in sensitivity for *BRCA1* mutation carriers but not *BRCA2* mutation carriers (35). This finding remains to be confirmed and, as noted above, MRI screening is currently recommended in both *BRCA1* and *BRCA2* mutation carriers. This differential sensitivity by mutation is thought to be related to the greater age-specific risk of breast cancer in *BRCA1* mutation carriers than *BRCA2* mutation carriers in the young population included in the MARIBS trial (age 35–49) (41).

False-positive MRI results also remain a significant concern. These generally require follow-up evaluation and may be associated with significant patient anxiety. However, screening breast MRI is less likely to be falsely positive in *BRCA1/2* mutation carriers than noncarriers, supporting the use of screening breast MRI in this population (15).

Finally, claustrophobia and the inability to perform MRI in patients with aneurysm clips and pacemakers may limit the use of screening breast MRI in select patients (42).

Despite the remaining unanswered questions about screening MRI and its limitations, its use is becoming widespread. Indeed the most recent National Comprehensive Cancer Network (NCCN) guidelines recommend annual MRI and mammography with CBE every six months starting at age 25 for breast cancer screening in women who meet criteria for the hereditary breast–ovarian cancer syndrome (41). In addition, the American Cancer Society now recommends annual MRI for women whose lifetime breast cancer risk exceeds 20–25% (40).

BREAST CANCER PREVENTION IN UNAFFECTED *BRCA1/2* MUTATION CARRIERS

Despite the advances in breast cancer screening for the early detection of breast cancer in high-risk women, many *BRCA1/2* mutation carriers also take steps to prevent the development of the disease. Prevention options available to *BRCA1/2* mutation carriers include both surgical and chemoprevention approaches.

Risk-Reducing Surgery

Risk-reducing surgical options for *BRCA1/2* mutation carriers at risk for breast cancer include prophylactic bilateral salpingo-oophorectomy (PBSO) and prophylactic bilateral mastectomy (PBM). Although it is not ethically possible to study the impact of these interventions in a randomized manner, there is substantial nonrandomized data to support their efficacy in reducing the risk of breast cancer in comparison to surveillance.

Prophylactic Bilateral Salpingo-Oophorectomy

Several studies have demonstrated that PBSO reduces the risk of breast cancer in *BRCA1/2* mutation carriers by approximately 50%. In a study of 241 unaffected *BRCA1/2* mutation carriers with a median followup of eight years, Rebbeck et al. found that 21 of 99 women undergoing PBSO developed breast cancer in comparison to 60 of 142 of those electing surveillance [hazard ratio (HR) 0.47; 95% confidence interval (CI): 0.29–0.77] (45). Similarly, a prospective single-institution study with a median followup of 24 months by Kauff et al. revealed that among 170 *BRCA1/2* carriers, breast cancer developed in 3 of 98 of those undergoing PBSO as compared to 8 of 72 choosing surveillance (HR 0.32; 95% CI: 0.08–1.20) (46). In a follow-up analysis of pooled data prospectively collected from these two groups, breast cancer was found to occur in 19 of 303 of those undergoing PBSO, as compared to 29 of 296 of those undergoing surveillance (HR 0.48; 95% CI: 0.26–0.90) (47).

Notably, this follow-up analysis suggested that the breast cancer risk reduction benefit offered by PBSO may be limited to *BRCA2* mutation carriers, a finding which may be explained by the higher frequency of estrogen receptor–positive breast cancer in *BRCA2* mutation–associated breast cancer than *BRCA1* mutation–associated breast cancer (47–49). However, a prior retrospective case-control study demonstrated a similar degree of risk reduction for *BRCA1* and *BRCA2* mutation carriers who had undergone PBSO (56% for *BRCA1*, 46% for *BRCA2*) (50). Thus, the potential for differential efficacy of PBSO for *BRCA1* and *BRCA2* mutation carriers requires further study and the procedure is currently considered to be an appropriate option for breast cancer risk reduction for both groups of women (51).

The breast cancer protection offered by PBSO varies with age and is the greatest when the procedure is performed in younger women. Indeed, PBSO does not offer any breast cancer protection if performed after the age of 50, suggesting that its efficacy may be due to the induction of premature menopause (45,50,52,53). Obviously, since it induces menopause, it is recommended that PBSO is deferred until the completion of childbearing (41).

Despite the fact that PBSO induces menopause, a recent study carried out in women with a hereditary predisposition to ovarian cancer suggested that this procedure does not have negative impact on overall quality of life. Not surprisingly, high-risk women choosing this procedure reported increased endocrine symptoms and worse sexual function than those choosing screening. However, those undergoing PBSO reported significantly fewer cancer-related worries (54).

In order to alleviate menopausal symptoms, some clinicians prescribe hormone replacement therapy (HRT) following PBSO. There are data indicating that such an approach does not negate the beneficial effect of PBSO on breast cancer risk reduction (55). However, little information exists on the impact of duration of use of HRT after PBSO on breast cancer risk. In cases in which HRT is utilized, most clinicians try to use it for the shortest period of time necessary to relieve menopausal symptoms and recommend that it be discontinued prior to the age of 50, the age after which it has been shown to increase breast cancer risk in the general population (56).

In addition to reducing the risk of breast cancer in *BRCA1/2* mutation carriers, a recent prospective observational study has suggested that PBSO may also provide a mortality benefit in this population. In this study, 271 *BRCA1/2* mutation carriers who had not undergone PBSO were matched with 155 *BRCA1/2* carriers who had undergone the procedure. With a median followup of approximately two years, PBSO was found to be associated with a 76% reduction in overall mortality (HR 0.24; 95% CI: 0.08–0.71) and a 90% reduction in breast cancer–specific mortality (HR 0.10; 95% CI: 0.02–0.71) (57).

PBSO is associated with a low complication rate provided that it is performed by an experienced surgeon (46). Approximately one-quarter of women found to have *BRCA1/2* mutations chose to undergo PBSO within one year of learning their mutation status (58). According to current guidelines, PBSO should be considered for breast cancer risk reduction in women with known or strongly suspected *BRCA1/2* mutations, who desire the procedure (51). Notably, PBSO is also a means of ovarian cancer prevention in *BRCA1/2* mutation carriers. A detailed discussion of the impact of PBSO on ovarian cancer risk is found in Chapter 16. In clinical practice, women with *BRCA1/2* mutations are strongly encouraged to undergo PBSO after the completion of childbearing, although this strong recommendation is more due to its substantial impact on ovarian cancer risk reduction than its weaker effect on breast cancer risk reduction.

Prophylactic Bilateral Mastectomy

PBM has also been shown to be an effective means of breast cancer risk reduction in *BRCA1/2* mutation carriers. Meijers–Heijboer et al. prospectively followed 139 *BRCA1/2* carriers, 76 of whom chose PBM, and 63 of whom elected to undergo intensive surveillance. Initial findings revealed a 95% reduction in the risk of breast cancer associated with

PBM (59). In a recent update with 5.2 years median followup, one of the women in the PBM group developed metastatic breast cancer, suggesting the presence of an occult malignancy at the time of her PBM, as compared with nine of the women in the surveillance group. Notably, three of the women in the surveillance arm chose to undergo PBM during the longer follow-up period and were censored at that time. The breast cancer risk reduction provided by PBM was 92% and was significant after adjusting for both age and whether or not PBSO was also performed (60).

A second study with a mixed prospective/retrospective design evaluated the effect of PBM in 483 *BRCA1/2* mutation carriers. Those undergoing PBM were followed for a median of 5.5 years after their surgeries and those electing surveillance (controls) had a median followup of 6.7 years. Two of the 105 carriers (1.9%) who underwent PBM developed subsequent breast cancer, as compared with 184 of the 378 controls (48.7%). PBM reduced the risk of breast cancer by approximately 90% in women with intact ovarian function and by approximately 95% in women who had also undergone PBSO (61).

Hartmann et al. reported a third study of PBM, which was not limited to *BRCA1/2* mutation carriers but which revealed a similar degree of breast cancer risk reduction. In this retrospective study, 214 women with family histories of breast cancer who underwent PBM were compared to sister controls who had not undergone PBM. Among this high-risk group, PBM reduced the risk of breast cancer by 90–94% (62). In a substudy, Hartmann et al. reported that *BRCA1/2* mutations were identified in 26 of the 214 high-risk women who had undergone PBM included in their original publication. Of these 26, none had developed breast cancer after 13.5 years median followup. However, three other women, two of whom did not harbor *BRCA1/2* mutations and one whose mutation status was not able to be determined, developed breast cancer after PBM. Analysis both assuming and not assuming that this woman had a *BRCA1/2* mutation revealed that PBM reduced the risk of breast cancer by 89.5% to 100% (63).

Although some view PBM as a radical surgical procedure, follow-up studies indicate women are generally satisfied with the procedure. Frost et al. reported a descriptive study in which women at risk for hereditary breast cancer who had undergone PBM completed a questionnaire. They identified a 70% satisfaction rate. Notably, 74% of the participants reported a reduction in worry about developing breast cancer after undergoing PBM. Few women reported adverse effects of the procedure on level of stress, self-esteem, sexual relationships, and feelings of femininity or emotional stability (64). In another similar questionnaire study, Bresser et al. reported a 60% satisfaction rate among women who underwent PBM with reconstruction; however, 44% reported a negative change in their sexual relationships as a result of the procedure. A negative impact on sexual relationships was associated with lack of information, emphasizing the importance of adequate preoperative counseling and informed consent prior to PBM (65).

It is imperative that PBM specimens undergo rigorous pathologic analysis as there is a substantial risk of identifying premalignant or occult malignant lesions. In one prospective study, occult invasive breast cancer was found in 1% of PBM specimens (62). The likelihood of identifying high-risk lesions and in situ malignancies is even higher, with studies demonstrating up to approximately 50% risk of identifying atypical ductal hyperplasia, atypical lobular hyperplasia, DCIS, or lobular carcinoma in situ (LCIS) in PBM specimens from high-risk women (59,66,67).

The type of surgical procedure to perform for PBM is somewhat controversial. Although it is associated with a better cosmetic outcome by preserving the nipple–areola complex, most do not recommend the subcutaneous mastectomy as it does not remove all at-risk tissue. One prospective study revealed that the only cases of breast cancer after

PBM occurred after subcutaneous mastectomy (61). Despite this, some have suggested that subcutaneous mastectomy be performed since the local failure rate is still low and cosmesis is superior (68). Indeed, the optimal surgical procedure is currently unknown and should be addressed on an individual level with each patient until clinical trials can settle the issue.

The decision to undergo PBM is an individual one, but it is appropriate to consider in any woman with a known *BRCA1/2* mutation. Such patients usually undergo evaluation with a surgeon and a reconstructive surgeon prior to the procedure. Psychological evaluation is also recommended in some cases. In addition, many physicians perform MRI prior to PBM in order to detect occult malignancies. Axillary lymph node assessment does not need to be performed at the time of PBM, although it is not unreasonable to consider a sentinel lymph node procedure in the event that an occult malignancy is detected (51).

Chemoprevention

The use of selective estrogen receptor modulators for breast cancer chemoprevention originated when studies of tamoxifen in the adjuvant setting demonstrated a reduction in the incidence of metachronous primary CBC (69). Despite these findings, results of studies of tamoxifen for breast cancer prevention in high-risk women have been variable.

Fisher et al. reported the largest study of tamoxifen chemoprevention performed to date—the National Surgical Breast and Bowel Project Breast Cancer Prevention (NSABP P1) trial. In this trial, a heterogeneous group of 13,388 high-risk women, only a small fraction of whom faced increased breast cancer risk due to strong family history, were randomized to tamoxifen 20 mg daily for five years or placebo. After 69 months median followup, tamoxifen was reported to reduce the risk of invasive breast cancer by 49% and the risk of noninvasive breast cancer by 50%. Notably, it reduced the risk of estrogen receptor–positive breast cancer by 69%, but had no impact on the risk of estrogen receptor–negative breast cancer. Tamoxifen also reduced the risk of osteoporotic fractures. Risks of endometrial cancer, stroke, deep vein thrombosis, and pulmonary embolism were all higher in the tamoxifen arm, although this was largely limited to women older than 50 (70). Despite the study being unblinded after publication of the initial results, a recent update, now with seven years median followup indicates similar reductions in invasive and noninvasive breast cancer risks [risk ratio (RR) 0.57 and 0.63, respectively] (71).

In contrast to the NSABP P1 study, two smaller European studies did not show a benefit of tamoxifen in reducing the risk of breast cancer. In the Italian Tamoxifen Prevention study, 5408 low-to-normal-risk women who had undergone hysterectomy were randomized to tamoxifen 20 mg daily for five years or placebo. Notably, concurrent HRT was permitted. With a median followup of 46 months, this underpowered trial did not identify a difference in breast cancer incidence between the two arms in the group as a whole, although there was a reduction in the incidence of breast cancer associated with tamoxifen in the women taking concurrent HRT (72). In the Royal Marsden Hospital Tamoxifen Chemoprevention trial, 2471 healthy women at increased breast cancer risk due to family history were randomized to tamoxifen 20 mg daily or placebo for up to eight years. No difference in the incidence of breast cancer was seen between the two arms (RR 1.06; 95% CI: 0.7–1.7; $p = 0.8$). Concurrent HRT was also permitted in this study (73).

The results of the most recent tamoxifen chemoprevention study, the International Breast Cancer Intervention Study I (IBIS-I), are concordant with those of the NSABP P1 study. In this trial, 7152 women at increased risk for breast cancer, largely based on family history although some were based on personal history of benign breast disease or LCIS, were randomized to tamoxifen 20 mg daily for five years or placebo. Concurrent HRT was also permitted in this trial. Initial results with a median followup of 50 months revealed a 32% reduction in the risk of breast cancer in the tamoxifen arm (74). A recently reported update of the IBIS-I study, now with median followup of 96 months, reveals that the reduction of breast cancer incidence associated with tamoxifen persists after the five years of therapy (RR 0.73; 95% CI: 0.58–0.91; $p = 0.004$). As with the NSABP P1 study, tamoxifen prevented only estrogen receptor–positive breast cancers in this trial (75).

The explanation for the different results reported to date regarding the ability of tamoxifen to prevent breast cancer is not clear. It is possible that no effect was seen in the Italian trial because a lower-risk population was studied, because it was underpowered, and because concurrent HRT was permitted. It is possible that the Royal Marsden Hospital study was also negative due to the confounding effect of concurrent HRT; however, the IBIS-I trial also allowed concurrent HRT and was not a negative study. In addition, the high-risk participants included in the NSABP P1, Royal Marsden Hospital, and IBIS-I trials differed, with the P1 participants largely at increased risk due to non-genetic factors and the Royal Marsden Hospital and IBIS-I participants largely at increased risk due to inherited factors. It is possible the effects of tamoxifen differ in these populations, although this would not explain the concordance of the NSABP P1 and IBIS-I trials. Based on these discordant results, the risk–benefit ratio for tamoxifen chemoprevention is unclear.

None of the tamoxifen prevention trials to date have been limited to women with known *BRCA1/2* mutations and there is significant controversy surrounding whether tamoxifen breast cancer chemoprevention is beneficial in this population. Genomic analysis for *BRCA1/2* mutations was performed in 288 breast cancer cases that occurred in the NSABP P1 study participant. This identified 8 *BRCA1* mutations and 11 *BRCA2* mutations. No reduction in the risk of breast cancer associated with tamoxifen was identified in the *BRCA1* mutation carriers (RR 1.67; 95% CI: 0.32–10.70), whereas a trend toward a reduction in the risk of breast cancer associated with tamoxifen was identified in the *BRCA2* mutation carriers (RR 0.38; 95% CI: 0.06–1.56). This difference was attributed to the fact that *BRCA2* mutation–associated breast cancers are more frequently estrogen-receptor positive than *BRCA1* mutation–associated breast cancers (76). It should be noted, however, that the numbers of *BRCA1/2* mutations identified in this substudy are small and the confidence intervals are broad; thus, one cannot draw conclusions from these findings.

In addition, the likelihood of carrying a *BRCA1/2* mutation was calculated using the Claus model for all 70 cases of breast cancer that developed in participants of the Royal Marsden Hospital tamoxifen chemoprevention trial. *BRCA1/2* mutation analysis was performed on 62 of the 70 breast cancer cases. There was a nonsignificant trend toward reduced risk of breast cancer developing in women taking tamoxifen, who had lower likelihood of carrying a *BRCA1/2* mutation but not in those with higher likelihood. However, only four *BRCA1/2* mutations were identified in the study, although some cases may have been missed due to technical issues (77). As with the NSABP P1 substudy described above, this substudy is limited by small numbers but does raise questions about the benefit of tamoxifen for chemoprevention in *BRCA1/2* mutation carriers. This questionable benefit is likely limited to *BRCA1* mutation carriers in whom breast cancers are more likely to be estrogen-receptor negative (78).

In addition to its questionable efficacy in *BRCA1/2* mutation carriers, such women must consider the potential side effects associated with tamoxifen that have been identified in the prevention trials to date. It should be noted, however, that the most significant of these, thromboembolism and endometrial cancer, are greatest in older women, and it is younger *BRCA1/2* mutation carriers who are most likely to consider tamoxifen chemoprevention. Given these uncertainties and risks, the true benefit of tamoxifen for chemoprevention in *BRCA1/2* mutation carriers is not known and the decision to undergo tamoxifen chemoprevention is a personal choice.

New agents for breast cancer prevention in high-risk women are currently being evaluated. After being observed to reduce breast cancer incidence during osteoporosis trials, raloxifene was compared to tamoxifen for breast cancer prevention in the NSABP P2 Study of Tamoxifen and Raloxifene (79). This trial compared tamoxifen 20 mg daily to raloxifene 60 mg daily in a heterogeneous population of postmenopausal women at increased risk for breast cancer. They found no difference in the risk of invasive breast cancer between the two arms (RR 1.02; 95% CI: 0.82–1.28), but there was a trend toward less noninvasive breast cancer in the tamoxifen arm (RR 1.40; 95% CI: 0.89–2.00). The explanation for this finding is unclear. The side-effect profile associated with raloxifene is superior, with fewer cases of venous thromboembolism and uterine cancer (80,81). Data regarding the efficacy of raloxifene for breast cancer prevention in *BRCA1/2* mutation carriers are not available.

Similar to tamoxifen, aromatase inhibitors have also been noted to reduce the incidence of new primary metachronous CBC in women treated in the adjuvant setting (82,83). As a result, anastrozole and exemestane are currently being evaluated for the prevention of breast cancer in high-risk women in the IBIS-II trial and MAP.3 trials, respectively (84,85).

Current NCCN guidelines recommend that tamoxifen or raloxifene (for postmenopausal women) be considered for breast cancer prevention in high-risk women (51). However, as noted above, data regarding the benefit in the *BRCA1/2* heterozygote population is minimal; thus, the choice regarding chemoprevention is personal and should be made with clinician guidance, considering both the risks and the benefits.

BREAST CANCER SCREENING AND PREVENTION IN AFFECTED *BRCA1/2* MUTATION CARRIERS

In addition to the risk posed by their breast cancers, affected *BRCA1/2* mutation carriers are at elevated risk for metachronous breast cancer. Multiple series have demonstrated that the risk of metachronous CBC in *BRCA1/2* mutation carriers is 25% to 40% after 10 to 20 years (4–8). This risk is particularly high in *BRCA1/2* mutation carriers diagnosed at a young age (6). Although results have varied, most studies have suggested that the risk of ipsilateral breast tumor recurrence (IBTR) in affected *BRCA1/2* mutation carriers treated with breast conserving therapy is approximately 10% to 20%, which is similar to that for women with sporadic breast cancer treated with breast conserving therapy (46–8,10,86–88). However, affected women with *BRCA1/2* mutations, who undergo breast conserving therapy have been noted to develop late ipsilateral recurrences that often occur in different quadrants from their original malignancies, suggesting that they are at elevated risk for developing new primary future ipsilateral breast cancers (7,9). These rates of metachronous ipsilateral and CBCs in affected *BRCA1/2* mutation carriers underscore the importance of continued screening and consideration of prevention interventions in affected *BRCA1/2* mutation carriers who retain breast tissue.

With regard to screening, no specific guidelines exist for *BRCA1/2* mutation carriers who have previously had breast cancer. However, women with prior breast cancer were included in many of the breast MRI screening trials for high-risk women (33,34,36,37). Thus, most clinicians recommend following the previously described screening guidelines, using MRI, mammography, and CBE for ongoing surveillance to detect metachronous ipsilateral and contralateral primary breast cancers in this population.

Due to the substantial risk of future breast cancer, some affected *BRCA1/2* mutation carriers choose to undergo mastectomy for their affected breast with concurrent prophylactic contralateral mastectomy (PCM) as an intervention to both treat their current breast cancer and prevent future breast cancer. Notably, PCM at the time of mastectomy for a diagnosis of breast cancer has not been shown to improve survival (4).

The decision to pursue mastectomy for the affected breast with PCM is an individual choice. As is the case with PBM, studies demonstrate that women who chose PCM are satisfied with the outcome and do not experience adverse effects on emotional well-being. A descriptive study of 583 women who underwent PCM identified an 83% satisfaction rate after a mean 10.3 years following the procedure. However, approximately 25% of women reported adverse effects of the procedure on feelings of femininity, sexual relationships, and satisfaction with physical appearance, emphasizing the need for careful discussion of the risks and benefits of the procedure with affected women making their surgical plans. Notably, in this study, the type of mastectomy impacted satisfaction with a higher dissatisfaction rate among those who underwent subcutaneous PCM than those who underwent simple PCM (89). Another recent study evaluated predictors and outcomes of PCM in 435 women within one year of *BRCA1/2* mutation testing. Among those found to have *BRCA1/2* mutations, 18% chose PCM. Younger age at diagnosis and higher baseline levels of cancer-specific distress also predicted for choosing PCM. The procedure did not have a negative impact on distress levels (90).

Since surgical decisions need to be made fairly quickly at the time of breast cancer diagnosis, some have advocated peri-diagnostic genetic counseling and testing for women at high risk for harboring *BRCA1/2* mutations, who have not undergone previous genetic testing. This approach has been shown to be feasible and to impact surgical decisions. In a prospective study of peri-diagnostic genetic testing and counseling in 194 women newly diagnosed with breast cancer, who had at least 10% likelihood of carrying a *BRCA1/2* mutation, 48% of those found to have *BRCA1/2* mutations chose PCM (91). As is the case with PCM performed in affected women previously identified as *BRCA1/2* mutation carriers, PCM performed in affected women who undergo peri-diagnostic genetic counseling and testing has been shown not to have a negative impact on quality of life or distress levels (92).

Despite the feasibility of peri-diagnostic genetic counseling and testing, the decision to perform PCM does not need to be made immediately at the time of breast cancer diagnosis in women at high risk for carrying *BRCA1/2* mutations or known mutation carriers. If peri-diagnostic genetic testing is not available or desired or known *BRCA1/2* mutation carriers do not wish to pursue immediate therapeutic mastectomy with PCM, it is possible to initially perform breast-conserving surgery and to then proceed with systemic chemotherapy. Such women can undergo genetic counseling and testing if necessary during their adjuvant chemotherapy and can then opt for mastectomy of the affected side plus PCM after the conclusion of their chemotherapy. This approach does not impact their breast cancer treatment and avoids the radiation that would be required to complete their breast conserving therapy. In one study, 17% of patients who initially chose breast conservation but who were then identified as *BRCA1/2* mutation carriers ultimately chose mastectomy of the affected side with PCM prior to radiation therapy (93).

BRCA1/2 mutation status does not currently impact decisions regarding systemic therapy for breast cancer. This topic is reviewed in detail in Chapter 21.

However, a remaining question is whether systemic chemotherapy influences the risk of metachronous CBC. One retrospective study suggested that adjuvant chemotherapy reduces the risk of metachronous CBC in *BRCA1/2* mutation carriers [odds ratio (OR) 0.40; 95% CI: 0.26–0.80] (12). In contrast, a prospective study of 491 *BRCA1/2* mutation carriers with Stage I–II breast cancer did not find an impact of adjuvant chemotherapy on risk of subsequent metachronous CBC (6). The risk of metachronous CBC is not currently considered in decisions regarding adjuvant chemotherapy in affected *BRCA1/2* mutation carriers.

Substantial data indicates that hormonal interventions (tamoxifen and oophorectomy) for the treatment of breast cancer in affected *BRCA1/2* mutation carriers impact their risk of metachronous contralateral and ipsilateral breast cancer. However, it must be noted that the choice to use adjuvant hormonal therapy is made based on the hormone receptor status of the breast cancer at hand and not on *BRCA1/2* mutation status.

Narod et al. reported a case control study in which 209 *BRCA1/2* mutation carriers with bilateral breast cancer were compared with 384 *BRCA1/2* mutation carriers with unilateral breast cancer. A history of tamoxifen treatment for the first breast cancer was associated with a 50% reduction in the odds of developing bilateral disease (OR 0.5; 95% CI: 0.28–0.89). Among the subset of patients diagnosed with their first breast cancer prior to the age of 50, oophorectomy reduced the odds of having bilateral breast cancer by 69% (OR 0.31; 95% CI: 0.15–0.67). As is the case with PBSO, the effect of oophorectomy for prevention of new primary breast cancers in affected older women was less profound than that in premenopausal women. Notably, the protective effect of tamoxifen observed in this study was evident regardless of whether oophorectomy had been performed. Unfortunately, estrogen receptor status was not available for most women included in this study (12).

More recently, Gronwald et al. reported a case-control study in 285 *BRCA1/2* mutation carriers with bilateral breast cancer and 751 *BRCA1/2* mutation carriers with unilateral breast cancer. This study confirmed an approximately 50% reduction in bilateral disease in both *BRCA1* and *BRCA2* mutation carriers who were treated with tamoxifen. However, they did not observe an additive protective effect of tamoxifen in women who had undergone oophorectomy, although this subgroup was small (OR 0.83; 95% CI: 0.24–2.89) (11).

In a recent prospective study, Metcalfe et al. identified factors that impact the risk of metachronous CBC in a cohort of 491 *BRCA1/2* mutation carriers with Stage I–II breast cancer. Similar to the above-described retrospective series, they identified a 41% reduction in risk with tamoxifen use (HR 0.59; 95% CI: 0.35–1.01; $p = 0.05$), although this was not significant on multivariate analysis. They also identified a 56% reduction in risk with a history of oophorectomy (HR 0.44; 95% CI: 0.21–0.91). The impact of oophorectomy on risk reduction was greatest in women diagnosed prior to age 50 (HR 0.24; 95% CI: 0.07–0.77). Again, information regarding hormone receptor status was not available for many subjects in this study (6).

Pierce et al. performed a retrospective cohort study assessing the rate of metachronous ipsilateral and CBC among 160 affected *BRCA1/2* mutation carriers and 445 controls with sporadic breast cancer. As expected, rates of CBC were greater among *BRCA1/2* mutation carriers than sporadic controls whereas rates of IBTR did not differ between the two groups as a whole. Among the *BRCA1/2* mutation carriers group, nonsignificant trends toward reduced risk of IBTR with oophorectomy and tamoxifen were observed (HR 0.55; $p = 0.44$ and HR 0.29; $p = 0.22$, respectively). With regard to CBC in the *BRCA1/2* mutation carrier group, tamoxifen was associated with a 69% reduction in risk ($p = 0.05$) and oophorectomy was associated with a nonsignificant reduction in risk (HR 0.46; $p = 0.15$) (7).

Although commonly used in the adjuvant treatment of breast cancer, there are no data as yet available regarding the impact of aromatase inhibitors on the risks of metachronous ipsilateral and CBCs in affected *BRCA1/2* mutation carriers.

FUTURE DIRECTIONS

Although progress in breast cancer screening and prevention for *BRCA1/2* mutation carriers has been substantial in recent years, the burden of breast cancer risk faced by this population calls for further improvements still.

With regard to screening, MRI in addition to mammography is rapidly becoming the standard of care for breast cancer screening in *BRCA1/2* mutation carriers. However, further research is required to optimize screening protocols such that the best approach to integrating MRI and other screening techniques can be determined.

Improving breast cancer prevention in *BRCA1/2* mutation carriers is an active area of ongoing research. Given that most *BRCA1* mutation–associated breast cancers are estrogen-receptor negative, current investigation focuses on non-hormonal approaches to the prevention of breast cancer in this high-risk population (48). Two avenues under active study are poly(ADP-ribose) polymerase (PARP-1) inhibitors and retinoids.

PARP-1 is an enzyme involved in the repair of single-strand DNA breaks. In the absence of PARP-1 activity, single-strand DNA breaks may go uncorrected and become double-strand DNA breaks. The repair of double-strand DNA breaks often occurs via homologous recombination, a process that is dependent on *BRCA1* and *BRCA2* function. Thus, in *BRCA1*- or *BRCA2*-deficient cells, the inhibition of PARP-1 activity may lead to double-strand DNA breaks that, upon accumulation, result in cell death. Preclinical data using *BRCA*-deficient nonmalignant cells demonstrated efficacy of PARP-1 inhibitors in causing cell death, although this finding has not been reproduced in *BRCA*-deficient malignant cells. It has been suggested that additional genetic mutations, which accumulate during the process of carcinogenesis, may result in insensitivity to PARP-1 inhibition in malignant as opposed to nonmalignant *BRCA*-deficient cells. This has led to the suggestion that PARP-1 inhibition may be a viable approach to breast cancer prevention in *BRCA1/2* mutation carriers. Further preclinical and clinical studies are required to assess this possibility (94–97).

Retinoids are derivatives of Vitamin A that have been shown to be effective in preventing multiple malignances. They act by binding to the retinoid acid receptor and the retinoid X receptor (RXR), leading to modulation of cellular transcription (98). Recently, it has been shown that bexarotene, an RXR-selective retinoid, prevents the development of mammary tumors in animal models (99). This is thought to occur via the inhibition of cyclo-oxygenase-2, the overexpression of which is thought to be involved in the development of breast cancer, especially of the estrogen receptor–negative phenotype (98). It has therefore been suggested that bexarotene may be an effective chemopreventive agent in *BRCA1/2* mutation carriers. A pilot clinical trial evaluating Bexarotene in women with known *BRCA1/2* mutations or those thought to be at high risk for harboring *BRCA1/2* mutations recently completed accrual.

CONCLUSION

The breast cancer risk faced by carriers of *BRCA1/2* mutations is high. There have been significant improvements in the early detection and prevention of these cancers in recent years. In addition, breast cancer therapies have been shown to reduce the risk of new primary breast malignancies in *BRCA1/2* mutation carriers already affected with breast cancer.

Advances in MRI technology have led to a change in the standard of care for breast cancer screening in *BRCA1/2* mutation carriers. It is hoped that the early detection afforded by MRI screening will ultimately lead to a decrease in the morbidity and mortality associated with breast cancer in this population.

Surgical prevention interventions using PBM and PBSO have proven to be effective means of risk reduction in women with *BRCA1/2* mutations. It is anticipated that further clarification regarding the optimal procedure for PBM will be obtained in upcoming years and that developments in the management of menopausal symptoms will further improve quality of life in women after PBSO. Although current options for chemoprevention for breast cancer in *BRCA1/2* mutation carriers are limited to hormonal therapies, ongoing research regarding nonhormonal prevention approaches is promising.

For women with *BRCA1/2* mutations who are already affected with breast cancer, it is important to note that the screening and prevention interventions presented in this chapter that are appropriate for unaffected women should also be applied to affected women for the early detection or prevention of metachronous breast cancers. It is hoped that improvements in adjuvant therapies and, perhaps, the application of new chemopreventive agents such as PARP-1 inhibitors to treatment in the adjuvant setting will further reduce the risk of metachronous primary breast cancers in this population.

Continued research into breast cancer screening and prevention in women with *BRCA1/2* mutations with the goal of minimizing the impact of breast cancer in this population is ongoing. Recent years have brought significant improvements and new avenues of research bring the promise of further hope.

REFERENCES

1. Claus EB, Schildkraut JM, Thompson WD, et al. The genetic attributable risk of breast and ovarian cancer. Cancer 1996; 77:2318–2324.
2. Ford D, Easton DF, Stratton M, et al. Genetic heterogeneity and penetrance analysis of the *BRCA1* and *BRCA2* genes in breast cancer families. The Breast Cancer Linkage Consortium. Am J Hum Genet 1998; 62:676–689.
3. Antoniou A, Pharoah PD, Narod S, et al. Average risks of breast and ovarian cancer associated with *BRCA1* or *BRCA2* mutations detected in case Series unselected for family history: a combined analysis of 22 studies. Am J Hum Genet 2003; 72:1117–1130.
4. Brekelmans CT, Seynaeve C, Menke-Pluymers M, et al. Survival and prognostic factors in *BRCA1*-associated breast cancer. Ann Oncol 2006; 17:391–400.
5. Haffty BG, Harrold E, Khan AJ, et al. Outcome of conservatively managed early-onset breast cancer by *BRCA1/2* status. Lancet 2002; 359:1471–1477.
6. Metcalfe K, Lynch HT, Ghadirian P, et al. Contralateral breast cancer in *BRCA1* and *BRCA2* mutation carriers. J Clin Oncol 2004; 22:2328–2335.
7. Pierce LJ, Levin AM, Rebbeck TR, et al. Ten-year multi-institutional results of breast-conserving surgery and radiotherapy in *BRCA1/2*–associated stage I/II breast cancer. J Clin Oncol 2006; 24:2437–2443.
8. Robson M, Levin D, Federici M, et al. Breast conservation therapy for invasive breast cancer in Ashkenazi women with *BRCA* gene founder mutations. J Natl Cancer Inst 1999; 91:2112–2117.
9. Turner BC, Harrold E, Matloff E, et al. *BRCA1/BRCA2* germline mutations in locally recurrent breast cancer patients after lumpectomy and radiation therapy: implications for breast-conserving management in patients with *BRCA1/BRCA2* mutations. J Clin Oncol 1999; 17:3017–3024.

10. Robson ME, Chappuis PO, Satagopan J, et al. A combined analysis of outcome following breast cancer: differences in survival based on *BRCA1/BRCA2* mutation status and administration of adjuvant treatment. Breast Cancer Res 2004; 6:R8–R17.

11. Gronwald J, Tung N, Foulkes WD, et al. Tamoxifen and contralateral breast cancer in *BRCA1* and *BRCA2* carriers: an update. Int J Cancer 2006; 118:2281–2284.

12. Narod SA, Brunet JS, Ghadirian P, et al. Tamoxifen and risk of contralateral breast cancer in *BRCA1* and *BRCA2* mutation carriers: a case-control study. Hereditary Breast Cancer Clinical Study Group. Lancet 2000; 356:1876–1881.

13. Burke W, Daly M, Garber J, et al. Recommendations for follow-up care of individuals with an inherited predisposition to cancer. II. *BRCA1* and *BRCA2*. Cancer Genetics Studies Consortium. JAMA 1997; 277:997–1003.

14. Tilanus-Linthorst M, Verhoog L, Obdeijn IM, et al. A *BRCA1/2* mutation, high breast density and prominent pushing margins of a tumor independently contribute to a frequent false-negative mammography. Int J Cancer 2002; 102:91–95.

15. Kriege M, Brekelmans CT, Obdeijn IM, et al. Factors affecting sensitivity and specificity of screening mammography and MRI in women with an inherited risk for breast cancer. Breast Cancer Res Treat 2006; 100:109–119.

16. Carney PA, Miglioretti DL, Yankaskas BC, et al. Individual and combined effects of age, breast density, and hormone replacement therapy use on the accuracy of screening mammography. Ann Intern Med 2003; 138:168–175.

17. Mitchell G, Antoniou AC, Warren R, et al. Mammographic density and breast cancer risk in *BRCA1* and *BRCA2* mutation carriers. Cancer Res 2006; 66:1866–1872.

18. McCormack VA, dos Santos Silva I. Breast density and parenchymal patterns as markers of breast cancer risk: a meta-analysis. Cancer Epidemiol Biomark Prev 2006; 15:1159–1169.

19. Haars G, van Noord PA, van Gils CH, et al. Measurements of breast density: no ratio for a ratio. Cancer Epidemiol Biomarkers Prev 2005; 14:2634–2640.

20. Buist DS, Porter PL, Lehman C, et al. Factors contributing to mammography failure in women aged 40–49 years. J Natl Cancer Inst 2004; 96:1432–1440.

21. Scheuer L, Kauff N, Robson M, et al. Outcome of preventive surgery and screening for breast and ovarian cancer in BRCA mutation carriers. J Clin Oncol 2002; 20:1260–1268.

22. Komenaka IK, Ditkoff BA, Joseph KA, et al. The development of interval breast malignancies in patients with BRCA mutations. Cancer 2004; 100:2079–2083.

23. Brekelmans CT, Seynaeve C, Bartels CC, et al. Effectiveness of breast cancer surveillance in *BRCA1/2* gene mutation carriers and women with high familial risk. J Clin Oncol 2001; 19: 924–930.

24. Sharan SK, Morimatsu M, Albrecht U, et al. Embryonic lethality and radiation hypersensitivity mediated by Rad51 in mice lacking *Brca2*. Nature 1997; 386:804–810.

25. Goss PE, Sierra S. Current perspectives on radiation-induced breast cancer. J Clin Oncol 1998; 16:338–347.

26. Andrieu N, Easton DF, Chang-Claude J, et al. Effect of chest x-rays on the risk of breast cancer among *BRCA1/2* mutation carriers in the international *BRCA1/2* carrier cohort study: a report from the EMBRACE, GENEPSO, GEO-HEBON, and IBCCS Collaborators' Group. J Clin Oncol 2006; 24:3361–3366.

27. Benson J. Is screening mammography safe for high-risk patients? Lancet Oncol 2006; 7: 360–362.

28. Narod SA, Lubinski J, Ghadirian P, et al. Screening mammography and risk of breast cancer in *BRCA1* and *BRCA2* mutation carriers: a case-control study. Lancet Oncol 2006; 7:402–406.

29. Goldfrank D, Chuai S, Bernstein JL, et al. Effect of mammography on breast cancer risk in women with mutations in *BRCA1* or *BRCA2*. Cancer Epidemiol Biomark Prev 2006; 15: 2311–2313.

30. Kerlikowske K, Grady D, Rubin SM, et al. Efficacy of screening mammography. A meta-analysis. JAMA 1995; 273:149–154.

31. Tilanus-Linthorst MM, Obdeijn IM, Bartels KC, et al. First experiences in screening women at high risk for breast cancer with MR imaging. Breast Cancer Res Treat 2000; 63:53–60.

32. Kriege M, Brekelmans CT, Boetes C, et al. Efficacy of MRI and mammography for breast-cancer screening in women with a familial or genetic predisposition. N Engl J Med 2004; 351: 427–437.

33. Warner E, Plewes DB, Hill KA, et al. Surveillance of *BRCA1* and *BRCA2* mutation carriers with magnetic resonance imaging, ultrasound, mammography, and clinical breast examination. JAMA 2004; 292:1317–1325.

34. Lehman CD, Blume JD, Weatherall P, et al. Screening women at high risk for breast cancer with mammography and magnetic resonance imaging. Cancer 2005; 103:1898–1905.

35. Leach MO, Boggis CR, Dixon AK, et al. Screening with magnetic resonance imaging and mammography of a UK population at high familial risk of breast cancer: a prospective multicentre cohort study (MARIBS). Lancet 2005; 365:1769–1778.

36. Kuhl CK, Schrading S, Leutner CC, et al. Mammography, breast ultrasound, and magnetic resonance imaging for surveillance of women at high familial risk for breast cancer. J Clin Oncol 2005; 23:8469–8476.

37. Sardanelli F, Podo F, D'Agnolo G, et al. Multicenter comparative multimodality surveillance of women at genetic-familial high risk for breast cancer (HIBCRIT study): interim results. Radiology 2007; 242:698–715.

38. Warner E, Causer PA. MRI surveillance for hereditary breast-cancer risk. Lancet 2005; 365: 1747–1749.

39. Robson ME, Offit K. Breast MRI for women with hereditary cancer risk. JAMA 2004; 292: 1368–1370.

40. American Cancer Society: guidelines for the early detection of cancer [accessed April 1, 2007]; available from: http://www.cancer.org/docroot/ped/content/ped_2_3x_acs_cancer_detection_guidelines_36.asp.

41. National Comprehensive Cancer Network Clinical Practice Guidelines in Oncology—v.1.2006: genetic/familial high-risk assessment: breast and ovarian [accessed September 1, 2006]; available from: http://www.nccn.org/professionals/physician_gls/PDF/genetics_screening.pdf.

42. Liberman L. Breast cancer screening with MRI—what are the data for patients at high risk? N Engl J Med 2004; 351:497–500.

43. Tilanus-Linthorst MM, Kriege M, Boetes C, et al. Hereditary breast cancer growth rates and its impact on screening policy. Eur J Cancer 2005; 41:1610–1617.

44. Plevritis SK, Kurian AW, Sigal BM, et al. Cost-effectiveness of screening *BRCA1/2* mutation carriers with breast magnetic resonance imaging. JAMA 2006; 295:2374–2384.

45. Rebbeck TR, Lynch HT, Neuhausen SL, et al. Prophylactic oophorectomy in carriers of *BRCA1* or *BRCA2* mutations. N Engl J Med 2002; 346:1616–1622.

46. Kauff ND, Satagopan JM, Robson ME, et al. Risk-reducing salpingo-oophorectomy in women with a *BRCA1* or *BRCA2* mutation. N Engl J Med 2002; 346:1609–1615.

47. Kauff N, Domcheck M, Friebel TM, et al. Multi-center prospective analysis of risk-reducing salpingo-oophorectomy to prevent BRCA-associated breast and ovarian cancer. ASCO annual meeting proceedings part I. J Clin Oncol 2006; 24:1003.

48. Eerola H, Heikkila P, Tamminen A, et al. Histopathological features of breast tumours in *BRCA1*, *BRCA2* and mutation-negative breast cancer families. Breast Cancer Res 2005; 7: R93–R100.

49. Verhoog LC, Brekelmans CT, Seynaeve C, et al. Survival in hereditary breast cancer associated with germline mutations of *BRCA2*. J Clin Oncol 1999; 17:3396–3402.

50. Eisen A, Lubinski J, Klijn J, et al. Breast cancer risk following bilateral oophorectomy in *BRCA1* and *BRCA2* mutation carriers: an international case-control study. J Clin Oncol 2005; 23:7491–7496.

51. National Comprehensive Cancer Network Clinical Practice Guidelines in Oncology—v.1.2007: breast cancer risk reduction [accessed February 4, 2007]; available from: http://www.nccn.org/professionals/physician_gls/PDF/breast_risk.pdf.

52. Kramer JL, Velazquez IA, Chen BE, et al. Prophylactic oophorectomy reduces breast cancer penetrance during prospective, long-term follow-up of *BRCA1* mutation carriers. J Clin Oncol 2005; 23:8629–8635.

53. Rebbeck TR, Levin AM, Eisen A, et al. Breast cancer risk after bilateral prophylactic oophorectomy in *BRCA1* mutation carriers. J Natl Cancer Inst 1999; 91:1475–1479.

54. Madalinska JB, Hollenstein J, Bleiker E, et al. Quality-of-life effects of prophylactic salpingo-oophorectomy versus gynecologic screening among women at increased risk of hereditary ovarian cancer. J Clin Oncol 2005; 23:6890–6898.

55. Rebbeck TR, Friebel T, Wagner T, et al. Effect of short-term hormone replacement therapy on breast cancer risk reduction after bilateral prophylactic oophorectomy in *BRCA1* and *BRCA2* mutation carriers: the PROSE Study Group. J Clin Oncol 2005; 23: 7804–7810.

56. Chlebowski RT, Hendrix SL, Langer RD, et al. Influence of estrogen plus progestin on breast cancer and mammography in healthy postmenopausal women: the Women's Health Initiative Randomized Trial. JAMA 2003; 289:3243–3253.

57. Domchek SM, Friebel TM, Neuhausen SL, et al. Mortality after bilateral salpingo-oophorectomy in *BRCA1* and *BRCA2* mutation carriers: a prospective cohort study. Lancet Oncol 2006; 7:223–229.

58. Schwartz MD, Kaufman E, Peshkin BN, et al. Bilateral prophylactic oophorectomy and ovarian cancer screening following *BRCA1/BRCA2* mutation testing. J Clin Oncol 2003; 21: 4034–4041.

59. Meijers-Heijboer H, van Geel B, van Putten WL, et al. Breast cancer after prophylactic bilateral mastectomy in women with a *BRCA1* or *BRCA2* mutation. N Engl J Med 2001; 345: 159–164.

60. Klijn JGM, Van Geel AN, Meijers-Heijboer H, et al. Long-term follow-up of the Rotterdam study on prophylactic mastectomy versus surveillance in *BRCA1/2* mutation carriers. ASCO annual meeting proceedings (post-meeting edition). J Clin Oncol 2004; 22:2004.

61. Rebbeck TR, Friebel T, Lynch HT, et al. Bilateral prophylactic mastectomy reduces breast cancer risk in *BRCA1* and *BRCA2* mutation carriers: the PROSE Study Group. J Clin Oncol 2004; 22:1055–1062.

62. Hartmann LC, Schaid DJ, Woods JE, et al. Efficacy of bilateral prophylactic mastectomy in women with a family history of breast cancer. N Engl J Med 1999; 340:77–84.

63. Hartmann LC, Sellers TA, Schaid DJ, et al. Efficacy of bilateral prophylactic mastectomy in *BRCA1* and *BRCA2* gene mutation carriers. J Natl Cancer Inst 2001; 93:1633–1637.

64. Frost MH, Schaid DJ, Sellers TA, et al. Long-term satisfaction and psychological and social function following bilateral prophylactic mastectomy. JAMA 2000; 284:319–324.

65. Bresser PJ, Seynaeve C, Van Gool AR, et al. Satisfaction with prophylactic mastectomy and breast reconstruction in genetically predisposed women. Plast Reconstr Surg 2006; 117: 1675–1682, discussion; 1683–1684.

66. Kauff ND, Brogi E, Scheuer L, et al. Epithelial lesions in prophylactic mastectomy specimens from women with BRCA mutations. Cancer 2003; 97:1601–1608.

67. Hoogerbrugge N, Bult P, de Widt-Levert LM, et al. High prevalence of premalignant lesions in prophylactically removed breasts from women at hereditary risk for breast cancer. J Clin Oncol 2003; 21:41–45.

68. Metcalfe KA, Semple JL, Narod SA. Time to reconsider subcutaneous mastectomy for breast-cancer prevention? Lancet Oncol 2005; 6:431–434.

69. Early Breast Cancer Trialists' Collaborative Group. Tamoxifen for early breast cancer: an overview of the randomised trials. Lancet 1998; 351:1451–1467.

70. Fisher B, Costantino JP, Wickerham DL, et al. Tamoxifen for prevention of breast cancer: report of the National Surgical Adjuvant Breast and Bowel Project P-1 study. J Natl Cancer Inst 1998; 90:1371–1388.

71. Fisher B, Costantino JP, Wickerham DL, et al. Tamoxifen for the prevention of breast cancer: current status of the National Surgical Adjuvant Breast and Bowel Project P-1 study. J Natl Cancer Inst 2005; 97:1652–1662.

72. Veronesi U, Maisonneuve P, Costa A, et al. Prevention of breast cancer with tamoxifen: preliminary findings from the Italian randomised trial among hysterectomised women. Italian Tamoxifen Prevention Study. Lancet 1998; 352:93–97.

73. Powles T, Eeles R, Ashley S, et al. Interim analysis of the incidence of breast cancer in the Royal Marsden Hospital tamoxifen randomised chemoprevention trial. Lancet 1998; 352: 98–101.

74. Cuzick J, Forbes J, Edwards R, et al. First results from the International Breast Cancer Intervention Study (IBIS-I): a randomised prevention trial. Lancet 2002; 360:817–824.

75. Cuzick J, Forbes JF, Sestak I, et al. Long-term results of tamoxifen prophylaxis for breast cancer—96-month follow-up of the randomized IBIS-I trial. J Natl Cancer Inst 2007; 99: 272–282.

76. King MC, Wieand S, Hale K, et al. Tamoxifen and breast cancer incidence among women with inherited mutations in *BRCA1* and *BRCA2*: National Surgical Adjuvant Breast and Bowel Project (NSABP-P1) Breast Cancer Prevention trial. JAMA 2001; 286:2251–2256.

77. Kote-Jarai Z, Powles TJ, Mitchell G, et al. *BRCA1/BRCA2* mutation status and analysis of cancer family history in participants of the Royal Marsden Hospital tamoxifen chemoprevention trial. Cancer Lett 2007; 247:259–265.

78. Lakhani SR, Van De Vijver MJ, Jacquemier J, et al. The pathology of familial breast cancer: predictive value of immunohistochemical markers estrogen receptor, progesterone receptor, HER-2, and p53 in patients with mutations in *BRCA1* and *BRCA2*. J Clin Oncol 2002; 20: 2310–2318.

79. Cummings SR, Eckert S, Krueger KA, et al. The effect of raloxifene on risk of breast cancer in postmenopausal women: results from the MORE randomized trial. Multiple outcomes of raloxifene evaluation. JAMA 1999; 281:2189–2197.

80. Vogel VG, Costantino JP, Wickerham DL, et al. Effects of tamoxifen vs raloxifene on the risk of developing invasive breast cancer and other disease outcomes: the NSABP Study of Tamoxifen and Raloxifene (STAR) P-2 trial. JAMA 2006; 295:2727–2741.

81. Vogel VG, Costantino JP, Wickerham DL, et al. The effects of tamoxifen versus raloxifene on the risk of developing noninvasive breast cancer in the NSABP study of tamoxifen and raloxifene (STAR) P-2 trial, San Antonio Breast Cancer Symposium, San Antonio, TX, 2006.

82. Howell A, Cuzick J, Baum M, et al. Results of the ATAC (arimidex, tamoxifen, alone or in combination) trial after completion of 5 years' adjuvant treatment for breast cancer. Lancet 2005; 365:60–62.

83. Coombes RC, Hall E, Gibson LJ, et al. A randomized trial of exemestane after two to three years of tamoxifen therapy in postmenopausal women with primary breast cancer. N Engl J Med 2004; 350:1081–1092.

84. Cuzick J. Aromatase inhibitors in prevention—data from the ATAC (arimidex, tamoxifen alone or in combination) trial and the design of IBIS-II (the second International Breast Cancer Intervention study). Recent Results Cancer Res 2003; 163:96–103, discussion; 264–266.

85. Ingle JN. Endocrine therapy trials of aromatase inhibitors for breast cancer in the adjuvant and prevention settings. Clin Cancer Res 2005; 11:900s–905s.

86. Robson M, Svahn T, McCormick B, et al. Appropriateness of breast-conserving treatment of breast carcinoma in women with germline mutations in *BRCA1* or *BRCA2*: a clinic-based series. Cancer 2005; 103:44–51.

87. Seynaeve C, Verhoog LC, van de Bosch LM, et al. Ipsilateral breast tumour recurrence in hereditary breast cancer following breast-conserving therapy. Eur J Cancer 2004; 40: 1150–1158.

88. Kirova YM, Stoppa-Lyonnet D, Savignoni A, et al. Risk of breast cancer recurrence and contralateral breast cancer in relation to *BRCA1* and *BRCA2* mutation status following breast-conserving surgery and radiotherapy. Eur J Cancer 2005; 41:2304–2311.

89. Frost MH, Slezak JM, Tran NV, et al. Satisfaction after contralateral prophylactic mastectomy: the significance of mastectomy type, reconstructive complications, and body appearance. J Clin Oncol 2005; 23:7849–7856.

90. Graves KD, Peshkin BN, Halbert CH, et al. Predictors and outcomes of contralateral prophylactic mastectomy among breast cancer survivors. Breast Cancer Res Treat 2006; Epub ahead of print October 26, 2006.

91. Schwartz MD, Lerman C, Brogan B, et al. Impact of *BRCA1/BRCA2* counseling and testing on newly diagnosed breast cancer patients. J Clin Oncol 2004; 22:1823–1829.

92. Tercyak KP, Peshkin BN, Brogan BM, et al. Quality of life after contralateral prophylactic mastectomy in newly diagnosed high-risk breast cancer patients who underwent *BRCA1/2* gene testing. J Clin Oncol 2007; 25:285–291.

93. Stolier AJ, Corsetti RL. Newly diagnosed breast cancer patients choose bilateral mastectomy over breast-conserving surgery when testing positive for a *BRCA1/2* mutation. Am Surg 2005; 71:1031–1033.

94. Bryant HE, Schultz N, Thomas HD, et al. Specific killing of *BRCA2*-deficient tumours with inhibitors of poly(ADP-ribose) polymerase. Nature 2005; 434:913–917.

95. Farmer H, McCabe N, Lord CJ, et al. Targeting the DNA repair defect in BRCA mutant cells as a therapeutic strategy. Nature 2005; 434:917–921.

96. De Soto JA, Deng CX. PARP-1 inhibitors: are they the long-sought genetically specific drugs for *BRCA1/2*-associated breast cancers? Int J Med Sci 2006; 3:117–123.

97. De Soto JA, Wang X, Tominaga Y, et al. The inhibition and treatment of breast cancer with poly(ADP-ribose) polymerase (PARP-1) inhibitors. Int J Biol Sci 2006; 2:179–185.

98. Kong G, Kim HT, Wu K, et al. The retinoid X receptor-selective retinoid, LGD1069, down-regulates cyclooxygenase-2 expression in human breast cells through transcription factor crosstalk: implications for molecular-based chemoprevention. Cancer Res 2005; 65: 3462–3469.

99. Wu K, Zhang Y, Xu XC, et al. The retinoid X receptor-selective retinoid, LGD1069, prevents the development of estrogen receptor-negative mammary tumors in transgenic mice. Cancer Res 2002; 62:6376–6380.

16

Ovarian Cancer Screening and Prevention Options: Ovarian Cancer Screening and Its Limitations. Who Should be Screened?

Karen H. Lu
Department of Gynecologic Oncology, University of Texas M.D. Anderson Cancer Center, Houston, Texas, U.S.A.

Steven J. Skates
Biostatistics Center, Massachusetts General Hospital, Boston, Massachusetts, U.S.A.

OVARIAN CANCER SCREENING AND PREVENTION STRATEGIES

Introduction

While risk of breast cancer for *BRCA* carriers is extremely high, risk of ovarian cancer is still significant. In general, the lifetime risk of ovarian cancer is 1 in 70; however, for *BRCA1* carriers, the risk is as high as 39% to 46% (1), and for *BRCA2* carriers, it is 12% to 22% (2,3). About 5% to 10% of ovarian cancers are due to inherited risk, and 90% of those are due to *BRCA1* or *BRCA2* mutations. Often, the first sign of a *BRCA* mutation (referring to either gene) in the family is multiple breast and ovarian cancers amongst close blood relatives. Following identification of these two genes (4,5) in the mid-1990s, genetic tests were developed that could identify carriers of *BRCA* mutations. The question then arises: What clinical interventions are advisable for reducing the risks of ovarian cancer following identification of a patient at higher risk than normal, either due to multiple familial breast or ovarian cancers or due to the presence of a *BRCA* mutation within the family? This chapter reviews the research, as of early 2007, for two approaches aimed at reducing the risk of ovarian cancer, namely prevention strategies and screening for early detection of ovarian cancer. However, it should be indicated at the outset that for women carrying a deleterious *BRCA* mutation, the current standard intervention is surgical removal of the ovaries following completion of child bearing. This standard is due to the high mortality from the late stage of diagnosis for most (75%) (6) ovarian cancers. Surgical removal of the ovaries is the most effective strategy for reducing mortality due to ovarian cancer (7).

Importance of Risk Assessment

When a patient consults a genetic counselor or other clinician, an important issue is to provide a perspective on the range of ovarian cancer risks. The lifetime risk of ovarian cancer in the general population is 1.4%, while for women with a personal history of breast cancer, it increases to 2.25%. A history of one first-degree relative (FDR)/second-degree relative (SDR) with breast cancer increases the risk by a factor of 1.1 to 1.7 (1.5–2.4%), and a history of two FDR/SDR breast cancers increases the risk by a factor of 1.1 to 2.8 (1.5–3.9%) (8). For carriers of a deleterious mutation in the *BRCA2* gene, the risk increases to 12% to 22%, and for carriers of a deleterious mutation in the *BRCA1* gene, the risk is 39% to 46%. Prior to information gained from genetic testing, women from families with a history of breast and ovarian cancers will have risks that vary between the risk in the normal population and the highest risk *BRCA1* population due to the different structures of their cancer pedigrees. This variation illustrates the vital role risk assessment plays in counseling the individual patient.

Multiple computer models have been developed for assessing the risk of being a *BRCA1* or *BRCA2* mutation carrier for a given family history of breast and ovarian cancer. Statistical models based on Mendelian inheritance, in particular, an autosomal dominant mode of inheritance for *BRCA* mutations, include Breast and Ovarian Analysis of Disease Incidence and Carrier Estimation Algorithm (BOADICEA) (2) and BRCA carrier PRObability (BRCAPRO) (9). These programs provide estimates of the probability of carrying a mutation in one of the *BRCA* mutations given the family pedigree of breast and ovarian cancers in FDRs and SDRs, and include the age at cancer diagnosis, current age or age at death of each member of the family, and relationship of the patient to each member of the family. They are used as an aid to genetic counselors to assist in decision making for genetic testing; however, they do not supplant genetic counseling, because among other considerations, they do not account for cancers in third-degree relatives (e.g., cousins) and embody only the knowledge at the time they were developed. In contradistinction, the genetic counselor can incorporate information from the most recent published research. Other chapters in this book address such programs and their use in clinical situations in much greater detail.

Modalities for Screening

The two primary modalities under investigation for ovarian cancer screening are blood tests for cancer biomarkers and ultrasound scans. The primary cancer biomarker for ovarian cancer is CA-125. The standard interpretation of CA-125 is whether it exceeds a level of 35 U/mL. CA-125 is approved for clinical use as a marker to evaluate recurrence of disease. Trials have been conducted examining CA-125 as a screening test and this research is ongoing. CA-125 at a single cutoff has limited utility. An alternative approach is to examine CA-125 values over time and determine whether a significant increase above an individual's baseline has occurred. A risk of ovarian cancer algorithm (ROCA) is one method that has been developed to investigate this approach (10) among others (11). ROCA may increase sensitivity without sacrificing the specificity of the CA-125 test. The most common method for scanning is transvaginal sonography (TVS). As compared with abdominal ultrasound, TVS allows for a more detailed view of the ovaries. While TVS with color Doppler may be helpful in evaluating pelvic or ovarian masses, its utility in ovarian cancer screening is unclear. We illustrate these modalities by describing ongoing studies with these modalities as the first-line tests, and then briefly describe research aimed at identifying additional markers to complement CA-125.

Screening Trials in Normal Risk Women

A definitive randomized screening trial is being conducted in the United Kingdom called the UK Collaborative Trial of Ovarian Cancer Screening (UKCTOCS) (12). Although it enrolls only normal risk women, it nonetheless addresses crucial issues that will be of importance to all women. The important aspects of this trial are its size (200,000 women are enrolled), the randomization between three arms [the first arm using ROCA (50,000) followed by TVS as a second-line test, the second arm using annual TVS (50,000) as a first-line test, and the third being a control arm of 100,000 women where no screening is performed], and the endpoint of ovarian cancer mortality. The trial has completed accrual and results are anticipated in 2012. It will provide a direct comparison between ROCA and TVS, and between screening and no screening, with ovarian cancer mortality as the hard endpoint. The prostate, lung, colorectal, and ovarian screening trial (13) is being conducted by the National Cancer Institute (NCI) in the United States, which is evaluating screening for these four malignancies. It began in 1993 and will last 21 years. In this trial, 75,000 men and 75,000 women have been enrolled and randomized to screening or no screening. For ovarian cancer screening, both CA-125 and TVS were used as first-line tests and were performed annually for five years. This trial met its accrual goals in 2000 and all enrolled subjects have now completed their screening studies.

At the University of Kentucky, van Nagel et al. have conducted a statewide ovarian cancer screening program using ultrasound as a first-line test since 1987 (14–16). In the first report, 3220 postmenopausal women were screened between 1987 and 1992, with 44 patients having a persistent abnormality on ultrasound leading to exploratory laparotomy. Three primary ovarian cancers were identified with two in stage IA and one in stage IIIB. Again sensitivity is encouraging but the positive predictive value (PPV) of TVS is low, with 14.5 surgeries performed for each ovarian cancer detected. In a subsequent report (16), after annual screening of 14,469 asymptomatic women between 1987 and 1999, 181 patients underwent surgery for suspected ovarian cancer. Seventeen cases were detected, resulting in a PPV of 9.4%, eleven were in stage I, three in stage II, and three in stage III. Four patients developed ovarian cancer within one year of screening, giving a sensitivity of 17/21 (81%). Since then, the algorithm for indication for surgery has changed and the PPV has increased above 10% (17). This program is ongoing and now includes premenopausal women at high risk.

Until such trials are completed, with two planning reports by 2014, no conclusion about the efficacy of ovarian cancer screening can be made. Given the unknown efficacy, screening normal risk women for ovarian cancer should be confined to clinical research trials.

Although CA-125 remains the best ovarian cancer biomarker to date, its limitations are well recognized, and much research is aimed at identifying additional biomarkers that will complement the sensitivity of CA-125 or find ovarian cancers earlier than CA-125. Candidate biomarkers are evaluated singly and in panels (18). Advanced proteomic techniques such as mass spectrometry are searching fluids from ovarian cancer cases and comparing the protein lists with similar lists from suitably matched control subjects to identify candidate proteins for evaluation as ovarian cancer biomarkers. This research is in its beginning stages, and NCI has recently funded the Clinical Proteomics Technology Assessment for Cancer (CPTAC) network to establish firmer scientific footings in this area.

Screening Trials in Women at Increased Risk

Because ovarian cancer screening is recommended for high-risk women (19), screening trials for ovarian cancer in high-risk women cannot be a comparison of screening to no screening. Often they are single arm trials designed to estimate an operating characteristic such as feasibility, specificity, or PPV.

A Norwegian study led by Dorum et al. (20) screened annually 745 women from hereditary breast/ovarian cancer families for an average of 2.7 years. A woman was eligible if she was an FDR of a woman with ovarian cancer who had another female FDR (or SDR through a male) with ovarian cancer or breast cancer diagnosed under age 60. Seven ovarian cancers were found on the prevalence (first) screen, six in late stage disease. Two were found on interval screens, one with borderline early stage disease and one with late stage disease. Only one ovarian cancer occurred under age 40, and based on the findings from this study, the authors' recommendations for ovarian cancer screening in high-risk women as defined by this study's eligibility criteria included annual screening with CA-125 and vaginal ultrasound beginning at age 35, and discussion of prophylactic oophorectomy at age 45.

A prospective screening study was conducted by the Gilda Radner Ovarian Cancer Detection Program in Los Angeles among 290 Ashkenazi Jewish women with one of three founder mutations (*BRCA1 185delAG* and *5382insC* and *BRCA2 6174delT*) (21). Screening occurred over 10 years, with an average duration of five years. For the first five years, screening with CA-125 and TVS occurred twice per year, and after July 1995, screening occurred once per year. Two ovarian and six peritoneal incident cancers were detected among 24 surgeries performed for abnormal ultrasound (20) or CA-125 (4) results. One ovarian cancer case was stage Ic, and one was stage IIc. The six peritoneal cancers were by definition late stage (IIIc) and all occurred in *BRCA1 185delAG* carriers. Of the four cancers diagnosed within six months of the last screen, one was stage Ic ovarian cancer and was detected by TVS, and three were peritoneal cancer, one detected by TVS, one detected by CA-125 > 35 U/mL, and one due to pain. The conclusions drawn from this trial were that neither intensive screening nor prophylactic oophorectomy would be helpful for peritoneal cancers or for ovarian cancer. However, the latter conclusion is based on two ovarian cancers detected, both in early stage (Ic, IIc), and it would appear further studies are required before a strong conclusion can be made.

Because of the sparseness of data on ovarian cancers detected in screening studies of high-risk women, additional studies are ongoing. Here we present a brief summary of three studies using CA-125 via ROCA and two studies using TVS as a first-line test. Analyses of CA-125 data from trials in the UK and Sweden (22) demonstrated that CA-125 rose rapidly in women subsequently diagnosed with ovarian cancer, while CA-125 had a relatively flat profile in women with no ovarian cancer detected. The rise over time was at least as important as the absolute level of CA-125 in distinguishing cases from controls. A statistical method was developed to implement this approach, termed the ROCA. Based on these results, the Cancer Genetics Network (CGN), a U.S. network sponsored by the NCI, and other collaborative groups including the NCI ovarian Specialized Program on Research Excellence (SPORE) groups and an NCI Early Detection Research Network (EDRN) site, instituted a prospective screening study beginning in 2001 of women at high risk using ROCA. Eligibility criteria included (*i*) the subject or FDR or SDR with a deleterious *BRCA* mutation, (*ii*) the family contains at least two ovarian or breast cancers diagnosed under age 50 among the subject or FDR or SDR blood relatives within the same lineage, or (*iii*) the subject is of Ashkenazi ethnicity with one FDR or two SDR with ovarian or breast cancer diagnosed between age 30 and 50. Since ovarian cancer is regarded as a rapidly arising disease, women in this study are screened frequently with CA-125 tests every three months and CA-125 values interpreted according to ROCA. An elevated risk results in referral to ultrasound. To date ROCA has accrued over 2300 women.

In 2003, the Gynecologic Oncology Group instituted a prospective study (GOG0199) of high-risk women using the same eligibility criteria as the CGN ROCA study with subjects choosing to undergo either risk reducing salpingo-oophorectomy (RRSO), or screening using ROCA with CA-125 testing occurring every three months. GOG0199 completed accrual in November 2006 and it is anticipated that results will be available at the end of 2011.

Finally, a study of women at high-risk has begun in the United Kingdom, termed the UK Familial Ovarian Cancer Screening Study (UKFOCSS) that tests women every four months for CA-125 values, with ROCA used to interpret the results and for decision making for referral to TVS. The eligibility criteria include that the subject is at least 35 years of age and must have an FDR with breast or ovarian cancer in a high-risk family, where the family contains (*i*) two or more individuals with ovarian cancer who are FDRs, or (*ii*) one individual with ovarian cancer and one individual with breast cancer diagnosed under age 50 who are FDRs, or (*iii*) one individual with ovarian cancer and two individuals with breast cancer diagnosed under age 60 years who are connected by first-degree relationships.

The U.K. study eligibility criteria are less broad than the ROCA study and less strict than the Norwegian study. The differences between the three screening studies using CA-125 as the first-line test indicate that consensus has not been reached on the frequency of CA-125 testing, the method of interpretation of the CA-125 test, and the definition of "high risk." Therefore all these aspects of ovarian cancer screening are under investigation and should still be considered under the research umbrella, with optimal choices remaining to be defined.

Until results from the prospective screening trials are reported, no firm conclusions can be made about the sensitivity of screening for ovarian cancer. Mortality reduction due to screening could then be tentatively projected from comparisons between the stage distributions of the screening studies with stage distributions from historical reports.

Two ovarian cancer screening studies with TVS as first-line testing have been conducted. In the United Kingdom, Campbell et al. (23) reported on a 10-year observational study of TVS in 2500 women (age ≥17) with at least one FDR with ovarian cancer. There were 4231 screens (2500 first screens, 998 second screens, 733 third or higher order screens) with 104 screens giving a positive result and 11 cancers detected, seven in stage I, and four of borderline malignancy. One additional ovarian cancer was identified within 12 months of a scan. This encouraging result indicates TVS has a high sensitivity for ovarian cancer, although the number of surgeries (9.5) required to detect one case borders on the acceptable PPV of 10% (24). The University of Kentucky has now included high-risk women in their screening program described above. As previously indicated, TVS as a first-line screen appears to have excellent sensitivity while the PPV is low though within the acceptable range. Work is ongoing to refine the algorithms leading to surgical decisions, aiming to improve the PPV without affecting sensitivity.

Prevention Strategies

Because the efficacy of ovarian cancer screening in high-risk patients is as yet unproven, women should also be counseled regarding options for ovarian cancer chemoprevention and surgical prevention.

Chemoprevention

In the general population, large case–control studies have shown that oral contraceptives decrease the risk of ovarian cancer by 50% (25). For women with *BRCA1* and *BRCA2* mutations, studies have shown mixed results. Narod et al. demonstrated a 50% reduction in ovarian cancer risk with use of the oral contraceptive in *BRCA1* and *BRCA2* mutation carriers (26). In a recent update of this cohort, their group examined 799 cases and 2424 controls and again found a significant reduction of risk for ovarian cancer due to oral contraceptive use. For *BRCA1* carriers, the odds ratio was 0.56 and for *BRCA2* carriers it was 0.39 (27). Whittemore et al. found similar results (28). However, although a study by Modan et al. from Israel did not report a negative effect of oral contraceptives on ovarian cancer risk, a protective benefit was not observed (29). Importantly, oral contraceptives may have a negative effect on breast cancer risk in *BRCA*1 mutation carriers. Narod et al. reported a slightly increased risk of breast cancer in women with *BRCA1* mutations who use oral contraceptives before age 30 and for more than five years (relative risk 1.2–1.3) (26).

There have been some small trials examining novel chemopreventive agents for ovarian cancer. *N*-(4-hydroxyphenyl)retinamide (4HPR), Cox 2 inhibitors, and progestins have all been proposed as possible ovarian chemopreventive agents in high-risk patients. However, data are preliminary.

Surgical Prevention

RRSO has definitively been shown to decrease the risk of ovarian cancer (7,30,31). In a multicenter prospective study of 1828 *BRCA1* or *BRCA2* mutation carriers, RRSO was associated with an 80% reduction in risk of ovarian cancer [hazard ratio (HR) = 0.20; confidence interval (CI) 0.07–0.58] (31). A single institution, prospective study of 170 women found a similar 85% reduction in risk (HR = 0.15; CI 0.02–1.31) (30). In a multicenter, retrospective study of 551 *BRCA1* or *BRCA2* mutation carriers, RRSO was associated with a 96% reduction of ovarian cancer risk (HR = 0.04; CI 0.01–0.16) (7). In all of these studies, RRSO is associated with a significant reduction in risk of ovarian cancer. A small risk of primary peritoneal cancer remains even after RRSO.

In addition to the 85% significant reduction in ovarian cancer risk afforded by RRSO, when performed in premenopausal women, it also decreases risk of breast cancer in *BRCA1* and *BRCA2* mutation carriers by approximately 50%. Rebbeck et al. reported a 53% reduction in breast cancer risk (HR = 0.47; CI 0.29–0.77) (7) and Kauff et al. reported a 68% reduction in breast cancer risk (HR = 0.32; CI 0.08–1.2) (30).

When prophylactic bilateral salpingo-oophorectomies were performed in known mutation carriers, early studies identified microscopic tumors arising in the ovaries and the fallopian tubes in some cases (32,33). Subsequent studies have confirmed that careful pathologic sectioning, including complete serial sectioning of the ovaries and fallopian tubes, is necessary in order to identify these early lesions (34). Standard routine processing of the specimens by pathologists does not include serial sectioning; therefore, the gynecologic surgeon needs to discuss the case with the pathologist to ensure that this special handling is performed. Additionally, in general, a CA-125 and transvaginal ultrasound immediately prior to the surgery may be helpful to identify an asymptomatic process. Women should be counseled prior to surgery that if a gross lesion is identified at the time of surgery, full cancer staging will be performed. Backup should be available for general gynecologists who perform this procedure. Patients also need to be notified that, even in the absent of gross lesions, there is still a possibility of finding occult cancers at the time of pathologic review.

With the identification of occult lesions in the ovaries and fallopian tubes, guidelines for the RRSO procedure have been published (35). The procedure can be performed via laparoscopy or laparotomy. In both instances, the pelvis and pelvic organs should be thoroughly visualized, and the abdomen including diaphragm, liver, omentum, bowel, paracolic gutters, and appendix should be carefully inspected. Any abnormal areas should be biopsied. Peritoneal washings should be taken. When the ovaries are removed, the gynecologic surgeon should be careful to remove the entire ovary by isolating and ligating the ovarian vessels proximal to the end of any identifiable ovarian tissue. The fallopian tubes should be removed in their entirety, up to the uterine cornual.

Although the efficacy of RRSO is proven, there are certainly specific clinical questions that remain. First, the question of what age RRSO should be performed is important. Current recommendations from consensus groups recommend RRSO at age 35, or when child bearing is completed (36). It is important to note that age of diagnosis of ovarian cancer differs for *BRCA1* and *BRCA2* mutations. Women with a *BRCA1* mutation have a 10% to 21% chance of developing ovarian cancer by age 50; while for *BRCA2* carriers, the risk is only 2% to 3% by age 50. Therefore, consideration can be made for recommending RRSO at a slightly later age to women with *BRCA2* mutations. However, there have certainly been reports of ovarian cancer under age 50 in women with *BRCA2* mutations, so patients must be carefully counseled. Additionally, the benefit of RRSO in decreasing breast cancer risk in premenopausal women must also be considered. This benefit increases the earlier the ovaries are removed, and therefore, this must be balanced with the desire to maintain ovarian function.

Second, there is debate as to whether the uterus should also be removed at the time of the RRSO. Data from some studies suggest an increased risk of uterine cancer in mutation carriers (37,38), whereas others show no increased risk (39,40). This topic is reviewed in greater detail in Chapter 4. In general, it is felt that this decision should be individualized. Given the lack of a clear increased risk of uterine cancer in *BRCA1/2* carriers, hysterectomy is not felt to be absolutely necessary as part of the RRSO procedure. However, for women who have other gynecologic indications to remove the uterus, including abnormal Pap smears or abnormal uterine bleeding, a hysterectomy can be considered. In addition, those women who have taken tamoxifen or plan to take tamoxifen may wish to consider removing their uterus due to the increased risk of uterine cancer with tamoxifen. Removing the uterus slightly increases the length and morbidity of the surgery.

A very relevant question for mutation carriers undergoing RRSO regards the subsequent use of hormone replacement therapy (HRT) to alleviate menopausal symptoms. A study by Rebbeck et al. has shown that short-term HRT after RRSO in *BRCA1* and *BRCA2* mutation carriers does not impact the benefits of the procedure on reducing breast cancer risks (41). Although more studies are necessary, premenopausal patients without a history of breast cancer may consider the option of short-term HRT until age 50 to lessen vasomotor symptoms.

In terms of surveillance for primary peritoneal cancer after RRSO, there are no studies currently available to guide recommendations. Signs and symptoms of primary peritoneal cancer should be reviewed annually as well as routine gynecologic exams. It is unclear whether an annual CA-125 is of benefit. Transvaginal ultrasounds are no longer recommended after women have their ovaries and fallopian tubes removed.

Finally, the role of RRSO in high-risk patients who do not have a documented *BRCA1* or 2 mutation should also be discussed. In the absence of a known mutation, risk of ovarian cancer should be assessed based on family history. Because current technology for identifying *BRCA1* and *BRCA2* mutation carriers does not allow identification of all mutations, patients with very strong family histories of breast and ovarian cancers should be counseled as if they are mutation carriers. For families who have family histories consistent with site-specific breast cancer, a recent study showed that risk for ovarian cancer is quite low (42). Each individual should be counseled not only as to their ovarian cancer risk, but also to the efficacy and limitations of ovarian cancer screening and prevention. This topic is reviewed in greater detail in Chapter 17.

Thus, preoperative counseling should include a discussion of the benefits of RRSO in reducing ovarian cancer risk as well as breast cancer risk. However, patients should understand the small but finite risk of primary peritoneal cancer even after RRSO. In addition, a careful discussion of the role of hysterectomy, cancer surveillance after RRSO, and HRT should also be done preoperatively. Finally, the risk of finding an occult ovarian cancer and the plan for staging should also be discussed.

Although the results of the retrospective case–control studies appear to be overwhelmingly in favor of RRSO, retrospective studies are prone to multiple biases such as ascertainment bias, recall bias, and selection bias. A prospective study enables biases either to be minimized or to be adjusted for in the analysis, and thus a prospective study is being conducted by Dr. Mark Greene of NCI through the GOG0199, comparing the outcomes of a high-risk cohort facing the choice between undergoing RRSO and screening for ovarian cancer for five years. The screening approach is the same as the CGN study outlined in the previous section and the eligibility criteria are the same as for ROCA. The study is ongoing and is due for completion in 2011. This prospective study will improve the knowledge of the trade-offs between RRSO and screening for ovarian cancer.

CONCLUSION

The availability of clinical genetic testing for *BRCA1* and *BRCA2* and the emergence of effective prevention strategies allow us to identify women at high risk for gynecologic cancers and prevent these cancers from occurring. Studies are ongoing to define the screening modalities, their frequency, mode of implementation, and population, which will suitably contribute to the overall care of women at increased risk of ovarian cancer. The current challenge for gynecologic oncologists is to have clear criteria for identifying which ovarian cancer patients should be referred for genetic counseling and testing. In addition, general gynecologists will begin to play a greater role in the management of these high-risk women. The importance of multidisciplinary management of these individuals at high risk for multiple cancers cannot be stressed enough. Gynecologic oncologists, gynecologists, and medical oncologists focusing on gynecologic tumors must work closely with breast medical oncologists, breast surgeons, and genetic counselors.

REFERENCES

1. King MC, Marks JH, Mandell JB. Breast and ovarian cancer risks due to inherited mutations in BRCA1 and BRCA2. Science 2003; 302(5645):643–646.
2. Antoniou AC, Pharoah PP, Smith P, Easton DF. The BOADICEA model of genetic susceptibility to breast and ovarian cancer. Br J Cancer 2004; 91(8):1580–1590.
3. Chen S, Iversen ES, Friebel T, et al. Characterization of BRCA1 and BRCA2 mutations in a large United States sample. J Clin Oncol 2006; 24(6):863–871.
4. Anderson LA, Friedman L, Osborne-Lawrence S, et al. High-density genetic map of the BRCA1 region of chromosome 17q12-q21. Genomics 1993; 17(3):618–623.
5. Wooster R, Bignell G, Lancaster J, et al. Identification of the breast-cancer susceptibility gene BRCA2. Nature 1995; 378(6559):789–792.

6. Carlson KJ, Skates SJ, Singer DE. Screening for ovarian cancer (see comments). Ann Intern Med 1994; 121(2):124–132.

7. Rebbeck TR, Lynch HT, Neuhausen SL, et al. Prophylactic oophorectomy in carriers of BRCA1 or BRCA2 mutations. N Engl J Med 2002; 346(21):1616–1622.

8. Kazerouni N, Greene MH, Lacey JV Jr, Mink PJ, Schairer C. Family history of breast cancer as a risk factor for ovarian cancer in a prospective study. Cancer 2006; 107(5):1075–1083.

9. Parmigiani G, Berry D, Aguilar O. Determining carrier probabilities for breast cancer-susceptibility genes BRCA1 and BRCA2. Am J Hum Genet 1998; 62(1):145–158.

10. Skates SJ, Pauler DK, Jacobs IJ. Screening based on the risk of cancer calculation from Bayesian hierarchical change-point and mixture models of longitudinal markers. J Am Stat Assoc 2001; 96(454):429–439.

11. McIntosh MW, Urban N. A parametric empirical Bayes method for cancer screening using longitudinal observations of a biomarker. Biostatistics 2003; 4(1):27–40.

12. Jacobs IJ, Menon U. Progress and challenges in screening for early detection of ovarian cancer. Mol Cell Proteomics 2004; 3(4):355–366.

13. Westhoff C. Current status of screening for ovarian cancer. Gynecol Oncol 1994; 55(3 Pt 2): S34–S37.

14. DePriest PD, van Nagell JR Jr, Gallion HH, et al. Ovarian cancer screening in asymptomatic postmenopausal women. Gynecol Oncol 1993; 51(2):205–209.

15. DePriest PD, Gallion HH, Pavlik EJ, Kryscio RJ, van Nagell JR. Transvaginal sonography as a screening method for the detection of early ovarian cancer. Gynecol Oncol 1997; 65(3): 408–414.

16. van Nagell JR Jr, DePriest PD, Reedy MB, et al. The efficacy of transvaginal sonographic screening in asymptomatic women at risk for ovarian cancer (see comments). Gynecol Oncol 2000; 77(3):350–356.

17. DePriest P, Skates SJ, eds. Personal communication. 2006: Boston.

18. Terry KL, Sluss PM, Skates SJ, et al. Blood and urine markers for ovarian cancer: a comprehensive review. Dis Markers 2004; 20(2):53–70.

19. National Institutes of Health Consensus Development Conference Statement. Ovarian cancer: screening, treatment, and follow-up. Gynecol Oncol 1994; 55(3 Pt 2):S4–S14.

20. Dorum A, Heimdal K, Lovslett K, et al. Prospectively detected cancer in familial breast/ovarian cancer screening. Acta Obstet Gynecol Scand 1999; 78(10):906–911.

21. Liede A, Karlan BY, Baldwin RL, Platt LD, Kuperstein G, Narod SA. Cancer incidence in a population of Jewish women at risk of ovarian cancer. J Clin Oncol 2002; 20(6): 1570–1577.

22. Skates SJ, Menon U, MacDonald N, et al. Calculation of the risk of ovarian cancer from serial CA-125 values for preclinical detection in postmenopausal women. J Clin Oncol 2003; 21(10 suppl):206–210.

23. Tailor A, Bourne TH, Campbell S, Okokon E, Dew T, Collins WP. Results from an ultrasound-based familial ovarian cancer screening clinic: a 10-year observational study. Ultrasound Obstet Gynecol 2003; 21(4):378–385.

24. Jacobs I, Bast RC Jr. The CA 125 tumour-associated antigen: a review of the literature. Hum Reprod 1989; 4(1):1–12.

25. The reduction in risk of ovarian cancer associated with oral-contraceptive use. The cancer and steroid hormone study of the centers for disease control and the national institute of child health and human development. N Engl J Med 1987; 316(11):650–655.

26. Narod SA, Dube MP, Klijn J, et al. Oral contraceptives and the risk of breast cancer in BRCA1 and BRCA2 mutation carriers. J Natl Cancer Inst 2002; 94(23):1773–1779.

27. McLaughlin JR, Risch HA, Lubinski J, et al. Reproductive risk factors for ovarian cancer in carriers of BRCA1 or BRCA2 mutations: a case-control study. Lancet Oncol 2007; 8(1): 26–34.

28. Whittemore AS, Balise RR, Pharoah PD, et al. Oral contraceptive use and ovarian cancer risk among carriers of BRCA1 or BRCA2 mutations. Br J Cancer 2004; 91(11): 1911–1915.

29. Modan B, Hartge P, Hirsh-Yechezkel G, et al. Parity, oral contraceptives, and the risk of ovarian cancer among carriers and noncarriers of a BRCA1 or BRCA2 mutation. N Engl J Med 2001; 345(4):235–240.

30. Kauff ND, Satagopan JM, Robson ME, et al. Risk-reducing salpingo-oophorectomy in women with a BRCA1 or BRCA2 mutation. N Engl J Med 2002; 346(21):1609–1615.

31. Finch A, Beiner M, Lubinski J, et al. Salpingo-oophorectomy and the risk of ovarian, fallopian tube, and peritoneal cancers in women with a BRCA1 or BRCA2 Mutation. JAMA 2006; 296 (2):185–192.

32. Lu KH, Garber JE, Cramer DW, et al. Occult ovarian tumors in women with BRCA1 or BRCA2 mutations undergoing prophylactic oophorectomy. J Clin Oncol 2000; 18(14): 2728–2732.

33. Colgan TJ, Murphy J, Cole DEC, Narod S, Rosen B. Occult carcinoma in prophylactic oophorectomy specimens—prevalence and association with BRCA germline mutation status. Am J Surg Pathol 2001; 25(10):1283–1289.

34. Powell CB, Kenley E, Chen LM, et al. Risk-reducing salpingo-oophorectomy in BRCA mutation carriers: role of serial sectioning in the detection of occult malignancy. J Clin Oncol 2005; 23(1):127–132.

35. Society of Gynecologic Oncologists Clinical Practice Committee Statement on prophylactic salpingo-oophorectomy. Gynecol Oncol 2005; 98(2):179–181.

36. Daly MB, Axilbund JE, Bryant E, et al. NCCN genetic/familial high-risk assessment: breast and ovarian. NCCN Clinical Practice Guidelines in Oncology 2006:1–30.

37. Lavie O, Ben-Arie A, Pilip A, et al. BRCA2 germline mutation in a woman with uterine serous papillary carcinoma—case report. Gynecol Oncol 2005; 99(2):486–488.

38. Biron-Shental T, Drucker L, Altaras M, Bernheim J, Fishman A. High incidence of BRCA1-2 germline mutations, previous breast cancer and familial cancer history in Jewish patients with uterine serous papillary carcinoma. Eur J Surg Oncol 2006; 32(10):1097–1100.

39. Cancer risks in BRCA2 mutation carriers. The breast cancer linkage consortium. J Natl Cancer Inst 1999; 91(15):1310–1316.

40. Risch HA, McLaughlin JR, Cole DE, et al. Prevalence and penetrance of germline BRCA1 and BRCA2 mutations in a population series of 649 women with ovarian cancer. Am J Hum Genet 2001; 68(3):700–710.

41. Rebbeck TR, Friebel T, Wagner T, et al. Effect of short-term hormone replacement therapy on breast cancer risk reduction after bilateral prophylactic oophorectomy in BRCA1 and BRCA2 mutation carriers: the PROSE Study Group. J Clin Oncol 2005; 23(31):7804–7810.

42. Kauff ND, Mitra N, Robson ME, et al. Risk of ovarian cancer in BRCA1 and BRCA2 mutation-negative hereditary breast cancer families. J Natl Cancer Inst 2005; 97(18): 1382–1384.

17

Management of *BRCA*-Negative Hereditary Breast Cancer Families

Noah D. Kauff

Clinical Genetics and Gynecology Services, Memorial Sloan-Kettering Cancer Center, New York, New York, U.S.A.

CAUSES OF *BRCA*-NEGATIVE HEREDITARY BREAST CANCER

In families with features of an autosomal-dominant inherited predisposition to early-onset breast cancer, full sequencing of the coding regions of *BRCA1* and *BRCA2* will only identify deleterious mutations in just over half of these families (Fig. 1) (1). Inherited mutations in other tumor suppressor genes, such as *p53* and *PTEN*, will account for less than 1% to 2% of the remaining families. There are several possible explanations for why these apparent hereditary breast cancer families do not demonstrate a deleterious *BRCA1* or *BRCA2* mutation including (*i*) the cluster of cancers is a chance event; (*ii*) the individual tested may be a phenocopy (i.e., an individual with a sporadic cancer unrelated to an inherited predisposition that exists within a family); (*iii*) the inherited predisposition is secondary to a mutation in an as yet unidentified cancer predisposition gene; or (*iv*) full sequencing of the coding region of *BRCA1* and *BRCA2* is unable to detect a deleterious mutation that is present in one of the genes.

Cluster of Cancers Is a Chance Event

Given that breast cancer is the single most common cancer in women with one in nine women developing breast cancer by age 85, having a cluster of two or even three breast cancers within a family is not a rare event, especially if there are multiple females in a lineage who live to an advanced age. However, the development of breast cancer is markedly less common at younger ages, with approximately 1 in 225 women developing breast cancer by age 40 and 1 in 50 women developing breast cancer by age 50 (2). Therefore, in families where multiple individuals (i.e., three or more) in a direct lineage develop breast cancers at earlier ages (prior to age 60), it becomes less likely that these are sporadic cases that have occurred in clusters by chance alone.

Tested Individual Is a Phenocopy

In families with multiple affected relatives where a single individual has been tested and no deleterious mutation in *BRCA1* or *BRCA2* is identified, a possibility that must be considered is that the individual tested is a phenocopy. In this situation, there is an

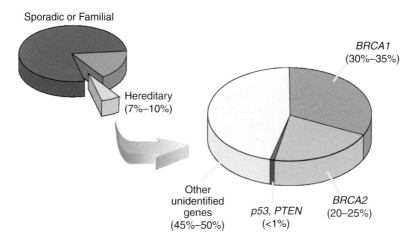

Figure 1 Causes of hereditary susceptibility to breast cancer. Approximately 7–10% of all cases of invasive breast cancer appear to be secondary to an inherited, autosomal dominant cancer susceptibility. Of these inherited cases, 50–55% are thought to be secondary to mutations in either *BRCA1* or *BRCA2*. Less than 1% of these cases are thought to be due to mutations in other identified cancer susceptibility genes such as *p53* and *PTEN*. The remaining 45–50% of inherited breast cancers are thought to be secondary to mutations in other, as yet to be identified, cancer susceptibility genes.

individual who has developed breast cancer within a family with an identifiable inherited predisposition, but the individual's breast cancer is not caused by this familial predisposition (an example is illustrated in Fig. 2).

Predisposition Is the Result of a Mutation in an as Yet Unidentified Cancer Susceptibility Gene

There is strong data from the Breast Cancer Linkage Consortium (BCLC) suggesting that there are genes, aside from *BRCA1* and *BRCA2*, associated with high-penetrance autosomal-dominant predisposition to breast cancer (3). This group conducted a linkage analysis in 237 families with at least four cases of breast cancer diagnosed prior to the age of 60. Linkage analysis is a method in which polymorphic markers that flank a putative gene of interest are typed to determine cosegregation with a specific phenotype (i.e., breast cancer). In the Linkage Consortium study, individuals with breast cancer were typed for markers that flanked *BRCA1* on chromosome 17 and *BRCA2* on chromosome 13. Using this methodology, 84% of these 237 families showed linkage to either *BRCA1* or *BRCA2*. However, when the cohort was limited to the 83 families who had four or five cases of female breast cancer but no ovarian or male breast cancer (which we refer to as site-specific breast cancer), linkage to *BRCA1* or *BRCA2* was only demonstrated in 33% of families. Even when families with six or more breast cancers were analyzed, 19% of these families did not cosegregate disease with *BRCA1* or *BRCA2* (Table 1).

Although the data from the Linkage Consortium provides compelling evidence for the existence of other genes associated with site-specific hereditary breast cancer, this same data set provides strong evidence against a significant contribution of genes other than *BRCA1* and *BRCA2* in hereditary breast–ovarian cancer. When the cohort was limited to families with at least four cases of breast cancer and only one case of ovarian

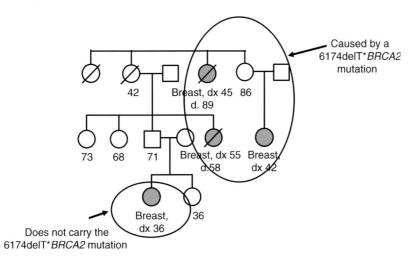

Figure 2   Proband is a phenocopy. In this example, the cluster of cancers in the proband's aunt at age 55, the proband's great aunt at age 45 and the proband's first cousin, once removed, at age 42 were caused by the 6174delT mutation in *BRCA2*. However, genetic testing demonstrated that the proband, with breast cancer at age 36, does not carry this mutation. Therefore the proband is a phenocopy as her breast cancer was caused by factors other than the known familial predisposition.

cancer, 90% of these families showed linkage to either *BRCA1* (69%) or *BRCA2* (21%). In the 52 families with two or more cases of ovarian cancer at any age and at least four cases of breast cancer diagnosed prior to age 60, 100% showed linkage to either *BRCA1* or *BRCA2* (Table 2).

Full Sequencing of *BRCA1* and *BRCA2* Is Unable to Detect a Deleterious Mutation That Is Present in One of These Genes

If essentially all of inherited breast–ovarian cancer is linked to *BRCA1* and *BRCA2*, why does a negative *BRCA* sequencing result in an inherited breast cancer family not rule out an inherited predisposition to ovarian cancer? The Linkage Consortium and others have demonstrated that even in families where linkage can be demonstrated to *BRCA1* or *BRCA2*, sequencing will only detect mutations in 63% to 85% of these families (3,4). The reason for this is that although polymerase chain reactionbased sequencing approaches

Table 1   Proportion of Site-Specific Breast Cancer Families Linked to *BRCA1* or *BRCA2*

		Proportion of linked families (95% CI)		
	N	*BRCA1*	*BRCA2*	Other
4–5 Breast cancers	83	0.28 (0.11–0.50)	0.05 (0.00–0.29)	0.67 (0.35–0.89)
≥6 Breast cancers	34	0.21 (0.08–0.42)	0.60 (0.34–0.83)	0.19 (0.01–0.45)

Abbreviation: CI, confidence interval.
Source: From Ref. 3.

Table 2   Proportion of Hereditary Breast Cancer Families with Ovarian Cancer in the Lineage Linked to *BRCA1* or *BRCA2*

		Proportion of linked families (95% CI)		
	N	*BRCA1*	*BRCA2*	Other
1 Ovarian cancer	42	0.69 (0.50–0.86)	0.21 (0.06–0.40)	0.10 (0.00–0.28)
≥2 Ovarian cancers	52	0.91 (0.76–0.99)	0.09 (0.01–0.24)	0.00 (0.01–0.11)

Abbreviation: CI, confidence interval.
Source: From Ref. 3.

are highly robust for the detection of single nucleotide substitutions as well as insertion or deletion of a few nucleotides, it is not robust for the detection of large deletions that include either the 3' or 5' end of an exon. Similarly, conventional sequencing will not detect genomic inversions or duplications (5,6). In 2006, Walsh et al. examined 300 hereditary breast cancer families in which conventional sequencing did not detect a deleterious mutation in either *BRCA1* or *BRCA2* (7). All families included in this study had at least four breast cancers diagnosed prior to age 60 in a single lineage. In this study, 35 (12%) of the families had previously undetected mutations in *BRCA1* or *BRCA2*. When the study was stratified according to the presence or absence of ovarian cancer in the lineage, 25 (18.5%) of 135 families demonstrated a structural rearrangement if ovarian cancer was present in the lineage. However, if no ovarian or male breast cancer was in the lineage, only 6 (4.3%) of 140 families demonstrated a genomic rearrangement. Additionally, although this study demonstrated that structural rearrangements account for at least a proportion of families in which linkage has been shown and no mutation has been identified on conventional sequencing, not all families in which there was a high probability of linkage to *BRCA1* or *BRCA2* have a deleterious mutation identified even using these enhanced mutation detection technologies. Many of these remaining families are likely explained by noncoding mutations in promoters, enhancers, and other regulatory regions that are beyond our ability to detect with current mutation detection methodologies.

WHAT IS KNOWN ABOUT CANCER RISKS IN *BRCA*-NEGATIVE HEREDITARY BREAST CANCER FAMILIES?

When discussing cancer risks and management in *BRCA*-negative hereditary breast cancer, it is important to distinguish those families with site-specific breast cancer from those with hereditary breast–ovarian cancer. The following discussions will address these situations individually.

BRCA-Negative Hereditary Breast–Ovarian Cancer Families

Given the limitations of *BRCA* sequencing, combined with the linkage data shown above, the possibility of an occult *BRCA* mutation likely should be considered if there are multiple cases (i.e., ≥3–4) of breast cancer prior to age 60 AND a family history of epithelial ovarian cancer or multiple other *BRCA* associated (pancreatic, prostate, melanoma) cancers in a lineage. Additionally, the possibility of an occult *BRCA* mutation should be considered if there are six or more breast cancers prior to age 60 in the lineage, even in the absence of nonbreast cancers in the lineage (Table 3).

Table 3 In Which Patients Should the Possibility of an Occult *BRCA1* or *BRCA2* Mutation Be Considered?

The possibility of an occult *BRCA1* or *BRCA2* mutation should be considered if there are
  Multiple cases (i.e., ≥3–4 cases of breast cancer before 60) AND
  Any epithelial ovarian cancer in the lineage
  Male breast cancer in lineage
  More than 6 breast cancers (prior to 60) in lineage
  Multiple *BRCA*-associated cancers (i.e., pancreatic prostate, melanoma) in lineage

BRCA-Negative Site-Specific Breast Cancer Families

As discussed earlier, in site-specific breast cancer families where there are no more than four to five affected relatives and no ovarian or other *BRCA*-associated cancers present, only 33% of these families will show linkage to either *BRCA1* or *BRCA2* prior to genetic testing. If genetic testing further decreases the likelihood of a *BRCA1* or *BRCA2* mutation in these families by 63% to 85%, it is not clear how much incremental benefit individuals from these families will derive from participating in intensive breast and gynecologic cancer risk-reduction strategies.

In order to provide data relevant to this issue, Kauff et al. recently conducted a prospective study to examine the risk of breast and ovarian cancer in *BRCA*-negative, site-specific breast cancer kindreds (8). In this study, there were 165 *BRCA*-negative, site-specific hereditary breast cancer kindreds identified in which there were at least three cases of breast cancer (mean 4.14, range 3–9) in a lineage with at least one breast cancer diagnosed prior to age 50. All probands had undergone *BRCA* mutation screening by either full sequencing or, in individuals of exclusively Ashkenazi Jewish heritage, founder mutation testing, as this has been shown to detect approximately 95% of detectable mutations in this population (9,10). Probands, along with their first- and second-degree relatives, were followed prospectively for a mean of 3.4 years to determine the incidence of new breast and ovarian cancer in these kindreds. The observed rates of breast and ovarian cancer were then compared to the expected population rates obtained from the Surveillance, Epidemiology, and End Results database (2).

As expected, a threefold increased risk of subsequent breast cancer was observed in this cohort [standardized incidence rations (SIR) 3.13, 95% confidence Interval (CI): 1.88–4.89, $p < 0.001$]. However, there was no increased risk of ovarian cancer observed in 2534 women years of followup with 1 case observed and 0.66 expected (SIR 1.52, 95% CI: 0.02–8,46), $p = 0.04$) (Table 4).

These results, if confirmed, suggest that women from *BRCA*-negative site-specific breast cancer families may not be at significantly increased risk of ovarian cancer.

Table 4 Cancers Developing During 3.4 Years Prospective Followup in 165 *BRCA*-Negative Site-Specific Hereditary Breast Cancer Kindreds

Cancer	Observed cancers	Expected cancers	Standardized incidence rations	p-Value
Breast	19	6.07	3.13	<0.001
Ovary	1	0.66	1.52	0.48

Source: From Ref. 8.

MANAGEMENT OF *BRCA*-NEGATIVE HEREDITARY BREAST CANCER FAMILIES

BRCA-Negative Hereditary Breast–Ovarian Cancer Families

In families meeting the criteria in Table 3 that are suspicious for having an occult *BRCA1* or *BRCA2* mutation despite normal *BRCA1* and *BRCA2* sequencing, affected individuals likely should be managed similarly to women where a *BRCA* mutation has been detected. Specific management strategies appropriate to this group are described in Chapters 15 and 16.

It may also be appropriate to manage unaffected individuals in these families with intensive breast and gynecologic risk-reduction approaches including, in select instances, risk-reducing surgeries. It should, however, be kept in mind that, in most cases, these individuals will have no more than a 50% chance of having the inherited predisposition that is present in the family. Unaffected individuals from such families are best managed by a multidisciplinary team experienced in the care of women who may be at inherited risk.

BRCA-Negative Site-Specific Breast Cancer Families

BRCA-negative women with strong family histories of breast cancer but no family history of other *BRCA*-associated cancer (i.e., ovarian cancer, male breast cancer, or pancreatic cancer) need to be followed up closely for breast cancer risk. At Memorial Sloan-Kettering Cancer Center, it is believed that screening for these individuals should include monthly self-exam; clinical breast exam two times per year; and annual mammography starting 5 to 10 years prior to the earliest age of breast cancer in the family (though not prior to age 25). Investigational screening with breast ultrasound or magnetic resonance imaging may also be appropriate. Risk-reducing mastectomy is also considered in select cases, though it is important to consider that data from the BCLC has suggested that the breast cancers in these families are more likely to be of lower grade and have less nuclear pleomorphism than either *BRCA1*- or *BRCA2*-associated breast cancers (11).

Participation in ovarian cancer risk-reduction screening should be considered investigational, given both the unclear evidence that these women are at increased risk and the limited evidence that ovarian cancer screening is efficacious in any risk group (12). Similarly, it is not clear what role risk-reducing salpingo-oophorectomy has for the prevention of ovarian cancer in women from *BRCA*-negative site-specific breast cancer kindreds as they may not be at increased risk of ovarian cancer compared to the general population. Importantly, there still may be a role for surgical ovarian ablation to decrease the risk of breast cancer in this group. Several studies have suggested that premenopausal oophorectomy is associated with a reduction in subsequent breast cancer risk in carriers of both *BRCA1* and *BRCA2* mutations (13,14) and in women with familial breast cancer without a known mutation (15). However, definitive information regarding the relative risks and benefits of this approach awaits the results of future studies.

CONCLUSIONS

BRCA-negative hereditary breast cancer will account for approximately half of the 15,000 to 22,000 inherited breast cancers that will be diagnosed in the United States in 2007. Despite this substantial public health impact, there remains a paucity of information regarding the evaluation and management of this syndrome. Well-designed prospective studies evaluating women from these families are desperately needed so that we can better learn how to reduce the risk of breast and related cancers in these women while simultaneously minimizing the sequelae of our risk-reducing approaches.

ACKNOWLEDGMENTS

Much of the work described in this review was supported by Department of Defense Breast Cancer Research Program (DAMD17-03-1-0375 to N.D.K.), the Koodish Fellowship Fund, the Danzinger Foundation, the Frankel Foundation, and the Prevention Control and Population Research Program of Memorial Sloan-Kettering Cancer Center.

Parts of this text have been adapted from the following publication: Isaacs C, Kauff ND, Domchek SM. In: Perry MC, ed. Beyond *BRCA1* and *BRCA2* Breast Cancer Genetics. Alexandria: American Society of Clinical Oncology 2006 Educational Book; American Society of Clinical Oncology 2006:57–62.

REFERENCES

1. Robson ME, Boyd J, Borgen PI, Cody HS 3rd. Hereditary breast cancer. Curr Probl Surg 2001; 38:387–480.
2. Ries LAG, Harkins D, Krapcho M, et al. SEER Cancer Statistics Review, 1975–2003. Bethesda, MD: National Cancer Institute, 2006.
3. Ford D, Easton DF, Stratton M, et al. Genetic heterogeneity and penetrance analysis of the *BRCA1* and *BRCA2* genes in breast cancer families. The Breast Cancer Linkage Consortium. Am J Hum Genet 1998; 62:679–689.
4. Unger MA, Nathanson KL, Calzone K, et al. Screening for genomic rearrangements in families with breast and ovarian cancer identifies *BRCA1* mutations previously missed by conformation-sensitive gel electrophoresis or sequencing. Am J Hum Genet 2000; 67: 841–850.
5. Gad S, Caux-Moncoutier V, Pages-Berhouet S, et al. Significant contribution of large *BRCA1* gene rearrangements in 120 French breast and ovarian cancer families. Oncogene 2002; 21: 6841–6847.
6. Montagna M, Dalla Palma M, Menin C, et al. Genomic rearrangements account for more than one-third of the *BRCA1* mutations in northern Italian breast/ovarian cancer families. Hum Mol Genet 2003; 12:1055–1061.
7. Walsh T, Casadei S, Coats KH, et al. Spectrum of mutations in *BRCA1*, *BRCA2*, *CHEK2*, and *TP53* in families at high risk of breast cancer. JAMA 2006; 295:1379–1388.
8. Kauff ND, Mitra N, Robson ME, et al. Risk of ovarian cancer in *BRCA1* and *BRCA2* mutation-negative hereditary breast cancer families. J Natl Cancer Inst 2005; 97:1382–1384.
9. Frank TS, Deffenbaugh AM, Reid JE, et al. Clinical characteristics of individuals with germline mutations in *BRCA1* and *BRCA2*: analysis of 10,000 individuals. J Clin Oncol 2002; 20:1480–1490.
10. Kauff ND, Perez-Segura P, Robson ME, et al. Incidence of non-founder *BRCA1* and *BRCA2* mutations in high risk Ashkenazi breast and ovarian cancer families. J Med Genet 2002; 39: 611–614.
11. Lakhani SR, Gusterson BA, Jacquemier J, et al. The pathology of familial breast cancer: histological features of cancers in families not attributable to mutations in *BRCA1* or *BRCA2*. Clin Can Res 2000; 6:782–789.
12. U.S. Preventive Services Task Force. Screening for ovarian cancer: recommendation statement. Ann Fam Med 2004; 2:260–262.

13. Kauff ND, Satagopan JM, Robson ME, et al. Risk-reducing salpingo-oophorectomy in women with a *BRCA1* or *BRCA2* mutation. N Engl J Med 2002; 346:1609–1615.
14. Rebbeck TR, Lynch HT, Neuhausen SL, et al. Prophylactic oophorectomy in carriers of *BRCA1* or *BRCA2* mutations. N Engl J Med 2002; 346:1616–1622.
15. Olson JE, Sellers TA, Iturria SJ, et al. Bilateral oophorectomy and breast cancer risk reduction among women with a family history. Cancer Detect Prev 2004; 28:357–360.

18

Pathology of Breast Tumors in Hereditary Breast Cancer

William D. Foulkes

Departments of Medicine, Human Genetics, and Oncology, McGill University, Montreal, Quebec, Canada

Lars A. Akslen

The Gade Institute, Section for Pathology, Haukeland University Hospital, University of Bergen, Bergen, Norway

SUMMARY

Over the last few years, it has become apparent that B1BCs have a rather specific phenotype, i.e., these infiltrating breast cancers show expression of proteins that are usually only found in basally situated cells in the normal breast. This phenotype is negatively associated with expression of both estrogen receptor and the oncogene *erbB*-2, also known as *HER2*. The tumors are often of high histological grade and show a high degree of aneuploidy. By contrast, it has been much harder to identify a specific phenotype for B2BCs, although these cancers can usually be distinguished from B1BCs. The clinical implications of the pathological features of B1BCs and B2BCs are beginning to be used clinically by cancer geneticists, and to a lesser extent, by oncologists.

INTRODUCTION

BRCA1 (OMIM 113705) was identified in 1994 (1), followed a year later by *BRCA2* (OMIM 600185) (2). It was not immediately apparent that the breast cancers (BCs) occurring in *BRCA1* and *BRCA2* mutation carriers differed, but early studies indicated that *BRCA1*-related breast cancers (B1BCs) were often high-grade infiltrating ductal BCs with marked aneuploidy (3). Subsequent studies confirmed and extended these observations, the most notable being the Breast Cancer Linkage Consortium (BCLC) paper on differences between B1BC, *BRCA2*-related breast cancers (B2BCs) and so-called sporadic (age-matched) BC. This study showed that B1BC was more distinct from sporadic BC than was B2BC, and notably, medullary or atypical medullary BCs were much more common (13%) in B1BC than in B2BC (3%) or in controls (2%) ($p < 0.0001$). More specifically, by microscopic examination, BCs with *BRCA1* germline mutations have been associated with increased frequency of medullary features such as pushing margins, marked nuclear atypia, high mitotic frequency, areas of necrosis, and often significant lymphocytic infiltration (4). Two of these features (clear demarcation and lymphoid infiltrates) are among the defining features of medullary carcinoma. Other studies have confirmed that typical medullary carcinomas have been observed in 8% to 13% of B1BC compared with 3% for sporadic BC (5), whereas individual medullary features have been found in around 35% to 60% of all B1BCs. In contrast, BCs associated with *BRCA2* germline mutations appear to be less specific morphologically. In their study from 1998, Lakhani et al. reported that B2BC tumors had less tubular differentiation, some tendency for pushing margins, and less mitotic activity than the population of sporadic BC (4), but others have reported higher mitotic rates and marked nuclear pleomorphism in these tumors (6). Both B1BC and B2BC are often well demarcated, but significant differences have been indicated with respect to mitotic frequency and lymphocytic invasion. More studies are needed to further explore the B2BC phenotype. Ductal carcinoma in situ (DCIS) was also noted to be less commonly present adjacent to the cancer in B1BC than in controls (7). This study was then followed up by an analysis of a larger number of cases (4) that found that the only factor common to both B1BC and B2BC that stood out in a multivariable analysis was a continuous pushing tumor margin, which is a defining feature of medullary carcinomas. This is a notable, and to this date, unconfirmed finding. It is interesting because, as stated above, (atypical) medullary BCs are not common in B2BC, so the pushing margin of B2BC cannot be attributed to these features of the cancer. Although the BCLC did not find an excess of lobular BCs in B2BC, Armes et al. did report an excess (8), and there have been anecdotal reports of families containing many cases of lobular B2BC (9). Certainly, it is rare to find a B1BC that has a lobular phenotype.

Following these largely morphological studies, immunohistochemical analyses showed that B1BCs were much more likely than all other BCs to not express estrogen receptor (ER), progesterone receptor (PgR) (10,11), or erythroblastic bacteria oncogen homology 2/herstatin (erbB-2/HER2) (10). This phenotype has more recently come to be referred to as the "triple negative phenotype." Notable, even in these early studies, was that ER levels (measured either biochemically or immunohistochemically) in B1BC were usually either negative or (if the breast tumors were reported as ER positive), only low levels of ER could be found in the tumors. Some thought that this was because B1BC was diagnosed at a younger-than-average age and were often of high grade, but it soon became apparent that even considering the younger age of onset of B1BC, there was a clear underrepresentation of ER-positive BCs in this group. More recent studies have shown that B1BCs are four to five times more likely to be ER negative than are high-grade cancers occurring in noncarriers (12) (Table 1). In early studies, B2BCs already appeared to be different from B1BCs, in that they were frequently ER positive (11).

Table 1 ER Status in Grade 3 non-B12BC, B1BC, and B2BC

Class	N	ER+%
1) Noncarriers	65	46.2
2) BRCA1	138	15.2
3) BRCA2	36	63.9

P-values[a] *P1/2* < 0.0001 *P1/3* = 0.065 *P2/3* < 0.0001

Note: $P_{a/b}$ represents the *P* value for the *t*-test of ER+% in classes a and b.
Abbreviations: B12BC, BRCA1/2-related breast cancer; B1BC, *BRCA1*-related breast cancers; B2BC, *BRCA2*-related breast cancers; ER, estrogen receptor.
Source: From Ref. 12.

These findings have been confirmed in much larger studies (13). There have been scores of papers focusing on the pathology of *BRCA1/2*-related breast cancer (B12BC). What follows is a distillation of these papers, with a focus on clinically relevant themes. Table 2 summarizes some of the key differences between B1BC and B2BC.

BRCA1-RELATED BC

Preneoplastic Lesion in B1BC

When considering morphology, there have been several studies, with largely conflicting results (15–17). Overall, it seems that if there is a subtle heterozygote phenotype in the breasts of *BRCA1* carriers; it is too subtle to be reliably detected using standard morphological tools. Using immunohistochemistry, several groups have noted abnormalities of the PgR (with predominance of subtype A and lack of subtype B) (18) or overexpression of PgR in general (19) in apparently normal breast tissue obtained at the time of cancer surgery or at prophylactic surgery. These studies require confirmation, particularly as they do not seem to have measured precisely the same proteins.

Noninvasive Cancers in B1BC

There is very little strong evidence in support of an increased frequency of DCIS in B1BC (16,17,20). One study that focused on women with DCIS only found that 3/369

Table 2 Differences and Similarities Between *BRCA1*- and *BRCA2*-Related Breast Cancers: A Brief Overview

	BRCA1	*BRCA2*
Morphology	Ductal, no special type (75%), typical medullary ~5%, atypical medullary 10–30%	Ductal, no special type (75%), atypical medullary <5%, lobular/ductal with lobular features more common than in *BRCA1* (~10%)
Grade	High (grade 3, 75%)	Medium/high (grade 2, 45%; grade 3, 45%)
ER	Negative (75%)	Positive (75%)
HER2	Negative (95%)	Negative (95%)
P53	Positive (50%)	Positive (40%)
CK5	Positive (50%)	Negative (90%)
BCL2[a]	Low	High
"TNP"[a,b,c]	Half	Zero
"CBP"[a,c,d]	Three-quarters	Zero
CDKN2A[a]	Low	High
Cyclin D1	Negative (90%)	Positive (60%)
Carcinoma in situ[a]	Not commonly associated	Commonly associated

[a] Three studies or less, so no percentages added.
[b] TNP: ER, PR, and HER2 negative.
[c] Based on unpublished data from Foulkes, Akslen and Brunet, *P* value for TNP association with *BRCA1*: 6.7×10^{-5}, for CBP association with *BRCA1*: 4.1×10^{-7}
[d] CBP: ER and HER2 negative, CK5/6 and/or EGFR positive.
Abbreviations: BCL2, B-cell leukemia/lymphoma 2; CBP, core basal phenotype; CDKN2A, Cyclin dependent kinase inhibitor 2A; CK, cytokeratin; EGFR, epidermal growth factor receptor; ER, estrogen receptor; HER2, herstatin; PgR, progesterone receptor PR; TNP, triple negative phenotype;
Source: From Ref. 14.

women with DCIS carried a *BRCA1* mutation (21), but with no current control group (either negative, no cancer, or positive, invasive cancer); the clearest message from this paper was, as can be gleaned from previous publications (17), that DCIS is more common in B2BC than in B1BC (they found 9 *BRCA2* carriers among the 369 women with DCIS). As has been pointed out by others (22), this may be more a feature of the "snapshot" nature of pathological analysis than any reflection on the biological processes: it makes sense that B1BC may well "destroy the evidence" of their origins by virtue of their fast growth. B2BCs probably grow slightly more slowly and therefore "biological archeology" is easier; nevertheless, when DCIS does occur in ER-negative B1BC, it is usually ER-negative as well (23). Some have argued that, in fact, B1BC arises from an ER-negative stem cell (24), but there is currently little or no evidence one way or another (25).

Invasive Cancers in B1BC

The Basal Phenotype of B1BC

In 2000, Perou et al. showed that morphologically similar BCs could be divided into several subgroups, based on their gene expression profile (26). One of these molecularly defined subgroups was found to contain BCs that did not stain for either ER or HER2/neu (also known as erbB-2) proteins in the tumor cells. This is an unusual combination, as ER and HER2 staining are often inversely associated. As some of the genes differentially expressed in these cancers are usually only expressed in the basal cells of the breast [such as cytokeratin (CK)5/6 and annexin VIII], they called these BCs "basal BCs." In contrast, "luminal" BCs were mainly ER positive, and expressed CK8/18 (most BCs express CK8/18), a protein seen in breast cells adjacent to the lumen of the duct. These findings were not meant to imply that basal cancers arose from basal cells (or indeed any type of cell) but that they expressed proteins normally found in these cells in the adult female breast. Immunohistochemical assays using antibodies raised against CK5/6 and CK8/18 showed that these basal BCs tended to have high levels of CK5/6 and low levels of CK8/18, consistent with the gene expression studies (Fig. 1A).

Most BCs can be divided into those that express luminal keratins, the so-called simple epithelial type keratins such as CKs 7, 8, 18, and 19 and those that also feature high levels of expression of genes that are characteristic of the basal epithelial cells of the normal mammary gland, the stratified epithelial CKs, such as CKs 5, 6, 14, 15, and 17. Other markers, such as smooth muscle actin, glial fibrillary acidic protein, calponin, and P-cadherin may also be present in basal-like BCs (Fig. 1B). Basal BCs are not frequent, comprising between 5% and 15% of all invasive ductal BCs of no special type. Conventional histopathological as well as molecular studies of BCs with "basaloid" cell differentiation have shown that these tumors are often high grade (27), have areas of necrosis (28), may have a typical or atypical medullary morphology (29), and have a distinct pattern of genetic alterations (27), including frequent *TP53* mutations (30). Around half of typical medullary BCs have a mixed basal/luminal phenotype and less than 15% are pure basal (31).

As B1BC are often both ER negative and HER2 negative, these findings immediately suggested that B1BC might fall into the so-called basal group. This was subsequently shown in a study of 72 BCs diagnosed in Ashkenazi Jewish women under 65 years of age where B1BC were nine times more likely to express CK5/6 than tumors not arising in B12BC ($p = 0.002$) (32). Expression array studies also showed that the B1BC were overwhelmingly basal in phenotype (33). Further studies have refined and extended these original findings, showing that epidermal growth factor receptor (EGFR)

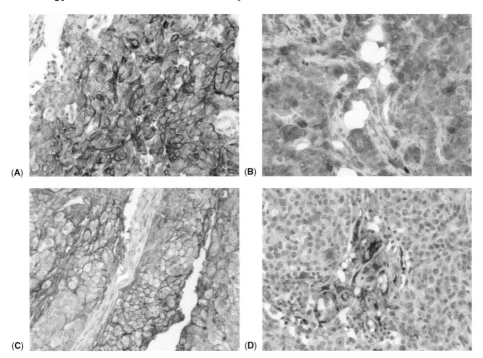

Figure 1   Typical immunohistochemical findings in a *BRCA1*-related breast cancer. (**A**) (*top left*) CK5/6: Strong expression of CK5/6 in a poorly differentiated breast carcinoma with lymphocytic infiltration (Nottingham grade III) (×400). (**B**) (*top right*) P-cadherin: Strong membrane and cytoplasmic expression of P-cadherin in an invasive ductal carcinoma (Nottingham grade III) (×400). (**C**) (*bottom left*) EGFR: Strong membrane expression of EGFR in a poorly differentiated ductal carcinoma (Nottingham grade III) (×400). (**D**) (*bottom right*) GMP: Presence of GMP within a high-grade ductal breast carcinoma (Nottingham grade III) (×400). *Abbreviations*: CK, cytokeratin; EGFR, epidermal growth factor receptor; GMP, glomeruloid microvascular proliferation.

(Fig. 1C) (34), P-cadherin (35,36), fascin (37), annexin VIII (38), caveolin-1 (39), and other basal-related proteins (40) are all overrepresented in B1BC and could form the basis of a clinical assay for B1BC (for a review of this and other aspects of the pathology of B12BC, see Ref. 41). The BCLC studied this in some detail. They showed in a much larger series of cases that ER-negative, CK5/6- and CK14-positive breast tumors were approximately 35 times more likely to carry a *BRCA1* mutation compared to controls; almost one-half of all *BRCA1* cancers had this phenotype, whereas it was seen in only 1.6% of the *BRCA1/2*-negative controls (42). Overall, the profile of B1BCs is remarkably similar to that of basal BCs (43) but it should be remembered that over 50% of B1BCs do not have the full basal phenotype, and B1BC can be an ER-positive, grade 1 BC.

Other Basal-Related Phenotypes of B1BC

Proteins connected to proliferation/cell cycle regulation have been shown to be abnormally expressed in B1BC. In particular, cyclin E has been found to be overexpressed in B1BC at both mRNA (44) and protein levels (40,45); this is often seen with loss of kinase-inhibitory protein 1 (KIP1) (also known as p27, encoded by *CDKN1B*). Interestingly, although these proteins are clearly related to proliferation, among high-grade BCs, they are more likely to be overexpressed in basal than in HER2-overexpressing cancers and therefore are not solely linked to the grade of the cancer. *TP53* is more frequently mutated and/or overexpressed in B1BC than in controls (46,47) and interestingly, these mutations have a somewhat different spectrum than has been observed for non-B12BC (47). The significance of this is not clear but may mean that some of the mutations observed are "passengers" and do not have a pathogenic role.

The oncoprotein myelocyto-matosis oncogene (MYC) is also frequently over-expressed in B1BC, as measured by fluorescent in situ hybridization (FISH), and MYC amplification may be one of the mechanisms by which B1BCs demonstrate genomic instability (48,49). The antiapoptotic protein B-cell leukemia/lymphoma 2 (BCL-2) is generally found at low levels in high-grade cancers, and B1BCs are no exception (50): the balance between high rates of proliferation and high rates of apoptosis and/or tumor necrosis may be a fine one in B1BC. In several studies, features of B1BC that are not definitely "basal-associated," such as overexpression of cyclin E, T-box 2 (TBX2), and MYC, and lack of expression of KIP1 have been used to identify B1BC (45,49).

Vascular Phenotypes in B1BC

Recent studies have indicated that B1BC might develop a particular angiogenic phenotype. Glomeruloid microvascular proliferation (GMP) is characterized by nests of closely associated microvessels resembling renal glomeruli (51,52). In BC, presence of GMP has been associated with high nuclear grade ER negativity and HER2 expression and is thought to represent an aggressive vascular phenotype (53) (Fig. 1D). GMP was found to be an independent prognostic indicator by multivariate analysis, thus providing additional information beyond traditional tumor characteristics. Further studies of BC revealed that presence of GMP was significantly associated with germline *BRCA1* mutations [odds ratio (OR) 2.6] (54). In B1BC, 32% of the tumors were GMP positive, compared with 15% in non-B12BC. Also, the frequency of GMP was significantly increased among the CK5/6 expressing basal BCs (55). These findings indicate that the *BRCA1* genotype, the basal-like tumor phenotype, and the vascular phenotype of GMP are all closely related, and GMP might represent a novel prognostic or possibly predictive marker of particular interest for novel treatment strategies. Thus far, the relationship between B1BC and the GMP phenotype has not been studied in detail. BRCA1 protein was previously associated with inhibition of vascular endothelial growth factor (VEGF) transcription and secretion in BC cells (56), indicating that BRCA1 impairment leads to VEGF increase. Notably, VEGF expression was recently shown to be stronger in basal-like BC (57). More recently, deficiency of BRCA1 in a murine system resulted in an aggressive, vascular phenotype of the resulting breast tumors (58).

Defects in X-Inactivation in B1BC

BRCA1 binds to unpaired X-chromosomes in pachytene spermatocytes, mainly localizing to the XY body, which contains the unpaired, densely heterochromatic and silenced X-chromosome (59). This suggested a role for BRCA1 in X-inactivation. Subsequently, in female somatic cells, BRCA1 protein was found to co-localize on the inactive X-chromosome with the RNA X inactive specific transcript (XIST). Interestingly, cells lacking BRCA1 appear to have defects in X-chromosome structure, and when BRCA1 expression was reconstituted in the cells, focal XIST staining was found (60). Additionally, when basal-like BCs were studied, they showed the same loss of X-inactivation that was seen in B1BC. To add a further twist, BRCA1 protein levels were completely normal in these BCs (61), suggesting at least two pathways to this aspect of the basal phenotype BC. Whether this loss of control of silent heterochromatin is a more general genomic consequence of loss of BRCA1 protein (and/or loss of proteins related to the basal phenotype of BC) or whether it is restricted to the X-chromosome remains in question. The biological significance of loss of X-inactivation is also uncertain.

The Involvement of *BRCA1* in Nonhereditary BC

Somatic *BRCA1* mutations are rarely found in sporadic BC (62) but *BRCA1* expression is often reduced in carcinomas. This may be explained by *BRCA1* promoter methylation, which has been demonstrated in 7% to 31% of sporadic cancers (63) or loss of heterozygosity (LOH) of the *BRCA1* locus, which occurs in 15% to 45% of sporadic BC (64). Studies looking at the relationship between *BRCA1* methylation, *BRCA1* LOH, and clinical features of the breast tumors have been inconsistent (65–67) and there does not seem to be a clear correlation between *BRCA1* methylation and histopathological phenotype. In one study, tumors with LOH of *BRCA1* had high mitotic indices, few tubules, and a very little DCIS (68). It is an attractive hypothesis that somatic inactivation of BRCA1 by promoter methylation and LOH leads to *BRCA1*-like basal BC, but recent studies (discussed above) have found that the majority of sporadic basal-like tumors do not exhibit *BRCA1* promoter methylation and, in fact, have high levels of BRCA1 protein consistent, with normal regulation of *BRCA1* expression (61,69). Therefore, it does not seem that *BRCA1* inactivation is a general characteristic of sporadic basal-like tumors and that inactivation of other genes aside from *BRCA1* can result in a basal phenotype.

BRCA2-RELATED BC

Preneoplastic Lesion in B2BC

As for B1BC, there have been several studies of early lesion in *BRCA2* carriers, with conflicting results (15–17). Interpretation of the work has not been helped by the combining of *BRCA1* and *BRCA2* carriers in most studies. Currently, there is no accepted heterozygote phenotype in the breasts of *BRCA2* carriers.

Noninvasive Cancers in B2BC

DCIS is more common in B2BC than in B1BC. In the only large study performed in a population of 369 women with pure DCIS unselected for family history, 9 (2.4%) were *BRCA2* carriers and 3 (0.8%) were *BRCA1* carriers (17). This finding is mirrored by the observation in the U.K. screening study comparing magnetic resonance imaging (MRI) and mammography that the latter may have a greater role in detecting B2BC than B1BC, because in most centers, mammography appears superior to MRI for the detection of DCIS (70). In the few studies that have been carried out, DCIS occurring in *BRCA2* carriers shows LOH at markers adjacent to *BRCA2* (71). The presence of DCIS in and around invasive B2BC probably means that these cancers have a longer sojourn time in the breast than do invasive B1BC, rather than suggesting that B1BC do not arise from DCIS.

Invasive Cancers in B2BC

Searching for a Specific BRCA2 Phenotype

In general, this search has so far been unsuccessful, as no specific set of markers has been able to reliably pick out B2BC from nonhereditary controls. Like most BCs,

B2BCs are ER positive (11,13), HER2 negative (13,40), and CK8 positive (40,72). They express cyclin D1 (CCND1), but amplification of CCND1 may be more frequent in B2BC than in controls (40). Additionally, *TP53* mutations/overexpressions are more frequent in B2BC than in controls; however, most studies have been limited by small sample size (47). Notably, although one study found that B2BC tumors were more likely than controls to express the basal marker EGFR (34), most others have found that B2BC is rarely basal in nature (13,40). Again, unlike B1BC, but like nonhereditary BC, BCL-2 expression is usually high in B2BC, although not statistically significantly higher than controls (40). DNA repair proteins are differentially expressed in B1BC and B2BC: the latter are more likely than the former to show nuclear *RAD51* expression (73). However, these proteins cannot distinguish between B2BC and nonhereditary BC, and this failure has also been observed in comparative genomic hybridization (CGH) studies (74). Only one study found a discriminator between B2BC and nonhereditary cancers. This study was based on only 21 BC cases and the *BRCA2* classifier used correctly identified only 5 of 8 B2BC. This classifier was better at identifying tumors without *BRCA2* mutations (13 out of 14 correct) but seven of these were B1BC, and as has been shown, it is relatively easy to distinguish B1BC from B2BC. A reanalysis of these data using phylogenetic methods (75) to provide a relatively simple way of imposing a hierarchical structure on the data (with branch lengths in the classification tree representing the degree of separation observed) found that all three types of BC could be distinguished. One of the practical difficulties with interpreting and then using these types of data are the small numbers, the lack of validation, and the need for RNA. Nevertheless, they suggest that real differences between B2BC and nonhereditary BC do exist.

Interestingly, it has been argued that there are two basic proliferation pathways in BC: one, mainly among ER-positive BCs shows KIP1 and cyclin D1 overexpression resulting in cell proliferation via an intact retinoblastoma protein (RB) pathway, whereas the other, which is RB independent, involves cyclin E and occurs in cells with low ER and KIP1 levels (76). Clearly, B2BC falls into the first group and B1BC into the second.

The Involvement of BRCA2 in Nonhereditary BC

In contrast to *BRCA1*, there has been much less work on the role of somatic alterations of *BRCA2* in the etiology of nonhereditary BC. LOH has been reported in several series, but this does not necessarily implicate BRCA2 in tumorigenesis. Additionally, somatic mutations in B2BC are very rare (77–79) and promoter methylation is absent (80). These findings suggest that *BRCA2* has a limited role in nonhereditary BC. This is interesting because the phenotype of B2BC more closely resembles the majority of nonhereditary BCs than does B1BC (ER positive, HER2 negative). Perhaps B1BC, B2BC, and non-B12BC are three completely different molecular entities, and the similarities are more apparent than they are real.

CLINICAL IMPLICATIONS OF PATHOLOGICAL FEATURES OF *BRCA1/2*-RELATED CANCERS

One of the most important implications of the "new pathology" of B12BC is whether this has treatment implications, and whether this extends to similar BC phenotypes that arise as a result of somatic mutations. This matter will be dealt with in greater detail in Chapter 21, by Mark Robson.

IMPLICATIONS OF THE SHAPE OF THE SURVIVAL CURVE FOR B1BC AND BASAL-LIKE BCS

From a gene expression point of view, ER-positive and ER-negative BCs are very different (81) and may even be derived from different cells of origin (25). Interestingly, many studies have shown that the three-year survival for basal-like BCs is particularly poor, but that the survival curves for these cancers and luminal types of BCs meet at 15 to 20 years and may even cross over. The implication is that for basal-like BCs, surviving the first three years or so is particularly important. A related implication is that durable responses to adjuvant chemotherapy are possible and may even be more likely in basal-like BCs, as long as the early losses seen in the first three years are avoided. Thus, B1BC and basal-like BCs can be seen as an acute form of BC, where death is not rare, but if a response to chemotherapy is obtained that persists beyond three years, it is likely to be sustained, and thus cures are obtainable. In contrast, ER-positive BC has more of the characteristic of a progressive, chronic disease, where death is rare, but convincing cures are more difficult of obtain. However, in order to reduce the high recurrence rate of B1BC in the first three years, urgent attempts to identify new biologically targeted agents are warranted.

FUTURE DIRECTIONS

One of the most practical uses of the distinctive pathology of B1BC is to use it to improve the specificity of genetic testing, which is an expensive process. For example, among ER- and HER2-negative BCs, CK5/6 positivity was associated with an OR of 9 for the presence of a germline *BRCA1* mutation (32) and in a follow-up study, the BCLC found that if a BC is ER negative, CK5 and CK14 positive, it is 150 times more likely to be a B1BC than if the cancer is ER positive and CK5 and CK14 positive. Another approach is to use CGH; several studies have noted global differences between B1BC, B2BC, and nonhereditary cancers (82,83), and one Dutch group have identified a potential classifier of B1BC involving loss of chromosomes 3p and 5q and gain of 3q (84). In the near future, the pathological features of B1BC will be used on routine basis to select and exclude individuals for *BRCA1* gene testing.

As discussed above, identifying B2BC is difficult, but if testing for B12BC is to be done sequentially, then identifying B2BC first could be of use. For example, these cancers are more likely than B1BC to show cytoplasmic but not nuclear RAD51 staining (OR 4.25; $p = 0.002$) (73). Refining a robust B2BC CGH classifier that could distinguish B2BC from non-B12BC would be of considerable help; such work is under way in Amsterdam.

From an oncologist's perspective, an important question is whether having a *BRCA1/2* mutation would make a difference to treatment. As both *BRCA1* and *BRCA2* are clearly implicated in DNA repair, and deficient DNA repair in a tumor may mean that errors introduced by chemotherapeutic agents cannot be repaired, it is plausible that chemotherapy use in B12BC could result in preferential activation of programmed cell death pathways. For this reason, there is some reason to believe that B12BC, lacking efficient DNA repair, may be particularly susceptible to agents that act directly on DNA, e.g., platinum and mitomycin C. The real excitement comes, however, from the possibility that "triple negative" BCs (i.e., ER, PgR, and HER2 negative) may be susceptible to new biological therapies, just as bronchoalveolar adenocarcinomas (for some reason, mainly in Asian nonsmoking women) are susceptible to gefitinib because of intragenic EGFR mutations (84,85). The vascular phenotype of B1BC (54) (see above) offers special opportunities for antiangiogenic therapies.

ACKNOWLEDGMENT

I would like to thank Jean-Sébastien Brunet M.Sc. for his help with preparing this chapter.

REFERENCES

1. Miki Y, Swensen J, Shattuck-Eidens D, et al. A strong candidate for the breast and ovarian cancer susceptibility gene BRCA1. Science 1994; 266(5182):66–71.
2. Wooster R, Bignell G, Lancaster J, et al. Identification of the breast cancer susceptibility gene BRCA2. Nature 1995; 378(6559):789–792.
3. Marcus JN, Watson P, Page DL, et al. Hereditary breast cancer: pathobiology, prognosis, and BRCA1 and BRCA2 gene linkage. Cancer 1996; 77(4):697–709.
4. Lakhani SR, Jacquemier J, Sloane JP, et al. Multifactorial analysis of differences between sporadic breast cancers and cancers involving BRCA1 and BRCA2 mutations. J Natl Cancer Instit 1998; 90(15):1138–1145.
5. Honrado E, Osorio A, Palacios J, Benitez J. Pathology and gene expression of hereditary breast tumors associated with BRCA1, BRCA2 and CHEK2 gene mutations. Oncogene 2006; 25(43):5837–5845.
6. Agnarsson BA, Jonasson JG, Bjornsdottir IB, Barkardottir RB, Egilsson V, Sigurdsson H. Inherited BRCA2 mutation associated with high grade breast cancer. Breast Cancer Res Treat 1998; 47(2):121–127.
7. Breast Cancer Linkage Consortium. Pathology of familial breast cancer: differences between breast cancers in carriers of BRCA1 or BRCA2 mutations and sporadic cases. Lancet 1997; 349:1505–1510.
8. Armes JE, Egan AJ, Southey MC, et al. The histologic phenotypes of breast carcinoma occurring before age 40 years in women with and without BRCA1 or BRCA2 germline mutations: a population-based study. Cancer 1998; 83(11):2335–2345.
9. Thiffault I, Hamel N, Pal T, et al. Germline truncating mutations in both MSH2 and BRCA2 in a single kindred. Br J Cancer 2004; 90(2):483–491.
10. Johannsson OT, Idvall I, Anderson C, et al. Tumour biological features of BRCA1-induced breast and ovarian cancer. Eur J Cancer 1997; 33(3):362–371.
11. Karp SE, Tonin PN, Begin LR, et al. Influence of BRCA1 mutations on nuclear grade and estrogen receptor status of breast carcinoma in Ashkenazi Jewish women. Cancer 1997; 80(3): 435–441.
12. Foulkes WD, Metcalfe K, Sun P, et al. Estrogen receptor status in *BRCA1*- and *BRCA2*-related breast cancer: the influence of age, grade, and histological type. Clin Cancer Res 2004; 10(6): 2029–2034.
13. Lakhani SR, van de Vijver MJ, Jacquemier J, et al. The pathology of familial breast cancer: predictive value of immunohistochemical markers estrogen receptor, progesterone receptor, HER-2, and p53 in patients with mutations in BRCA1 and BRCA2. J Clin Oncol 2002; 20(9): 2310–2318.
14. Narod SA, Foulkes WD. BRCA1 and BRCA2: 1994 and beyond. Nat Rev Cancer 2004; 4(9): 665–676.
15. Hoogerbrugge N, Bult P, Widt-Levert LM, et al. High prevalence of premalignant lesions in prophylactically removed breasts from women at hereditary risk for breast cancer. J Clin Oncol 2003; 21(1):41–45.
16. Adem C, Reynolds C, Soderberg CL, et al. Pathologic characteristics of breast parenchyma in patients with hereditary breast carcinoma, including BRCA1 and BRCA2 mutation carriers. Cancer 2003; 97(1):1–11.
17. Kauff ND, Brogi E, Scheuer L, et al. Epithelial lesions in prophylactic mastectomy specimens from women with BRCA mutations. Cancer 2003; 97(7):1601–1608.

18. Mote PA, Leary JA, Avery KA, et al. Germ-line mutations in BRCA1 or BRCA2 in the normal breast are associated with altered expression of estrogen-responsive proteins and the predominance of progesterone receptor A. Genes Chromosomes Cancer 2004; 39(3): 236–248.

19. King TA, Gemignani ML, Li W, et al. Increased progesterone receptor expression in benign epithelium of BRCA1-related breast cancers. Cancer Res 2004; 64(15):5051–5053.

20. Sun CC, Lenoir G, Lynch H, Narod SA. In-situ breast cancer and BRCA1. Lancet 1996; 348(9024):408.

21. Claus EB, Petruzella S, Matloff E, Carter D. Prevalence of BRCA1 and BRCA2 mutations in women diagnosed with ductal carcinoma in situ. JAMA 2005; 293(8):964–969.

22. Adem C, Jenkins RB, Capron F, Stoppa-Lyonnet D. High-risk lesions in high-risk women: a high-risk formalin-based biology. J Clin Oncol 2004; 22(6):1159–1161.

23. Osin P, Crook T, Powles T, Peto J, Gusterson B. Hormone status of in-situ cancer in BRCA1 and BRCA2 mutation carriers [letter]. Lancet 1998; 351(9114):1487.

24. Foulkes WD. BRCA1 functions as a breast stem cell regulator. J Med Genet 2004; 41(1):1–5.

25. Dontu G, El-Ashry D, Wicha MS. Breast cancer, stem/progenitor cells and the estrogen receptor. Trends Endocrinol Metab 2004; 15(5):193–197.

26. Perou CM, Sorlie T, Eisen MB, et al. Molecular portraits of human breast tumours. Nature 2000; 406(6797):747–752.

27. Jones C, Nonni AV, Fulford L, et al. CGH analysis of ductal carcinoma of the breast with basaloid/myoepithelial cell differentiation. Br J Cancer 2001; 85(3):422–427.

28. Tsuda H, Takarabe T, Hasegawa F, Fukutomi T, Hirohashi S. Large, central acellular zones indicating myoepithelial tumor differentiation in high-grade invasive ductal carcinomas as markers of predisposition to lung and brain metastases. Am J Surg Pathol 2000; 24(2): 197–202.

29. Tot T. The cytokeratin profile of medullary carcinoma of the breast. Histopathol 2000; 37(2): 175–181.

30. Sorlie T, Perou CM, Tibshirani R, et al. Gene expression patterns of breast carcinomas distinguish tumor subclasses with clinical implications. Proc Natl Acad Sci USA 2001; 98(19):10869–10874.

31. Jacquemier J, Padovani L, Rabayrol L, et al. Typical medullary breast carcinomas have a basal/myoepithelial phenotype. J Pathol 2005; 207(3):260–268.

32. Foulkes WD, Stefansson IM, Chappuis PO, et al. Germline BRCA1 mutations and a basal epithelial phenotype in breast cancer. J Natl Cancer Inst 2003; 95:1482–1485.

33. Sorlie T, Tibshirani R, Parker J, et al. Repeated observation of breast tumor subtypes in independent gene expression data sets. Proc Natl Acad Sci U S A 2003; 100(14): 8418–8423.

34. van der GP, Bouter A, van der ZR, et al. Re: germline BRCA1 mutations and a basal epithelial phenotype in breast cancer. J Natl Cancer Inst 2004; 96(9):712–713.

35. Arnes JB, Brunet JS, Stefansson I, et al. Placental cadherin and the basal epithelial phenotype of BRCA1-related breast cancer. Clin Cancer Res 2005; 11(11):4003–4011.

36. Palacios J, Honrado E, Osorio A, et al. Immunohistochemical characteristics defined by tissue microarray of hereditary breast cancer not attributable to BRCA1 or BRCA2 mutations: differences from breast carcinomas arising in BRCA1 and BRCA2 mutation carriers. Clin Cancer Res 2003; 9(10):3606–3614.

37. Rodriguez-Pinilla SM, Sarrio D, Honrado E, et al. Prognostic significance of basal-like phenotype and fascin expression in node-negative invasive breast carcinomas. Clin Cancer Res 2006; 12(5):1533–1539.

38. Stein T, Price KN, Morris JS, et al. Annexin A8 is up-regulated during mouse mammary gland involution and predicts poor survival in breast cancer. Clin Cancer Res 2005; 11(19 Pt 1): 6872–6879.

39. Pinilla SM, Honrado E, Hardisson D, Benitez J, Palacios J. Caveolin-1 expression is associated with a basal-like phenotype in sporadic and hereditary breast cancer. Breast Cancer Res Treat 2006; 99(1):85–90.

40. Palacios J, Honrado E, Osorio A, et al. Phenotypic characterization of BRCA1 and BRCA2 tumors based in a tissue microarray study with 37 immunohistochemical markers. Breast Cancer Res Treat 2005; 90(1):5–14.

41. Honrado E, Benitez J, Palacios J. The molecular pathology of hereditary breast cancer: genetic testing and therapeutic implications. Mod Pathol 2005; 18(10):1305–1320.

42. Lakhani SR, Reis-Filho JS, Fulford L, et al. Prediction of BRCA1 status in patients with breast cancer using estrogen receptor and basal phenotype. Clin Cancer Res 2005; 11(14): 5175–5180.

43. Korsching E, Packeisen J, Agelopoulos K, et al. Cytogenetic alterations and cytokeratin expression patterns in breast cancer: Integrating a new model of breast differentiation into cytogenetic pathways of breast carcinogenesis. Laboratory Invest 2002; 82(11): 1525–1533.

44. Van't Veer LJ, Dai HY, van de Vijver MJ, et al. Gene expression profiling predicts clinical outcome of breast cancer. Nature 2002; 415(6871):530–536.

45. Chappuis PO, Donato E, Goffin JR, et al. Cyclin E expression in breast cancer: predicting germline BRCA1 mutations, prognosis and response to treatment. Ann Oncol 2005; 16(5): 735–742.

46. Crook T, Crossland S, Crompton MR, Osin P, Gusterson BA. p53 mutations in BRCA1-associated familial breast cancer. Lancet 1997; 350(9078):638–639.

47. Greenblatt MS, Chappuis PO, Bond JP, Hamel N, Foulkes WD. TP53 mutations in breast cancer associated with BRCA1 or BRCA2 germ-line mutations: distinctive spectrum and structural distribution. Cancer Res 2001; 61(10):4092–4097.

48. Grushko TA, Dignam JJ, Das S, et al. MYC is amplified in BRCA1-associated breast cancers. Clin Cancer Res 2004; 10(2):499–507.

49. Adem C, Soderberg CL, Hafner K, et al. ERBB2, TBX2, RPS6KB1, and MYC alterations in breast tissues of BRCA1 and BRCA2 mutation carriers. Genes Chromosomes Cancer 2004; 41(1):1–11.

50. Freneaux P, Stoppa-Lyonnet D, Mouret E, et al. Low expression of bcl-2 in Brca1-associated breast cancers. Br J Cancer 2000; 83(10):1318–1322.

51. Pettersson A, Nagy JA, Brown LF, et al. Heterogeneity of the angiogenic response induced in different normal adult tissues by vascular permeability factor/vascular endothelial growth factor. Lab Invest 2000; 80(1):99–115.

52. Wesseling P, Vandersteenhoven JJ, Downey BT, Ruiter DJ, Burger PC. Cellular components of microvascular proliferation in human glial and metastatic brain neoplasms. A light microscopic and immunohistochemical study of formalin-fixed, routinely processed material. Acta Neuropathol (Berl) 1993; 85(5):508–514.

53. Straume O, Chappuis PO, Salvesen HB, et al. Prognostic importance of glomeruloid microvascular proliferation indicates an aggressive angiogenic phenotype in human cancers. Cancer Res 2002; 62(23):6808–6811.

54. Goffin JR, Straume O, Chappuis PO, et al. Glomeruloid microvascular proliferation is associated with p53 expression, germline BRCA1 mutations and an adverse outcome following breast cancer. Br J Cancer 2003; 89(6):1031–1034.

55. Foulkes WD, Brunet JS, Stefansson IM, et al. The prognostic implication of the basal-like (cyclin E high/p27 low/p53+/glomeruloid-microvascular-proliferation+) phenotype of BRCA1-related breast cancer. Cancer Res 2004; 64(3):830–835.

56. Kawai H, Li H, Chun P, Avraham S, Avraham HK. Direct interaction between BRCA1 and the estrogen receptor regulates vascular endothelial growth factor (VEGF) transcription and secretion in breast cancer cells. Oncogene 2002; 21(50):7730–7739.

57. Ribeiro-Silva A, Ribeiro do Vale F, Zucoloto S. Vascular endothelial growth factor expression in the basal subtype of breast cancer. Am J Clin Pathol 2006.

58. Furuta S, Wang JM, Wei S, et al. Removal of BRCA1/CtIP/ZBRK1 repressor complex on ANG1 promoter leads to accelerated mammary tumor growth contributed by prominent vasculature. Cancer Cell 2006; 10(1):13–24.

59. Scully R, Chen J, Plug A, et al. Association of BRCA1 with Rad51 in mitotic and meiotic cells. Cell 1997; 88(2):265–275.

60. Ganesan S, Silver DP, Greenberg RA, et al. BRCA1 supports XIST RNA concentration on the inactive X chromosome. Cell 2002; 111(3):393–405.

61. Richardson AL, Wang ZC, De NA, et al. X chromosomal abnormalities in basal-like human breast cancer. Cancer Cell 2006; 9(2):121–132.

62. Futreal PA, Liu Q, Shattuck-Eidens D, et al. BRCA1 mutations in primary breast and ovarian carcinomas. Science 1994; 266(5182):120–122.

63. Catteau A, Harris WH, Xu CF, Solomon E. Methylation of the BRCA1 promoter region in sporadic breast and ovarian cancer: correlation with disease characteristics. Oncogene 1999; 18(11):1957–1965.

64. Rio PG, Maurizis JC, Peffault de LM, Bignon YJ, Bernard-Gallon DJ. Quantification of BRCA1 protein in sporadic breast carcinoma with or without loss of heterozygosity of the BRCA1 gene. Int J Cancer 1999; 80(6):823–826.

65. Esteller M, Silva JM, Dominguez G, et al. Promoter hypermethylation and BRCA1 inactivation in sporadic breast and ovarian tumors [see comments]. J Natl Cancer Inst 2000; 92(7):564–569.

66. Staff S, Isola J, Tanner M. Haplo-insufficiency of BRCA1 in sporadic breast cancer. Cancer Res 2003; 63(16):4978–4983.

67. Wei M, Grushko TA, Dignam J, et al. BRCA1 promoter methylation in sporadic breast cancer is associated with reduced BRCA1 copy number and chromosome 17 aneusomy. Cancer Res 2005; 65(23):10692–10699.

68. Hanby AM, Kelsell DP, Potts HW, et al. Association between loss of heterozygosity of BRCA1 and BRCA2 and morphological attributes of sporadic breast cancer. Int J Cancer 2000; 88(2):204–208.

69. Matros E, Wang ZC, Lodeiro G, Miron A, Iglehart JD, Richardson AL. BRCA1 promoter methylation in sporadic breast tumors: relationship to gene expression profiles. Breast Cancer Res Treat 2005; 91(2):179–186.

70. Leach MO, Boggis CR, Dixon AK, et al. Screening with magnetic resonance imaging and mammography of a UK population at high familial risk of breast cancer: a prospective multicentre cohort study (MARIBS). Lancet 2005; 365(9473):1769–1778.

71. Thomassen M, Kruse TA, Olsen KE, Borg A, Gerdes AM. Loss of heterozygosity at BRCA2 in a ductal carcinoma in situ and three invasive breast carcinomas in a family with a germline BRCA2 mutation. Breast Cancer Res Treat 2004; 87(3):273–276.

72. Hedenfalk I, Duggan D, Chen Y, et al. Gene-expression profiles in hereditary breast cancer. N Engl J Med 2001; 344(8):539–548.

73. Honrado E, Osorio A, Palacios J, et al. Immunohistochemical expression of DNA repair proteins in familial breast cancer differentiate BRCA2-associated tumors. J Clin Oncol 2005; 23(30):7503–7511.

74. van Beers EH, van WT, Wessels LF, et al. Comparative genomic hybridization profiles in human BRCA1 and BRCA2 breast tumors highlight differential sets of genomic aberrations. Cancer Res 2005; 65(3):822–827.

75. Desper R, Khan J, Schaffer AA. Tumor classification using phylogenetic methods on expression data. J Theor Biol 2004; 228(4):477–496.

76. Loden M, Stighall M, Nielsen NH, et al. The cyclin D1 high and cyclin E high subgroups of breast cancer: separate pathways in tumorogenesis based on pattern of genetic aberrations and inactivation of the pRb node. Oncogene 2002; 21(30):4680–4690.

77. Lancaster JM, Wooster R, Mangion J, et al. BRCA2 mutations in primary breast and ovarian cancers. Nature Genet 1996; 13(2):238–240.

78. Teng DH, Bogden R, Mitchell J, et al. Low incidence of BRCA2 mutations in breast carcinoma and other cancers. Nature Genet 1996; 13(2):241–244.

79. Janatova M, Zikan M, Dundr P, Matous B, Pohlreich P. Novel somatic mutations in the BRCA1 gene in sporadic breast tumors. Hum Mutat 2005; 25(3):319.

80. Collins N, Wooster R, Stratton MR. Absence of methylation of CpG dinucleotides within the promoter of the breast cancer susceptibility gene BRCA2 in normal tissues and in breast and ovarian cancers. Br J Cancer 1997; 76(9):1150–1156.

81. Gruvberger S, Ringner M, Chen YD, et al. Estrogen receptor status in breast cancer is associated with remarkably distinct gene expression patterns. Cancer Res 2001; 61(16): 5979–5984.

82. Tirkkonen M, Johannsson O, Agnarsson BA, et al. Distinct somatic genetic changes associated with tumor progression in carriers of BRCA1 and BRCA2 germ-line mutations. Cancer Res 1997; 57(7):1222–1227.

83. Wessels LFA, van Welsem T, Hart AAM, Van't Veer LJ, Reinders MJT, Nederlof PM. Molecular classification of breast carcinomas by comparative genomic hybridization: a specific somatic genetic profile for BRCA1 tumors. Cancer Res 2002; 62(23):7110–7117.

84. Lynch TJ, Bell DW, Sordella R, et al. Activating mutations in the epidermal growth factor receptor underlying responsiveness of non-small-cell lung cancer to Gefitinib. N Engl J Med 2004; 350(21):350.

85. Paez JG, Janne PA, Lee JC, et al. EGFR mutations in lung cancer: correlation with clinical response to gefitinib therapy. Science 2004; 304(5676):1497–1500.

19
Pathology of Ovarian Tumors in Mutation Carriers

Frédérique Penault-Llorca
Département de Pathologie, Centre Jean Perrin, Clermont-Ferrand Cedex, France

Sunil R. Lakhani
Molecular and Cellular Pathology, School of Medicine, University of Queensland, Queensland Institute of Medical Research & The Royal Brisbane & Women's Hospital, Herston, Queensland, Australia

INTRODUCTION

Epithelial ovarian cancer (EPC) is a heterogeneous disease. Ovarian neoplasms can be subdivided into three main groups: epithelial/stromal, germ cell, or sex cord/stromal. Among epithelial tumors, different tumor subtypes present with different clinical and morphological features reflecting their underlying distinctive molecular characteristics. EPC has a poor outcome in part due to the fact that at the time of diagnosis, 75% of the patients have disease advanced beyond the ovary. Patients with early-stage disease, limited to the ovary or pelvis (Stages I and II, respectively), have survival in the 80% to 95% range, whereas the survival of patients with disease involving the upper abdomen or beyond (Stages III and IV, respectively) is 10% to 30% (1). In the United States, 10% to 20% of patients with ovarian cancer have a first- or second-degree relative with breast and/or ovarian cancer (2). The lifetime risk for developing ovarian cancer in the general population is 1.6% whereas it rises up to 7% if women have two first-degree relatives affected with this disease.

EPIDEMIOLOGY

Three clinical manifestations of hereditary ovarian cancer have been recognized: (*i*) "site-specific" ovarian cancer, (*ii*) the breast and ovarian cancer syndrome, and (*iii*) the hereditary nonpolyposis colorectal cancer (HNPCC; Lynch II syndrome). The first two groups are associated with germline mutations in the *BRCA1* and *BRCA2* tumor suppressor genes, whereas HNPCC is associated with germline mutations in the DNA mismatch repair genes, primarily *hMLH1* and *hMSH2* (3). Approximately 10% of all EPCs are hereditary, with mutations in the *BRCA* genes accounting for approximately 90% of cases. Most of the available information relates to *BRCA1*-linked disease given that *BRCA1* germline mutations are approximately four times more common in ovarian cancer patients than *BRCA2* mutations. A minority (probably fewer than 10%) results from germline mutations in the genes responsible for HNPCC or Lynch syndrome (4). In Israel, up to 40% of women with ovarian cancer with a family history of this disease and 13% of sporadic cases have been shown to carry germline *BRCA1* mutations.

BRCA1 AND *BRCA2* MUTATIONS AND LIFETIME CANCER RISK

The risk of an individual with a mutation developing cancer of the ovary appears to be influenced by the position of the mutation within the *BRCA* gene, the presence of allelic variants of modifying genes, and the hormonal exposure of the carrier (5). The risk of breast cancer for a woman with *BRCA1* or two mutations ranges from 56% to 87%. In contrast, the cumulative lifetime risk of ovarian cancer is 40% to 50% for *BRCA1* mutation carriers and 20% to 30% for *BRCA2* mutation carriers. This compares to a 1.6% risk in the general population. Interestingly, for *BRCA2* carriers, ovarian cancer seems to occur more commonly in individuals with mutations in exon 11, "the ovarian cancer cluster region" (6). The basis for the range in risks of ovarian cancer in mutation carriers is likely due to both environmental and genetic factors affecting penetrance. For example, oral contraceptives' use and tubal ligation exert a protective effect and *HRAS1* tandem repeat are associated with an increased risk. Moreover, differences in gene penetrance have been observed among different families with identical *BRCA1* mutations.

Mutations of *BRCA* genes are rare in sporadic ovarian cancers. It is postulated that the high rates of loss heterozygosity in the *BRCA1* and two loci in sporadic tumors may play a role in the development of sporadic ovarian tumors. Nevertheless, such loss of heterozygotie (LOH) may also be a late event in somatic ovarian cancer (7).

PATHOLOGY AND CLINICAL MANIFESTATIONS

Hereditary ovarian cancers exhibit distinct clinicopathologic features compared with sporadic cancers. Hereditary ovarian cancers are epithelial whereas malignancies of sex cord-stromal origins or of germ cells are not seen in association with mutations in these genes. The breast and ovarian cancer phenotypes associated with mutations in *BRCA1* and *BRCA2* are similar, confirming that the two proteins exert common functions in ovaries. Most ovarian cancers associated with germline *BRCA* mutations are diagnosed at a younger age (mean age 53 vs. 64 for sporadic) and are high-grade and advanced-stage serous carcinomas. Most studies have reported that papillary serous adenocarcinoma is the predominant type to occur in *BRCA1* or *BRCA2* carriers (5).

In a large collaborative study carried out on behalf of the Breast Cancer Linkage Consortium, we characterized the histopathological features of breast cancers arising in patients harboring germline mutations in the *BRCA1* and *BRCA2* genes (8). In this study, a systematic blinded detailed review of more than 200 *BRCA*-associated ovarian cancers was performed and compared with population-based controls. We confirmed the greater frequency of serous carcinomas in *BRCA1*-associated tumors (Fig. 1A), consistent with previous studies by Rubin et al. (9), Berchuck et al. (10), and more recently by Shaw et al. (11).

Our study and others have also shown that malignant mucinous carcinoma (Fig. 2A) is underrepresented in *BRCA1* mutation carriers (8,12), suggesting that mutations in this gene do not generally play a role in the development of this subtype of epithelial neoplasm.

The frequencies of endometrioid and clear cell (Fig. 1B) carcinomas were similar to, or slightly lower than, their frequencies in controls, in accordance with other

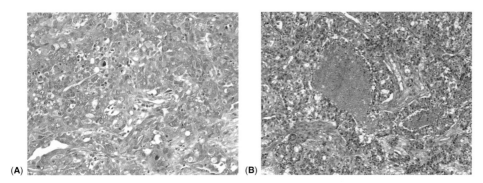

Figure 1 *BRCA1*-associated histopathological type: (**A**) High-grade serous carcinoma (HESX10) (**B**) endometrioid carcinoma.

reports (9). These types therefore represent a significant fraction of tumors in *BRCA1* carriers (36% and 18%, respectively). We found that borderline tumors (Fig. 2B) are much more rare (as a proportion of all ovarian tumors) in *BRCA1* carriers, in accordance with previous observations (13).

Furthermore, we showed that *BRCA1*-associated tumors are of higher grade ($p < 0.0001$), on an average, than control tumors. This difference has been found in several other studies (3,9,11). We also found a greater proportion of solid tumors in the *BRCA1* group ($p = 0.001$), indicating poor differentiation, an effect also seen by Shaw et al. (11). The other morphological features, such as vascular invasion, necrosis, and mitotic count, were not significantly associated with *BRCA1* mutations in this study. Consistent with the association with grade, we found a higher frequency of strong *p53* staining in *BRCA1* and *BRCA2* tumors ($p = 0.018$). In contrast, our study did not reveal any difference in human epidermal growth factor receptor 2 (HER2) expression between *BRCA1* and *BRCA2* ovarian cancers or controls. This contrasts with the pattern in breast cancer, in which HER2 overexpression is less frequent in *BRCA*-associated cancers than in controls (14).

The distribution of histological features in *BRCA2* carriers is very similar to those seen in *BRCA1* carriers, with a very low frequency of borderline and mucinous tumors, a higher-than-average frequency of serous tumors, and smaller but significant frequencies of endometrioid and giant-cell tumors. *BRCA2* tumors are also of higher-than-average grade and more frequently have a solid component.

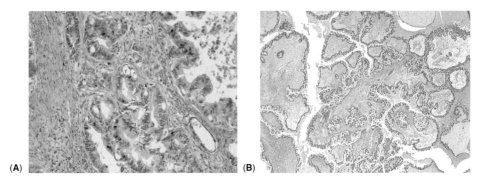

Figure 2 *BRCA1* nonassociated ovarian tumors: (**A**) Invasive mucinous carcinoma (HESX10) (**B**) serous borderline tumor.

Table 1   Features of *BRCA1/2*-Associated Ovarian Cancer

Younger age (10 yr younger than sporadic)
Similar features in *BRCA1* and *BRCA2* mutations carriers
Epithelial tumors, predominantly serous, high grade (solid, numerous mitosis), *p53+*
No difference for HER2 overexpression between *BRCA*-associated and controls
Are not usually mucinous or borderline

This similarity in ovarian cancer pathology between *BRCA1* and *BRCA2* carriers contrasts with the breast cancer pathology, where there is a very marked contrast between *BRCA1*- and *BRCA2*-associated diseases. The only notable differences between *BRCA1*- and *BRCA2*-related ovarian cancers are the much lower risk in *BRCA2* carriers and the different age distributions, with *BRCA2*-associated disease occurring later in life.

MICROARRAY DATA ON *BRCA1/2* OVARIAN TUMORS

Recent microarray studies from Marquez et al. showed that the different ovarian subtypes were associated with distinct gene expression profiles. This finding supports the long-held belief that histotypes of ovarian cancers come to resemble normal fallopian tube and endo-metrial and colonic epithelium (15). Several potential molecular markers for serous, endometrioid, clear cell, and mucinous ovarian cancers have been identified. Other microarray studies have found different profiles associated with tumor grade, prognosis, and response to therapy (16–18).

Complementary (cDNA) microarrays were used to compare gene expression patterns in ovarian cancers associated with *BRCA1* or *BRCA2* mutations with gene expression patterns in sporadic EPCs and to identify patterns common to both hereditary and sporadic tumors. Jazaeri et al. (19) showed that mutations in *BRCA1* and *BRCA2* may lead to carcinogenesis through distinct molecular pathways. In their study, the greatest contrast in gene expression was observed between tumors with *BRCA1* mutations and those with *BRCA2* mutations; 110 genes showed statistically significantly different expression levels ($p < 0.0001$). Furthermore, these distinct pathways also appeared to be involved in sporadic cancers. Sporadic carcinogenic pathways may result from epigenetic aberrations of *BRCA1* and *BRCA2* or their downstream effectors as this group of genes could segregate sporadic tumors into two subgroups, "*BRCA1*-like" and "*BRCA2*-like," suggesting that *BRCA1*-related and *BRCA2*-related pathways are also involved in sporadic ovarian cancers. Fifty-three genes were differentially expressed between tumors with *BRCA1* mutations and sporadic tumors; 6 of the 53 mapped to *Xp11.23* and were expressed at higher levels in tumors with *BRCA1* mutations than in sporadic tumors. Compared with the immortalized ovarian surface epithelial cells used as reference, several interferon-inducible genes were overexpressed in the majority of tumors with a *BRCA* mutation and in sporadic tumors.

EVALUATION OF THE RISK: DOES PATHOLOGY PLAY A ROLE IN WHO TO TEST?

The National Institutes of Health consensus statement is quite broad and states that a woman with one first-degree relative with ovarian cancer may choose to be screened for ovarian cancer (20). Additionally, it is recommended that women with two or more family members affected by ovarian cancer should have counseling by a gynecologic oncologist or other qualified specialist about her individual risk. Morphological and immunohistochemical features of a tumor have also been shown to be powerful predictors of *BRCA1* mutation status that could aid in identifying individuals who should be referred for genetic counseling and testing. Even in the absence of information on family history, the mutation prevalence in women with poorly differentiated and undifferentiated serous tumors exceeds 10% in most age groups, whereas the prevalence in those with mucinous and well-differentiated tumors is low (8). The addition of *p53* staining further improves prediction of mutation status. Similar predictions can be made for *BRCA2* tumors. Thus, the use of pathological features of ovarian tumors may substantially improve the targeting of predictive genetic testing.

OTHER GYNECOLOGICAL TUMOR SITES ASSOCIATED WITH *BRCA* MUTATIONS

BRCA1 and *BRCA2* carriers also have elevated risks of fallopian tube (21) and primary peritoneal carcinomas (22). Schorge et al. found that 26% of papillary serous adenocarcinomas of the peritoneum were associated to *BRCA1* mutations. These tumors had higher level of *p53* mutations and were less likely to overexpress HER2 than wild-type *BRCA1* subjects (22).

PROGNOSIS AND TREATMENT

Women with hereditary ovarian cancers have a distinctly better clinical outcome with longer overall survival and recurrence-free interval after chemotherapy than is seen in those with sporadic cancers, and this is particularly true if they received platinum-based therapy. This difference is thought to be due to a chemosensitivity of the *BRCA*-deficient tumor cells to DNA damaging agent such as cisplatin (23). Nevertheless, in some studies, these results might be influenced by survival bias, as only women who had survived long enough to be tested were included. Such a bias would select against mutation carriers with a poor prognosis, and could thereby skew the findings.

RISK REDUCTION OPTION

Women with a family history including two or more first- or second-degree relatives with either ovarian cancer alone or both breast and ovarian cancers should undertake prophylactic salpingo-oophorectomy immediately after childbearing has been completed to reduce the risk of ovarian cancer (20,24). Screening procedures have proven highly ineffective in the general population and the consensus is that the current screening methodologies (pelvic ultrasound, CA-125 levels) do not perform any better in the setting of hereditary ovarian cancer.

Women carrying a *BRCA* mutation are more prone to undergo prophylactic oophorectomy (PO) than prophylactic mastectomy, with more than 50% of the carriers opting for oophorectomy as compared to 8% to 28% undergoing mastectomy (25). The evidence of a predisposition to tubal carcinoma in *BRCA* mutation carriers has raised the question whether an oophorectomy alone would be enough. It is now a standard practice to perform a prophylactic bilateral salpingo-oophorectomy (PSO), although some authors advocate the inclusion of hysterectomy for the management of such patients in order to remove interstitial and isthmic portion of the tubes (26).

PSO reduces the risk of ovarian, fallopian tube, or primary peritoneal cancers by 98% and the risk of breast and ovarian cancer by 54%. The risk of developing peritoneal carcinoma remains. It has been variably estimated ranging from 1.8% 1 to 27 years after PO in the Gilda Radner registry (27), to 10.7% in the National Cancer Institute (NCI) registry of cancer-prone families (28). In a series from Casey et al. (29), a 3.5% cumulative risk for all mutation carriers and a 3.9% cumulative risk for *BRCA1* mutation carriers were calculated through 20 years of followup after PSO. The calculated cumulative risks of developing intra-abdominal carcinomatosis after PO in members of hereditary breast and ovarian cancer syndrome families, specifically those who carry deleterious mutations, are well below the estimated risks of ovarian cancer published previously from the NCI registry for similar patients (29). Some cases of presumed peritoneal cancer following PO in the old studies could represent peritoneal spread of an undiagnosed primary ovarian cancer due to sampling error. PSO also reduces the risk of subsequent breast cancer if performed premenopausally.

PATHOLOGICAL FINDINGS IN PSO SPECIMEN

In ovaries removed from patients undergoing PO or PSO, putative precursors of ovarian carcinoma or occult ovarian carcinoma have been observed. Ovarian dysplasia has been described in prophylactic oophorectomies' specimens by Deligdisch et al. (30,31) and identified (*i*) in ovarian surface epithelium and in epithelial inclusion cyst, (*ii*) adjacent to overt carcinoma, and incidentally often in the patients with family history. Data from Salazar et al. (32) have shown changes such as metaplasia, surface papillomatosis (Fig. 3), deep cortical invaginations (Fig. 4), inclusion cysts (Fig. 5), and epithelial hyperplasia and atypia (Fig. 6) were significantly more frequent in specimens from POs associated with *BRCA* mutations. Atypia and hyperplasia have also been described in the fallopian tubes (Fig. 7) (33).

Those data remain controversial; as such, changes have also been observed, to a lesser extent, in normal ovaries removed, for instance, during total hysterectomy (TAH) for fibromas. Nevertheless, few microscopic or tiny gross carcinomas have been reported,

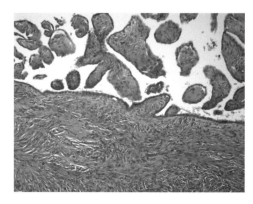

Figure 3   Surface papillomatosis.

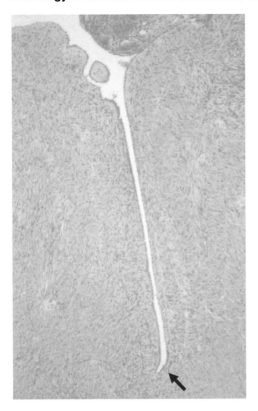

Figure 4 Deep cortical invaginations.

mainly in PO specimens from patients at high risk for the development of ovarian carcinoma with occult carcinoma including ovarian, fallopian, and peritoneal carcinomas detected in 1.7% to 17% of cases.

Only a small number of studies have examined the molecular genetic features of such lesions (34). We have performed a study evaluating cancer-prone phenotypes in 31 prophylactic specimens' oophorectomy (PSO) (*18* from the Mount Sinai School of Medicine, NY and *13* from Centre Jean Perrin) (35). Patients were eligible if they had a known *BRCA* mutation, and/or a family history of ovarian cancer, and/or a family or personal history of breast cancer (median age 50) (PSO group). The control group was composed of 21 normal ovaries from patients with no known risk for ovarian cancer, undergoing TAH-BSO for uterine leiomyoma, and seven cases of Stage III to IV ovarian invasive serous papillary carcinoma. Our results showed a progressive increased expression of Ki67 and *p53* between normal, PSO, and ovarian carcinoma ($p = 0.01$). A similar trend was observed for cytoplasmic CA-125 expression.

An increased level of morphologic abnormalities of ovarian surface epithelium and inclusion glands has been shown to be associated with expression of *p53* in normal ovaries, suggesting that abnormalities of *p53* may be an early event in carcinogenesis (8, for review). Moreover, *p53* mutations have been observed in normal epithelium and inclusion glands adjacent to invasive serous carcinomas. These data suggest that *p53* mutations are an early event and might be present prior to stromal invasion and correspond to an early event in serous tumor carcinogenesis (34). Additionally, mutations in *p53* are associated with loss of *BRCA1* or *BRCA2* function in the majority of tumors.

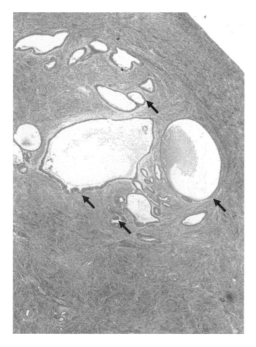

Figure 5 Inclusion cysts.

Thus, these findings suggest that PSO specimens from high-risk women should by thoroughly sampled (ovaries and fallopian tubes) as they may harbor preinvasive lesions or occult carcinomas. Additionally, *p53* mutations have been noted to arise in preinvasive epithelium and appear to be associated with loss of *BRCA1/2* function.

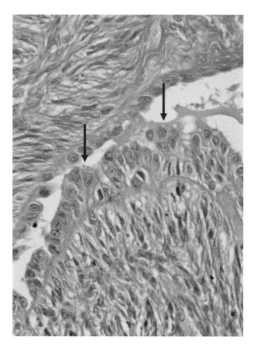

Figure 6 Epithelial hyperplasia and atypia.

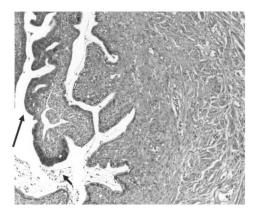

Figure 7   Tubal dysplasia.

HEREDITARY NONPOLYPOSIS COLORECTAL CANCER

Two genes in particular, *MLH1* and *MSH2*, account by far for most of HNPCC. The cumulative risk of ovarian cancer in HNPCC families is more than 12%. Ovarian cancer in HNPCC syndrome is diagnosed at younger age than in the general population. Most tumors are low-stage and well-differentiated or moderately differentiated carcinomas. Annual followup is recommended for these patients and includes concurrent CA-125 screening and transvaginal ultrasound every 6 to 12 months as well as consideration for prophylactic TAH and PSO once childbearing is complete (36,37).

CONCLUSION

Individuals carrying germline mutations in one allele of the *BRCA1* or *BRCA2* genes are at significantly increased risk of developing ovarian and fallopian tube cancer. Once cancer has developed, the pathology and clinical behavior of *BRCA*-associated tumors is distinct from sporadic cases. The tumors occur earlier than sporadic ovarian tumors (on average 10 years younger). They are typically epithelial tumors, predominantly of serous subtype, and high grade (solid architecture, numerous mitosis). Frequent *p53* mutations are noted. Borderline and mucinous tumors are rare in mutation carriers. Bilateral prophylactic salpingo-oophorectomy is recommended for women with known mutations immediately after childbearing has been completed to reduce the risk of ovarian and breast cancers. Given the frequency of preinvasive lesions, it is recommended that the PSO specimens be carefully and thoroughly processed.

REFERENCES

1. Berkenblit A, Cannistra SA. Advances in the management of epithelial ovarian cancer. J Reprod Med 2005; 50(6):426–38.
2. Wooster R, Weber BL. Breast and ovarian cancer. Genomic medicine. N Engl J Med 2003; 348:2339–2347.
3. Prat J, Ribe A, Gallardo A. Hereditary ovarian cancer. Hum Pathol 2005; 36(8):861–870.
4. Boyd J. Specific keynote: hereditary ovarian cancer: what do we know. Gynecol Oncol 2003; 88:S8–S10.

5. Sowter HM, Ashworth A. *BRCA1* and *BRCA2* as ovarian cancer susceptibility genes. Carcinogenesis 2005; 26(10):1651–1656.

6. Gayther SA, Mangion J, Russel P, et al. Variation of risks of breast and ovarian cancer associated with different germline mutations of the *BRCA2* gene. Nat Genet 1997; 15: 103–105.

7. Coukos G, Rubin SC. *BRCA1* and *BRCA2* mutations in ovarian carcinoma. In: Altechk, Deligdisch, Kase, eds. Diagnosis and Management of Ovarian Disorders. San Diego: Academic Press, Elsevier, 2003:201–208.

8. Lakhani SR, Manek S, Penault-Llorca F, et al. Pathology of ovarian cancers in *BRCA1* and *BRCA2* carriers. Clin Cancer Res 2004; 10(7):2473–2481.

9. Rubin SC, Benjamin I, Behbakht K, et al. Clinical and pathological features of ovarian cancer in women with germ-line mutations of *BRCA1*. N Engl J Med 1996; 335:1413–1416.

10. Berchuck A, Heron KA, Carney ME, et al. Frequency of germline and somatic *BRCA1* mutations in ovarian cancer. Clin Cancer Res 1998; 4:2433–2437.

11. Shaw PA, McLaughlin JR, Zweemer RP, et al. Histopathologic features of genetically determined ovarian cancer. Int J Gynecol Pathol 202; 21:407–411.

12. Stratton JF, Gayther SA, Russell P, et al. Contribution of *BRCA1* mutations to ovarian cancer. N Engl J Med 1997; 336:1125–1130.

13. Gotlieb WH, Friedman E, Bar-Sade RB, et al. Rates of Jewish ancestral mutations in *BRCA1* and *BRCA2* in borderline ovarian tumors. J Natl Cancer Inst (Bethesda) 1998; 90: 995–1000.

14. Lakhani SR, Van De Vijver MJ, Jacquemier J, et al. The pathology of familial breast cancer: predictive value of immunohistochemical markers estrogen receptor, progesterone receptor, HER-2, and *p53* in patients with mutations in *BRCA1* and *BRCA2*. J Clin Oncol 2002; 20: 2310–2318.

15. Marquez RT, Baggerly KA, Patterson AP, et al. Patterns of gene expression in different histotypes of epithelial ovarian cancer correlate with those in normal fallopian tube, endometrium, and colon. Clin Cancer Res 2005; 11(17):6116–6126.

16. Goto T, Takano M, Sakamoto M, et al. Gene expression profiles with cDNA microarray reveals RhoGDI as a predictive marker for paclitaxel resistance in ovarian cancers. Oncol Rep 2006; 15(5):1265–1271.

17. Ouellet V, Guyot MC, Le Page C, et al. Tissue array analysis of expression microarray candidates identifies markers associated with tumor grade and outcome in serous epithelial ovarian cancer. Int J Cancer 2006; 119(3):599–607.

18. De Smet F, Pochet NL, Engelen K, et al. Predicting the clinical behavior of ovarian cancer from gene expression profiles. Int J Gynecol Cancer 2006; 16(suppl 1):147–151.

19. Jazaeri AA, Yee CJ, Sotiriou C, Brantley KR, Boyd J, Liu ET. Gene expression profiles of *BRCA1*-linked, *BRCA2*-linked, and sporadic ovarian cancers. J Natl Cancer Inst 2002; 94(13): 990–1000.

20. Ovarian cancer: screening, treatment, and follow-up. NIH Consens State 1994; 12(3):30.

21. Sobol H, Jacquemier J, Bonaiti C, Dauplat J, Birnbaum D, Eisinger F. Fallopian tube cancer as a feature of *BRCA1*-associated syndromes. Gynecol Oncol 2000; 78(2):263–264.

22. Schorge JO, Muto MG, Lee SJ, et al. *BRCA1*-related papillary serous carcinoma of the peritoneum has a unique molecular pathogenesis. Cancer Res 2000; 60(5):1361–1364.

23. Foulkes WD. *BRCA1* and *BRCA2*: chemosensitivity, treatment outcomes and prognosis. Fam Cancer 2006; 5(2):135–142.

24. Eisinger F, Bressac B, Castaigne D, et al. Identification and management of hereditary breast-ovarian cancers (2004 update). Pathol Biol (Paris) 2006; 54(4):230–250.

25. Wagner TM, Moslinger R, Langbauer G, et al. Attitude towards prophylactic surgery and effects of genetic counselling in families with *BRCA* mutations. Austrian Hereditary Breast and Ovarian Cancer Group. Br J Cancer 2000; 82(7):1249–1253.

26. Paley PJ, Swisher EM, Garcia RL, et al. Occult cancer of the fallopian tube in *BRCA1* germline mutation carriers at prophylactic oophorectomy: a case for recommending hysterectomy at surgical prophylaxis. Gynecol Oncol 2001; 80(2):176–180.

27. Piver MS, Baker TR, Jishi MF, et al. Familial ovarian cancer. A report of 658 families from the Gilda Radner Familial Ovarian Cancer Registry 1981–1991. Cancer 1993; 71(2 suppl): 582–588.

28. Tobacman JK. Intra abdominal carcinomatosis after PO in ovarian-cancer-prone families. Lancet 1982; ii:795–779.

29. Casey MJ, Synder C, Bewtra C, Narod SA, Watson P, Lynch HT. Intra-abdominal carcinomatosis after prophylactic oophorectomy in women of hereditary breast ovarian cancer syndrome kindreds associated with *BRCA1* and *BRCA2* mutations. Gynecol Oncol 2005; 97 (2):457–467.

30. Deligdisch L, Miranda C, Barba J, Gil J. Ovarian dysplasia: nuclear texture analysis. Cancer 1993; 72(11):3253–3257.

31. Deligdisch L, Gil J, Kerner H, Wu HS, Beck D, Gershoni-Baruch R. Ovarian dysplasia in prophylactic oophorectomy specimens: cytogenetic and morphometric correlations. Cancer 1999; 86(8):1544–1550.

32. Salazar H, Godwin AK, Daly MB, et al. Microscopic benign and invasive malignant neoplasms and a cancer-prone phenotype in prophylactic oophorectomies. J Natl Cancer Inst 1996; 88(24):1810–1820.

33. Rabban JT, Bell DA. Current issues in pathology of ovarian cancer. J Reprod Med 2005; 50: 467–474.

34. Bell DA. Origins and molecular pathology of ovarian cancer. Mod Pathol 2005; 18(suppl 2): S19–S32.

35. Schlosshauer PW, Cohen CJ, Penault-Llorca F, et al. Prophylactic oophorectomy: a morphologic and immunohistochemical study. Cancer 2003; 98(12):2599–2606.

36. Malander S, Rambech E, Kristoffersson U, et al. The contribution of the hereditary nonpolyposis colorectal cancer syndrome to the development of ovarian cancer. Gynecol Oncol 2006; 101(2):238–243.

37. NCCN: Clinical Practice Guidelines in Oncology: v.1.2006. Colorectal Cancer Screening. Available at: http://www.nccn.com/professionals/physician_gls/PDF/genetics_screening.pdf, 2006.

20

Local Treatment Issues in Women with Hereditary Breast Cancer

Merav A. Ben-David and Lori J. Pierce

Department of Radiation Oncology, Comprehensive Cancer Center, University of Michigan, Ann Arbor, Michigan, U.S.A.

INTRODUCTION

Through carefully designed randomized trials for early stage breast cancer, breast-conserving surgery followed by whole breast radiation therapy (RT) has been shown to result in survival equivalent to that achieved with modified radical mastectomy while affording a woman the opportunity to preserve her breast (1–6). However, in women with hereditary breast cancer, outcomes following mastectomy versus breast-conserving therapy have not been directly compared. Thus, comparability of rates of local control, disease-specific survival, overall survival, and toxicity by treatment is unproven. In addition, questions have been raised as to whether the baseline elevated breast cancer risk in women with hereditary disease will be further increased due the use of radiotherapy to the breast for treatment of the index cancer. Given the limited number of patients diagnosed with hereditary breast cancer each year and the uncertainty whether these women would consent to a randomization between mastectomy and breast conservation, it is doubtful whether a randomized comparison will ever occur. Thus, our current knowledge of ipsilateral breast tumor recurrence (IBTR) following the use of breast-conserving surgery and RT and the risk of developing a contralateral breast cancer in women with hereditary breast cancer is based upon single and multi-institutional retrospective analyses and prospective nonrandomized studies, primarily in women who are known carriers of a *BRCA1/2* breast cancer susceptibility gene. The potential implications of a conservative approach and actual clinical results, with emphasis upon women with a known deleterious *BRCA1/2* mutation, will be presented in this chapter.

THE ROLE OF THE *BRCA1* AND *BRCA2* GENES AND IMPLICATIONS FOR RADIOTHERAPY

It has been over a decade since the *BRCA1* and *BRCA2* genes were identified, and yet the precise function of these proteins has not been fully revealed. Tumors arising in carriers who are heterozygous for deleterious germline *BRCA1/2* mutations are associated with the loss of the wild-type allele and therefore express a damaged, truncated, inactive protein. It appears that both *BRCA1* and *BRCA2* are involved in the double-strand break repair of DNA (7). Ionizing radiation causes double-strand breaks, among other lesions,

345

and those occurring in S/G2 phases of the cell cycle are repaired in part by homologous recombination. *BRCA1* has a role in the regulation and promotion of the DNA double-strand break repair process, and loss of breast cancer1 (*BRCA1*) protein function has been shown to result in a reduction in the frequency of homologous recombination events in irradiated cells (8). This, in turn, may lead to increased radiation sensitivity. Other implicated functions of the *BRCA1* gene include nonhomologous end joining DNA repair (9); S-phase and G2M cell-cycle checkpoint repair (10); and participation in the apoptotic process (10) and in the repair of single-stranded DNA damage (10). The *BRCA2* protein interacts with the RAD51 protein to facilitate homologous recombination following DNA breakdown (11,12). A truncated *BRCA2* protein will not allow the essential connection between these two proteins, thus leading to a reduction in homologous recombination and, in vitro, an increase in radiation sensitivity (11,12).

Because the *BRCA1/2* genes hold a valuable role in maintaining genomic integrity, a possible consequence of a defective protein in cancers of patients with *BRCA1/2* mutations could be the development of a highly radiation-sensitive tumor. Moreover, since *BRCA1* and *2* are both tumor-suppressor genes and the somatic cells of mutation carriers are already lacking one normal copy of the gene, it has been suggested that radiotherapy following breast-conserving surgery could increase the rate of second cancers in the treated breast from direct radiation exposure and further increase the rates of contralateral breast cancers beyond the elevated baseline risk as a consequence of scattered low-dose radiation. Clinical data addressing each of these hypothetical concerns will be discussed in the text to follow.

LOCAL CONTROL RESULTS IN *BRCA1/2* CARRIERS WITH EARLY-STAGE BREAST CANCER

Impact of *BRCA1/2* Testing upon Surgical Choice at Breast Cancer Diagnosis

Recent studies have examined the impact of genetic cancer risk assessment upon surgical choices at the time of breast cancer diagnosis (13,14). In a study by Schwartz et al. of 194 newly diagnosed breast cancer patients at high risk for having a mutation, who subsequently underwent genetic testing, 48% of patients found to carry a *BRCA1/2* mutation chose bilateral mastectomy (13). Upon multivariate analysis of predictors for bilateral mastectomy, positive test results were associated with a threefold increase in pursuing bilateral mastectomy. Equal numbers of *BRCA1/2* carriers chose breast conservation therapy as bilateral surgery; however, *BRCA1/2* carriers were less likely to undergo a unilateral mastectomy when compared to patients who declined testing or received an uninformative test result (*BRCA1/2* negative or ambiguous result). In a study from City of Hope by Weitzel et al., 32 women enrolled in a hereditary cancer registry underwent genetic cancer risk assessment including *BRCA1/2* testing at the time of their breast cancer diagnosis (14). Of the patients, 7 were found to have a deleterious *BRCA1/2* mutation, 22 tested negative, and 3 had a variant of uncertain significance. In this small series, all seven patients with a deleterious mutation opted for bilateral mastectomy rather than unilateral surgery compared to only 2/22 women (9%) who tested negative for a mutation. Although it is not clear exactly what the surgical preferences are in the majority of breast cancer patients who are found to be *BRCA1/2* carriers, it appears that there is interest in both bilateral mastectomy and breast conservation. Thus, information regarding likely outcomes by surgical approach would be important when counseling these women. It is also important to perform genetic risk assessments in these cancer patients prior to definitive local therapy using treatment algorithms that coordinate testing into the overall treatment plan (13–15).

Results in *BRCA1/2* Carriers Treated with Mastectomy

Recent reports have documented the reduction in risk of developing breast cancer with the use of prophylactic mastectomy in known *BRCA1/2* carriers (16–18). Both prospective trials and retrospective cohort studies have demonstrated risk reductions of 90% or greater with up to a median followup of 13 years with the use of prophylactic mastectomy. However, these results must be distinguished from outcomes in women with a *BRCA1/2* breast cancer susceptibility gene, who have a known diagnosis of breast cancer. To our knowledge, there are only limited data of outcomes of women with *BRCA1/2*-associated breast cancer treated with mastectomy. In the series by El-Tamer et al., there was no significant difference in the rate of local-regional recurrence in the 30 *BRCA1/2* carriers treated with mastectomy compared to mastectomy in 216 noncarriers (i.e., 5.9% in *BRCA1* and 0% in *BRCA2* carriers vs. 3.7% in noncarriers, respectively, $p = $ ns) with a median followup of four years for the overall study (19). This compares to the significant difference found upon univariate analysis between 21 *BRCA1/2* carriers and 220 noncarriers (23.1% in *BRCA1* and 12.5% in *BRCA2* carriers vs. 5.9% in noncarriers, $p = 0.05$) treated with breast conservation that was not significant upon multivariate analysis. In the study by Eccles et al. of familial breast cancer of the 70 patients with a positive family history who underwent mastectomy, 14.3% experienced a local recurrence compared to a 16.5% failure rate in 79 women with a negative family history ($p = $ ns) (20). When the outcome specifically in 39 known *BRCA1* mutation carriers was compared to that in negative controls, again there was no significant difference in rates of recurrence (10.3% vs. 16.5%, $p = $ ns). Furthermore, there were no significant differences between rates of local control at 10 years in *BRCA1/2* carriers treated with either breast conservation or mastectomy, with estimates of 16.7% and 10.3%, respectively ($p = $ ns). Therefore, although published results are limited, rates of local-regional control following mastectomy in *BRCA1/2* carriers with breast cancer appear to be comparable to those observed with sporadic breast cancer. Additional studies, however, are needed to confirm these findings.

Results in *BRCA1/2* Carriers Treated with Breast-Conserving Surgery and Radiotherapy

In contrast to the limited published results in *BRCA1/2* carriers treated with mastectomy, multiple series have been reported providing outcomes following breast-conserving surgery and RT, specifically comparing rates of IBTR in *BRCA1/2* carriers with rates in women with sporadic disease. Many of the breast conservation series in *BRCA1/2* carriers are presented in Table 1.

In comparison to consistent estimates of IBTR in breast conservation trials of (presumably) sporadic breast cancer patients of approximately 0.75% to 1% per year, IBTR rates in *BRCA1/2* carriers have varied by series. The majority of the studies have not shown a significant difference in the rates of IBTR between known *BRCA1/2* carriers and noncarriers, whereas others have demonstrated significantly higher rates of in-breast tumor failure in *BRCA1/2* carriers. Factors that have likely contributed to these differences will be discussed.

One of the first studies of breast conservation in a known *BRCA1/2* carrier population was reported by Robson et al. from Memorial Sloan–Kettering Cancer Center

Table 1 Rates of Ipsilateral Breast Tumor Recurrence Following Breast-Conserving Surgery and RT for *BRCA1/2*-Associated Early-Stage Breast Cancer

Author (Refs.)	Patients (*n*)		Breast cancer (%)		*p*-Value	Followup (Yr)
	BRCA1/2	Sporadic	*BRCA1/2*	Sporadic		
Haffty et al.[a] (21)	22	105	49	21	0.007	12
Metcalfe et al. (22)	188	–	11.5	–	–	10
Pierce et al. (23)	160	445	12	9	0.19	10
Robson et al. (24)	87	–	14	–	–	10
Robson et al. (25)	56	440	12	8	0.68	10
Delaloge et al. (26)	53	43	9 (*BRCA1*) 37 (*BRCA2*)	12	0.07	10
Eccles et al. (20)	36	83	17	24	0.63	10
Kirova et al. (27)	27	261	24	19	0.47	9
Seynaeve et al. (28)	26	174	15	12	0.76	6
Chappuis et al. (29)	–	–	6	7	0.93	5
El-Tamer et al. (19)	21	207	19	6	0.05	4

[a] All patients ≤42 years of age at diagnosis.
Abbreviations: IBTR, ipsilateral breast tumor recurrence; RT, radiation therapy.

(30). Using clinical samples tested for three founder mutations (*BRCA1 185delAG*, *BRCA1 5382 insC*, and *BRCA2 6174delAT*) in women of Ashkenazi Jewish descent, women with a *BRCA1/2* mutation had a nonsignificant increase in IBTR compared to women of Ashkenazi Jewish descent who were not mutation carriers; however, mutation status was not a significant predictor for recurrence in univariate or multivariate analyses. Only patient age (<50 years) significantly predicted for a 2.5-fold increased risk of IBTR. In a subsequent report by Robson et al. in collaboration with McGill University, age under 50 years was the only significant predictor of metachronous IBTR in women with and without germline *BRCA1/2* founder mutations (25). Recently, in a report by Robson et al. of 87 carriers identified either through complete coding sequence analysis or through targeted analysis of founder mutations, rates of IBTR in carriers were shown to be similar to those reported in young women without known mutations (24). Of note, 67% of the IBTR in *BRCA1/2* carriers were ductal carcinoma in situ only without an invasive component as compared to 85% with invasive histologies at the contralateral breast. This finding, in addition to the excess of subsequent cancer events in the contralateral breast relative to the ipsilateral breast (37.6% vs. 13.6%, respectively) is consistent with an altered progression of disease in the irradiated breast when compared to the untreated contralateral breast presumably from sterilization of subclinical disease with radiation.

In a report from the United Kingdom by Eccles et al. (20), the incidence of IBTR was neither increased at 10 years in patients with a significant family history and/or known *BRCA1* mutation compared to the patients with a negative family history (i.e., 22% with a positive family history vs. 24% in patients with a negative family history) nor was there a difference observed in rates of IBTR between known *BRCA1* carriers and negative history controls (i.e., 17% vs. 24%, respectively). However, the baseline rate of IBTR in the negative history controls was considerably higher than generally reported in the published literature, which may, in part, reflect the criteria for inclusion in this cohort, i.e., that the calculated heterozygote risk for the index case only had to be less than 20%.

In any regard, in their series, the presence of a *BRCA1* mutation did not confer a higher rate of IBTR compared to women with sporadic breast cancer as defined in their study.

Seynaeve et al. recently updated their results from the Daniel den Hood Cancer Centre in the Netherlands (28). In a series of 87 women with hereditary breast cancer treated with breast conservation, 26 were found to have a *BRCA1/2* mutation. With a median followup of six years, 15% of *BRCA1/2* carriers experienced an IBTR compared to 12% in sporadic controls matched by age and year of diagnosis (p = ns). Upon multivariate analysis for IBTR, after correction for age at diagnosis and tumor size, no increased risk of recurrence was found for *BRCA1/2* carriers.

In contrast to these and other series showing no significant differences in rates of IBTR between *BRCA1/2* carriers and matched noncarriers, once analyses have been corrected for confounding variables, a minority of studies have demonstrated higher rates of IBTR in *BRCA1/2* carriers when compared to noncarriers. In a report by El-Tamer et al. from Columbia-Presbyterian Hospital, 21 *BRCA1/2* carriers who were treated with breast conservation were identified from a registry of 739 women of Jewish descent with breast cancer under the age of 65 years (19). Upon univariate analysis, the authors reported a significantly higher crude risk of IBTR for *BRCA1/2* carriers compared to noncarriers at five years (p = 0.05); however log-rank comparisons of Kaplan–Meier estimates did not demonstrate significant differences over time between the two groups, a result consistent with a limited number of absolute events and power at five years. Similarly, an abstract by Bremer et al. detailing outcomes in nine known *BRCA1/2* carriers, the majority of whom were treated with breast conservation, reported three local recurrences in nine *BRCA1/2* patients (33%) with bilateral cancer versus 8 recurrences out of 101 patients (8%) in the noncarrier group also with bilateral breast cancer, at a median followup of 72 months from diagnosis of the first primary and 30 months from the second primary (31). Again, the number of events was limited and conclusions are tentative at best.

Haffty et al. reported the outcome of 22 patients with *BRCA1/2*-associated breast cancer and compared this to results of 105 women with sporadic breast cancer; all patients were treated with breast conservation and were diagnosed at age 42 years or younger (21). The age of the genetic cohort was significantly younger than patients with sporadic breast cancer (33 and 37 years, respectively). With 12-year followup, the rate of IBTR was 49% in the genetic group compared to 21% in the sporadic group (p = 0.007), (Fig. 1). The authors noted that none of the carriers had undergone a prophylactic oophorectomy or had received tamoxifen.

The results of a multi-institutional collaboration previously reported by Pierce et al. were recently updated (23). The outcome of 160 patients with a *BRCA1/2* deleterious mutation was compared to the outcome in noncarriers matched in a 1:3 ratio by age and date of diagnosis (23). With a median followup of 7.9 years for carriers and 6.7 years for women with sporadic disease, a nonsignificant 37% increase in IBTR was observed in the *BRCA1/2* carriers relative to the rate in the control group (p = 0.19). The rate of IBTR was significantly higher among *BRCA1/2* mutation carriers who did not undergo oophorectomy compared to controls [hazard ratio (HR) 1.94; p = 0.03] (Fig. 2). However, when the outcome in only those mutation carriers who underwent bilateral oophorectomy was compared to that of sporadic controls, the risk of IBTR was similar (p = 0.39) (Fig. 3). Tamoxifen treatment was associated with 58% reduction in IBTR in both carriers and controls. When tamoxifen use was analyzed in *BRCA1/2* carriers who had not undergone oophorectomy, no local failures were observed in carriers following tamoxifen compared to IBTR rates of 8%, 17%, and 31% at 5, 10, and 15 years, respectively, in carriers who did not receive tamoxifen. Thus, these data

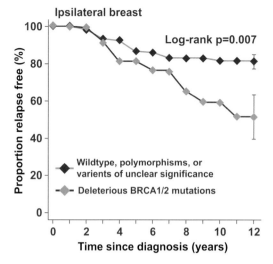

Figure 1 Proportion of women free of ipsilateral breast tumor recurrence by genetic predisposition. *Source*: From Ref. 21.

suggest a reduction in the risk of IBTR in *BRCA1/2* carriers treated with breast conservation with both tamoxifen use and prophylactic oophorectomy.

Thus, it appears that factors that account for the discordant findings among breast conservation series in *BRCA1/2* carriers are complex and include limitations in study design; variable penetrance of the genes; qualitative differences in phenotypic expression by site of mutation; and differences in treatment such as whether hormonal interventions are a part of the management strategy. Clearly, studies have shown that both prophylactic bilateral oophorectomy and tamoxifen use can reduce the risk of breast cancer in known *BRCA1/2* carriers, with risk reductions of approximately 40% to 50% (22,33–35). Therefore, it is not surprising that these interventions could also reduce the risk of IBTR in known carriers with breast cancer who opt to be treated with breast conservation, as shown in the

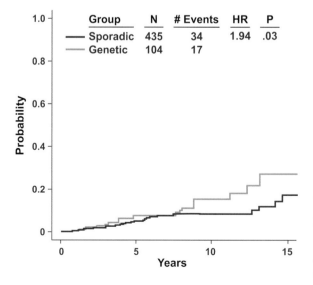

Figure 2 In-breast tumor recurrence in *BRCA1/2* mutation carriers and sporadic controls who have not undergone bilateral prophylactic oophorectomy. *Abbreviation*: HR, hazard ratio. *Source*: From Ref. 23.

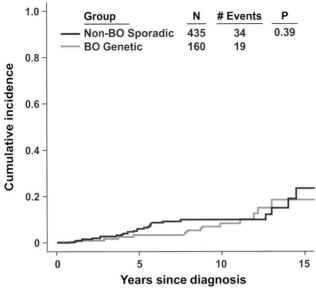

Figure 3 Ipsilateral breast tumor recurrence among *BRCA1/2* mutation carriers who have undergone BO versus sporadic controls who have not undergone oophorectomy. The number of events for the BO genetic mutation carrier groups is predicted based on respective time-dependent covariate models under the assumption that the BO occurred at the time of the breast cancer diagnosis for each patient. *Abbreviation*: BO, bilateral prophylactic oophorectomy. *Source*: From Ref. 23.

collaborative series. Thus, hormonal interventions such as tamoxifen use and prophylactic oophorectomy should be taken into account when comparing results across series.

POTENTIAL RADIATION-ASSOCIATED TOXICITIES FOLLOWING BREAST CONSERVATION

Because of the involvement of the *BRCA1* and *BRCA2* genes in the maintenance of genomic integrity, it has been suggested that mutation carriers would be at greater risk of acute and chronic radiation-associated toxicities due to incomplete repair of radiation-induced damage compared to patients with two normal copies of the genes. To study the potential side effects of RT in a known *BRCA1/2* cohort, Gaffney et al. reported toxicity in 21 carriers treated with RT either following breast-conserving surgery or mastectomy (36). Patients were treated with a variety of RT treatment techniques and dose regimens. Acute toxicity consisting of moist desquamation and moderate erythema was reported in approximately one-third of the patients, a rate higher than generally reported following standard radiation field and doses in patients with sporadic disease. There were no reported late sequelae of RT with a mean followup of approximately 8.5 years. In the series by Pierce et al. (32), acute radiation toxicity in *BRCA* carriers was graded using the Radiation Therapy Oncology Group Acute Radiation Morbidity Criteria (37). Toxicity results in *BRCA1/2* carriers were compared to those observed in a matched sporadic cohort. No excess skin toxicity was demonstrated in the genetic cohort. Only 1% and 3% of cases in the genetic and sporadic cohort, respectively, had confluent areas of moist desquamation ($p = 0.9$); there were no cases of Grade 4 skin toxicity. There was no difference in pulmonary symptoms or breast pain between the groups. The incidence of chronic RT-associated adverse events, specifically chronic sequelae in the skin, subcutaneous tissues, lung, and bone was the same for both groups.

A recent report by Shanley et al. also compared rates of acute and late toxicities in *BRCA1/2* carriers treated with breast radiotherapy to those observed in matched breast cancer controls (38). With median followups of 6.75 years for carriers and 7.75 years for controls, 55 matched case-control pairs were evaluated using patient interviews, photographs, and the Late Effects on Normal Tissues–Subjective, Objective, Management and Analytic (LENT-SOMA) scale, which assesses late effects on normal tissues (39). With respect to acute toxicities, while more carriers noted some degree of breast pain with RT (21.1% difference, $p = 0.03$), no significant differences were noted in degree of breast erythema, moist desquamation, or fatigue. Chronic toxicity, as measured by rates of rib fractures, lung fibrosis, soft-tissue/bone necrosis, and cardiac fibrosis did not differ by group. Similarly, rates of edema, fibrosis, telangiectasia, and atrophy were comparable between *BRCA1/2* carriers and controls using LENT-SOMA scoring.

Therefore, in the reports of acute toxicity in which carriers and noncarriers were matched, rates of acute radiation-associated morbidity were comparable between *BRCA1/2* carriers and controls, and data from all three series demonstrated similar rates of chronic RT-associated events in mutation carriers and noncarriers with up to seven years of followup. As the latency period for the potential complication of radiation-induced malignancies has been shown to be 10 years and longer, additional followup will be needed to ensure there is no increase in the incidence of second cancers beyond baseline levels observed in *BRCA1/2* carriers following RT.

CONTRALATERAL BREAST CANCER

The baseline risk of developing bilateral breast cancer in *BRCA1/2* carriers is significantly greater compared to noncarriers, with the development of metachronous disease in the contralateral breast reported to be as high as 40% in *BRCA1/2* carriers at 10 years after treatment of the index breast cancer with RT (Table 2).

Whether this elevated baseline risk could be further increased as a result of scattered radiation following definitive treatment of the initial breast cancer has been questioned. To our knowledge, there are no published studies prospectively comparing rates of contralateral breast cancer in known carriers who have received breast RT compared to rates in carriers who have not received radiation. Several investigators have, however, reported their experience in retrospective analyses. Eccles et al. reported similar rates of contralateral breast cancer in patients with a positive family history of breast cancer (approximately half were *BRCA1* positive), who received adjuvant RT compared to patients who did not receive radiation, i.e., 27/81 (33.3%) and 24/61 (39.3%), respectively, $p = 0.95$ (20). In a series by Metcalfe et al., the 5- and 10-year actuarial estimates of contralateral breast cancer were 16.9% and 29.5%, respectively (22). When factors potentially impacting rates of contralateral breast cancer were analyzed, RT was not associated with an elevated risk of contralateral breast cancer (HR 0.86; $p = 0.51$). Thus, at present, there are no data to suggest that the risk of contralateral breast cancer is further increased beyond baseline rates in carriers who have received breast irradiation. These patients will, however, continue to be followed up over time. Despite the lack of evidence that scatter radiation can increase the rate of contralateral breast cancers, it is always prudent to minimize scatter to the contralateral breast when possible. Treatment planning measures such as omission of the medial wedge and use of intensity

Table 2 Rates of Contralateral Breast Cancer in *BRCA1/2*-Associated Breast Cancer

Author (Refs.)	Patients (*n*)		Breast cancer (%)		*p*-Value	Followup (Yr)
	BRCA1/2	Sporadic	*BRCA1/2*	Sporadic		
Haffty et al. (21)	22	105	42	9	0.007	12
Metcalfe et al. (22)	491	–	29.5	–	–	10
Pierce et al. (23)	160	445	26	3	<0.0001	10
Robson et al. (24)	87	–	38	–	–	10
Eccles[a] et al. (20)	75	162	40	11	<0.001	10
Kirova et al. (27)	27	261	37	7	0.0003	9
Seynaeve[a] et al. (28)	26	174	23	6	0.06	6
El-Tamer et al. (19)	51	436	23 (*BRCA1*) 19 (*BRCA2*)	12	0.05	4

[a]*p*-Value for difference between total hereditary breast cancer group and sporadic group.

modulated RT have been shown to reduce scatter to the contralateral breast. Incorporation of these and other technical modifications into routine treatment planning should be encouraged.

Consistent with the reduction in risk of contralateral breast cancers with adjuvant tamoxifen following treatment for sporadic breast cancer (40), Narod et al. demonstrated a reduction in risk of contralateral breast cancer using tamoxifen in *BRCA1/2* carriers (33). In a case control study, *BRCA1/2* carriers with bilateral breast cancer were matched and compared to carriers with unilateral disease. In this study, adjuvant tamoxifen was associated with a 50% reduction in the occurrence of contralateral breast cancer compared to the group without adjuvant tamoxifen treatment. Similar results were observed in the collaborative study from the Hereditary Cancer Clinical Study Group, in which tamoxifen use was associated with a 50% reduction in risk of contralateral breast cancer in known *BRCA1* carriers ($p = 0.01$) and a 58% reduction in *BRCA2* carriers ($p = 0.05$) (34). Bilateral salpingo-oophorectomy has also been shown to significantly reduce breast cancer risk in known *BRCA1/2* carriers. In an analysis of 99 *BRCA1/2* mutation carriers who underwent oophorectomy and 142 who did not, the risk of a subsequent breast cancer was reduced by 53% after oophorectomy (35). In the recent report by Metcalfe et al. (22), oophorectomy was associated with a 59% reduction in risk of contralateral breast cancer, and when multiple factors were considered in a multivariate analysis, only oophorectomy was found to significantly protect against the development of contralateral breast cancer.

Despite the reductions in risk afforded by tamoxifen use and oophorectomy, the risk of contralateral breast cancer still appears to exceed the risk observed in women with sporadic breast cancer following breast-conserving surgery and RT. In the collaborative series by Pierce et al., using a time-dependent covariate model to study the impact of bilateral oophorectomy upon risk of contralateral breast cancer in *BRCA1/2* carriers relative to noncarriers, breast cancer rates remained significantly higher in *BRCA1/2* carriers despite oophorectomy compared to controls, with 10 and 15 estimates 16% and 26% for carriers versus 4% and 11% for noncarriers, respectively ($p = 0.007$) (23), as shown in Figure 4.

Thus, additional strategies are needed in *BRCA1/2* mutation carriers to reduce their contralateral breast cancer risk to levels observed in women with early-stage sporadic disease.

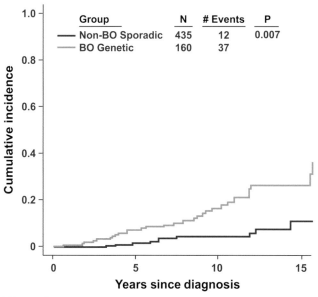

Figure 4 Contralateral breast cancers among *BRCA1/2* mutation carriers who have undergone BO versus sporadic controls who have not undergone oophorectomy. The number of events for the BO genetic mutation carrier groups is predicted based on respective time-dependent covariate models under the assumption that the BO occurred at the time of the breast cancer diagnosis for each patient. *Abbreviation*: BO, bilateral prophylactic oophorectomy. *Source*: From Ref. 23.

SALVAGE OF AN IBTR

An IBTR occurs in approximately 8% to 15% of women at 10 to 20 years after the treatment of sporadic breast cancer following breast-conserving surgery and RT (1–6). The potential for long-term survival after an isolated local recurrence highlights the importance of effective salvage therapy for these women. Currently, mastectomy is the standard surgical salvage for an isolated IBTR and, following mastectomy, survival rates have been reported between 57% and 69% at 10 years (41).

   Approximately 90% of in-breast tumor recurrences in sporadic breast cancer are in the same quadrant of the breast and are of similar histology as the original cancer, consistent with a true recurrence of the primary tumor rather than a new primary cancer (1,42,43). However, for *BRCA1/2* mutation carriers, it appears that new cancers rather than true recurrences constitute the majority of lesions that have collectively been considered as in-breast tumor recurrences. The median time to recurrence in *BRCA1/2* carriers generally exceeds that observed in sporadic disease. In the collaborative study, the median time to IBTR was 8.7 years in *BRCA1/2* carriers compared to 4.7 years in women with sporadic cancer (23), and Kirova et al. reported a 6.7 year time to recurrence in carriers versus 3.8 years with sporadic disease (27). Haffty et al. reported that for *BRCA1/2* carriers younger than 42 years of age at diagnosis, median time to IBTR was 8 years (21). The location and histologies of these "recurrences" are often distinctly different than those after treatment for sporadic disease. Haffty et al. observed that 9/11 (82%) *BRCA1/2* carriers with breast cancer, who experienced an IBTR, had lesions at different locations and/or were of different histologies than their original lesions (21). In the collaborative series, 60% of the "recurrences" in *BRCA1/2* carriers were located in a quadrant other than the quadrant of the primary lesion versus 29% in the control sporadic group ($p = 0.04$) (23). All recurrences/new primaries in the *BRCA1/2* carriers were successfully salvaged with surgery and with 3.3-year median followup, all patients are free of recurrence locally and systemically. Thus, the increased median time to recurrence, differences in location and histology of the recurrent lesion compared to the primary, and the successful surgical salvage are all more consistent with a new primary in the treated breast rather than a true recurrence. Confirmation will require comparison of molecular markers between the recurrence/new primary and the original cancer; these studies are under way.

LOCAL TREATMENT OPTIONS IN HIGH-RISK WOMEN

For women with breast cancer with family histories consistent with hereditary disease, who have either not undergone testing for a *BRCA1/2* mutation or have tested negatively for a deleterious *BRCA1/2* mutation, recommendations for local treatment are unclear. Options include both breast-conserving therapy with close observation of the contralateral breast or definitive unilateral mastectomy and a prophylactic contralateral mastectomy, the same options as in women with *BRCA1/2*-associated breast cancer. Published results following breast-conserving therapy in women with hereditary breast cancer suggest somewhat contradictory findings. In a study by Eccles et al., the outcome following breast-conserving therapy was compared in women with known *BRCA1* mutations ($n = 36$), women with an unknown mutation status and a positive family history (defined as having a minimum of one first-degree relative under age 60 years or one paternal second-degree relative under age 60 with breast cancer) ($n = 36$) and women with a negative family history ($n = 83$) (20). When the risk of IBTR following breast-conserving surgery and RT was compared between patients who did and did not have a family history of breast cancer, results were not significantly different, with the risk of ipsilateral recurrence at 10 years of 22% and 24%, respectively ($p = 0.77$). However, when rates were compared within the positive family history group by whether patients were known to be a *BRCA1* mutation carrier or of unknown mutation status, results differed with the 10-year IBTR of 16.7% in *BRCA1* carriers versus 27.8% in those of unknown mutation status, suggesting less favorable in-breast tumor control with breast conservation in the positive family history group when known *BRCA1* carriers were excluded from analysis. Similarly, Seynaeve et al. reported a statistically nonsignificant increase in local failures in patients with a strong family history of breast cancer (defined as three or more first-degree relatives with breast and/or ovarian cancer) and an unknown mutation status compared to rates in known *BRCA1/2* carriers, with crude rates of 24% in unspecified cases of hereditary breast cancer versus 15% in *BRCA1/2* carriers (compared to 12% in women with sporadic disease, $p = 0.14$) (28). After correction for age at onset and tumor size, multivariate analysis for IBTR for *BRCA1/2* carriers and unspecified hereditary breast cancer patients versus sporadic controls revealed no increased risk of IBTR for *BRCA1* carriers and a significantly increased twofold risk of IBTR for unspecified hereditary breast cancer patients compared to sporadic controls (HR 2.31; $p = 0.02$). Thus, these results suggest less favorable results with breast conservation in patients with unspecified hereditary breast cancer when compared to known *BRCA1/2* carriers.

However, these results differ from those published by Kirova et al. from the Institut Curie (27). In this report, genetic testing was performed in patients with histories consistent with either two first-degree relatives affected with cancer with at least either one with invasive breast cancer before 41 years or one with ovarian cancer at any age or at least three first- or second-degree relatives from the same lineage affected with invasive breast cancer or ovarian cancer at any age. Analysis of IBTR revealed comparable rates of recurrence in known *BRCA1/2* carriers ($n = 29$), patients with a family history who tested negative for a deleterious *BRCA1/2* mutation ($n = 107$), and patients with sporadic disease ($n = 271$), with crude rates of 24%, 22%, and 19%, respectively with nine-year median followup. In addition, the median time to IBTR of 39 months in patients with a family history who were not *BRCA1/2* carriers was similar to that in noncarriers (i.e., 46 months) but different from *BRCA1/2*-associated breast cancers (i.e., 80 months).

Patients of unknown mutation status may harbor breast cancer susceptibility genes yet to be identified that may respond differently to RT and/or other treatment modalities. Furthermore, the heterogeneity of patients with otherwise unspecified hereditary breast cancer further complicates the comparison of results between series and the suggestion of common treatment guidelines. Until additional breast cancer susceptibility genes can be identified and correlated with risk modifiers and associated clinical outcomes, individualized genetic counseling and followup are needed for these women.

FOLLOWUP OF *BRCA1/2* CARRIERS AFTER BREAST-CONSERVING SURGERY AND RT

The majority of local breast cancer recurrences occur within the first five years after breast-conserving surgery and RT (41). Therefore, current guidelines suggest that women with early-stage breast cancer, who are treated with breast conservation, have a breast examination by an oncologist at least once every six months in the first five years following diagnosis and annually thereafter with the goal of identifying recurrent disease or second breast cancers as early as possible (44,45). However, as previously discussed, studies in *BRCA1/2* carriers with breast cancer treated with conservative surgery and RT have shown that recurrences/new primaries occur later in mutation carriers compared to patients treated for sporadic disease. These data would suggest that clinical followup should continue every six months beyond five years in carriers with a history of breast cancer, perhaps up to 10 years following diagnosis. Published guidelines also recommend that all women with a prior diagnosis of breast cancer have yearly mammographic evaluation (45). To our knowledge, however, there are no published guidelines recommending the appropriate follow-up management of *BRCA1/2* carriers with breast cancer treated with breast conservation. Mammography has been reported to be relatively insensitive among *BRCA1/2* carriers for several reasons including increased breast density observed in younger women (46,47), the benign mammographic appearance of some *BRCA*-associated cancers (46) and the rapid growth pattern of some *BRCA1/2* associated cancers (44). The rate of "interval cancers" in *BRCA1/2* carriers undergoing surveillance with mammogram only has been reported to be 26% to 50% (48–50), and 25% to 35% have associated positive axillary nodes at diagnosis (49,50). Magnetic resonance imaging (MRI) has recently been tested as a screening tool for high-risk women and known *BRCA1/2* carriers. MRI compares favorably to mammography with respect to improved sensitivity and specificity, with rates of sensitivity of 71% to 100% and 90% to 95% specificity compared to sensitivity and specificity with mammography of 36% to 43% and 94% to 99%, respectively (46,51–53). However, MRI study performance has declined on later incident screens, suggesting that some of the apparent early benefit over mammography was likely related to prevalent (at initial screening) versus incident (at follow-up screening) detection bias (54). In the series by Warner et al., sensitivity with MRI was 85% on the first year of screening and decreased to 50% by the third year (51), and in the series by Kriege et al., the sensitivity was 79% at first screen and 62% at the second year (52). This study also included 139 patients with a personal history of breast cancer. In this group, MRI had the best sensitivity, specificity, and positive predictive value (67%, 96%, and 44%, respectively) compared to mammogram, ultrasound, or a combination of both techniques in detecting a recurrence/new primary and contralateral breast cancer. Furthermore, when women at high risk for breast cancer and *BRCA1/2* carriers were screened with mammography alone, a high rate of positive axillary lymph nodes (25–35%) at diagnosis was found (49,50) that was reduced to 13% to 21% using multimodality screening (51,52).

Although positive data regarding the use of MRI in surveillance for healthy carriers are emerging, data are insufficient to recommend routine MRI for *BRCA1/2* carriers with a personal history of breast cancer. Further studies are needed to address the value of MRI in the irradiated breast and to estimate its yield in diagnosing recurrent/new disease.

SUMMARY

For women with early-stage breast cancer, who are known to harbor a *BRCA1/2* mutation, there is no established "gold standard" local treatment of the involved breast. Therefore, the full range of treatment options, i.e., bilateral mastectomy, unilateral mastectomy with observation of the contralateral breast; and breast-conserving surgery and radiotherapy, with observation of the opposite breast must be considered for each patient and the choice individualized based upon patient preference. If breast conservation is seriously considered, it should be noted that although most retrospective series suggest comparable rates of local control between *BRCA1/2* carriers and noncarriers following breast-conserving surgery and RT, other studies suggest differences in risk of recurrence, which, in part, may be due to patient selection and/or absence of the integration of hormonal risk-reduction strategies into patient management. Furthermore, women treated conservatively have an increased risk of breast cancer in the untreated contralateral breast compared to women with sporadic disease. Due to the spectrum of *BRCA1/2*-associated breast cancers and the complexities of the management of women who are known carriers, breast cancer patients who have a *BRCA1/2* mutation and chose breast conservation should be carefully followed up in high-risk clinics, with surveillance focused not only upon the treated breast but also the untreated contralateral breast.

REFERENCES

1. Veronesi U, Cascinelli N, Mariani L, et al. Twenty-year follow-up of a randomized study comparing breast-conserving surgery with radical mastectomy for early breast cancer. N Engl J Med 2002; 347(16):1227–1232.
2. Fisher B, Anderson S, Bryant J, et al. Twenty-year follow-up of a randomized trial comparing total mastectomy, lumpectomy, and lumpectomy plus irradiation for the treatment of invasive breast cancer. N Engl J Med 2002; 347(16):1233–1241.
3. Blichert-Toft M, Rose C, Andersen JA, et al. Danish randomized trial comparing breast conservation therapy with mastectomy: six years of life-table analysis. Danish Breast Cancer Cooperative Group. J Natl Cancer Inst Monogr 1992; (11):19–25.
4. Jacobson JA, Danforth DN, Cowan KH, et al. Ten-year results of a comparison of conservation with mastectomy in the treatment of stage I and II breast cancer. N Engl J Med 1995; 332(14):907–911.
5. Sarrazin D, Le MG, Arriagada R, et al. Ten-year results of a randomized trial comparing a conservative treatment to mastectomy in early breast cancer. Radiother Oncol 1989; 14(3): 177–184.

6. van Dongen JA, Voogd AC, Fentiman IS, et al. Long-term results of a randomized trial comparing breast-conserving therapy with mastectomy: European Organization for Research and Treatment of Cancer 10801 trial. J Natl Cancer Inst 2000; 92(14):1143–1150.

7. Narod S, Foulkes W. *BRCA1* and *BRCA2*: 1994 and beyond. Nat Rev Cancer 2004; 4(9): 665–676.

8. Scully R, Ganesan S, Vlasakova K, et al. Genetic analysis of *BRCA1* function in a defined tumor cell line. Mol Cell 1999; 4(6):1093–1099.

9. Xu B, Kim S, Kastan MB. Involvement of *BRCA1* in S-phase and G(2)-phase checkpoints after ionizing irradiation. Mol Cell Biol 2001; 21(10):3445–3450.

10. Gowen LC, Avrutskaya AV, Latour AM, et al. *BRCA1* required for transcription-coupled repair of oxidative DNA damage. Science 1998; 281(5379):1009–1012.

11. Chen CF, Chen PL, Zhong Q, et al. Expression of *BRC* repeats in breast cancer cells disrupts the *BRCA2–Rad51* complex and leads to radiation hypersensitivity and loss of G(2)/M checkpoint control. J Biol Chem 1999; 274(46):32931–32935.

12. Xia F, Taghian DG, DeFrank JS, et al. Deficiency of human *BRCA2* leads to impaired homologous recombination but maintains normal nonhomologous end joining. Proc Natl Acad Sci USA 2001; 98(15):8644–8649.

13. Schwartz M, Lerman C, Brogan B, et al. Impact of *BRCA1/BRCA2* counseling and testing on newly diagnosed breast cancer patients. J Clin Oncol 2004; 22(10):1823–1829.

14. Weitzel J. McCaffrey S, Nedelcu R, et al. Effect of genetic cancer risk assessment on surgical decisions at breast cancer diagnosis. Arch Surg 2003; 138:1323–1328.

15. Stolier A, Fuhrman G, Mauterer L, et al. Initial experience with surgical treatment planning in the newly diagnosed breast cancer patient at high risk for *BRCA1* or *BRCA2* mutation. The Breast J 2004; 10(6):475–480.

16. Hartmann LC, Sellers TA, Schaid DJ, et al. Efficacy of bilateral prophylactic mastectomy in *BRCA1* and *BRCA2* gene mutation carriers. J Natl Cancer Inst 2001; 93(21):1633–1637.

17. Rebbeck TR, Friebel T, Lynch HT, et al. Bilateral prophylactic mastectomy reduces breast cancer risk in *BRCA1* and *BRCA2* mutation carriers: the PROSE Study Group. J Clin Oncol 2004; 22(6):1055–1062.

18. Meijers-Heijboer H, van Geel B, van Putten WL, et al. Breast cancer after prophylactic bilateral mastectomy in women with a *BRCA1* or *BRCA2* mutation. N Engl J Med 2001; 345 (3):159–164.

19. El-Tamer M, Russo D, Troxel A, et al. Survival and recurrence after breast cancer in *BRCA1/2* mutation carriers. Ann Surg Oncol 2003; 11(2):157–164.

20. Eccles D, Simmonds P, Goddard J, et al. Familial breast cancer: an investigation into the outcome of treatment for early stage disease. Fam Cancer 2001; 1(2):65–72.

21. Haffty BG, Harrold E, Khan AJ, et al. Outcome of conservatively managed early-onset breast cancer by *BRCA1/2* status. Lancet 2002; 359(9316):1471–1477.

22. Metcalfe K, Lynch HT, Ghadirian P, et al. Contralateral breast cancer in *BRCA1* and *BRCA2* mutation carriers. J Clin Oncol 2004; 22(12):2328–2335.

23. Pierce LJ, Levin A, Rebbeck TR, et al. Ten-year multi-institutional results of breast-conserving surgery and radiotherapy in *BRCA1/2*–associated stage I/II breast cancer. J Clin Oncol 2006; 24(16):2437–2443.

24. Robson M, Svahn T, McCormick B, et al. Appropriateness of breast-conserving treatment of breast carcinoma in women with germline mutations in *BRCA1* or *BRCA2*: a clinic-based series. Cancer 2005; 103(1):44–51.

25. Robson ME, Chappuis PO, Satagopan J, et al. A combined analysis of outcome following breast cancer: differences in survival based on *BRCA1/BRCA2* mutation status and administration of adjuvant treatment. Breast Cancer Res 2004; 6(1):R8–R17.

26. Delaloge S, Kloos I, Ariane D, et al. Young age is the major predictor of local relapse among conservatively treated *BRCA1*-, or *BRCA2*-, or non *BRCA*-linked hereditary breast cancer (BC). Abstracts of Papers, Vol. 22(41). 39th Annual Meeting of the American Society of Clinical Oncology, Chicago, IL, May 31–June 3, 2003

27. Kirova YM, Stoppa-Lyonnet D, Savignoni A, et al. Risk of breast cancer recurrence and contralateral breast cancer in relation to BRCA1 and BRCA2 mutation status following breast-conserving surgery and radiotherapy. Eur J Cancer 2005; 41(15):2304–2311.

28. Seynaeve C, Verhoog LC, van de Bosch LM, et al. Ipsilateral breast tumour recurrence in hereditary breast cancer following breast-conserving therapy. Eur J Cancer 2004; 40(8): 1150–1158.

29. Chappuis P, Kapusta L, Begin L, et al. Germline BRCA1/2 mutations and p27^{Kip1} protein levels independently predict outcome after breast cancer. J Clin Oncol 2000; 18(24):4045–4052.

30. Robson M, Levin D, Federici M, et al. Breast conservation therapy for invasive breast cancer in Ashkenazi women with BRCA gene founder mutations. J Natl Cancer Inst 1999; 91(24): 2112–2117.

31. Bremer M, Doerk T, Sohn C, et al. Local relapse after postoperative radiotherapy in patients with bilateral breast cancer by BRCA1/2 status. Abstracts of Papers, Vol. 22(42). 39th Annual Meeting of the American Society of Clinical Oncology, Chicago, IL, May 31–June 3, 2003.

32. Pierce LJ, Strawderman M, Narod SA, et al. Effect of radiotherapy after breast-conserving treatment in women with breast cancer and germline BRCA1/2 mutations. J Clin Oncol 2000; 18(19):3360–3369.

33. Narod SA, Brunet JS, Ghadirian P, et al. Tamoxifen and risk of contralateral breast cancer in BRCA1 and BRCA2 mutation carriers: a case-control study. Hereditary Breast Cancer Clinical Study Group. Lancet 2000; 356(9245):1876–1881.

34. Gronwald J, Tung N, Foulkes W, et al. Tamoxifen and contralateral breast cancer in BRCA1 and BRCA2 carriers: an update. Int J Cancer 2006; 118:2281–2284.

35. Rebbeck T, Lunch H, Neuhausen S, et al. Prophylactic oophorectomy in carriers of BRCA1 or BRCA2 mutations. N Eng J Med 2002; 346:1616–1622.

36. Gaffney DK, Brohet RM, Lewis CM, et al. Response to radiation therapy and prognosis in breast cancer patients with BRCA1 and BRCA2 mutations. Radiother Oncol 1998; 47(2): 129–136.

37. Cox JD, Stetz J, Pajak TF. Toxicity criteria of the Radiation Therapy Oncology Group (RTOG) and the European Organization for Research and Treatment of Cancer (EORTC). Int J Radiat Oncol Biol Phys 1995; 31(5):1341–1346.

38. Shanley S, McReynolds K, Ardem-Jones A, et al. Late toxicity is not increased in BRCA1/ BRCA2 mutation carriers undergoing breast radiotherapy in the United Kingdom. Clin Cancer Res 2006; 12(23):7025–7032.

39. Pavy J, Denekamp J, Letschert J, et al. Late effects toxicity scoring: the SOMA scale. Radiotherr Oncol 1995; 35:11–15.

40. Early Breast Cancer Trialists' Collaborative Group. Effects of chemotherapy and hormonal therapy for early breast cancer on recurrence and 15-year survival: an overview of the randomised trials. Lancet 2005; 365(9472):1687–1717.

41. Harris JH, Lippman ME, Morrow M, Osborn CK. Diseases of the Breast. 3rd ed. Lippincott Williams & Wilkins, 2004:719–744.

42. Fisher B, Anderson S, Redmond CK, et al. Reanalysis and results after 12 years of follow-up in a randomized clinical trial comparing total mastectomy with lumpectomy with or without irradiation in the treatment of breast cancer. N Engl J Med 1995; 333(22):1456–1461.

43. Clark RM, Whelan T, Levine M, et al. Randomized clinical trial of breast irradiation following lumpectomy and axillary dissection for node-negative breast cancer: an update. Ontario Clinical Oncology Group. J Natl Cancer Inst 1996; 88(22):1659–1664.

44. NCCN Breast Cancer Panel. Breast cancer treatment clinical guidelines in oncology. Version 1, 2005. J Natl Compr Cancer Netw 2005; 3(3):238–289.

45. Smith TJ, Davidson NE, Schapira DV, et al. American Society of Clinical Oncology 1998 update of recommended breast cancer surveillance guidelines. J Clin Oncol 1999; 17(3):1080.

46. Tilanus-Linthorst M, Verhoog L, Obdeijn IM, et al. A BRCA1/2 mutation, high breast density and prominent pushing margins of a tumor independently contribute to a frequent false-negative mammography. Int J Cancer 2002; 102(1):91–95.

47. Ziv E, Shepherd J, Smith-Bindman R, Kerlikowske K. Mammographic breast density and family history of breast cancer. J Natl Cancer Inst 2003; 95(7):556–558.

48. Komenaka IK, Ditkoff BA, Joseph KA, et al. The development of interval breast malignancies in patients with BRCA mutations. Cancer 2004; 100(10):2079–2083.

49. Brekelmans CT, Seynaeve C, Bartels CC, et al. Effectiveness of breast cancer surveillance in *BRCA1/2* gene mutation carriers and women with high familial risk. J Clin Oncol 2001; 19(4): 924–930.

50. Scheuer L, Kauff N, Robson M, et al. Outcome of preventive surgery and screening for breast and ovarian cancer in *BRCA* mutation carriers. J Clin Oncol 2002; 20(5):1260–1268.

51. Warner E, Plewes DB, Hill KA, et al. Surveillance of *BRCA1* and *BRCA2* mutation carriers with magnetic resonance imaging, ultrasound, mammography, and clinical breast examination. JAMA 2004; 292(11):1317–1325.

52. Kriege M, Brekelmans CTM, Boetes C, et al. Efficacy of MRI and mammography for breast-cancer screening in women with a familial or genetic predisposition. N Engl J Med 2004; 351(5):427–437.

53. Kuhl CK, Schrading S, Leutner CC, et al. Mammography, breast ultrasound, and magnetic resonance imaging for surveillance of women at high familial risk for breast cancer. J Clin Oncol 2005; 23(33):8469–8476.

54. Helvie MA. Surveillance of *BRCA1* and *BRCA2* carriers. JAMA 2005; 293(8):931.

21

Systemic Therapy for *BRCA*-Associated Breast Cancer

Mark Robson

Clinical Genetics Service, Memorial Sloan-Kettering Cancer Center, New York, New York, U.S.A.

INTRODUCTION

Treatment of hereditary breast cancer, as that of all types of breast cancer, can be broadly divided into local and systemic phases. In a preceding chapter, the influence of germline predisposition on local management decisions, particularly the appropriateness of breast conserving treatment, is considered. In this chapter, we will consider the question of whether women with hereditary breast cancer should be approached differently when it comes to decision-making about systemic adjuvant therapy.

The presence of a germline predisposition could influence systemic adjuvant therapy decisions in one of two ways. First, if hereditary breast cancer has a different prognosis from nonhereditary cancer, then providers and patients may be more or less likely to consider systemic treatment in a given clinical circumstance. Hence, the question of whether women with hereditary breast cancers have a different prognosis than women with nonhereditary cancers assumes importance. Second, even without a prognostic effect, it is possible that hereditary breast cancers are either more or less sensitive to specific therapeutic agents. If this is the case, then women may benefit from "tailoring" of treatment through selection of specific treatment regimens based upon the etiology of their cancer.

PROGNOSIS IN HEREDITARY BREAST CANCER

As noted in earlier chapters, germline mutations in several genes may confer an autosomal dominant predisposition to breast cancer. For most of these syndromes (e.g., Li-Fraumeni, Cowden, Peutz-Jeghers), there are essentially no studies describing histopathology or breast cancer outcomes. Therefore, the focus of the remainder of this chapter will be largely on hereditary breast cancer due to mutations in *BRCA1* or *BRCA2*, with comments on other syndromes when data are available.

Prognostic Factors

Foulkes et al. describe the distribution of traditional breast cancer prognostic factors in hereditary breast cancer, especially those associated with *BRCA1/*2 mutations in Chapter 18 of this book. The reader is referred to this chapter and other recent reviews (1,2) for detailed discussion. *BRCA1*-associated breast cancers (B1BC) are typically high grade and hormone receptor negative (about 80–90% of cases) and do not overexpress human epidermal growth factor receptor (HER)2(3). Mutations in *P53* are often detected (1,3–6). As described in Chapter 18, these tumors frequently have a basal-like pattern of gene expression. *BRCA2*-associated breast cancers (B2BC), on the other hand, are less distinct from sporadic disease with similar rates of hormone receptor positivity. B2BC, like B1BC, are usually "HER2 negative" (3).

Thus, several adverse prognostic factors are observed with increased frequency in hereditary breast cancer, particularly that due to mutations in *BRCA1*. The recent gene expression studies briefly mentioned above and described in detail by Foulkes et al. would suggest that this is because *BRCA1* mutation carriers are prone to develop a specific subtype of breast cancer (basal-like) that manifests many of these adverse features simultaneously. *BRCA2* carriers, on the other hand, have not been shown, as yet, to have a tendency to develop a cancer with a specific immunophenotypic profile. As a result, other than some suggestions that *BRCA2*-associated cancers may be generally of higher histologic grade than nonassociated cancers, there is little evidence that the distribution of prognostic factors in *BRCA2*-associated disease is any different than that of noncarriers.

Studies of Outcome in *BRCA*-Associated Breast Cancer

A number of studies compare outcomes in hereditary and nonhereditary breast cancer (Table 1). Nearly all of these reports examine the prognosis of breast cancer associated with germline *BRCA1* and *BRCA2* mutations, rather than with other types of hereditary breast cancer. Unfortunately, none can be considered definitive. In most of these studies, germline mutation carriers are identified within groups of women who have already survived their breast cancer for some period of time, so-called "prevalent cohorts." This introduces a survival bias, also known as Neyman bias, because some women will have died before having had the opportunity to be tested. If the factor of interest (in this case, germline mutation) is associated with early death, then the effect of the survival bias will be to obscure such an effect, as these women will not undergo testing and their adverse outcome will not be recognized. The comparator groups in these studies are usually untested hospital or population registry controls, matched for age and year of diagnosis but not for survival for the time period from diagnosis to testing in the cases. Survival bias is a particular issue in clinic-based ascertainments, where hereditary breast cancer cases are identified after referral to a risk identification service, as the delay from diagnosis to testing may be measured in decades. Such ascertainments are also subject to a referral bias, since most women are referred because of either early-onset disease or strong family history and may not be completely representative of the pool of all mutation carriers. Even hospital-based ascertainments that attempt to evaluate all women with, for instance, early-onset breast cancer (13,21) may not completely avoid this problem if testing is not performed on all members of the incident cohort. Retrospective cohort designs have been developed by our group (16,21) and others (9,27) to circumvent these ascertainment biases, but are limited by the requirement that the studies be performed on women from founder populations, where testing can be performed on archival pathology material. Even in studies in founder populations, where mutation prevalence may be as high as 10% in unselected women with breast cancer, the number of mutation carriers is often too small to ensure robust conclusions, especially at the limits of the follow-up period. As described in the Introduction, there have been a large number of studies of

Table 1 Studies of Outcome in Hereditary Breast Cancer Due to Mutations in *BRCA1* or *BRCA2*

Author	Country	Ascertainment type	Years of diagnosis	N carriers	Source of comparison group(s)	Comments
Porter et al. (7)	Scotland	P, F	1942–1992	35 *BRCA1*	Age-matched BC patients from population	Linkage families
Marcus et al. (8)	United States	P, F	NS	72 *BRCA1*	Hospital tumor registry	Linkage families
Foulkes et al. (9)[a]	Canada	RC	1990–1995	12 *BRCA1*	Cohort members w/o mutation	All AJ
Verhoog et al. (10)	The Netherlands	P, F	1969–1995	49 *BRCA1*	Hospital tumor registry	30 proven carriers
Johannsson et al. (11)	Sweden	P, F	1958–1995	33 *BRCA1*	Population registry 1958–1995 (unmatched and matched)	
Robson et al. (12)	United States	P, E	1992–1995	23 *BRCA1* 7 *BRCA2*	Cohort members w/o mutation	All AJ
Ansquer et al. (13)[b]	France	P, E	1990–1995	15 *BRCA1*	Early-onset w/o mutation	
Lee et al. (14)	United States	–	–	58 (1 and 2)	FDR of noncarriers	Cases FDR of known carriers
Verhoog et al. (15)	The Netherlands	P, F	NS	28 *BRCA2*	Hospital tumor registry	20 proven carriers
Robson et al. (16)[c]	United States	RC	1980–1990	28 (1 and 2)	Cohort members w/o mutation	All AJ
Pierce et al. (17)[d]	North America	P, F	NS	71 (1 and 2)	Hospital registries	All breast conservation
Loman et al. (18)	Sweden, Denmark	P, F	Ascertained 1995–1999	54 *BRCA2*	Population tumor registry	36 proven carriers
Foulkes et al. (19)[a]	Canada	RC	1986–1995	16 *BRCA1*	Cohort members w/o mutation	All AJ
Hamann and Sinn (20)	Germany	P, F	1961–1994	36 *BRCA1*	Familial BC testing (-)	
Stoppa-Lyonnet et al. (21)[b]	France	P, E	1991–1998	40 *BRCA1*	Early-onset w/o mutation	
Chappuis et al. (22)[a]	Canada	RC	1986–1996	32 (1 and 2)	Cohort members testing (-)	All AJ

(Continued)

Table 1 Studies of Outcome in Hereditary Breast Cancer Due to Mutations in *BRCA1* or *BRCA2* (*Continued*)

Author	Country	Ascertainment type	Years of diagnosis	N carriers	Source of comparison group(s)	Comments
Eerola et al. (23)	Finland	P, F	1953–1995	75 (1 and 2)	Population tumor registry *BRCA* (-) families	
Eccles et al. (24)	U.K.	P, F, and E	1959–1996	75 *BRCA1*	Familial BC from clinic Nonfamilial hospital controls	
Goffin et al. (4)[a]	Canada	P	1980–1995	30 *BRCA1*	Cohort members testing (-)	All AJ
Veronesi et al. (25)	Italy	P, F	NS	39 (1 and 2)	Familial testing (-)	
Chappuis et al. (26)[a]	Canada	P	1980–1995	30 *BRCA1*	Cohort members testing (-)	All AJ
El-Tamer et al. (27)	United States	RC	1989–1999	51 (1 and 2)	Cohort members testing (-)	All AJ
Robson et al. (28)[a,c]	United States, Canada	RC	1980–1995	55 (1 and 2)	Cohort members testing (-)	All AJ
Musolino et al. (29)	Italy	P, F	1976–2003	8 *BRCA1*	Familial testing (-) "Low risk," untested	
Brekelmans et al. (30)	The Netherlands	P, F	1980–2001	223 *BRCA1*	Hospital registry controls	27 not tested
Pierce et al. (31)[d]	North America	P, F	NS	160 (1 and 2)	Hospital registries	All breast conservation
Arnes et al. (32)[a]	Canada	RC	1980–1995	35 (1 and 2)	Cohort members testing (-)	All AJ

[a] Overlapping ascertainment (Canada).
[b] Overlapping ascertainment (France).
[c] Overlapping ascertainment (United States).
[d] Overlapping ascertainment (North America).

Note: AJ, Ashkenazi Jewish; E, early age at diagnosis; F, family history; P, prevalent; RC, retrospective cohort; Ascertainment types.

Abbreviations: BC, breast cancer; FDR, first degree relative; NS, not stated.

outcome in *BRCA*-associated breast cancer. Because of various design limitations, whether a germline *BRCA* mutation constitutes an adverse prognostic factor remains unresolved.

Ascertainment by Family History

A large number of studies compare outcomes in mutation carriers who were identified on the basis of clinical suspicion, usually raised by the presence of a significant family history of breast cancer, with or without ovarian cancer (7,8,10,11,15,17,18,20,23–25,29–31). Several of these studies include individuals who are presumed to be mutation carriers, but not documented as such. For instance, the earliest studies (7,8) described outcomes in women who were members of families in which the apparent predisposition was shown by linkage analysis to be due to *BRCA1*. A number of other studies included not only those women who were shown to carry a *BRCA* mutation, but also untested affected family members (10,15,18,20,23,30). One study (14) is completely based on the description of survival in affected first degree relatives of known mutation carriers. While most women with breast cancer in these families are likely to be carriers of the family mutation, there may be some dilution of a prognostic effect of mutation status by the inclusion of phenocopies.

Varied comparison groups were also used for these studies. Most commonly, women with mutations were compared with women from either hospital (8,10,15,17,24,30,31) or population (7,11,18,23) tumor registries. In most cases, carriers and their comparison groups were matched for age at diagnosis. In several studies, matching was also performed for year of diagnosis. Other studies compared mutation carriers with women who were evaluated for *BRCA* mutations but were found not to carry one (20,23–25,29).

The great majority of these studies found no significant difference in survival between mutation carriers and the comparison groups (10,11,15,17–20,23–25,30). One early study of women from *BRCA1* linked families found an improved outcome among women from linked families when compared with the broad survival experience of all women in the Scottish population over a different time period (7). Another study found decreased survival among *BRCA2* carriers (18), but women presenting with stage IV disease were included and there was no significant difference after adjustment for stage at diagnosis. Taken together, these studies suggest that *BRCA* status is not associated with worse outcome. The nature of the ascertainment in most of these studies introduces a possible survival bias, in that mutation carriers suffering early death may not be identified, leading to an underestimation of any negative prognostic effect. Various approaches were employed to reduce the impact of this ascertainment bias, such as evaluating all affected family members, excluding probands for the calculation, and limiting analyses to individuals undergoing testing within a limited period of time after diagnoses. Germline status was not shown to be a negative prognostic factor in those studies that employed these adjustments.

Ascertainment by Age at Onset

A smaller number of studies identified mutation carriers by testing groups of women with early-onset breast cancer without regard to family history (12,13,21). Other studies (24) included early-onset cancer as an ascertainment criterion but did not separately describe outcomes in women ascertained in this way. In all studies, outcomes in mutation carriers were compared with outcomes in women from the cohorts who were not shown to have a mutation on testing. These were not incident cohorts, as women underwent testing some period of time after their diagnosis, and these studies are therefore subject to the possibility of a survival bias as described previously. Germline *BRCA* mutations did not have an adverse effect on survival in the New York (12) and U.K. (24) studies. In the studies from the Institut Curie (13,21), germline *BRCA1* mutations were associated with a significantly worse overall survival, even after adjustment for tumor size, clinical nodal status, histopathologic grade, and estrogen receptor status.

Retrospective Cohort Studies

To address the problem of survival bias, three groups have described results of retrospective cohort studies performed in Ashkenazi Jewish women with breast cancer. In these studies, breast cancer patients were identified as potential subjects based solely on Jewish religious preference. All women with available tissue, surviving or dead, were included in these ascertainments. After gathering clinical information and outcome data, de-identified paraffin embedded archival tissues were tested for the presence of the Ashkenazi founder mutations (*BRCA1* 185delAG and 5382insC and *BRCA2* 6174delT) and genotype linked to the clinical data by means of a unique study identifier. While these studies avoid survival bias, they are somewhat limited by the small number of carriers identified, the hospital-based nature of the ascertainment, and the question of whether the results are necessarily applicable to women from different ethnic groups.

The group from McGill University/Jewish General Hospital in Montreal has utilized the retrospective cohort design to elucidate factors associated with outcome on Ashkenazi Jewish women with breast cancer diagnosed before the age of 65 (4,9,19,22,26,32,33). In aggregate, these studies described a significantly worse outcome in *BRCA1* carriers than in women without *BRCA1* mutations. The impact of *BRCA1* mutations was particularly evident in women without axillary nodal metastases. This group described the association between germline *BRCA1* mutations and immunohistochemical features that are frequently seen in breast cancers with the "basal-like" or gene expression profile, such as expression of cytokeratin 5/6 (34), p53 (4), cyclin E (26), and P-cadherin (32), and low levels of expression of p27 (22). In some of these reports, the significance of *BRCA1* mutation was independent of individual factors such as p53 (4) and p27 (22). However, when the aggregate phenotype was considered, *BRCA1* was no longer an independent factor (33).

A similar design has been employed by investigators at Columbia University and Memorial Sloan-Kettering (16,27). Like the Canadian studies, the Memorial study also showed a negative impact of *BRCA* mutation status on outcome. In a combined series with the Montreal group, this negative impact was shown to be associated with *BRCA1*, but not *BRCA2*, mutations, to be independent of stage, and to be most significant in women not receiving chemotherapy (28). In contrast, the Columbia series did not find any difference in 5- or 10-year breast cancer specific or overall survival between women with and without mutations.

This group of studies seems to indicate that breast cancers that arise in *BRCA1* carriers often manifest a particular immunophenotype, and that this immunophenotype is associated with an adverse outcome, particularly in early stage disease. The negative impact may be more evident in node negative patients because these women are less likely to receive adjuvant chemotherapy, and adjuvant chemotherapy may mitigate the adverse prognosis associated with this particular phenotype. There was no indication of an adverse effect of the *BRCA2* 6174delT mutation. This lack of influence from the *BRCA2* founder mutation may explain the negative finding of the Columbia study, as 40% of the mutations in that study were in *BRCA2*.

Conclusion

The impact of *BRCA1* and *BRCA2* on prognosis should be considered separately. Breast cancer arising as the result of a germline *BRCA2* mutation does not appear to be more likely to manifest adverse prognostic features than sporadic cancer, and it appears that *BRCA2* mutations are not associated with a worse outcome. B1BC, on the other hand, have often been associated with a variety of negative histopathologic and immunohistochemical prognostic factors. Furthermore, several studies designed to minimize ascertainment biases have described a worse outcome in women with B1BC. Recent reports indicate that B1BC are often similar to cancers manifesting a "basal epithelial-like" gene expression profile. This type of breast cancer simultaneously manifests many of the negative features observed in B1BC. Hence, it seems likely that germline *BRCA1* mutations are associated with an adverse prognosis when the cancer that arose as a result of that mutation manifests this phenotype. However, the germline mutation probably does not have an independent negative effect on outcome. As a corollary to this, B1BC that do not manifest this phenotype may have a prognosis similar to that of disease that is not associated with mutations.

GERMLINE *BRCA* MUTATIONS AS PREDICTORS OF RESPONSE TO CHEMOTHERAPY

The exact process through which mutation of *BRCA1* and *BRCA2* leads to an increased risk of breast cancer has not yet been defined. However, a large body of evidence suggests that the products of these genes are intimately involved in the cellular response to DNA damage. It is presumed, although not proven, that disruption of this function leads to the observed cancer susceptibility. A review of these issues is beyond the scope of this chapter, and the reader is referred to several recent summaries for more information (35–38). For the purposes of this discussion, it is sufficient to note that one piece of evidence that *BRCA1* and *BRCA2* are involved in the response to DNA damage is the observation of increased sensitivity to ionizing radiation in cells lacking the products of these genes. As the induction of DNA damage is hypothesized to be the mechanism of cytotoxicity for several chemotherapy drugs, several groups have investigated the hypothesis that *BRCA*-deficient cells may also be sensitive to particular cytotoxic agents (39). Indeed, some authors have suggested that germline *BRCA* status may become useful as a factor to be considered when choosing specific chemotherapy regimens for women with *BRCA*-associated breast cancer (40,41). However, most of the evidence that *BRCA*-deficient cells respond differently to chemotherapy than do cells with intact function comes from preclinical studies with various in vitro systems (many of which were not human in origin), interventions, and endpoints.

Preclinical Studies

Cis-Platinum and Related Compounds

Platinum compounds are believed to induce primarily intrastrand DNA cross-links, with a small proportion of adducts being associated with interstrand links (42). The failure to repair these cross-links results in cell death. Early work by Husain et al. indicated that acquired platinum resistance in the human breast cancer cell line MCF-7 and human ovarian cancer line SK-OV3 was associated with increased expression of *BRCA1*, and that introduction of a *BRCA1* antisense plasmid into the resistant ovary cancer line was associated with a significant decrease in the IC50 of *cis*-platinum (43). Other groups have demonstrated significantly greater sensitivity to *cis*-platinum in mouse embryonic stem cells (44) or mouse mammary epithelial cells (45) that are lacking functional *BRCA1*. Few studies have evaluated the effect of *cis*-platinum on *BRCA2*-deficient cells. One group has developed a mouse model with targeted disruption of *BRCA2* in the small intestine (46). The apoptotic response in small intestinal crypts after treatment with *cis*-platinum was not significantly increased, but there was a reduction in clonogenic survival measured by crypt number. A recent study has described *cis*-platinum sensitivity in a *BRCA2*-deficient human pancreatic cancer cell line, CAPAN-1 (47).

Anthracyclines

Anthracyclines and anthracenediones are among the most commonly used agents in breast cancer. Studies examining the sensitivity of *BRCA*-deficient cells to anthracyclines (usually doxorubicin) have been inconclusive with some reporting increased sensitivity (48,49) and some decreased sensitivity (50).

There are no studies evaluating sensitivity to doxorubicin in *BRCA2*-deficient cell lines.

Taxanes and Vinca Alkaloids

Whether *BRCA1* or 2 deficiency results in resistance to agents that interfere with microtubule polymerization and depolymerization is a topic of considerable discussion. Some groups have suggested that *BRCA1* is involved in effecting apoptosis in cells with disrupted mitotic spindle formation, and loss of that function would therefore be hypothesized to be associated with decreased apoptosis (resistance) (41). In support of this hypothesis, Mullan et al. noted increased sensitivity to paclitaxel and vincristine when *BRCA1* was overexpressed in the human breast cancer cell line MDA435 (51). In addition, the same group described a significant increase in the IC50 of paclitaxel when *BRCA1* expression was reduced by siRNA in the T47D breast cancer cell line and a significant increase in sensitivity to paclitaxel and vinorelbine when *BRCA1* function was partially reconstituted in HCC1937 cells, a *BRCA1* deficient cell line (52). Another group has also described comparative resistance to paclitaxel in HCC1937 cells, which was reversed after transfection of *BRCA1* (53). Finally, Lafarge et al. described resistance to paclitaxel and vincristine in HBL-100 human breast cancer cells in which *BRCA1* was inhibited by transfection of a ribozyme (54). Other studies have been less supportive of the hypothesis. Tassone et al. reported that HCC1937 cells were more sensitive to vincristine than MCF-7 or MDA-MB468 human breast cancer cells, and similar with respect to sensitivity to docetaxel (55). This group also described a decrease in sensitivity to vincristine after transfection of *BRCA1*, with no significant change in response to docetaxel. Other groups have reported no difference in sensitivity to paclitaxel in *Brca1* null mouse embryonic fibroblasts (MEFs) compared with MEF with functional *BRCA1* (48), and either decreased sensitivity or no change after transfection of *BRCA1* into mouse (56) or human (50) ovarian cancer lines with defective *BRCA1* function.

Studies of the *BRCA2* deficient line CAPAN-2 did not demonstrate a significant degree of resistance to paclitaxel (57). Differential paclitaxel sensitivity was also not described in a study of cell lines with other defects in the Fanconi anemia (FA)/*BRCA2* pathway (58).

Mitomycin C

Mitomycin C (MMC) is a prototypical DNA cross-linking agent, inducing double strand DNA breaks that are most effectively repaired by homologous recombination. *BRCA1* and *BRCA2* appear to be critical to this type of DNA repair, and one would therefore hypothesize that cells lacking *BRCA1/2* function would be hypersensitive to MMC. Moynahan et al. (59) reported that *BRCA1* negative mouse embryonic stem cells were exquisitely sensitive to MMC. This sensitivity was partially reversed by transfection of wild-type *BRCA1* and essentially completely reversed after correction of the *BRCA1* mutation through gene targeting.

MMC sensitivity has not been evaluated in other studies of *BRCA1* deficient cell lines. However, sensitivity has been clearly shown in BRCA2 deficient cells, including the human pancreatic cancer line CAPAN-1 (57), the Chinese hamster ovary line VC-8 (49), and the targeted mouse small intestine model described above (46). These observations are perhaps not surprising given the relationship between *BRCA2* and FA, and the long-known hypersensitivity of FA cells to MMC. This was confirmed again in a recent study of pancreatic cancer cell lines with various FA/BRCA2 pathway defects (58).

Other Drugs

Evaluation of the interaction between *BRCA* status and sensitivity to agents other than those described has not been extensive. Several studies have suggested an increased sensitivity to etoposide in *BRCA1* (48,52,54) or *BRCA2* (57) deficient cell lines. Two studies have suggested increased sensitivity to topoisomerase I inhibition by camptothecin or topotecan in *BRCA1* deficient MEFs (48) and *BRCA2* deficient Chinese hamster ovary cells (60). One study described an increased sensitivity to bleomycin in *BRCA1*-deficient HCC1937 (52). There does not appear to be any differential sensitivity to antimetabolites such as fluorouracil or gemcitabine (48,52).

Clinical Studies

Few clinical studies have directly evaluated the impact of *BRCA1* or *BRCA2* expression on responsiveness to chemotherapy. The constraints on design of these types of studies are significant, as for studies of outcomes in general. In terms of general responsiveness to chemotherapy, it is worth noting that two retrospective cohort studies describing a worse survival for *BRCA1* mutation carriers than noncarriers only found a significant influence of germline status in women not receiving adjuvant chemotherapy (4,28,52). This suggests that the worse outcome associated with the *BRCA1* "phenotype" can be mitigated by treatment. Of course, this does not resolve the question of whether *BRCA*-associated breast cancers are more or less sensitive to specific chemotherapeutic agents.

A suggestion that *BRCA*-associated breast cancers may be clinically sensitive to at least some types of chemotherapy was provided by Chappuis et al. in their description of superior clinical and pathologic responses to neoadjuvant chemotherapy (anthracycline/ cyclophosphamide-based) in *BRCA1/2* carriers (4,28,61). In their series of 11 *BRCA1/2* carriers, 10 of 11 women achieved a clinical complete response after neoadjuvant treatment, and 4 of 9 (44%) who went to surgery achieved a pathologic complete response (pCR). This was significantly greater than the results achieved by controls matched for age and stage at presentation. Delaloge et al. also reported a 53% pCR rate in 15 *BRCA1* carriers receiving neoadjuvant anthracycline-based chemotherapy compared with 0% of 5 BRCA2 carriers and 14% of matched sporadic controls (62). While encouraging, these studies did not describe long-term follow-up for survival. Hereditary cancers, especially due to *BRCA1* mutations, tend to have a high proliferative rate, and this correlates with chemotherapy response in other studies. While the results are consistent with chemosensitivity related to the germline predisposition, they are by no means conclusive. Interestingly, one study suggests that "basal-like" breast cancers are also more likely to respond to neoadjuvant chemotherapy (63), which suggests this may be a more generic effect of phenotype rather than a specific consequence of germline mutation.

Several studies have indicated an improved outcome for *BRCA*-associated ovarian cancer compared with sporadic disease (64–67). It has been suggested that this difference results from an increased sensitivity to the *cis*-platinum-based therapy that is routinely given to patients with advanced ovarian cancer. However, other factors may be involved. For instance, *BRCA*-associated cancers are more likely to be optimally debulked (65).

Summary

Preclinical studies suggest that *BRCA*-associated breast cancers may be sensitive to certain agents (especially *cis*-platinum and MMC, and possibly anthracyclines and etoposide). Preclinical studies have also raised the possibility of relative paclitaxel resistance, at least in *BRCA1* deficient cells, but this is less clear. Much of the evidence for differential chemosensitivity is derived from experiments which may or may not reflect clinical realities, and the outcomes of preclinical studies are frequently discordant with the results of clinical trials. The few clinical studies conducted are limited in various ways, but do suggest improved responses in *BRCA*-associated breast cancer and ovarian cancer. Whether these differences are due to differential chemosensitivity or to other clinical factors is not clear. Therefore, there is insufficient evidence at present to modify systemic chemotherapy recommendations in either the adjuvant or metastatic setting based upon germline *BRCA* status.

FUTURE DIRECTIONS

Aside from the potential clinical trials mentioned above, there are several new approaches in development targeted toward women with hereditary breast cancer.

PARP Inhibition

Poly(ADP)-ribose polymerases (PARPs) are a family of enzymes with varying functions. Some members of the family appear to be critical to the repair of single-strand DNA breaks through base excision repair (BER) pathways. Cells lacking *BRCA1* or *2* function have relatively intact BER pathways and can therefore competently repair this type of DNA damage. If PARP function is inhibited, single-strand breaks convert to double strand breaks (DSBs) and are repaired by the DSB repair pathways. In *BRCA*-deficient cells, of course, these pathways are deficient. In theory, then, disruption of PARP function (either with or without a DNA-damaging stimulus) would result in accumulating DSBs in *BRCA*-deficient cells, eventually resulting in apoptosis, while DSB repair-competent cells would survive the insult (68). Two proof-of-principle experiments were recently published describing sensitivity to PARP inhibition in *BRCA2*-deficient Chinese hamster ovary VC-8 cells (69), *BRCA1* or *BRCA2*-deficient mouse embryonic stem cells (70), and human breast cancer cell lines with *BRCA2* "knocked down" by siRNA (69). These results have generated considerable interest in developing PARP inhibitors as specific targeted therapies for women with germline *BRCA* mutations, and phase I clinical trials are underway (71). It is important to remember, however, that *BRCA*-associated breast cancer cells contain many acquired genetic abnormalities, and it remains to be seen if the exciting preclinical studies accurately presage the results of properly designed clinical trials (72).

EGFR Inhibition

As noted by Foulkes et al. in Chapter 18 of this book and described above, B1BC often have an immunohistochemical phenotype that overlaps that noted in cancers with the so-called "basal-like" or "basal epithelial-like" gene expression profile. Epidermal growth factor receptor (EGFR, HER1) overexpression is commonly noted in this subtype. EGFR expression has also been reported in 67% of *BRCA1*-associated tumors (73). Clinical trials evaluating the impact of EGFR inhibition in "triple negative" breast cancer with cetuximab are in progress. If these are successful, similar approaches may be of use for a significant proportion of *BRCA1*-associated cancers.

Antiangiogenic Therapy

Glomeruloid microvascular proliferation (GMP) is a specific morphologic finding of focal proliferative buddings of endothelial cells, resembling a renal glomerulus. They appear to be related to vascular endothelial growth factor (VEGF) levels (74), but are not completely correlated with microvessel density. GMP appears to be part of the *BRCA1* phenotype described previously (33). If these GMPs reflect an angiogenic phenotype in B1BC, then interference with angiogenesis (e.g., with bevacizumab) may be a productive strategy.

CONCLUSION

Hereditary breast cancer due to germline mutations in *BRCA1* and *BRCA2* has been a subject of intense study since the discovery of these genes. Many studies of outcome have been performed. It is still not clear whether a diagnosis of hereditary breast cancer is associated with a worse prognosis, although there are suggestions that the "typical" B1BC may be associated with increased risk of death. While B1BC may have a worse prognosis, there is not yet sufficient evidence to use germline status as an independent indicator of the need for systemic therapy. Similarly, there are theoretical grounds and some preclinical evidence for sensitivity or resistance to certain chemotherapeutic agents. However, in the absence of firmer clinical trial data, it is premature to select (or avoid) certain agents based upon the genetic etiology of the tumor. Such trials are desperately needed, given the intriguing in vitro experimental results, but are devilishly hard to accomplish given the relative rarity of *BRCA*-associated breast cancer. Although these comments are made with *BRCA*-associated disease in mind, the same applies to cancer associated with germline *p53* mutations. Concerns have been raised that women with Li-Fraumeni-associated breast cancer may be at increased risk for anthracycline-induced leukemia or radiation-induced sarcoma, and that primary and adjuvant treatment should be modified on this basis. While this may certainly be true, at the present time it remains a hypothesis that needs to be either proven or disproved.

REFERENCES

1. Honrado E, Benitez J, Palacios J. The molecular pathology of hereditary breast cancer: genetic testing and therapeutic implications. Mod Pathol 2005; 18(10):1305–1320.
2. Honrado E, Benitez J, Palacios J. Histopathology of BRCA1- and BRCA2-associated breast cancer. Crit Rev Oncol Hematol 2006; 59(1):27–39.
3. Lakhani SR, Van DV, Jacquemier J, et al. The pathology of familial breast cancer: predictive value of immunohistochemical markers estrogen receptor, progesterone receptor, HER-2, and p53 in patients with mutations in BRCA1 and BRCA2. J Clin Oncol 2002; 20(9):2310–2318.
4. Goffin JR, Chappuis PO, Begin LR, et al. Impact of germline BRCA1 mutations and overexpression of p53 on prognosis and response to treatment following breast carcinoma: 10-year follow up data. Cancer 2003; 97(3):527–536.

5. Palacios J, Honrado E, Osorio A, et al. Immunohistochemical characteristics defined by tissue microarray of hereditary breast cancer not attributable to BRCA1 or BRCA2 mutations: differences from breast carcinomas arising in BRCA1 and BRCA2 mutation carriers. Clin Cancer Res 2003; 9(10 Pt 1):3606–3614.

6. Palacios J, Honrado E, Osorio A, et al. Phenotypic characterization of BRCA1 and BRCA2 tumors based in a tissue microarray study with 37 immunohistochemical markers. Breast Cancer Res Treat 2005; 90(1):5–14.

7. Porter DE, Cohen BB, Wallace MR, et al. Breast cancer incidence, penetrance and survival in probable carriers of BRCA1 gene mutation in families linked to BRCA1 on chromosome 17q12-21. Br J Surg 1994; 81(10):1512–1515.

8. Marcus JN, Watson P, Page DL, et al. Hereditary breast cancer: pathobiology, prognosis, and BRCA1 and BRCA2 gene linkage. Cancer 1996; 77(4):697–709.

9. Foulkes WD, Wong N, Brunet JS, et al. Germ-line BRCA1 mutation is an adverse prognostic factor in Ashkenazi Jewish women with breast cancer. Clin Cancer Res 1997; 3(12 Pt 1): 2465–2469.

10. Verhoog LC, Brekelmans CT, Seynaeve C, et al. Survival and tumour characteristics of breast-cancer patients with germline mutations of BRCA1. Lancet 1998; 351(9099):316–321.

11. Johannsson OT, Ranstam J, Borg A, Olsson H. Survival of BRCA1 breast and ovarian cancer patients: a population-based study from southern Sweden. J Clin Oncol 1998; 16(2):397–404.

12. Robson M, Gilewski T, Haas B, et al. BRCA-associated breast cancer in young women. J Clin Oncol 1998; 16(5):1642–1649.

13. Ansquer Y, Gautier C, Fourquet A, Asselain B, Stoppa-Lyonnet D. Survival in early-onset BRCA1 breast-cancer patients. Institut Curie Breast Cancer Group. Lancet 1998; 352(9127):541.

14. Lee JS, Wacholder S, Struewing JP, et al. Survival after breast cancer in Ashkenazi Jewish BRCA1 and BRCA2 mutation carriers. J Natl Cancer Inst 1999; 91(3):259–263.

15. Verhoog LC, Brekelmans CT, Seynaeve C, et al. Survival in hereditary breast cancer associated with germline mutations of BRCA2. J Clin Oncol 1999; 17(11):3396–3402.

16. Robson M, Levin D, Federici M, et al. Breast conservation therapy for invasive breast cancer in Ashkenazi women with BRCA gene founder mutations. J Natl Cancer Inst 1999; 91(24): 2112–2117.

17. Pierce LJ, Strawderman M, Narod SA, et al. Effect of radiotherapy after breast-conserving treatment in women with breast cancer and germline BRCA1/2 mutations. J Clin Oncol 2000; 18(19):3360–3369.

18. Loman N, Johannsson O, Bendahl P, et al. Prognosis and clinical presentation of BRCA2-associated breast cancer. Eur J Cancer 2000; 36(11):1365–1373.

19. Foulkes WD, Chappuis PO, Wong N, et al. Primary node negative breast cancer in BRCA1 mutation carriers has a poor outcome. Ann Oncol 2000; 11(3):307–313.

20. Hamann U, Sinn HP. Survival and tumor characteristics of German hereditary breast cancer patients. Breast Cancer Res Treat 2000; 59(2):185–192.

21. Stoppa-Lyonnet D, Ansquer Y, Dreyfus H, et al. Familial invasive breast cancers: worse outcome related to BRCA1 mutations. J Clin Oncol 2000; 18(24):4053–4059.

22. Chappuis PO, Kapusta L, Begin LR, et al. Germline BRCA1/2 mutations and p27(Kip1) protein levels independently predict outcome after breast cancer. J Clin Oncol 2000; 18(24): 4045–4052.

23. Eerola H, Vahteristo P, Sarantaus L, et al. Survival of breast cancer patients in BRCA1, BRCA2, and non-BRCA1/2 breast cancer families: a relative survival analysis from Finland. Int J Cancer 2001 Aug 1; 93(3):368–372.

24. Eccles D, Simmonds P, Goddard J, et al. Familial breast cancer: an investigation into the outcome of treatment for early stage disease. Fam Cancer 2001; 1(2):65–72.

25. Veronesi A, de GC, Magri MD, et al. Familial breast cancer: characteristics and outcome of BRCA 1-2 positive and negative cases. BMC Cancer 2005; 5:70.

26. Chappuis PO, Donato E, Goffin JR, et al. Cyclin E expression in breast cancer: predicting germline BRCA1 mutations, prognosis and response to treatment. Ann Oncol 2005; 16(5): 735–742.

27. El-Tamer M, Russo D, Troxel A, et al. Survival and recurrence after breast cancer in BRCA1/2 mutation carriers. Ann Surg Oncol 2004; 11(2):157–164.

28. Robson ME, Chappuis PO, Satagopan J, et al. A combined analysis of outcome following breast cancer: differences in survival based on BRCA1/BRCA2 mutation status and administration of adjuvant treatment. Breast Cancer Res 2004; 6(1):R8–R17.

29. Musolino A, Michiara M, Bella MA, et al. Molecular profile and clinical variables in BRCA1-positive breast cancers. A population-based study. Tumori 2005; 91(6):505–512.

30. Brekelmans CT, Seynaeve C, Menke-Pluymers M, et al. Survival and prognostic factors in BRCA1-associated breast cancer. Ann Oncol 2006; 17(3):391–400.

31. Pierce LJ, Levin AM, Rebbeck TR, et al. Ten-year multi-institutional results of breast-conserving surgery and radiotherapy in BRCA1/2-associated stage I/II breast cancer. J Clin Oncol 2006; 24(16):2437–2443.

32. Arnes JB, Brunet JS, Stefansson I, et al. Placental cadherin and the basal epithelial phenotype of BRCA1-related breast cancer. Clin Cancer Res 2005; 11(11):4003–4011.

33. Foulkes WD, Brunet JS, Stefansson IM, et al. The prognostic implication of the basal-like (cyclin E high/p27 low/p53+/glomeruloid-microvascular-proliferation+) phenotype of BRCA1-related breast cancer. Cancer Res 2004; 64(3):830–835.

34. Foulkes WD, Stefansson IM, Chappuis PO, et al. Germline BRCA1 mutations and a basal epithelial phenotype in breast cancer. J Natl Cancer Inst 2003; 95(19):1482–1485.

35. Deng CX. BRCA1: cell cycle checkpoint, genetic instability, DNA damage response and cancer evolution. Nucl Acids Res 2006; 34(5):1416–1426.

36. Rudkin TM, Foulkes WD. BRCA2: breaks, mistakes and failed separations. Trends Mol Med 2005; 11(4):145–148.

37. Venkitaraman AR. Cancer susceptibility and the functions of BRCA1 and BRCA2. Cell 2002; 108(2):171–182.

38. Venkitaraman AR. Tracing the network connecting the BRCA and Fanconi Anaemia proteins. Nat Rev Cancer 2004; 4(4):266–276.

39. Foulkes WD. BRCA1 and BRCA2: chemosensitivity, treatment outcomes and prognosis. Fam Cancer 2006; 5(2):135–142.

40. Kennedy RD, Quinn JE, Mullan PB, Johnston PG, Harkin DP. The role of BRCA1 in the cellular response to chemotherapy. J Natl Cancer Inst 2004; 96(22):1659–1668.

41. Mullan PB, Gorski JJ, Harkin DP. BRCA1–A good predictive marker of drug sensitivity in breast cancer treatment? Biochim Biophys Acta 2006; 1766(2):205–216.

42. Reed E. Cisplatin, carboplatin, and oxaliplatin. In: Chabner BA, Longo DL, eds. Cancer Chemotherapy: Principles and Practice. 3 ed. Philadelphia: Lippincott, Williams, and Wilkins, 2001:332–341.

43. Husain A, He G, Venkatraman ES, Spriggs DR. BRCA1 up-regulation is associated with repair-mediated resistance to *cis*-diamminedichloroplatinum(II). Cancer Res 1998; 58(6):1120–1123.

44. Bhattacharyya A, Ear US, Koller BH, Weichselbaum RR, Bishop DK. The breast cancer susceptibility gene BRCA1 is required for subnuclear assembly of Rad51 and survival following treatment with the DNA cross-linking agent cisplatin. J Biol Chem 2000; 275(31):23899–23903.

45. Sgagias MK, Wagner KU, Hamik B, et al. BRCA1-deficient murine mammary epithelial cells have increased sensitivity to CDDP and MMS. Cell Cycle 2004; 3(11):1451–1456.

46. Hay T, Patrick T, Winton D, Sansom OJ, Clarke AR. BRCA2 deficiency in the murine small intestine sensitizes to p53-dependent apoptosis and leads to the spontaneous deletion of stem cells. Oncogene 2005; 24(23):3842–3846.

47. van der Heijden MS, Brody JR, Gallmeier E, et al. Functional defects in the fanconi anemia pathway in pancreatic cancer cells. Am J Pathol 2004; 165(2):651–657.

48. Fedier A, Steiner RA, Schwarz VA, Lenherr L, Haller U, Fink D. The effect of loss of BRCA1 on the sensitivity to anticancer agents in p53-deficient cells. Int J Oncol 2003; 22(5): 1169–1173.

49. Kraakman-van der ZM, Overkamp WJ, van Lange RE, et al. BRCA2 (XRCC11) deficiency results in radioresistant DNA synthesis and a higher frequency of spontaneous deletions. Mol Cell Biol 2002; 22(2):669–679.

50. Zhou C, Smith JL, Liu J. Role of BRCA1 in cellular resistance to paclitaxel and ionizing radiation in an ovarian cancer cell line carrying a defective BRCA1. Oncogene 2003; 22(16): 2396–2404.

51. Mullan PB, Quinn JE, Gilmore PM, et al. BRCA1 and GADD45 mediated G2/M cell cycle arrest in response to antimicrotubule agents. Oncogene 2001; 20(43):6123–6131.

52. Quinn JE, Kennedy RD, Mullan PB, et al. BRCA1 functions as a differential modulator of chemotherapy-induced apoptosis. Cancer Res 2003; 63(19):6221–6228.

53. Tassone P, Tagliaferri P, Perricelli A, et al. BRCA1 expression modulates chemosensitivity of BRCA1-defective HCC1937 human breast cancer cells. Br J Cancer 2003; 88(8):1285–1291.

54. Lafarge S, Sylvain V, Ferrara M, Bignon YJ. Inhibition of BRCA1 leads to increased chemoresistance to microtubule-interfering agents, an effect that involves the JNK pathway. Oncogene 2001; 20(45):6597–6606.

55. Tassone P, Blotta S, Palmieri C, et al. Differential sensitivity of BRCA1-mutated HCC1937 human breast cancer cells to microtubule-interfering agents. Int J Oncol 2005; 26(5): 1257–1263.

56. Sylvain V, Lafarge S, Bignon YJ. Dominant-negative activity of a BRCA1 truncation mutant: effects on proliferation, tumorigenicity in vivo, and chemosensitivity in a mouse ovarian cancer cell line. Int J Oncol 2002; 20(4):845–853..

57. Abbott DW, Freeman ML, Holt JT. Double-strand break repair deficiency and radiation sensitivity in BRCA2 mutant cancer cells. J Natl Cancer Inst 1998; 90(13):978–985.

58. van der Heijden MS, Brody JR, Dezentje DA, et al. In vivo therapeutic responses contingent on Fanconi anemia/BRCA2 status of the tumor. Clin Cancer Res 2005; 11(20):7508–7515.

59. Moynahan ME, Cui TY, Jasin M. Homology-directed DNA repair, mitomycin-c resistance, and chromosome stability is restored with correction of a BRCA1 mutation. Cancer Res 2001; 61(12):4842–4850.

60. Rahden-Staron I, Szumilo M, Grosickaz E, Kraakman van der ZM, Zdzienicka MZ. Defective BRCA2 influences topoisomerase I activity in mammalian cells. Acta Biochim Pol 2003; 50(1):139–144.

61. Chappuis PO, Goffin J, Wong N, et al. A significant response to neoadjuvant chemotherapy in BRCA1/2 related breast cancer. J Med Genet 2002; 39(8):608–610.

62. Delaloge S, Pelissier P, Kloos I, et al. BRCA1-linked breast cancer (BC) is highly more chemosensitive than its BRCA2-linked or sporadic counterparts. Program and Abstracts of the 27th Congress of the European Society for Medical Oncology. 2002.

63. Rouzier R, Perou CM, Symmans WF, et al. Breast cancer molecular subtypes respond differently to preoperative chemotherapy. Clin Cancer Res 2005; 11(16):5678–5685.

64. Cass I, Baldwin RL, Varkey T, Moslehi R, Narod SA, Karlan BY. Improved survival in women with BRCA-associated ovarian carcinoma. Cancer 2003; 97(9):2187–2195.

65. Boyd J, Sonoda Y, Federici MG, et al. Clinicopathologic features of BRCA-linked and sporadic ovarian cancer. JAMA 2000; 283(17):2260–2265.

66. Ben DY, Chetrit A, Hirsh-Yechezkel G, et al. Effect of BRCA mutations on the length of survival in epithelial ovarian tumors. J Clin Oncol 2002; 20(2):463–466.

67. Ramus SJ, Fishman A, Pharoah PD, Yarkoni S, Altaras M, Ponder BA. Ovarian cancer survival in Ashkenazi Jewish patients with BRCA1 and BRCA2 mutations. Eur J Surg Oncol 2001; 27(3):278–281.

68. Brody LC. Treating cancer by targeting a weakness. N Engl J Med 2005; 353(9):949–950.

69. Bryant HE, Schultz N, Thomas HD, et al. Specific killing of BRCA2-deficient tumours with inhibitors of poly(ADP-ribose) polymerase. Nature 2005; 434(7035):913–917.

70. Farmer H, McCabe N, Lord CJ, et al. Targeting the DNA repair defect in BRCA mutant cells as a therapeutic strategy. Nature 2005; 434(7035):917–921.

71. Fong PC, Spicer J, Reade S, et al. Phase I pharmacokinetic (PK) and pharmacodynamic (PD) evaluation of a small molecule inhibitor of poly ADP-ribose polymerase (PARP), Ku-0059436 in patients (p) with advanced solid tumors. J Clin Oncol 2006; 24:3022.

72. De Soto JA, Wang X, Tominaga Y, et al. The inhibition and treatment of breast cancer with Poly (ADP–ribose) polymerase (PARP-1) inhibitors. Int J Biol Sci 2006; 2(4):179–185.

73. Lakhani SR, Reis-Filho JS, Fulford L, et al. Prediction of BRCA1 status in patients with breast cancer using estrogen receptor and basal phenotype. Clin Cancer Res 2005; 11(14): 5175–5180.
74. Brat DJ, Van Meir EG. Glomeruloid microvascular proliferation orchestrated by VPF/VEGF: a new world of angiogenesis research. Am J Pathol 2001; 158(3):789–796.

Index